Thyroid Disorders: A Case Study Approach

Thyroid Disorders: A Case Study Approach

Editor: Gordon Knight

AMERICAN
MEDICAL PUBLISHERS
www.americanmedicalpublishers.com

AMERICAN
MEDICAL PUBLISHERS
www.americanmedicalpublishers.com

Cataloging-in-Publication Data

Thyroid disorders: a case study approach / edited by Gordon Knight.
p. cm.
Includes bibliographical references and index.
ISBN 979-8-88740-660-2
1. Thyroid gland--Diseases. 2. Thyroid gland--Diseases--Diagnosis.
3. Thyroid gland--Diseases--Treatment. I. Knight, Gordon.
RC655 .T49 2023
616.44--dc23

American Medical Publishers,
41 Flatbush Avenue,
1st Floor, New York,
NY 11217, USA

ISBN 979-8-88740-660-2 (Hardback)

Contents

Preface

The gland in the body which produces the hormones that regulate the utilization of energy by the body is known as the thyroid gland. The disorders related to this gland may lead to the production of too less of this hormone or too much, which can result in hypothyroidism or hyperthyroidism respectively. This in turn can cause symptoms such as weight loss, weight gain, irritability and fatigue. Some of the other disorders of the thyroid gland are goiter, thyroid cancer and thyroiditis. Different approaches, evaluations and case studies on thyroid disorders have been included in this book. Those in search of information to further their knowledge will be greatly assisted by it.

All of the data presented henceforth, was collaborated in the wake of recent advancements in the field. The aim of this book is to present the diversified developments from across the globe in a comprehensible manner. The opinions expressed in each chapter belong solely to the contributing authors. Their interpretations of the topics are the integral part of this book, which I have carefully compiled for a better understanding of the readers.

At the end, I would like to thank all those who dedicated their time and efforts for the successful completion of this book. I also wish to convey my gratitude towards my friends and family who supported me at every step.

Editor

1

Delayed Hypoparathyroidism following Thyroidectomy, a Diagnostic Conundrum: A Report of Three Cases from Sri Lanka

Piyumi Sachindra Alwis Wijewickrama[1] and Henry N. Rajaratnam[2]

[1]Endocrinology Unit, National Hospital of Sri Lanka, Colombo 10, 00700, Sri Lanka
[2]Nawaloka Hospitals PLC, 23, Deshamanya H. K Dharmadasa Mawatha, Colombo 2, 00200, Sri Lanka

Correspondence should be addressed to Piyumi Sachindra Alwis Wijewickrama; psw8624@gmail.com

Academic Editor: Suat Simsek

Introduction. Hypoparathyroidism, which is a common complication following total thyroidectomy can be transient in majority and permanent in 1.5% of the patients and usually occurs secondary to an inadvertent removal of parathyroid glands, mechanical or thermal injury or disruption of the vasculature. In some patients, it is observed that symptoms of hypocalcemia can occur for the first time several years after the surgery, which is known as "delayed hypoparathyroidism." We report three cases of delayed hypoparathyroidism from Sri Lanka, presenting several years after total thyroidectomy. *Case Presentation.* Case 1- a 60-year-old Sri Lankan woman who presented with symptomatic hypocalcemia for the first time, 30 years after total thyroidectomy for follicular thyroid carcinoma. Case 2- a 53-year-old Sri Lankan woman presenting with neuropsychiatric manifestations of hypocalcemia for the first time, 12 years after total thyroidectomy for papillary thyroid carcinoma. Case 3- a 49-year-old Sri Lankan woman developing symptoms of hypocalcemia for the first time, 11 years after completion of thyroidectomy for papillary thyroid carcinoma. All these patients were detected to have low parathyroid hormone levels, without an alternative etiology for hypoparathyroidism, hence leading to a diagnosis of delayed post-thyroidectomy hypoparathyroidism. *Conclusion.* Delayed hypoparathyroidism is a rare phenomenon, which is secondary to progressive atrophy of parathyroid glands and slowly progressive hypovascularization of parathyroids due to scar tissue retraction following thyroidectomy. The nonspecific nature of hypocalcemic symptoms and lack of continuous follow-up for a long time after thyroidectomy could contribute to a further delay in diagnosis. However, it is an important diagnosis to consider in any patient with a history of neck surgery presenting with hypocalcemia, irrespective of the time duration of surgery, as timely diagnosis and treatment can prevent long-term complications of hypocalcemia and improve the quality of life.

1. Introduction

Hypoparathyroidism is the most common complication following total thyroidectomy, occurring in 7.6% following anterior neck surgeries. The majority (19–38%) of postoperative hypoparathyroidism is transient, resolving within 6 months, and permanent hypoparathyroidism is observed in 1.5% after total thyroidectomy, increasing to 6.4% in patients undergoing total thyroidectomy with prophylactic neck dissection [1]. The short half-life of parathyroid hormone (PTH) and the delicate nature of the parathyroid glands make them more prone to injury, resulting in immediate clinical manifestations shortly after or during thyroidectomy.

The underlying mechanisms for hypoparathyroidism following thyroidectomy are disruption of vascularity, thermal or electrical injury, and mechanical damage or partial/complete removal of the parathyroid glands [2]. Following surgery, a significant injury should occur before hypoparathyroidism develops, as even one normal gland is adequate to carry out normal function. Parathyroid glands are mainly supplied by the inferior thyroid artery, and the blood supply is complex, needing close attention to preserve the blood supply during thyroidectomy. Usually, hypoparathyroidism manifests immediately after surgery, and if it persists for more than 6 months, it is defined as "permanent hypoparathyroidism" [3].

Presenting symptoms of hypoparathyroidism are those of hypocalcemia, which include perioral and fingertip paresthesia, muscle stiffness and cramps, seizures, and psychiatric manifestations. Elicitable signs of hypocalcemia include the Chvostek sign, which is due to the increased irritability of the facial nerve, and the Trousseau sign, which is the carpopedal spasm secondary to induced ischemia. The Chvostek sign is known to be absent in 1/3rd of patients with hypocalcemia, making it less specific than the Trousseau sign, which is present in 94% of patients with hypocalcemia [4].

Rarely, it is observed that patients can manifest features of hypoparathyroidism for the first time after several years of a thyroidectomy, which is known as "delayed hypoparathyroidism." We report three cases of delayed hypoparathyroidism from Sri Lanka, presenting several years after total thyroidectomy.

2. Case presentation

2.1. Case 1. A 60-year-old Sri Lankan unmarried woman presented with worsening hand, feet, and perioral numbness for 6 months duration and muscle cramps of the lower limbs for 3 years. There were no seizures, headache, chest pain, or features of heart failure. She did not have features supportive of thyrotoxicosis including loose stools, sweating, or palpitations. She did not have limb weakness.

She gave a history of reduced appetite and unintended weight loss of 4 kg over 4 months. She did not have evidence of other endocrine abnormalities, including adrenal insufficiency, and there were no features supportive of an autoimmune process, to suggest a polyglandular autoimmune syndrome. She did not have chronic cough, joint symptoms, or skin rash to suggest a granulomatous or infiltrative disorder. She was consuming an average diet with adequate amounts of fish, meat, and milk and getting adequate exposure to sunlight. She did not have a history of diarrhoea or steatorrhoea or a family history of celiac disease to suggest an ongoing malabsorptive process. Her urine output was normal, and she did not have features of uremia. She was not on any drugs such as bisphosphonates or chemotherapeutic agents such as cisplatin which could lead to hypocalcemia.

She was diagnosed with follicular carcinoma of the thyroid at the age of 27 for which she underwent total thyroidectomy with lymph node excision 33 years ago. Histology revealed well-differentiated follicular carcinoma with multifocal capsular invasion and lymph node metastases. Operative notes indicate that parathyroid glands had been identified and preserved during the surgery. She was given Iodine-131 treatment once after the surgery. Her records did not reveal an immediate postoperative hypocalcemia. However, she was empirically treated with calcium and calcitriol in the immediate postoperative period for 3 months, after which it was stopped. Following surgery, she was regularly followed up and managed at an oncology unit, and there was no recurrence of the malignancy. She does not give a history of hypocalcemia for 30 years after surgery, until she developed the current symptoms 3 years back. She was on thyroxine 250 μg daily.

On examination, she had a body mass index (BMI) of 18 kg/m^2. Her mucosae were pink. There was no neck mass or lymphadenopathy. She had no dental abnormalities. She had no carpopedal spasms, and the Trousseau sign was positive, but with an absence of the Chvostek sign. Her cardiovascular system examination was normal with a pulse rate of 88 beats per minute (bpm), blood pressure of 130/80 mmHg, and without features of heart failure. Her respiratory and abdominal examinations were normal.

Her higher functions were normal, and she was oriented in time, place, and person. Her cranial nerves, upper limb, and lower limb examinations were within normal limits. There were no abnormal movements. She did not have cataracts, and the fundi were normal without papilledema. Her joint examination and the spine were normal.

Her psychiatric assessment on presentation revealed reduced sleep, lack of interest, and low mood, suggestive of depressive features, without any suicidal ideas. She did not have significant memory impairment.

At this point, after considering the history and examination, a possibility of hypocalcemia was suspected. Table 1 summarizes her investigation results. The serum-ionized calcium was 1.1 nmol/l, in the low normal range. Serum inorganic phosphate was 4.8 mg/dl, in the upper normal limit, suggestive of hypoparathyroidism. Her intact PTH level was 12.2 pg/ml, at low normal limit. Her serum magnesium level was within the normal range. Her 25 (OH) Vitamin D level was normal at 32 ng/ml, where >30 ng/ml of Vitamin D is widely accepted to be at a sufficient range [1]. Table 1 summarizes her important investigations at the current presentation, as well as during periodic follow-ups after surgery, which indicates that the calcium and phosphate levels had been within the normal range until the current presentation.

She did not have evidence of an alternative etiology for the hypoparathyroidism, including features of autoimmunity. Thus, she was diagnosed with late onset hypoparathyroidism following thyroidectomy, manifesting 30 years after the surgery. Her thyroxine dose was reduced to 200 μg daily. As she was clearly symptomatic for hypoparathyroidism, with the current calcium level, she was started on calcium carbonate, a total dose of 1500 mg daily with alphacalcidol 0.5 μg three times daily, aiming to keep calcium at a low normal range. At the follow-up visit, one month after her initial presentation, her symptoms showed a remarkable improvement, and the serum-ionized calcium level had normalized to 1.2 mmol/l.

2.2. Case 2. A 53-year-old Sri Lankan mother of two presented with pins and needle sensations of fingers, muscle pains, and cramps for 3 months duration. She did not have perioral numbness, and there was no history of seizures or limb weakness.

She had a significant psychiatric history with low mood and lack of interest in day-to-day activities for which she was treated with fluoxetine by her psychiatrist for 3 months. Her mood disorder had responded to this treatment, but she developed paranoid delusions regarding her relatives.

TABLE 1: Summary of investigations of case 1.

Investigation	Immediately after surgery	12 years after op	24 years after op	30 years after op	Normal range
Serum-ionized calcium	1.13 mmol/l	1.26 mmol/l	1.2 mmol/l	1.1 mmo/l	1.12–1.32 mmo/l
Serum phosphate	4.3 mg/dl	3.5 mg/dl	3.6 mg/dl	4.8 mg/dl	2.7–4.5 mg/dl
Serum potassium				4.6 mmo/l	3.5–5.1 mmol/l
Serum sodium				142 mmo/l	136–146 mmol/l
Serum magnesium				0.9 mmol/l	0.85–1.1 mmol/l
Intact PTH				12.2 pg/ml	10–69 pg/ml
S. 25(OH) vitamin D level				32 ng/ml	30–100 ng/ml
Thyroid stimulation hormone (TSH)	25 mIU/l	0.003 mIU/l	0.02 mIU/l	0.004 mIU/l	0.4–4 mIU/l
Fasting blood sugar (FBS)				88 mg/dl	

However, she did not have suicidal ideas or significant memory impairment. She also gave a history of fatigue, lethargy, and inertia, mainly early in the morning. Her other systemic inquiries were normal, and she did not have features of adrenal insufficiency or an ongoing autoimmune process.

She was diagnosed with papillary carcinoma of thyroid 12 years ago, at the age of 41 years, and underwent total thyroidectomy, followed by ablative Iodine-131 therapy. Since then, she had been on thyroxine 150 μg/day. She did not give a history suggestive of hypocalcemia immediately after surgery and had not been on calcium or calcitriol treatment. She did not develop symptoms suggestive of hypocalcemia after surgery until the current presentation. The patient attained menopause at 50 years of age.

On examination, she was averagely built with a BMI of 23 kg/m^2. She was not pale. She had examination features suggestive of hypothyroidism, including puffy face, dry skin, coarse hair, mild bilateral pitting ankle edema, and delayed relaxation of ankle jerks. Her Chvostek sign and Trousseau sign were negative. Her pulse rate was 64 bpm, and the blood pressure was 120/70 mmHg. Her neck examination was normal apart from the thyroidectomy scar. Neurological examination was normal. Fundi were normal without papilledema.

The initial investigations revealed Hb 11 g/dl, with normal renal functions. However, her TSH was 17.5 mIU/L and free thyroxine was 0.4 ng/dl, confirming our clinical diagnosis of hypothyroidism.

Thereafter, her thyroxine dose was optimized by gradually increasing the dose to 225 μg daily over 3 months, following which her TSH was found to be 0.7 mIU/L. With this, her lethargy, inertia, and numbness of fingers improved to some extent, but still were not normalized. Her low mood also persisted, and fluoxetine dose was increased to 40 mg/day. Despite these measures, symptoms were the same even after 3 months. At this stage, the patient was reassessed and found to have silent mild bilateral cataracts. The Chvostek sign and Trousseau sign were positive at this point.

Her electrocardiogram (ECG) was normal with normal QT interval. Serum-ionized calcium was low with phosphate in the upper normal range, with high urinary excretion of calcium, suggestive of hypoparathyroidism. Her vitamin D level was within the sufficient range. The PTH level was found to be low at 7 pg/ml, confirming the diagnosis of hypoparathyroidism. Her CT scan of the brain did not reveal basal ganglia calcification. Table 2 summarizes her investigations at periodic follow-up visits and current presentations, indicating that ionized calcium had been within the normal range in the previous visits.

She did not have evidence to suggest an alternative etiology for the hypoparathyroidism. Thus, she was diagnosed with late onset post-thyroidectomy hypoparathyroidism manifesting 12 years after surgery.

She was treated with calcium carbonate 1 g daily with calcitriol 0.25 μg twice daily. After 1 month of treatment, her fatigue, lethargy, and dry skin improved and mood normalized. Ionized calcium became normal at 1.21 mmol/l, and her 24 hour urine calcium was normal.

2.3. Case 3. A 49-year-old Sri Lankan female presented with severe aches and pains with spasms of the hands and feet for 2 years duration. She first started to experience vague aches and pains with stiffness of shoulders 2 years ago, and she also noticed episodic cramps and spasms of the hands and feet. She did not have associated memory impairment, change in behavior, or seizures. Her appetite, weight, and bowel habits remained unchanged during this time. There was no lethargy or cold intolerance.

She had a history of toxic multinodular goiter 13 years back, for which she underwent subtotal thyroidectomy. As histology revealed papillary carcinoma of the thyroid, she had undergone completion thyroidectomy, followed by I-131 treatment. Since then, she was on long-term thyroxine replacement of 200 μg daily with close follow-up and remained well until 2 years ago. She did not have records of low calcium levels after the surgery, and she had never been on calcium or calcitriol treatment until the current presentation.

On examination, she was well-looking and of average build. She had no alopecia, fungal infections, or vitiligo. The thyroidectomy scar was present, and there were no neck lumps or cervical lymphadenopathy. She did not have papilloedema or cataracts, and her upper limb and lower limb examinations were normal. She had positive Chvostek sign and Trousseau sign. Her abdominal, respiratory, and cardiovascular examinations were normal, with a normal pulse rate of 80 bpm.

Her available current and past investigations are summarized in Table 3. She had a TSH of 0.4, with normal free

TABLE 2: Summary of investigations of case 2.

Investigation	Immediately after surgery	1 year after op	5 years after op	12 years after op- 3 months before	12 years after op- current presentation	Normal range
Serum-ionized calcium	1.1 mmol/l	1.2 mmol/l	1.2 mmol/l		0.8 mmo/l	1.12–1.32 mmo/l
Serum phosphate	4.2 mg/dl	3 mg/dl	3.2 mg/dl		4.5 mg/dl	2.7–4.5 mg/dl
Alkaline phosphatase					123 IU/L	44–147 IU/l
24 hour urinary calcium excretion					270 mg/24 hours	100–300 mg/24 hours
24 hour urine phosphate excretion					400 mg/24 hours	500–1500 mg/24 hours
Serum magnesium					0.9 mmol/l	0.85–1.1 mmol/l
Intact PTH					7 pg/ml	10–69 pg/ml
S. 25(OH) vitamin D level					38 ng/ml	30–100 ng/ml
Thyroid stimulation hormone (TSH)		0.056 mIU/L	0.9 mIU/L	17.5 mIU/L	0.7 mIU/l	0.4–4 mIU/l
Free T4 (FT4)				0.4 ng/dl		0.89–1.76 ng/dl

TABLE 3: Summary of investigations of case 3.

Investigation	Immediately after surgery	1 year after op	5 years after op	13 years after op- current presentation	Normal range
Serum-ionized calcium	1.13 mmol/l	1.2 mmol/l	1.15 mmol/l	0.8 mmo/l	1.12–1.32 mmo/l
Serum phosphate	4.3 mg/dl			4.8 mg/dl	2.7–4.5 mg/dl
Alkaline phosphatase				130 IU/L	44–147 IU/l
24 hour urinary calcium excretion				280 mg/24 hours	100–300 mg/24 hours
24 hour urine phosphate excretion				550 mg/24 hours	500–1500 mg/24 hours
Serum magnesium				1.4 meq/l	1.3–2.1 meq/l
Intact PTH				9 pg/ml	10–69 pg/ml
S. 25(OH) vitamin D level				33 ng/ml	30–100 ng/ml
Thyroid stimulation hormone (TSH)		0.04 mIU/L	0.2 mIU/L	0.4 mIU/l	0.4–4 mIU/l
Free T4 (FT4)				1.4 ng/dl	0.89–1.76 ng/dl

T4. Her serum calcium was low with marginally high serum phosphate. The PTH level was low at 9 pg/ml. Her Vitamin D was within the sufficient range.

She did not have evidence to suggest an alternative cause for hypoparathyroidism. Therefore, she was diagnosed with delayed post-thyroidectomy hypoparathyroidism with onset 11 years after the surgery.

She was started on calcium and calcitriol, and her symptoms improved with normalization of the calcium level. Currently, she is on follow-up without complications.

3. Discussion

This series describes 3 cases of post-thyroidectomy hypoparathyroidism, which presented several years after thyroidectomy. The main risk factors for permanent hypoparathyroidism following thyroidectomy are total thyroidectomy, advanced age at surgery, female gender, Graves' disease, and retrosternal goiter [3, 4]. All these patients were females who had undergone total thyroidectomies for thyroid malignancies. As the posterior capsule of the thyroid is usually removed during thyroidectomy for thyroid malignancy, parathyroid glands are at high risk of injury, leading to an increased risk of hypoparathyroidism in these patients [5]. Furthermore, thyroid cancer is known to have an increased risk for hypoparathyroidism when central lymph node dissection is performed, which would have added to the risk in the patient in Case 1 [3]. Risk of hypoparathyroidism after reoperation is known to be higher than the first surgery, which would have made the patient in Case 3 more vulnerable [6].

Few studies have suggested a transient hypocalcemia following radioactive iodine (RAI) treatment in high doses for thyroid cancer. One small study which enrolled 19 patients undergoing RAI treatment at 100–150 mci found that serum calcium reduced by 6 months after RAI treatment with inappropriately normal PTH levels [7]. As all these patients were treated by postoperative I-131 treatment, it could also have been a contributory factor for her hypoparathyroidism; however, there is no adequate evidence to support this hypothesis.

These patients were not on calcium or calcitriol supplements and did not give a history suggestive of hypocalcemia for 30 years, 12 years, and 11 years, respectively, following thyroidectomy. In all these cases, no clear precipitating factors of hypocalcemia could be identified and there was no evidence of alternative etiology for hypoparathyroidism such as autoimmune, granulomatous, or infiltrative disorders.

This phenomenon of delayed hypoparathyroidism is usually thought to occur secondary to progressive atrophy of the parathyroid glands. Another possible explanation is scar tissue formation in the parathyroid glands causing late onset retraction of scar tissue leading to worsening of hypovascularization and slowly progressive ischemia [8, 9]. Parathyroid vasculature undergoing arteriosclerotic changes in an elderly patient leading to infarction or atrophy of the remaining parathyroid tissue has also been described as a possible underlying mechanism for this late occurrence of the condition [10].

This can also be associated with other known causes for hypoparathyroidism, such as autoimmune hypoparathyroidism and infiltrating diseases of the parathyroid gland. As the symptoms of hypocalcemia could be nonspecific and vague, they could very well be attributed to other diseases, causing the diagnosis of hypocalcemia to be further delayed. Furthermore, it is observed that some patients can tolerate hypocalcemia for several years without severe symptoms, further delaying the diagnosis [11, 12]. These patients might not be on regular follow-up for so long after surgery, which further contributes to a late detection of this phenomenon, as seen in our patients. As the symptoms could be precipitated due to a superadded vitamin D deficiency, which is highly prevalent in Sri Lanka, it should always be looked for and corrected in these patients.

Only a few cases of delayed hypoparathyroidism following thyroidectomy have been reported in the literature. Simões et al. reported a patient with hypocalcemia presenting 33 years after a thyroidectomy, with a seizure [10]. Kamath and Rao reported a patient who developed features of hypoparathyroidism after 15 years of a thyroidectomy which was diagnosed further 10 years later when the patient presented with a seizure [11]. Halperin et al. reviewed 4 patients with delayed hypoparathyroidism who presented 5–23 years after total thyroidectomy with paresthesia, seizures, and psychiatric manifestations [12]. Bellamy and Kendall-Taylor reported a case of hypoparathyroidism presented for the first time 36 years following a total thyroidectomy for papillary thyroid carcinoma and suggested that latent hypocalcemia following thyroidectomy could be more common than it actually appears to be [13].

These cases highlight the rare occurrence of delayed hypoparathyroidism following thyroidectomy and add to the body of the existing literature regarding this poorly understood phenomenon. Moreover, it is important to consider delayed hypoparathyroidism in any patient with a history of neck surgery, presenting with mild, vague symptoms or severe symptoms of hypocalcemia, despite the time duration after the surgery, as well as to monitor the patients undergoing thyroidectomy for symptoms of hypocalcemia for several years after surgery.

4. Conclusions

Hypoparathyroidism following thyroidectomy is a well-known phenomenon which is transient or permanent. Late-onset hypoparathyroidism after several years of thyroidectomy is rare and occurs due to underlying progressive ischemia or atrophy of the parathyroid glands which were identified and preserved during surgery, but gives rise to hypocalcemia several years after the surgery. This diagnosis can easily be missed in these patients, as the symptoms are relatively vague and may mimic many other diseases. They might also not be regularly followed up long enough for the suspicion to be aroused. However, the correct diagnosis and treatment can effectively alleviate symptoms and prevent long-term complications of hypocalcemia. Therefore, although rare, this is an important phenomenon which clinicians should have in mind when evaluating patients with a history of neck surgery, irrespective of the timing of surgery.

References

[1] C. Gambardella, R. Patrone, F. Di Capua et al., "The role of prophylactic central compartment lymph node dissection in elderly patients with differentiated thyroid cancer: a multicentric study," *BMC Surgery*, vol. 18, p. 110, 2019.

[2] O. E. Anastasiou, M. P. Yavropoulou, T. S. Papavramidis et al., "Secretory capacity of the parathyroid glands after total thyroidectomy in normocalcemic subjects," *The Journal of Clinical Endocrinology & Metabolism*, vol. 97, no. 7, pp. 2341–2346, 2012.

[3] L. A. Orloff, S. M. Wiseman, V. J. Bernet et al., "American thyroid association statement on postoperative hypoparathyroidism: diagnosis, prevention, and management in adults," *Thyroid*, vol. 28, no. 7, pp. 830–841, 2018.

[4] J. E. Jesus and A. Landry, "Chvostek's and trousseau's signs," *New England Journal of Medicine*, vol. 367, no. 11, p. e15, 2012.

[5] M. Testini, L. Rosato, N. Avenia et al., "The impact of single parathyroid gland autotransplantation during thyroid surgery on postoperative hypoparathyroidism: a multicenter study," *Transplantation Proceedings*, vol. 39, no. 1, pp. 225–230, 2007.

[6] J. H. Lefevre, C. Tresallet, L. Leenhardt, C. Jublanc, J.-P. Chigot, and F. Menegaux, "Reoperative surgery for thyroid disease," *Langenbeck's Archives of Surgery*, vol. 392, no. 6, pp. 685–691, 2007.

[7] A. Guven, S. Salman, H. Boztepe et al., "Parathyroid changes after high dose radioactive iodine in patients with thyroid cancer," *Annals of Nuclear Medicine*, vol. 23, no. 5, pp. 437–441, 2009.

[8] C. A. Simões, M. K. Costa, L. B. Comerlato et al., "A case of "late" postsurgical hypoparathyroidism," *Case Reports in Endocrinology*, vol. 2017, Article ID 3962951, 2 pages, 2017.

[9] R. E. Cox, "Hypoparathyroidism: an unusual cause of seizures," *Annals of Emergency Medicine*, vol. 12, no. 5, pp. 314-315, 1983.

[10] B. M. Blanchard, "Focal hypocalcemic seizures 33 years after thyroidectomy," *Archives of Internal Medicine*, vol. 110, no. 3, pp. 382–385, 1962.

[11] S. D. Kamath and B. S. Rao, "Delayed post-surgical hypoparathyroidism: the forgotten chameleon!" *Journal of Clinical and Diagnostic Research*, vol. 11, no. 2, pp. OD07–OD09, 2017.
[12] I. Halperin, A. Nubiola, J. Vendrell, and E. Vilardell, "Late-onset hypocalcemia appearing years after thyroid surgery," *Journal of Endocrinological Investigation*, vol. 12, no. 6, pp. 419-420, 1989.
[13] R. J. Bellamy and P. Kendall-Taylor, "Unrecognized hypocalcaemia diagnosed 36 years after thyroidectomy," *Journal of the Royal Society of Medicine*, vol. 88, no. 12, pp. 690-691, 1995.

2

Pituitary Hyperplasia in Severe Primary Hypothyroidism: A Case Report and Review of the Literature

Prateek Shukla[1] **, Ketan R. Bulsara,**[2,3] **and Pooja Luthra**[2,4]

[1]*Division of Internal Medicine, UConn Health Center, Farmington, CT 06030, USA*
[2]*University of Connecticut School of Medicine, Farmington, CT 06030, USA*
[3]*Division of Neurosurgery, UConn Health Center, Farmington, CT 06030, USA*
[4]*Division of Endocrinology and Metabolism, UConn Health Center, Farmington, CT 06030, USA*

Correspondence should be addressed to Prateek Shukla; shukla@uchc.edu

Academic Editor: Mihail A. Boyanov

Pituitary hyperplasia is commonly present but remains largely undiagnosed in primary hypothyroidism. It is easily reversible with thyroid replacement therapy. If imaging is performed prior to biochemical evaluation, then patients may undergo pituitary surgery. We present the case of a 34-year-old female with profound primary hypothyroidism and secondary pituitary hyperplasia that resolved after thyroid hormone supplementation. We will discuss the current literature regarding pituitary hyperplasia in primary hypothyroidism in adults.

1. Introduction

Pituitary hyperplasia is a relatively common condition that occurs in both physiological and pathological states. Pregnancy is the most common condition associated with physiological pituitary enlargement, associated primarily with lactotroph hyperplasia [1, 2]. Pathological hyperplasia has been shown to be associated with end organ insufficiency from primary gonadal insufficiency [3, 4], primary adrenal insufficiency [5], and primary hypothyroidism [2, 6–50]. Although traditionally thought to be uncommon [44], pituitary enlargement is common in primary hypothyroidism and has now been well documented in the literature [2, 6–50].

We present an interesting case of a 34-year-old female with no prior diagnosis of hypothyroidism but a long history of hypothyroid symptoms, who presented with sudden onset of neurologic symptoms and an enlarged pituitary gland secondary to profound primary hypothyroidism. We will also review the published literature on pituitary hyperplasia secondary to primary hypothyroidism.

2. Case Report

Our patient is a 34-year-old Caucasian female with a past history of attention deficit hyperactivity disorder, hypertension, irritable bowel syndrome, and anxiety disorder who had a long standing history of dry skin and abnormal menstrual periods. She is nulligravida and had menorrhagia with irregular menses and increasing polymenorrhea, several months prior to presentation. She also had a history of chronic diarrhea alternating with constipation but had experienced a recent 20 lb weight gain. 1 month prior to presentation, she developed galactorrhea with breast enlargement and tenderness. 3 weeks prior to presentation, evaluation by her gynecologist revealed a thyroid stimulating hormone (TSH) >150 mIU/mL (0.5-5.5) free thyroxine (FT4) 0.4 ng/dL (0.61-1.82) and prolactin 29.4 ng/mL (3.34-26.72). An MRI of the pituitary at an outside facility revealed an enlarged pituitary gland measuring 14x12 mm, abutting the optic chiasm (Figures 1(a) and 1(b)). She presented to the hospital with a 1-day history of transient blurry vision, apraxia and aphasia, transient chest tightness, and increasing anxiety. The vision changes were described as an inability to focus on near objects with no reported loss of visual fields. She denied any pain or swelling in her neck, recent viral infections, excessive iodine intake, exposure to iodinated contrast agents, lithium or amiodarone, and any history of prolonged steroid use. She denied any increasing skin tags, changes in appearance or changes in ring or shoe size. There

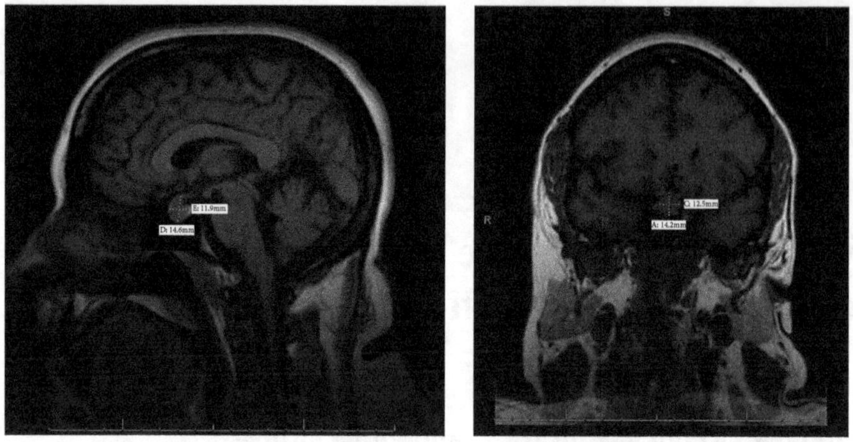

(a) Precontrast sagittal T-1 MRI. 2 weeks prior to presentation

(b) Precontrast coronal T-1 MRI. 2 weeks prior to presentation

FIGURE 1

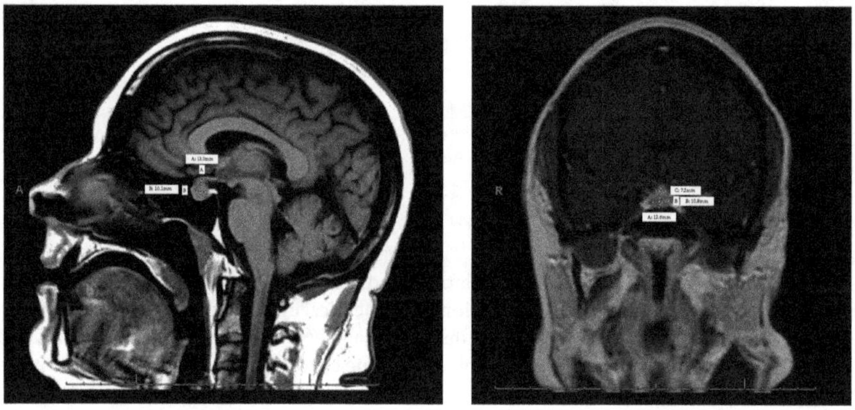

(a) Sagittal T1 MRI on admission

(b) Coronal T1 MRI from hospital admission

FIGURE 2

were no symptoms suggestive of adrenal insufficiency. Her medications included amphetamine, nebivolol, clonazepam, citalopram, hydrochlorothiazide, polyethylene glycol, and levocetirizine. Family history was significant for hyperthyroidism in her sister but was otherwise unremarkable for any pituitary disorders.

On physical exam, she had a body mass index of 41.53 kg/m^2, blood pressure of 110/89 mmHg, heart rate being regular at 62 beats per minute, and breathing 14 breaths per minute with oxygen saturations of 96% on ambient air. She was obese and in no distress, and oriented to time, place, and person. There was no obvious thyromegaly. No abdominal stria was noted and overall exam was unremarkable other than dry skin. Her neurological exam was normal and there were no obvious visual field deficits on bedside examination. Laboratory evaluation showed a (Table 1) TSH of 251.21 mIU/mL (0.5-5.5), total T4 of 2.07 μg/dL (4.87-11.72), FT4 of 0.44 ng/dL (0.61-1.82), free triiodothyronin (FT3) of 1.5 pg/mL (2.2-4.2), prolactin of 29.48 ng/mL (3.34-26.72) (23.5 ng/ml by dilution), estradiol 20 pg/mL, Luteinizing Hormone (LH) 2.52 mIU/mL, Follicle Stimulating Hormone (FSH) 5.03 mIU/mL, morning cortisol 8 μg/dL, adrenocorticotrophic hormone (ACTH) 10 pg/mL (6-58), insulin-like growth factor-1 (IGF-1) 109 ng/mL (108-368), Thyroglobulin antibody 4.9 IU/mL (0-4), thyroglobulin 159 ng/mL (1.3-31.8), Microsomal Antibody 1096.2 IU/mL (0-9), and Alpha subunit- 3.4 ng/mL (reference range <1.02). A repeat MRI of the pituitary at the time of admission showed an enlarged pituitary, 13x10.1 mm, which appeared slightly improved from the MRI 3 weeks prior to presentation, with decreased involvement of the optic chiasm (Figures 2(a) and 2(b)).

She was initially evaluated for surgery, for presumed diagnoses of pituitary macroadenoma; however prompt recognition of severe primary hypothyroidism causing pituitary hyperplasia prevented any unnecessary surgical intervention. She was started on levothyroxine and liothyronine replacement therapy. Six weeks after her initial presentation, laboratory evaluation showed improvement in thyroid function test with a (Table 1) TSH of 11.23 mIU/mL, FT4- 1.25 ng/dL, Total T3- 95 ng/dL (48-178), free T3 5.7 pg/mL, and Alpha subunit 0.53 ng/mL. A repeat MRI of the pituitary also showed decrease in the height of the pituitary gland to 10.5 mm and

Table 1: Thyroid function profile trend.

	TSH mIU/mL	Free T4 (ng/dL)	Free T3 (pg/mL)	Total T3 (ng/dL)
Baseline	251.21	0.44	1.5	-
6 weeks	11.23	1.25	-	95
4 months	0.77	1.63	-	141

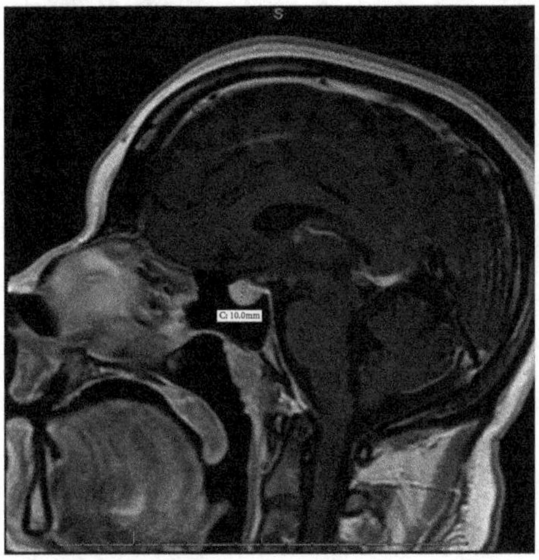

(a) Postcontrast T1 MRI image at 6 weeks from presentation

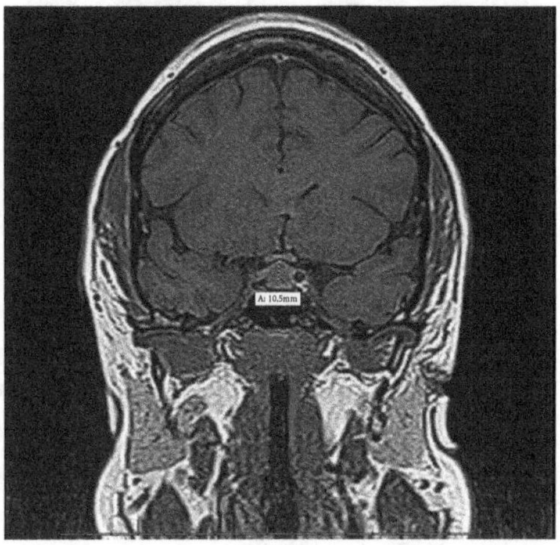

(b) Postcontrast coronal T2 MRI image at 6 weeks from presentation

Figure 3

with less involvement of the optic chiasm (Figures 3(a) and 3(b)). Within the pituitary gland, there was a 3 mm hypoenhancing focus in the right adenohypophysis suggestive of a microadenoma. She is currently doing well with significant improvement in her symptoms. Repeat laboratory evaluation 3 months after her initial presentation showed complete normalization of thyroid function tests (Table 1) with TSH 0.77 mIU/mL, Total T3 141 ng/dL, and FT4 1.63 ng/dL.

MRI of the pituitary 3 months after presentation shows that the pituitary measures 9.5 mm with a persistent 5 mm hypoenhancing focus in the right adenohypophysis (Figures 4(a) and 4(b)). The rest of the anterior pituitary hormone levels continue to be within reference range. The small microadenoma is thought to be an incidentaloma and is being monitored.

3. Discussion

Pituitary hyperplasia in profound and severe primary hypothyroidism was first recognized from the autopsy of a cretin in 1851 [51]. We performed a review of literature of all the case reports, case series, and reviews of adult patients with primary hypothyroidism and pituitary hyperplasia published in the English language (Supplement: Table 2) [2, 6–50]. We excluded case reports, case series, and reviews that only include pediatric cases or were published in a language other than English. The incidence of pituitary hyperplasia in primary hypothyroidism has not been clearly identified, but recent literature suggests that it may be more common than previously accepted. Autopsy studies, by Scheithauer et al. [52] in patients with primary hypothyroidism, have shown diffuse and nodular thyrotropic cell hyperplasia in 69% and 25% of glands, respectively, and a crude correlation was observed between the degree of thyrotropic cell hyperplasia and the relative lack of thyroid hormone replacement therapy. While all patients with pituitary hyperplasia due to primary hypothyroidism will exhibit some signs or symptoms of hypothyroidism, only 38% present with a chief complaint suggestive of hypothyroidism on initial presentation. Additionally up to 25% of the patients with primary hypothyroidism and associated pituitary hyperplasia will present with "tumoral signs" or presence of pituitary enlargement and 36% will present with signs or symptoms of hyperprolactinemia on initial presentation [53]. This is similar to our patient, who although had classic symptoms of primary hypothyroidism, sought medical attention primarily for headache and neurological symptoms.

Prolonged primary hypothyroidism leads to pituitary hyperplasia due to loss of negative feedback from lack of circulating thyroxine (T4) and triiodothyronine (T3), leading to excessive thyrotropin releasing hormone (TRH) secretion from the hypothalamus. Pituitary "tumorous" hyperplasia due to primary hypothyroidism occurs most frequently, accounting for approximately 33.3% of cases of secondary pituitary hyperplasia from end organ insufficiencies [40]. It is interesting to note that thyrotrophs comprise only 5%-10% of the adenohypohysial cells but can still cause significant pituitary enlargement [29, 53]. This can partly be explained by the fact that the number of thyrotrophs can increase substantially to up to 34% of the all adenohypophysial cells in patients with hypothyroidism [53]. This has been confirmed by histologic examination of the pituitary gland in cases

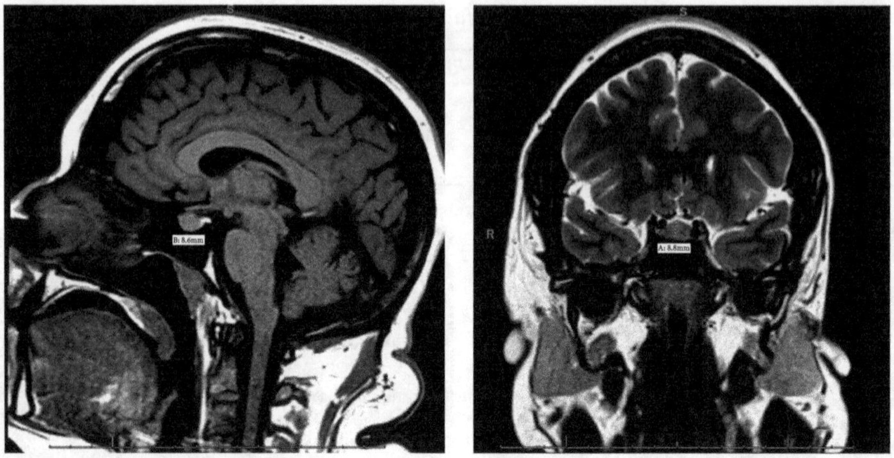

(a) Postcontrast sagittal T1 MRI image. 3 months from presentation

(b) Postcontrast coronal T2 MRI image. 3 months from presentation

FIGURE 4

where surgery was inadvertently performed [10, 21, 29]. As early as 1976, Yamada et al. [54] suggested that there was pituitary enlargement in patients with primary hypothyroidism. They showed evidence that 81% of patients with hypothyroidism have an abnormal increase in the volume of the sella turcica. In addition, the volume of sella turcica was directly related to the level of TSH and inversely related to the circulating thyroxine levels, suggesting that hyperplasia causes an increase in pituitary size [54].

Other observational studies also show a correlation between serum TSH level and the degree of pituitary enlargement. In an observational study by Khawaja et al. [37] which enrolled patients with TSH greater than 50 μIU/mL, pituitary enlargement on MRI was found in 37 of the 53 patients (70%), with 31 of the 37 patients (84%) having TSH levels of $\geq$100 μIU/mL. In the same study, younger patients, mostly females, with primary hypothyroidism tended to have higher incidence of pituitary enlargement [37]. A review of the current literature of several pediatric cases and most cases in adults also suggest the same, which is similar to our patient.

Another common theme, in patients with profound primary hypothyroidism and pituitary hyperplasia, is the presence of clinical and/or biochemical hyperprolactinemia. Profoundly hypothyroid patients will have concomitant hyperprolactinemia related to the elevated TRH level. In a study by Honbo et al. [55] in 1978, the serum prolactin level was found to be elevated in 39% of patients with untreated primary hypothyroidism. A significant correlation was found between serum prolactin and TSH, suggesting that the elevated serum prolactin level in primary hypothyroidism is mediated by TRH through negative feedback from hypothyroidism and not primarily by stalk effect [55]. The response of prolactin to TRH is also exaggerated in hypothyroid states vs. euthyroid states and is blunted in hyperthyroid states [56]. This has been highlighted in the literature in several instances, confounding the diagnosis and patients may be mislabeled with a pituitary adenoma or prolactinoma [6, 14–24, 28, 29, 35, 41, 49]. This was also the case in our patient, where she had clinical symptoms of hyperprolactinemia and mild elevation of serum prolactin levels. Moreover, pituitary lactotroph hyperplasia has also been identified on histology in patients with primary hypothyroidism [52].

The presence of pituitary enlargement and elevated TSH levels raises the possibility of a thyrotropin producing pituitary adenoma. However, those tend to be exceedingly rare, accounting for about 0.5% of all pituitary adenomas [53]. It is very important to make an accurate diagnosis to avoid devastating consequences of inappropriate pituitary surgery. The differential diagnosis for our patient included a pituitary adenoma, pituitary hyperplasia, thyroid hormone resistance, or hypophysitis. The presence of biochemical hypothyroidism and response to thyroid hormone replacement made the diagnosis of pituitary hyperplasia in our patient. Biochemical excess or deficiency for other pituitary hormones was ruled out. Appropriate response to thyroid hormone replacement therapy ruled out thyroid hormone resistance. Our patient had a mildly elevated alpha subunit initially which was likely related with profound hypothyroidism and subsequent testing revealed normal levels. In other reported cases, chronic untreated primary hypothyroidism with pituitary hyperplasia has caused long term sequelae, with complete pituitary failure and panhypopituitarism with appearance of empty sella syndrome [7, 44]. Other confounding clinical scenarios have been reported with "pseudoacromegaly," where patients had clinical signs and symptoms suggestive of acromegaly and imaging suggestive of pituitary adenoma; however a complete clinical history and biochemical evaluation revealed primary hypothyroidism [43, 50].

Although there are certain imaging characteristics that are traditionally associated with either pituitary hyperplasia or an adenoma, even with the use of modern imaging techniques like computed tomography (CT) and magnetic resonance imaging (MRI) with contrast injection, it is still challenging to distinguish between a pituitary adenoma and hyperplasia. The traditional CT criteria for pituitary macroadenoma include homogeneous enlargement of the gland to a height of greater than 10 mm, with or without erosion of the floor of the sella and deviation of the stalk [27]. Although an MRI offers better delineation of adenohypophyseal anatomy, its use cannot always reliably differentiate one from the other. Pituitary hyperplasia is often characterized as a homogeneously enhancing lesion [57] or a midline prominence of a pituitary mass with smooth contours (the "nipple sign") on a MRI [27]. While MRI findings suggestive of a TSH-secreting adenoma, include a central enhancing mass with a rim of normal compressed pituitary tissue, this can also be seen in pituitary hyperplasia [26, 27].

Appropriate biochemical testing is needed to guide management in such situations. Our case echoes previous case reports, where MRI of the brain was unable to rule out what was considered a symptomatic pituitary adenoma as the cause of pituitary enlargement. As a result, surgical intervention involving removal of the pituitary mass via transphenoidal approach was planned. Surgery was however avoided since thyroid hormone replacement demonstrated regression of the pituitary size on follow-up imaging. This response to therapy suggests TRH-related hyperplasia as the primary cause of pituitary enlargement. It also demonstrates the importance of approaching surgical management of pituitary enlargement in cases of profound primary hypothyroidism with caution. However, it should be noted that increased cell multiplication in cases of hyperplasia may lead to neoplastic transformation of thyrotropin cells and formation of independent TSH producing adenomas, where surgery may be necessary [58]. As a result, early response to hormone replacement therapy does not rule out an underlying neoplasm, and patients should continue to be followed by serial imaging, to track future changes in pituitary size and to evaluate for any adenomas that may be masked by the hyperplasia.

In patients who did undergo pituitary surgery, usually no adenomas were found and histologic examination revealed thyrotrophs that were large, oval with eccentric nucleus, and abundant slightly acidophilic cytoplasm and resemble those seen in the hypothyroid rat pituitary [29]. In addition, in a case series of 3 patients who underwent surgeries for suspected pituitary adenomas, there was combined hyperplasia of both thyrotrophs and lactotrophs. Histologically, no adenomas were identified; however these were suspected clinically, radiologically and in 2 cases, and identified operatively as well [21]. In the previously mentioned autopsy study by Scheithauer et al. [52] on patients with primary hypothyroidism, 94% of the glands showed thyrotroph hyperplasia without significant mass formation and almost 20% demonstrated lactotroph hyperplasia.

It has been shown that pituitary hyperplasia can progress rapidly following the induction of a hypothyroid state. In a series of 14 patients by Shimono et al. [57] who underwent radioactive iodine ablation for distant metastasis for thyroid cancer, the hypothyroid patients had significantly larger pituitary volume both quantitatively and visually on MRI, in comparison to healthy euthyroid volunteers within 3-5 weeks of induction of hypothyroid state. Conversely, replacement with thyroid hormones has also been shown to decrease pituitary size, even as early as 1 week [27]. The rapid response within 1 week was hypothesized by the authors of this study to have been related with the use of high triiodothyronine load used to investigate for thyroid hormone resistance and replacement with high doses of supplemental thyroid hormone [27]. In the study by Shimono et al. [57], the pituitary size decreased 5 weeks after thyroid hormone replacement. Khawaja et al. [37] reported regression of pituitary hyperplasia in 85% of patients who had a follow-up MRI. Most patients will tend to respond anywhere between 4 weeks to 3 months, with documented regression in almost all cases. The same was true for our patient, who had a good response to replacement with thyroid hormone within 6 weeks. The molecular mechanisms underlying this effect of thyroid hormone causing regression of pituitary hyperplasia remains unknown and speculative. However, it may likely be similar to that of dopamine agonist therapy induced reduction in pituitary volume in prolactinomas [59].

4. Conclusion

Pituitary hyperplasia in primary hypothyroidism is not uncommon and pituitary enlargement can be frequently observed on imaging. However, imaging with CT or MRI may not be able to reliably differentiate between an adenoma and hyperplasia and biochemical testing should guide diagnosis and management. Both radiographic imaging results and biochemical testing results are essential prior to proceeding with surgical intervention. Patients with hypothyroidism, who have pituitary enlargement incidentally diagnosed on brain imaging for other reasons, should be treated with thyroid hormone replacement and close follow-up and with repeat imaging.

Acknowledgments

The authors acknowledge Devin Bagec (University of Connecticut School of Medicine, Farmington CT 06030), Sai Aparna Nelakanti, and MBBS (Division of Endocrinology and Metabolism, UConn Health Center, Farmington CT 06030) who assisted in the writing of this article.

References

[1] E. Horvath, K. Kovacs, and B. Scheithauer, "Pituitary hyperplasia," *Pituitary*, vol. 1, no. 3/4, pp. 169–179, 1999.

[2] S. M. C. De Sousa, P. Earls, and A. I. McCormack, "Pituitary hyperplasia: case series and literature review of an under-recognised and heterogeneous condition," *Endocrinology, Diabetes & Metabolism Case Reports*, vol. 1, 2015.

[3] N. A. Samaan, A. V. Stepanas, J. Danziger, and J. Trujillo, "Reactive pituitary abnormalities in patients with Klinefelter's and Turner's syndromes," *JAMA Internal Medicine*, vol. 139, no. 2, pp. 198–201, 1979.

[4] B. W. Scheithauer, M. Moschopulos, K. Kovacs, B. S. Jhaveri, T. Percek, and R. V. Lloyd, "The pituitary in Klinefelter syndrome," *Endocrine Pathology*, vol. 16, no. 2, pp. 133–138, 2005.

[5] S. J. Winters, T. Vitaz, M. R. Nowacki, D. C. Craddock, C. Silverman, and F. A. Lopez, "Addison's disease and pituitary enlargement," *The American Journal of the Medical Sciences*, vol. 349, no. 6, pp. 526–529, 2015.

[6] W. R. Keye, B. H. Yuen, R. F. Knopf, and R. B. Jaffe, "Amenorrhea, hyperprolactinemia, and pituitary enlargement secondary to primary hypothyroidism: successful treatment with thyroid replacement," *Obstetrics & Gynecology*, vol. 48, no. 6, pp. 697–702, 1976.

[7] A. G. Vagenakis, K. Dole, and L. E. Braverman, "Pituitary enlargement, pituitary failure, and primary hypothyroidism," *Annals of Internal Medicine*, vol. 85, no. 2, pp. 195–198, 1976.

[8] M. H. Jawadi, L. B. Ballonoff, J. C. Stears, and F. H. Katz, "Primary hypothyroidism and pituitary enlargement: radiological evidence of pituitary regression," *Archives of Internal Medicine*, vol. 138, no. 10, pp. 1555–1557, 1978.

[9] J. C. Pita, S. Shafey, and R. Pina, "Diminution of large pituitary tumor after replacement therapy for primary hypothyroidism," *Neurology*, vol. 29, no. 8, p. 1169, 1979.

[10] M. S. Katz, R. I. Gregerman, E. Horvath, K. Kovacs, and C. Ezrin, "Thyrotroph cell adenoma of the human pituitary gland associated with primary hypothyroidism: clinical and morphological features," *Acta Endocrinologica*, vol. 95, no. 1, pp. 41–48, 1980.

[11] B. J. Silver, J. L. Kyner, A. R. Dick, and C. H. J. Chang, "Primary hypothyroidism: suprasellar pituitary enlargement and regression on computed tomographic scanning," *Journal of the American Medical Association*, vol. 246, no. 4, pp. 364-365, 1981.

[12] R. S. Gup, L. R. Sheeler, M. C. Maeder, and J. M. Tew, "PituitaRy enlargement and primary hypothyroidism: a report of two cases with sharply contrasting outcomes," *Neurosurgery*, vol. 11, no. 6, pp. 792–794, 1982.

[13] L. J. Valenta, J. Tamkin, R. Sostrin, A. N. Elias, and H. Eisenberg, "Regression of a pituitary adenoma following levothyroxine therapy of primary hypothyroidism," *Fertility and Sterility*, vol. 40, no. 3, pp. 389–392, 1983.

[14] A. Khalil, K. Kovacs, A. A. Sima, G. N. Burrow, and E. Horvath, "Pituitary thyrotroph hyperplasia mimicking prolactin-secreting adenoma," *Journal of Endocrinological Investigation*, vol. 7, no. 4, pp. 399–404, 1984.

[15] T. R. Groff, B. L. Shulkin, R. D. Utiger, and L. M. Talbert, "Amenorrhea-galactorrhea, hyperprolactinemia, and suprasellar pituitary enlargement as presenting features of primary hypothyroidism," *Obstetrics & Gynecology*, vol. 63, no. 3, pp. 86S–89S, 1984.

[16] L. T. Bilaniuk, T. Moshang, J. Cara et al., "Pituitary enlargement mimicking pituitary tumor," *Journal ofNeurosurgery*, vol. 63, no. 1, pp. 39–42, 1985.

[17] P. J. Heyburn, O. M. Gibby, M. Hourihan, R. Hall, and M. F. Scanlon, "Primary hypothyroidism presenting as amenorrhoea and galactorrhoea with hyperprolactinaemia and pituitary enlargement," *British Medical Journal (Clinical Research Ed.)*, vol. 292, no. 6536, pp. 1660-1661, 1986.

[18] C. Christopoulos, "Primary hypothyroidism presenting as amenorrhoea and galactorrhoea with hyperprolactinaemia and pituitary enlargement," *British Medical Journal (Clinical Research Ed.)*, vol. 293, no. 6547, pp. 624-625, 1986.

[19] M. R. Grubb, D. Chakeres, and W. B. Malarkey, "Patients with primary hypothyroidism presnting as prolactinomas," *American Journal of Medicine*, vol. 83, no. 4, pp. 765–769, 1987.

[20] T. Fujii, S. Misumi, K. Onoda, H. Fukuda, and Y. Ibuki, "Pituitary enlargement with target organ deficiency: hypothyroidism and hypogonadism," *World Neurosurgery*, vol. 28, no. 5, pp. 390–394, 1987.

[21] E. P. Pioro, B. W. Scheithauer, E. R. Laws Jr., R. V. Randall, K. T. Kovacs, and E. Horvath, "Combined thyrotroph and lactotroph cell hyperplasia simulating prolactin-secreting pituitary adenoma in long-standing primary hypothyroidism," *World Neurosurgery*, vol. 29, no. 3, pp. 218–226, 1988.

[22] M. Ahmed, M. Banna, N. Sakati, and N. Woodhouse, "Pituitary gland enlargement in primary hypothyroidism: a report of 5 cases with follow-up data," *Hormone Research*, vol. 32, no. 5-6, pp. 188–192, 1989.

[23] W. W. Hutchins, J. V. Crues III, P. Miya, and K. W. Pojunas, "MR demonstration of pituitary hyperplasia and regression after therapy for hypothyroidism," *American Journal of Neuroradiology*, vol. 11, no. 2, p. 410, 1990.

[24] A. W. Chan, I. A. Macfarlane, P. M. Foy, and J. B. Miles, "Pituitary enlargement and hyperprolactinaemia due to primary hypothyroidism: errors and delays in diagnosis," *British Journal of Neurosurgery*, vol. 4, no. 2, pp. 107–112, 1990.

[25] G. Fulcher, J. Roche, and A. McElduff, "Primary hypothyroidism with pituitary enlargement and a visual field abnormality," *Journal of Medical Imaging and Radiation Oncology*, vol. 36, no. 1, pp. 37–39, 1992.

[26] L. J. Wolansky, G. D. Leavitt, B. J. Elias, H. J. Lee, A. Dasmahapatra, and W. Byrne, "MRI of pituitary hyperplasia in hypothyroidism," *Neuroradiology*, vol. 38, no. 1, pp. 50–52, 1995.

[27] N. J. Sarlis, F. Brucker-Davis, J. L. Doppman, and M. C. Skarulis, "MRI-demonstrable regression of a pituitary mass in a case of primary hypothyroidism after a week of acute thyroid hormone therapy," *The Journal of Clinical Endocrinology & Metabolism*, vol. 82, no. 3, pp. 808–811, 1997.

[28] N. Özbey, E. Sariyildiz, L. Yilmaz, Y. Orhan, E. Sencer, and S. Molvalilar, "Primary hypothyroidism with hyperprolactinaemia and pituitary enlargement mimicking a pituitary macroadenoma," *International Journal of Clinical Practice*, vol. 51, no. 6, pp. 409–411, 1997.

[29] A. M. Alkhani, M. Cusimano, K. Kovacs, J. M. Bilbao, E. Horvath, and W. Singer, "Cytology of pituitary thyrotroph hyperplasia in protracted primary hypothyroidism," *The Pituitary Society*, vol. 1, no. 3-4, pp. 291–295, 1999.

[30] M. Young, K. Kattner, and K. Gupta, "Pituitary hyperplasia resulting from primary hypothyroidism mimicking macroadenomas," *British Journal of Neurosurgery*, vol. 13, no. 2, pp. 138–142, 1999.

[31] S. Yamagishi and M. Yokoyama-Ohta, "A rare case of pituitary hyperplasia with suprasellar extension due to primary myxoedema: case report," *Journal of International Medical Research*, vol. 27, no. 1, pp. 49–52, 1999.

[32] W. C. Nicholas and W. F. Russell, "Primary hypothyroidism presenting as a pituitary mass," *Journal of the Mississippi State Medical Association*, vol. 41, no. 3, pp. 511–514, 2000.

[33] S. M. Manocha, N. D. Moulick, and N. S. Shah, "Primary hypothyroidism presenting as a pituitary gland enlargement with regression following thyroxine therapy," *Journal of the Association of Physicians of India*, vol. 48, no. 6, p. 651, 2000.

[34] K. Hoogenberg and K. van Tol, "Pituitary hyperplasia during primary hypothyroidism," *Thyroid*, vol. 13, no. 8, pp. 831-832, 2003.

[35] J. M. Kroese, A. F. Grootendorst, and L. J. D. M. Schelfhout, "Postpartum amenorrhoea-galactorrhoea associated with hyperprolactinaemia and pituitary enlargement in primary hypothyroidism," *The Netherlands Journal of Medicine*, vol. 62, no. 1, pp. 28–30, 2004.

[36] A. S. Joshi and P. D. Woolf, "Pituitary hyperplasia secondary to primary hypothyroidism: a case report and review of the literature," *The Pituitary Society*, vol. 8, no. 2, pp. 99–103, 2005.

[37] N. M. Khawaja, B. M. Taher, M. E. Barham et al., "Pituitary enlargement in patients with primary hypothyroidism," *Endocrine Practice*, vol. 12, no. 1, pp. 29–34, 2006.

[38] E. Passeri, A. Tufano, M. Locatelli, A. G. Lania, B. Ambrosi, and S. Corbetta, "Large pituitary hyperplasia in severe primary hypothyroidism," *The Journal of Clinical Endocrinology & Metabolism*, vol. 96, no. 1, pp. 22-23, 2011.

[39] A. Agrawal and S. Diwan, "Pituitary hyperplasia resulting from primary hypothyroidism," *Asian Journal of Neurosurgery*, vol. 6, no. 2, pp. 99-100, 2011.

[40] L. Han, J. Wang, K. Shu, and T. Lei, "Pituitary tumorous hyperplasia due to primary hypothyroidism," *Acta Neurochirurgica*, vol. 154, no. 8, pp. 1489–1492, 2012.

[41] R. Rajput, A. Sehgal, and D. Gahlan, "Reversible thyrotroph hyperplasia with hyperprolactinemia: A rare presenting manifestation of primary hypothyroidism," *Indian Journal of Endocrinology and Metabolism*, vol. 16, no. 6, p. 1037, 2012.

[42] L. Eiland, N. M. Oyesiku, J. C. Ritchie, S. Isaacs, and A. G. Ioachimescu, "Pathogenesis of marked pituitary enlargement and increased serum thyroid-stimulating hormone in primary hypothyroidism," *Thyroid*, vol. 22, no. 1, pp. 101-102, 2012.

[43] K. H. Kumar, A. Shaikh, I. Anwar, and P. Prusty, "Primary hypothyroidism presenting as pseudoacromegaly," *Pituitary*, vol. 15, no. S1, pp. 49–52, 2012.

[44] D. Dutta, I. Maisnam, S. Ghosh et al., "Panhypopituitarism with empty sella a sequel of pituitary hyperplasia due to chronic primary hypothyroidism," *Indian Journal of Endocrinology and Metabolism*, vol. 16, Supplement 2, p. S282, 2012.

[45] C. P. Neves, E. T. Massolt, R. P. Peeters et al., "Pituitary hyperplasia: an uncommon presentation of a common disease , Endocrinology," *Endocrinology, Diabetes & Metabolism Case Reports*, no. 1, 2015.

[46] A. Moumen and A. Meftah, "An unusual pituitary mass revealing a primary hypothyroidism!," *Clinics and Practice*, vol. 5, no. 1, 2015.

[47] A. I. Siddiqi, J. Grieve, K. Miszkiel, and S. E. Baldeweg, "Tablets or scalpel: Pituitary hyperplasia due to primary hypothyroidism," *Radiology Case Reports*, vol. 10, no. 2, p. 1099, 2015.

[48] A. L. Pappy, N. Oyesiku, and A. Ioachimescu, "Severe TSH elevation and pituitary enlargement after changing thyroid replacement to compounded T4/T3 therapy," *Journal of Investigative Medicine High Impact Case Reports*, vol. 4, no. 3, Article ID 2324709616661834, 2016.

[49] M. S. Ansari and M. H. Almalki, "Primary hypothyroidism with markedly high prolactin," *Frontiers in Endocrinology*, vol. 7, no. 35, 2016.

[50] P. P. Chakraborty, R. Bhattacharjee, A. Roy, and S. Chowdhury, "Pseudoacromegaly: an unusual presenting manifestation of long-standing undiagnosed primary hypothyroidism," *Postgraduate Medical Journal*, vol. 93, no. 1104, pp. 639-640, 2017.

[51] B. Niepce, "Traité du goitre et du crétinisme," *Baillère*, 1851.

[52] B. W. Scheithauer, K. Kovacs, R. V. Randall, and N. Ryan, "Pituitary gland in hypothyroidism. Histologic and immunocytologic study," *Archives of Pathology & Laboratory Medicine*, vol. 109, no. 6, pp. 499–504, 1985.

[53] P. Beck-Peccoz, F. Brucker-Davis, L. Persani, R. C. Smallridge, and B. D. Weintraub, "Thyrotropin-secreting pituitary tumors," *Endocrine Reviews*, vol. 17, no. 6, pp. 610–638, 1996.

[54] T. Yamada, T. Tsukui, K. Ikejiri, Y. Yukimura, and M. Kotani, "Volume of sella turcica in normal subjects and in patients with primary hypothyroidism and hyperthyroidism," *The Journal of Clinical Endocrinology & Metabolism*, vol. 42, no. 5, pp. 817–822, 1976.

[55] K. S. Honbo, A. J. Van Herle, and K. A. Kellett, "Serum prolactin levels in untreated primary hypothyroldism," *American Journal of Medicine*, vol. 64, no. 5, pp. 782–787, 1978.

[56] P. J. Snyder, L. S. Jacobs, R. D. Utiger, and W. H. Daughaday, "Thyroid hormone inhibition of the prolactin response to thyrotropin-releasing hormone," *The Journal of Clinical Investigation*, vol. 52, no. 9, pp. 2324–2329, 1973.

[57] T. Shimono, H. Hatabu, K. Kasagi et al., "Rapid progression of pituitary hyperplasia in humans with primary hypothyroidism: demonstration with MR imaging," *Radiology*, vol. 213, no. 2, pp. 383–388, 1999.

[58] M. Langlois, J. B. Lamarche, and D. Bellabarba, "Long-standing goiter and hypothyroidism: an unusual presentation of a TSH-secreting adenoma," *Thyroid*, vol. 6, no. 4, pp. 329–335, 1996.

[59] G. T. Tindall, K. Kovacs, E. Horvath, and M. O. Thorner, "Presence of human prolactin-producing adenomas and bromocriptine: a histological, immunocytochemical, ultrastructural, and morphometric study," *The Journal of Clinical Endocrinology & Metabolism*, vol. 55, no. 6, pp. 1178–1183, 1982.

3

COVID-19 Infection-Related Thyrotoxic Hypokalemic Periodic Paralysis

Fadlila Fitriani,[1] Vina Yanti Susanti,[2] and Mohammad Robikhul Ikhsan[2]

[1]Study Program of Specialty, Department of Internal Medicine, Dr. Sardjito General Hospital/ Faculty of Medicine, Public Health and Nursing, Universitas Gadjah Mada, Jl. Kesehatan No. 1 Sekip Sinduadi DIY, Yogyakarta 55284, Indonesia
[2]Division of Endocrinology, Department of Internal Medicine, Dr. Sardjito General Hospital/ Faculty of Medicine, Public Health and Nursing, Universitas Gadjah Mada, Jl. Kesehatan No. 1 Sekip Sinduadi DIY, Yogyakarta 55284, Indonesia

Correspondence should be addressed to Mohammad Robikhul Ikhsan; m_robikhul@ugm.ac.id

Academic Editor: Toshihiro Kita

SARS-CoV-2 infection induces the dysfunction of many organs including the thyroid gland through the role of ACE2 receptors as well as the consequences of the cytokine storm. Thyroid diseases such as subacute thyroidism, Graves' disease, thyrotoxicosis, and Hashimoto's thyroiditis have been documented in patients with SARS-CoV-2 infection. However, there are limited reports about the consequences of SARS-CoV-2 infection-related thyroid complications. We describe a case of man who was admitted to the emergency department due to repeated lower limb weakness since diagnosed with COVID-19. He had refractory hypokalemia and was treated with potassium replacement therapy for 2 months. However, the complaints continued. The patient has no history of thyroid disease, yet the laboratory result showed hyperthyroidism. Accordingly, he received oral thiamazole. As the laboratory parameters of the thyroid hormones improved, potassium levels returned to normal and the limb weakness stopped. This unusual thyroid complication should be considered in SARS-CoV-2 infection. The prompt diagnosis and appropriate therapy can reduce the burden of the disease.

1. Introduction

Coronavirus disease 2019 (COVID-19) caused by the severe acute respiratory syndrome coronavirus 2 (SARS-CoV-2) infection exhibits a broad range of clinical conditions, ranging from asymptomatic to severe organ damage [1]. The SARS-CoV-2 enters the human cell mediated by the angiotensin-converting enzyme 2 (ACE2) receptors which express in numerous organs, including the thyroid gland [2]. These interactions induce inflammation of follicular cells which alter both the structure and function of the thyroid gland [3]. Higher incidence of hyperthyroidism was reported in patients with COVID-19 infection, presumably due to immune response to the infection [4, 5]. Hyperthyroidism stimulates the Na-K ATPase pumps in skeletal muscles which in turn promotes the cellular K^+ shifting, causing hypokalemia paralysis [6]. Thyroid function was shown to improve when the infection was resolved [7]. However, persistent hyperthyroid and hypokalemia were reported in case reports after COVID-19 infection [8, 9]. Thus, further understanding of SARS-CoV-2 infection-related thyrotoxic hypokalemic periodic paralysis is necessary to prevent the complications and determine the prognosis of these patients with COVID-19 infection.

2. Case Presentation

A 42-year-old male patient presented to the emergency department with weakness in his four extremities since a day before admission. The patient could stand but was too weak to walk. Tingling and pain sensations were occasionally reported in both the hands and the legs. He denied any trauma, paresthesia, or incontinence of the urinary or bowel systems. He has had cough and fever for the past five days without vomiting, diarrhea, or excessive sweating. Three months prior to admission, the patient had a COVID-19 infection. He experienced limb weakness and hypokalemia during hospitalization. He denied having any neck pain, and there was no swelling of the neck nor thyroid gland. He has no history of thyroid disease, hypertension, stroke, diabetes, nor malignancy. The patient had normal vital signs and underwent an electrocardiogram at the time of presentation. Crackles were found in both the lungs during a physical examination. There were no tumors or masses in his neck. A neurological examination indicated a bilateral upper and lower extremity motor impairment with similar strength of 4/5 and normal sensory function (Table 1). On laboratory finding, potassium level was 1.59 mmol/L, magnesium level was 2.23 mg/dL, free T4 (fT4) level was 3.75 ng/dL, and thyroid-stimulating hormone (TSH) level was <0.005 μIU/mL. The potassium urine concentration was 5.05 mmol/L, with a potassium excretion fraction of 2.34%. Proteinuria was negative from urine analysis, and the renal function was normal (Table 2). Patient was diagnosed with thyrotoxic hypokalemic periodic paralysis. The patient received potassium chloride 50 mEq intravenously and oral thiamazole 5 mg twice a day for potassium correction. After potassium was restored to a normal level of 3.48 mmol/L, the extremities' weakness improved, with motor strength of 5/5 in all extremities. The patient was then discharged and advised to continue taking thiamazole 5 mg twice daily as well as oral potassium supplements twice daily. He had no weakness in his upper or lower extremities during the two-month follow-up, and his potassium, fT4, and TSH levels were normal. We stopped the medication and continue to give a monthly evaluation. The symptoms did not return and the thyroid hormone and potassium levels remained normal at the fourth month even without therapy (Figure 1).

Table 1: Demographic and clinical findings of the patient.

Demography	
Age	42 years
Sex	Male
Race	Asian, Indonesian
Residence	Urban
Clinical manifestation	
Symptoms	
Acute paralysis	Yes
Symptom of hyperthyroid	
Palpitation	No
Weight loss	No
Tremor	No
Heat intolerance	No
Physical sign	
Paralysis without sensory abnormality	Yes
Exophthalmos	No
Goitre	No
ECG finding	
Sinus tachycardia	No
Fibrillation	No

Table 2: Summary of the laboratory test.

Laboratory test	Patient level	Reference range
Total leucocyte count	$12.40 \times 10^3/\mu$L	4.5–11.5
Hemoglobin	12.4 g/dL	13–18
Thrombocyte	$414 \times 10^3/\mu$L	150–450
BUN	13.9 mg/dL	6–20
Creatinine	0.91 mg/dL	0.7–1.2
Sodium	146 mmol/L	136–145
Potassium	1.59 mmol/L	3.5–5.1
Magnesium	2.23 mg/dL	1.6–2.4
Calcium	2.25 mmol/L	2.15–2.55
Urine creatinine	56.56 mg/dL	39–259
Urine potassium	5.05 mmol/L	32–83
Potassium excretion fraction	2, 34%	—
fT4	3.75 ng/dL	1–1.7
TSH	<0.005 μIU/mL	0.27–4.2
Urine routine test	Normal	

3. Discussion

The SARS-CoV-2 infection has been linked to thyroid dysfunction through a complex interplay of hormonal and immunomodulatory signaling molecules [2]. ACE 2 receptors and transmembrane protein serine 2 (TMPRSS2), which are highly expressed in the thyroid gland, play a key role in virus entrance into the cells. The entry of the virus induces immune activation, producing proinflammatory cytokines and destroying the follicular cells of the thyroid [10]. Other mechanisms include indirect pathways caused by the virus's systemic inflammatory response, which causes thyroid gland destruction [2]. Subacute thyroiditis (SAT), a self-limited thyroidal disease usually induced by viruses, has been reported in several case reports of COVID-19 patients [11–13]. SAT is typically characterized by painful tender thyroid glands radiating to the ear, as well as systematic symptoms of fever, malaise, or anorexia. The disease usually consists of three phases, including thyrotoxic phase, hypothyroidism, and recovery into euthyroid over weeks to months. In a systematic review conducted by Trimboli et al., the median interval time for SAT development of patients with COVID-19 was 30 days [12]. However, the marked sign of a painful neck was absent in our patient during his COVID-19 infection course as well as in the months after the recovery. Muller et al. and Lania et al. reported cases of atypical thyroiditis without any complaint of neck pain [4, 14]. Patients with destructive thyroiditis are unlikely to have neck pain. This might be due to lymphopenia, which limits the inflammatory cell infiltration to the thyroid gland causing a lack of inflammatory reaction and capsular tension inside the thyroid [15]. Painless thyroiditis also occurs in autoimmune thyroid disease (AITD). The two major disorders of AITD are Graves' disease and Hashimoto's thyroiditis. Both diseases are characterized by the presence of specific antibodies such as TSH receptor antibody (TRAb), which is expressed in Graves' disease, and thyroglobulin autoantibody (Tg Ab) and thyroperoxidase autoantibody (TPO-Ab), which are expressed in Hashimoto's thyroiditis. Unfortunately, we did not conduct the antibody test on our patient.

The thyroid function alterations were observed in 50 COVID-19 patients with no history of thyroid disease. Low TSH and free T3 (fT3) were found in both COVID-19 and

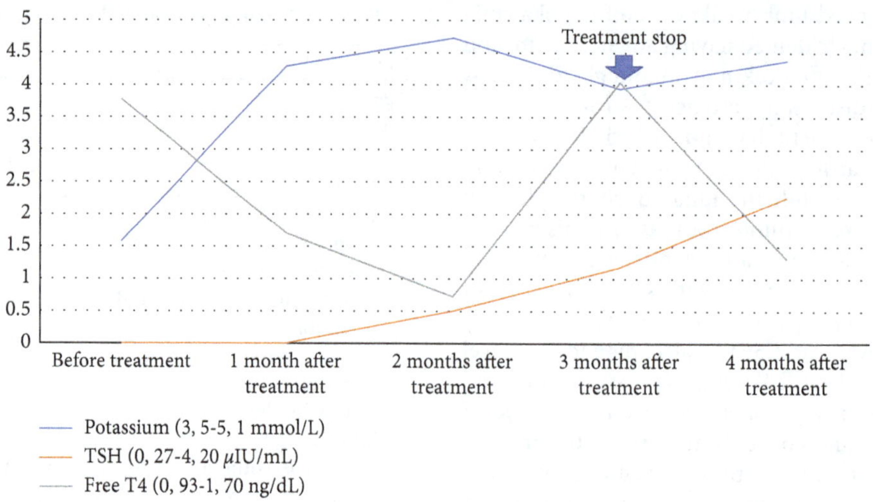

FIGURE 1: The changes of potassium, TSH, and free T4 before and after therapy of potassium replacement and thyroid hormone.

non-COVID-19 pneumonia. However, the declining levels of TSH and fT3 were positively correlated with the severity of pneumonia only in patients with COVID-19, thus suggesting the role of SARS-CoV infection in thyroid function alteration [16]. Another study conducted by Lania et al. reported a low level of TSH in 58 (20.2%) patients with COVID-19, with 31 of them exhibiting thyrotoxicosis from the laboratory findings. The study also discovered an inverse relationship between interleukin 6 (IL6) and TSH levels. However, a progressive decline of fT4 level without any drug intervention leads to the hypothesis of "silent" destructive thyroiditis [4]. In a postmortem study, an extensive apoptosis process in follicular epithelium which alters the follicular morphology was observed in the SARS-CoV-1 infection [17]. The apoptosis of the follicular cells induces the release of the preformed hormone, the elevation of fT4 concentration, and low TSH. In severely ill patients, such as seen in severe SARS-Co2 infection, the fT3 concentration was low due to the inhibition of deiodinase activity, thus producing T4 thyrotoxicosis, which has a less apparent clinical symptom of thyrotoxicosis [15, 18]. A high level of fT4 and a low concentration of TSH were observed after three months of SARS-CoV-2 infection in our patient. It was noted that low concentrations of immune cells such as CD4+, CD8+ T cells, B cells, and granulocyte cells were detected in peripheral blood of recovered plasma convalescence donors after two months of infection, thus indicating the long duration of immune disruption in patients with COVID-19 [19].

Thyrotoxic periodic paralysis (TPP) is a distinct manifestation of thyrotoxicosis where the patient develops a transient motor deficit due to acute hypokalemia. Due to the role of testosterone in the Na-K ATPase activity, TPP is more common in males, in line with our patient's gender [20]. One of the possible precipitating factors for TPP is infection. Kaushik et al. reported a case of hypokalemic paralysis associated with COVID-19 infection [21]. However, the thyroid function was normal, unlike in our case. Thyroid hormones promote the expression of Na-K ATPase in skeletal muscle cell membranes, allowing K+ to enter the intracellular compartment and causing hypokalemia in hyperthyroid patients in patients with COVID-19 has been reported in several case reports [22, 23]. The risk factors for hypokalemia in patients with COVID-19 include gastrointestinal loss, urinary loss, and diuretic use [22]. Furthermore, persistent hypokalemia was also reported in COVID-19 recovered patients [9]. The direct and indirect effects of SARS-CoV infection on the renal tubules influence the renin-angiotensin system (RAS). The binding of SARS-CoV-2 with the ACE2 receptors diminishes the ability of ACE2 to regulate RAS. Increasing RAS activity enhances the distal delivery of sodium and water to the collecting tubule of the kidney and the excretion of potassium, resulting in hypokalemia [9, 22, 23]. In our case, we excluded gastrointestinal loss since the patient had no symptoms of diarrhea or vomiting. The potassium urine excretion in our patient was normal, as well as the serum magnesium. Thus, we suggested hypokalemia in our case was due to the high level of thyroid hormones, leading to a thyrotoxicosis condition. In our case, intravenous potassium replacement therapy was effective in treating acute hypokalemic paralysis. The antithyroid drug and oral potassium supplementation were also effective in reducing the thyroid hormone, maintaining the serum potassium level, and inhibiting the recurrent TPP in our patient.

In conclusion, thyroid hormones play a critical role in regulating multiple organ systems. Close monitoring of thyroid hormones should be done in patients who exhibit the signs and symptoms of thyroid dysfunction, particularly in those with a history of thyroid disease and those receiving the antithyroid drug. Patients with COVID-related thyroid disease should be treated ap-propriately to prevent long-term complications which would affect their quality of life.

Consent

Written informed consent was obtained from the patient for the publication of this case report and any accompanying images.

References

[1] M. A. Barek, M. A. Aziz, and M. S. Islam, "Impact of age, sex, comorbidities and clinical symptoms on the severity of COVID-19 cases: a meta-analysis with 55 studies and 10014 cases," *Heliyon*, vol. 6, 2020.

[2] L. Scappaticcio, F. Pitoia, K. Esposito, A . Piccardo, and P. Trimboli, "Impact of COVID-19 on the thyroid gland: an update," *Reviews in Endocrine and Metabolic Disorders*, vol. 22, 2020.

[3] L. H. Duntas and J. Jonklaas, "COVID-19 and thyroid diseases: a bidirectional impact," *Journal of the Endocrine Society*, vol. 5, 2021.

[4] A. Lania, M. T. Sandri, M. Cellini, M. Mirani, E. Lavezzi, and G. Mazziotti, "Thyrotoxicosis in patients with COVID-19: the thyrcov study," *European Journal of Endocrinology*, vol. 183, no. 4, pp. 381–387, 2020.

[5] M. Güven and H. Gültekin, "The prognostic impact of thyroid disorders on the clinical severity of COVID-19: results of single-centre pandemic hospital," *International Journal of Clinical Practice*, vol. 75, no. 6, Article ID e14129, 2021.

[6] S. H. Lin and C. L. Huang, "Mechanism of thyrotoxic periodic paralysis," *Journal of the American Society of Nephrology*, vol. 23, no. 6, pp. 985–988, 2012.

[7] B. Khoo, T. Tan, S. A. Clarke et al., "Thyroid function before, during, and after COVID-19," *Journal of Clinical Endocrinology and Metabolism*, vol. 106, no. 2, pp. E803–E811, 2021.

[8] E. Tjønnfjord, R. B. Moe, W. Ghanima, and S. Aballi, "Subacute thyroiditis after COVID-19," *Tidsskrift for den Norske laegeforening: Tidsskrift for Praktisk Medicin, Ny Raekke*, vol. 141, no. 10, 2021.

[9] M. O. A lnafiey, A . M. A langari, A . M. A lafi, and A . A bushara, "Persistent hypokalemia post SA RS-coV-2 infection, is it a life-long complication?: case report," *Annals of Medicine and Surgery*, vol. 62, pp. 358–361, 2021.

[10] R. M. Ruggeri, A . Campennì, D. Deandreis et al., "SARS-COV-2-related immune-inflammatory thyroid disorders: facts and perspectives," *Expert Review of Clinical Immunology*, vol. 17, pp. 737–759, 2021.

[11] A. Khatri, E. Charlap, and A. Kim, "Subacute thyroiditis from COVID-19 infection: a case report and review of literature," *European Thyroid Journal*, vol. 9, no. 6, pp. 324–328, 2020.

[12] P. Trimboli, C. Cappelli, L. Croce, L. Scappaticcio, L. Chiovato, and M. Rotondi, "COVID-19-associated subacute thyroiditis: evidence-based data from a systematic review," *Frontiers in Endocrinology*, vol. 12, 2021.

[13] S. A . M. Mattar, S. J. Q. Koh, S. Rama Chandran, and B. P. Z. Cherng, "Subacute thyroiditis associated with COVID-19," *BMJ Case Reports*, vol. 13, no. 8, A rticle ID e237336, 2020.

[14] I. Muller, D. Cannavaro, D. Dazzi et al., "SARS-CoV-2-related atypical thyroiditis," *Lancet Diabetes and Endocrinology*, vol. 8, pp. 739–741, 2020.

[15] P. Caron, "Thyroiditis and SARS-CoV-2 pandemic: a review," *Endocrine*, vol. 72, pp. 326–331, 2021.

[16] M. Chen, W. Zhou, and W. Xu, "Thyroid function analysis in 50 patients with COVID-19: a retrospective study," *Thyroid*, vol. 31, no. 1, pp. 8–11, 2021.

[17] L. Wei, S. Sun, C. H Xu et al., "Pathology of the thyroid in severe acute respiratory syndrome," *Human Pathology*, vol. 38, no. 1, pp. 95–102, 2007.

[18] E. Fliers, A. C. Bianco, L. Langouche, and A. Boelen, "Thyroid function in critically ill patients," *Lancet Diabetes and Endocrinology*, vol. 3, pp. 816–825, 2015.

[19] F. Gong, Y. Dai, T. Zheng et al., "Peripheral CD4+ T cell subsets and antibody response in COVID-19 convalescent individuals," *Journal of Clinical Investigation*, vol. 130, no. 12, pp. 6588–6599, 2020.

[20] J. T. Batch, M. U. Jahngir, and I. Rodriguez, "Thyrotoxic Periodic Paralysis: An Incidental Diagnosis!" *Cureus*, vol. 12, 2020.

[21] A. Kaushik, A. Garg, B. M. Singh, A. K. Agarwal, and S. N. Wani, "Hypokalaemic paralysis associated with COVID-19 infection," *Journal of The Association of Physician of India*, vol. 69, 2020.

[22] A. Gaetano, F. Annachiara, F. Francesco, R. Perrone, G. Mori, and A. Elisabetta, "Hypokalemia in patients with COVID-19," 2020, https://www.medrxiv.org/content/early/2020/06/18/2020.06.14.20131169.

[23] D. Chen, X. Li, Q. Song et al., "Assessment of hypokalemia and clinical characteristics in patients with coronavirus disease 2019 in Wenzhou, China," *JAMA Network Open*, vol. 3, no. 6, Article ID e2011122, 2020.

An Unusual Presentation of Thyrotoxicosis: Leg Weakness and Hypokalemia in a 21-Year-Old Male

Mario S. Campana, Maria Riofrio, Raja S. Jadav, and Mattan Rozenek

St. Barnabas Hospital, Department of Internal Medicine, SBH Health System, The Bronx, NY 10457, USA

Correspondence should be addressed to Mario S. Campana; sebastian.campana316@gmail.com

Academic Editor: Mihail A. Boyanov

Patients with hyperthyroidism or thyrotoxicosis present with an unspecific constellation of signs or symptoms such as palpitations, tremors, weight loss, or diarrhea. In some severe cases, hyperthyroidism can predispose patients to metabolic abnormalities and arrhythmias. Thyrotoxic periodic paralysis (TTP) is a rare, life-threatening complication or variant of hyperthyroidism associated with hypokalemia and muscle weakness that affects young Asian or Hispanic males between 20–40 years. TTP is reversible, and the management consists of beta-blockers, antithyroid therapy, and conservative potassium correction to prevent severe cardiovascular events such as ventricular arrhythmias with the improvement of transient muscle paralysis. We present a case of a 21-year-old Hispanic male complaining with symptoms of thyrotoxicosis, marked hypokalemia, and severe generalized muscle weakness. Physicians must be aware of this uncommon complication of thyrotoxicosis called thyrotoxic periodic paralysis (TTP) to avoid potassium overcorrection and all the endocrine associations with this pathology.

1. Introduction

Thyrotoxic periodic paralysis is a rare manifestation or complication of thyrotoxicosis that usually affects a young group of patients between 20 and 40 years [1, 2]. The incidence is approximately 2% in the Asian population and about 0.1–0.2% in North American. It appears to be more common in men than in women, with almost a 26 : 1 difference, which is unusual because thyrotoxicosis has a higher incidence among women. Association between testosterone levels and increased Na/K+ ATPase pump action explain this predilection to males [3].

TTP is described as an onset of sporadic episodes of weakness and muscle pains seen predominantly at resting periods, usually at night, that worsens with physical activity, high-carbohydrate meals, exercise, and stress. It mainly affects the lower extremities and, less commonly, the upper extremities depending on the severity [4].

Hypokalemia in TTP is secondary to an intracellular shift of potassium induced by the increased levels of thyroid hormones that sensitize the Na+/K+ ATPase pumps. Obesity, hyperinsulinemia, or excessive levels of testosterone have been associated as triggers of TTP in patients with hyperthyroidism, increasing the activity of Na+/K+ pump and giving more predisposition to males [3, 5, 6].

The diagnosis of TTP can be challenging and misdiagnosed with other genetic syndromes such as Familial Hypokalemic Periodic Paralysis (FHPP) because of their similar clinical presentation and electrolytes imbalance.

Unlike TTP, familial hypokalemic periodic paralysis is an autosomal dominant condition that develops in patients with positive family history without features of hyperthyroidism.

The treatment of TPP includes acute management of thyrotoxicosis with beta-blockers, antithyroid therapy, and cautious potassium correction. Once the patient is euthyroid and normokalaemia was reached, muscular symptoms will subside. On the other hand, FHPP treatment is based on potassium replacement [7–9]. An accurate diagnosis is important to prevent life-threatening complications such as ventricular arrhythmias, constant muscular paralysis, and potassium overcorrection.

2. Case Presentation

A 21-year-old Hispanic male patient without any past medical history presented to the emergency department with a persistent, gradual, and generalized muscle weakness and sprain of the lower and upper extremities that started one week ago but was progressing from 5 to 10/10 of intensity and worsening with physical activity. The patient reported proximal muscle weakness with difficulty walking, standing up, and lifting objects. He had similar symptoms in the past but never this severe. He reported mild palpitations without chest pain, shortness of breath, blurry vision, weight loss, nausea, vomiting, or diarrhea.

The patient denied any family history of electrolytes imbalance, diabetes, hypertension, or thyroid disease and denied allergies or surgeries in the past but used alcohol and marijuana occasionally.

On examination, he was anxious, agitated, and with moist skin; vital signs showed a blood pressure of 133/85 mm Hg, heart rate 115 beats/minute, RR 22 breaths/minute, and temperature of 98.0 Fahrenheit. Head exam did not show lids lag, retractions, exophthalmos, or thyromegaly. Cardiopulmonary exam showed regular heart sounds with tachycardia but negative for crackles or wheezing and good work of breathing. Neurologic exam revealed normal sensation and deep tendon reflex but mild fine tremors on his hands with decreased strength in both lower extremities 2/5 and 3/5 in the upper extremities with preserved respiratory muscles. Cranial nerves 2–12 preserved. Electrocardiogram (EKG) showed sinus tachycardia without ST changes or T-wave inversions but prolonged QT interval (Figure 1). Laboratory findings including troponin, glucose, bicarbonate, renal profile, sodium, and calcium were within normal limits. Serum potassium was 2.1 mEq/L, magnesium 1.4 mEq/L, VBG was with an LA of 2.9 mmol/L, and CPK 1569 IU/L. The thyroid function test showed T4 19.4 ug/L (normal: 5–12 ug/L) and TSH 0.01 IU/mL (normal: 0.35–5.60 IU/mL) with normal cortisol levels (Table 1). Urine potassium was 66 (2–300 mEq/L).

The patient was managed with intravenous fluids, propranolol (60 mg daily), PTU (100 mg every 8 hour), and potassium chloride of 120 mEq oral and 40 mEq intravenous doses on the day of admission to the intensive care unit.

On the second day of hospitalization, potassium levels had normalized, and the patient's weakness subsided. Subsequent EKG (Figure 2) showed resolution of the QT prolongation and tachycardia. The motor strength at this time was 5/5 in the upper and lower extremities. The endocrinology team was consulted and recommended continuing beta-blockers (60 mg daily) and started on methimazole (10 mg daily) with conservative potassium correction and monitoring every 12 hours.

On the last day of hospitalization, his weakness has totally resolved, and the potassium levels had normalized. The patient requested his discharge and stated he will follow-up in the endocrinology clinic for further hyperthyroidism work up as an outpatient. He was discharged with the same dose of methimazole and propranolol.

3. Discussion

Hyperthyroidism is associated with some muscular complications, including thyrotoxic myopathies, myasthenia gravis, exophthalmic ophthalmoplegia, and TTP. TTP is characterized by a triad of muscle weakness, hypokalemia, and hyperthyroidism. The etiology of TTP is related to the increased activity of NA+/K+ ATPase pumps on the skeletal muscle [3, 10]. TTP has more predispositions to men compared to women despite thyroid disease being more associated with female patients. This strong predilection that occurs in males showed a possible association between increased testosterone levels and hypokalemic paralysis in patients with hyperthyroidism [3]. Androgens can increase the expression and activity of the Na+/K+ ATPase, therefore correlating with the severity of hypokalemia [11, 12].

Patients with a history of hyperthyroidism, obesity, type 2 diabetes mellitus, or metabolic syndrome with an increased risk of insulin resistance and subsequent hyperinsulinemia are more likely to develop hypokalemic muscle paralysis in acute thyrotoxicosis, creating a potential relationship between insulin resistance and TTP. In the study by Soonthorpun et al. [13], they found that subjects with a history of TTP were more obese and had lower insulin sensitivity than those with a history of simple thyrotoxicosis; therefore, insulin resistance with compensatory hyperinsulinemia may be a key feature of the pathogenesis of TTP [4, 13, 14]. There is no clear risk factor or etiology for TTP, but hyperinsulinemia or conditions that increase the levels of testosterone and catecholamine can increase the likelihood of developing TTP in a patient with thyrotoxicosis. The clinical characteristic of TTP is recurrent transient episodes of proximal muscle weakness, usually more in the lower extremities with spared sensory function. Paralysis can last from a few hours up to 48–72 h, with almost complete recovery after beta-blocker and potassium therapy. Some of the features of this condition can mimic acute neurologic syndromes such as Guillen Barre, transverse myelitis, or spinal cord lesions, but TTP can lead to spared respiratory muscles paralysis. Most patients have decreased or absent deep tendon reflex, which is discordant to other forms of hyperthyroidism [3, 10]. TTP is related with a normal acid-base balance, but with some electrolytes abnormalities such as hypophosphatemia, hypomagnesemia, low potassium excretion rate, and low trans-tubular potassium gradient (TTKG) [14].

There are some genetic etiologies that can share the same pattern of muscle weakness and electrolyte abnormalities of TTP. Familial hypokalemic periodic paralysis (FHPP) is a rare autosomal dominant disease caused by a mutation in either the L-type calcium channel or voltage-gated sodium channel. FHPP, as well as TTP, can present with episodes of low serum potassium and proximal muscle weakness. This disorder has lower clinical expression in females compared to males, with a male predominance of 9 to 1 [3, 7, 14]. Except for the hyperthyroidism features on TTP and the strong family story in FHPP, both entities are difficult to differentiate because of their similar clinical presentation of transient muscle weakness and severe hypokalemia with

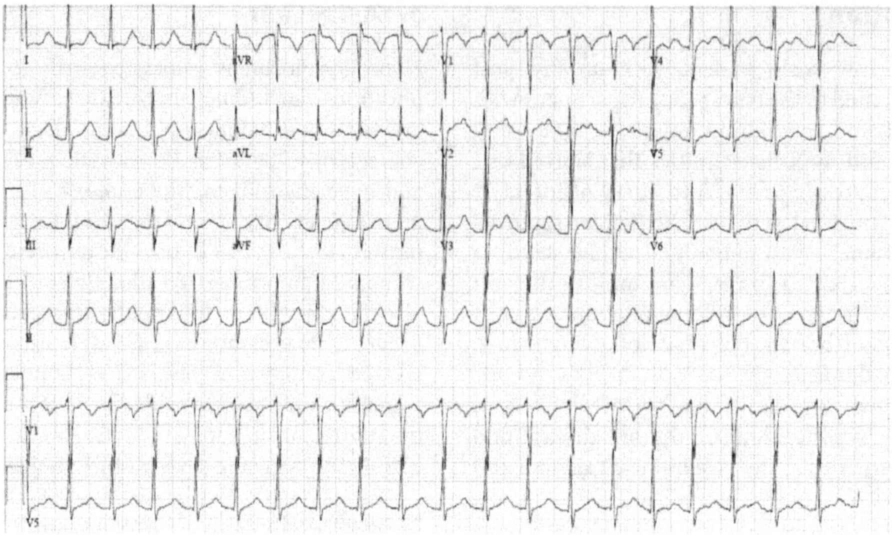

Figure 1: EKG on admission.

Table 1: Pertinent laboratory values on admission.

Labs	Value	Reference
Potassium	2.1 (mEq/L)	(3.5–5.3 mEq/L)
Magnesium	1.4 (mEq/L)	(1.3–2.1 mEq/L)
TSH	0.01 (IU/mL)	(0.34–5.60 IU/mL)
Total T4	19.4 (ug/L)	(6.0–12.0 ug/L)
T3	14.9 (pg/mL)	(2.0–4.4 pg/dL)
FT4	4.59 (ng/dL)	(0.82–1.77 ng/dL)
CPK	1569 IU/L	(38–174 IU/L)

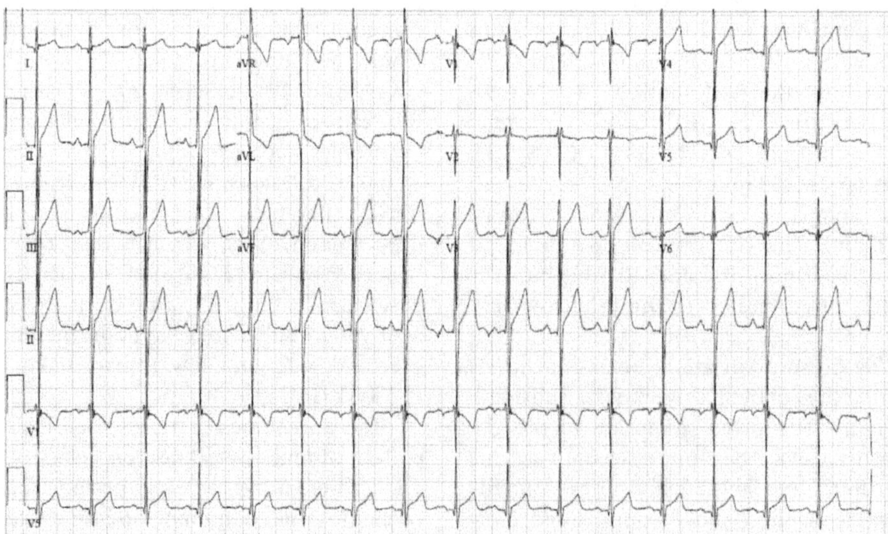

Figure 2: EKG on the second day of admission.

potential cardiogenic complication. However, both conditions have a different therapy approach. FHPP treatment consists of alleviating the symptoms, preventing acute attacks, and appropriate correction of potassium [14, 15].

On the other hand, the management of TTP consists of keeping the patient on a euthyroid state, with beta-blockers and thioamides, monitoring and avoiding life-threatening cardiogenic complications such as ventricular arrhythmias with a conservative correction of potassium to avoid paradoxical hypokalemia or rebound hyperkalemia. Propranolol inhibits the activity of Na+/K+ ATPase and, thus, increasing the levels of potassium, sometimes without the need for an aggressive replacement. Propranolol and high dose of antithyroid therapy allow a rapid resolution of symptoms and decrease the risk of rebound hyperkalemia.

4. Conclusions

TTP is a rare but potentially life-threatening complication of acute thyrotoxicosis.

It is important to assess patients with potential risk for developing TTP during clinical visits and identifying a history of obesity, metabolic syndrome, type 2 diabetes, or excessive testosterone levels. Propranolol and antithyroid therapy with a conservative and limited replacement of potassium are the key factors for appropriate management of TTP in the ICU.

This case report has a clinically and management relevance in patient with high risk of developing TTP and with atypical presentation of thyrotoxicosis. Endocrinologists, internists, and critical care physicians need to be aware and assess these complications during the admission.

Abbreviations

TTP: Thyrotoxic periodic paralysis
FHPP: Familial hypokalemic periodic paralysis
EKG: Electrocardiogram.

Consent

Consent was obtained during the admission.

References

[1] S. Bilha, O. Mitu, L. Teodoriu, C. Haba, and C. Preda, "Thyrotoxic periodic paralysis-a misleading challenge in the emergency department," *Diagnostics*, vol. 10, no. 5, p. 316, 2020.

[2] A. W. C. Kung, "Thyrotoxic periodic paralysis: a diagnostic challenge," *Journal of Clinical Endocrinology & Metabolism*, vol. 91, no. 7, pp. 2490-2495, 2006.

[3] M. Meseeha, B. Parsamehr, K. Kissell, and M. Attia, "Thyrotoxic periodic paralysis: a case study and review of the literature," *Journal of Community Hospital Internal Medicine Perspectives*, vol. 7, no. 2, pp. 103–106, 2017.

[4] M. A. Manoukian, J. A. Foote, and L. M. Crapo, "Clinical and metabolic features of thyrotoxic periodic paralysis in 24 episodes," *Archives of Internal Medicine*, vol. 159, no. 6, pp. 601–606, 1999.

[5] N. S. Neki, "Hyperthyroid hypokalemic periodic paralysis," *Pakistan Journal of Medical Sciences*, vol. 32, no. 4, pp. 1051-1052, 2016.

[6] S.-H. Lin and C.-L. Huang, "Mechanism of thyrotoxic periodic paralysis," *Journal of the American Society of Nephrology*, vol. 23, no. 6, pp. 985–988, 2012.

[7] A. Marx, J. P. Ruppersberg, C. Pietrzyk, and R. Rüdel, "Thyrotoxic periodic paralysis and the sodium/potassium pump," *Muscle & Nerve*, vol. 12, no. 10, pp. 810–815, 1989.

[8] H. Tassone, A. Moulin, and S. O. Henderson, "The pitfalls of potassium replacement in thyrotoxic periodic paralysis: a case report and review of the literature," *Journal of Emergency Medicine*, vol. 26, no. 2, pp. 157–161, 2004.

[9] K. Karndumri, Y. Thewjitcharoen, W. Chatchomchuan et al., "Impact of first-line treatment choice on long-term outcomes of hyperthyroid graves' disease patients with thyrotoxic periodic paralysis," *Journal of Clinical & Translational Endocrinology*, vol. 21, Article ID 100235, 2020.

[10] C.-C. Chang, C.-J. Cheng, C.-C. Sung et al., "A 10-year analysis of thyrotoxic periodic paralysis in 135 patients: focus on symptomatology and precipitants," *European Journal of Endocrinology*, vol. 169, no. 5, pp. 529–536, 2013.

[11] A. J. Patel, S. Tejera, S. P. Klek, and G. D. Rothberger, "Thyrotoxic periodic paralysis in a competitive bodybuilder with thyrotoxicosis factitia," *AACE Clinical Case Reports*, vol. 6, no. 5, pp. e252–e256, 2020.

[12] Y. Yao, L. Fan, X. Zhang, Z. Xiao, Y. Long, and H. Tian, "Episodes of paralysis in Chinese men with thyrotoxic periodic paralysis are associated with elevated serum testosterone," *Thyroid*, vol. 23, no. 4, pp. 420–427, 2013.

[13] S. Soonthornpun, W. Setasuban, and A. Thamprasit, "Insulin resistance in subjects with a history of thyrotoxic periodic paralysis (TPP)," *Clinical Endocrinology*, vol. 70, no. 5, pp. 794–797, 2009.

[14] L. Lam, R. J. Nair, and L. Tingle, "Thyrotoxic periodic paralysis," *Baylor University Medical Center Proceedings*, vol. 19, no. 2, pp. 126–129, 2006.

[15] D. P. Ryan, M. R. Dias da Silva, T. W. Soong et al., "Mutations in potassium channel Kir2.6 cause susceptibility to thyrotoxic hypokalemic periodic paralysis," *Cell*, vol. 140, no. 1, pp. 88–98, 2010.

5

An Adolescent Female with Bipolar Disorder Presenting with Lithium-Induced Hyperthyroidism

Pratibha Rana,[1] Patria Alba Aponte,[1] and Ghufran Babar[2]

[1]*Children's Mercy Hospital, 3101 Broadway Blvd., Kansas City, MO 64111, USA*
[2]*Department of Pediatric Endocrinology, Children's Mercy Hospital, 3101 Broadway Blvd., Kansas City, MO 64111, USA*

Correspondence should be addressed to Ghufran Babar; gbabar@cmh.edu

Academic Editor: Lucy Mastrandrea

Lithium therapy has been associated with several endocrine disorders including thyroid dysfunction, diabetes insipidus, and hyperparathyroidism. While its suppressive effect on thyroid function is well known, it is very rare to observe lithium-induced hyperthyroidism especially in the pediatric population. Here, we describe a case of lithium-induced hyperthyroidism in an adolescent female with bipolar disorder. The patient is a 17-year-old female who was treated with lithium for bipolar disorder and presented with symptoms and laboratory findings consistent with hyperthyroidism. Since thyroid autoantibodies were negative, thyroid dysfunction was attributed to lithium toxicity. Indeed, her clinical and biochemical hyperthyroid state resolved after stopping lithium therapy. Lithium-associated hyperthyroidism can occur in the pediatric population. We propose close monitoring of thyroid hormone levels in children on lithium therapy.

1. Case Report

Bipolar disorders are common in adolescents, with a lifetime prevalence of 2.5% [1] and 0.1% in children aged 9–13 years [2]. Lithium is commonly used for the treatment of bipolar disorders in children and adolescents [3]. It has been associated with several endocrine disorders including thyroid dysfunction, diabetes insipidus, and hyperparathyroidism. Its suppressive effect on thyroid function is well known; in contrast, lithium-induced hyperthyroidism is rare with a prevalence in the range of between 1% and 1.7% in the adult population [4, 5]. The first case of thyrotoxicosis in a patient treated with lithium was reported in 1974 [6]. Hyperthyroidism in lithium-treated patients has been associated with diffuse goiter, toxic multinodular goiter, and painless thyroiditis [7]. Lithium is also implicated in granulomatous thyroiditis, and it is reported to induce auto-antibody formation and autoimmunity in susceptible individuals [8]. There have not been any cases reported about lithium-induced hyperthyroidism in pediatric population. We are presenting an adolescent girl treated with lithium who presented with hyperthyroidism.

2. Methods

Retrospective chart review of the case study was carried out. Since it is a single case report, an approval from the Institutional Review Board (IRB) and consent are not required. However, when a new patient is seen in our clinic, the family signed a consent form for treatment and possible use of any clinical finding to report anonymously.

3. Case Presentation

Our patient is a 17-year-5-month-old female with bipolar disorder who was treated with lithium. She had been placed on Concerta, Abilify, and Lamictal before being switched to lithium monotherapy due to the limited success of these initial therapies. She responded well to lithium for two years until about 3-4 weeks prior to presentation, when she developed dizziness, heat intolerance, excessive sweating, tremors, and palpitations. Due to these symptoms, she stopped taking lithium and sought medical attention at her primary care provider's (PCP's) office. The PCP ordered laboratory tests which revealed a

Table 1: Hormonal profile of the patient with gradual improvements of thyroid hormone levels from being hyperthyroid to euthyroid.

Timeline	TSH (0.35–5.5 mcIU/mL)	Free T4 (0.9–1.9 ng/dL)	Total T3 (55–209 ng/dL)
Initial lab work	0.01	3.5	
2 days later	<0.02	3.7	351
2 weeks later	<0.02	2.0	
1 month later	<0.02	1.5	
2 months	<0.02	0.9	188
3 months	0.39	0.8	175
5 months	2.61	1.2	172
7 months	2.62	1.1	134

`suppressed TSH (<0.02 mcIU/mL, normal range: 0.35–5.50) and an elevated free T4 (3.5 ng/dL, normal range: 0.8–1.9), both consistent with hyperthyroidism. Her lithium level at that time was <0.3 (normal range: 0.6–1.2 mmol/L), likely due to noncompliance during the past two weeks. The PCP received these results on the weekend, and the patient was referred to the emergency department (ED) where, on examination, she was tachycardic (140 bpm), afebrile, and her blood pressure was 132/84 mmHg. Her thyroid exam revealed the presence of a nontender goiter; no nodules were palpable. Repeat laboratory tests at the ED confirmed biochemical hyperthyroidism (TSH: <0.02 mcIU/mL, total T3: 351 ng/dl, normal range: 55 to 209) and an elevated free T4 (3.7 ng/dL). There was a prolonged QT interval on her EKG. Of note, our patient had no family history of autoimmunity or thyroid disease. Thyroid suppressive therapy was initiated with methimazole, 10 mg PO 3 times a day (0.46 mg/kg/day) as advised by the endocrinologist. She was also started on propranolol (60 mg/day~0.92 mg/kg/day). The ESR, CRP, CBC, and BMP were normal. Thyroid autoantibodies (antithyroid peroxidase antibody, antithyroglobulin antibody, and thyroid stimulating immunoglobulin) were all negative. She was advised not to restart lithium and consult her psychiatrist. She was seen in the endocrine clinic about two weeks later, after being off-lithium for four weeks; her hyperthyroid symptoms had improved; however, she still had palpitations and heat intolerance, while her heart rate and blood pressure were still above the age appropriate ranges (101 bpm and 133/74 mm hg, respectively). She had mild tongue fasciculation but no exophthalmos. Repeat thyroid function tests showed a lower free T4 level (2.0 ng/dl) as compared with two weeks ago, while the TSH was still suppressed. A subsequent endocrine visit two weeks later showed a normalized free T4 (1.5 ng/dl) and improved clinical hyperthyroidism. As a result, propranolol was discontinued, while methimazole treatment was maintained. By three months after her initial presentation, the methimazole dose was reduced (10 mg b.i.d.) due to a borderline-low (0.8 ng/dl, normal range of 0.8 to 1.9 ng/dL), Methimazole was eventually discontinued after five months of initial presentation. At her last follow-up in the endocrine clinic (seven months after diagnosis of hyperthyroidism and several weeks after stopping methimazole), she was clinically and biochemically euthyroid (Table 1).

4. Discussion

The prevalence of bipolar disorders in adolescence ranges between 1.8% and 2.5% [9, 10]. They are considered as the fourth leading cause of disability among adolescent worldwide. In children with bipolar disorders, lithium is the only mood stabilizer approved by the FDA for acute mania and maintenance treatment [11]. In a recent meta-analysis of studies on the effects of lithium on thyroid function, the investigators compared the prevalence of hypothyroidism in patients treated with lithium with controls. The overall odds of clinical hypothyroidism were close to six times greater in lithium-treated subjects than in controls. Conversely, this study did not find any difference between patients and controls on lithium with respect to the prevalence of increased thyroid function [4]. On the contrary, lithium-induced hyperthyroidism is rare even in adults [12]; it is estimated to have the annual incidence of 0.1% [13]. Other studies have estimated the prevalence to be in the range of 1%–1.7% [5, 14]. Only a small number of children treated with lithium present with subclinical or clinical hypothyroidism, and/or goiter [15, 16], to our knowledge, ours is the first case of a pediatric patient with lithium-induced hyperthyroidism. The possible mechanism regarding lithium-induced hyperthyroidism is thought to be due to an expansion of the intrathyroidal iodine pool, induction of autoimmune hyperthyroidism (Graves' disease), and a toxic thyroid nodule or painless thyroiditis [7, 17]. In patients with primary affective disorders, thyroid autoantibodies were detected in 8 of 40 subjects treated with lithium, and only in 3 patients were treated with other psychotropic drugs. Furthermore, the lithium-treated patients exhibited significantly reduced numbers of suppressor and or cytotoxic T cells and increased B cell activity compared to those treated with drugs other than lithium [18]. Similar to amiodarone-induced toxic thyroiditis, painless thyroiditis may also be the result of a direct toxic effect of lithium on the thyroid, which seems to be the likely mechanism in our patient, in whom results of tests for thyroid antibodies remained negative. Furthermore, it has been reported that lithium-associated silent thyroiditis occurred with an incidence rate of approximately 1.3 cases per 1000 person-years, and lithium-associated thyrotoxicosis occurred with an incidence rate of approximately 2.7 cases per 1000 person-years, higher than the reported incidence rates of silent thyroiditis (<0.03–0.28 cases per 1000 person-years) and of thyrotoxicosis (0.8–1.2 cases per 1000 person-years) in the general population and calculated the odds of lithium exposure to be 4.7-fold higher in patients with thyroiditis [7]. Recently, a meta-analysis of 52 studies showed in nine of these that were cross-sectional or cohort studies describing around 2500 patients that 2.6% patients were hypothyroid [19]. Another cross-sectional study reported just one patient (1.2%) in their lithium-treated group [20]. The histopathological features of the thyroid gland showed an immunological phenomenon with lymphoid follicles and fibrosis in affected thyroid glands [21], and this autoimmune process was not detected in other prospective studies, pre- and postlithium treatment [22, 23]. In our patient, the thyroid antibodies were negative; CBC, C-reactive protein (CRP), and sedimentation rate (ESR) were normal, suggesting that a mild silent thyroiditis may have been the cause of hyperthyroidism. Miller and Daniels described that most hyperthyroid patients had serum lithium level in the therapeutic range [7]. However, our patient's lithium level was not elevated due to discontinuation of treatment 2 weeks before the levels were checked. The duration of lithium therapy in patients who develop hyperthyroidism and lithium-associated silent thyroiditis range between 6 days and 15 years. However, in some cases, thyrotoxicosis occurred 4 days to 5 months after withdrawal of lithium therapy [24], and in our patient, the duration of lithium therapy was about 2 years. In conclusion, lithium-induced hyperthyroidism is very rarely diagnosed in adults and has never been reported in children before our case. We believe it is necessary to increase awareness of the possibility of such drug-induced thyroid dysfunction in the pediatric population, especially in children with hyperthyroidism and negative thyroid autoantibodies. The transient nature of this disorder is associated with a better prognosis compared to patients with Graves' disease. Since lithium-induced hyperthyroidism may occur even after years of lithium therapy, it is advisable to regularly monitor the thyroid function in children during the whole duration of lithium treatment.

References

[1] K. R. Merikangas, H. S. Akiskal, J. Angst et al., "Lifetime and 12-month prevalence of bipolar spectrum disorder in the national comorbidity survey replication," *Archives of General Psychiatry*, vol. 64, no. 5, pp. 543–552, 2007.

[2] E. J. Costello, A. Angold, B. J. Burns et al., "The great smoky mountains study of youth," *Archives of General Psychiatry*, vol. 53, no. 12, pp. 1129–1136, 1996.

[3] B. Grant and J. A. Salpekar, "Using lithium in children and adolescents with bipolar disorder: efficacy, to lerability, and practical considerations," *Pediatric Drugs*, vol. 20, no. 4, pp. 303–314, 2018.

[4] R. F. McKnight, M. Adida, K. Budge, S. Stockton, G. M. Goodwin, and J. R. Geddes, "Lithium toxicity profile: a systematic review and meta-analysis," *The Lancet*, vol. 379, no. 9817, pp. 721–728, 2012.

[5] B. E. W. Brownlie and J. E. Wells, "The epidemiology of thyrotoxicosis in New Zealand: incidence and geographical distribution in north canterbury, 1983-1985," *Clinical Endocrinology*, vol. 33, no. 2, pp. 249–259, 1990.

[6] L. M. Franklin, "Thyrotoxicosis developing during lithium treatment: case report," *The New Zealand Medical Journal*, vol. 79, no. 511, p. 782, 1974.

[7] K. K. Miller and G. H. Daniels, "Association between lithium use and thyrotoxicosis caused by silent thyroiditis," *Clinical Endocrinology*, vol. 55, no. 4, pp. 501–508, 2001.

[8] M. J. Sinnott, H. D. McIntyre, and S. M. Pond, "Granulomatous thyroiditis and lithium therapy," *Australian and New Zealand Journal of Medicine*, vol. 22, no. 1, p. 84, 1992.

[9] A. R. Van Meter, A. L. R. Moreira, and E. A. Youngstrom, "Meta-analysis of epidemiologic studies of pediatric bipolar disorder," *The Journal of Clinical Psychiatry*, vol. 72, no. 9, pp. 1250–1256, 2011.

[10] K. R. Merikangas, L. Cui, G. Kattan, G. A. Carlson, E. A. Youngstrom, and J. Angst, "Mania with and without depression in a community sample of US adolescents," *Archives of General Psychiatry*, vol. 69, no. 9, pp. 943–951, 2012.

[11] J. McClellan, R. Kowatch, and R. L. Findling, "Practice parameter for the assessment and treatment of children and adolescents with bipolar disorder," *Journal of the American Academy of Child & Adolescent Psychiatry*, vol. 46, no. 1, pp. 107–125, 2007.

[12] M. L. Barclay, B. E. W. Brownlie, J. G. Turner, and J. E. Wells, "Lithium associated thyrotoxicosis: a report of 14 cases, with statistical analysis of incidence," *Clinical Endocrinology*, vol. 40, no. 6, pp. 759–764, 1994.

[13] A. Bocchetta and A. Loviselli, "Lithium treatment and thyroid abnormalities," *Clinical Practice and Epidemiology in Mental Health*, vol. 2, no. 1, pp. 23–28, 2006.

[14] R. Yassa, A. Saunders, C. Nastase, and Y. Camille, "Lithium-induced thyroid disorders: a prevalence study," *The Journal of Clinical Psychiatry*, vol. 49, no. 1, pp. 14–16, 1988.

[15] R. L. Findling, A. Robb, N. K. McNamara et al., "Lithium in the acute treatment of bipolar I disorder: a double-blind, placebo controlled study," *Pediatrics*, vol. 136, no. 5, pp. 885–894, 2015.

[16] G. R. DeLong and A. L. Aldershof, "Long-term experience with lithium treatment in childhood: correlation with clinical diagnosis," *Journal of the American Academy of Child & Adolescent Psychiatry*, vol. 26, no. 3, pp. 389–394, 1987.

[17] M. T. McDermott, K. D. Burman, F. D. Hofeldt, and G. S. Kidd, "Lithium-associated thyrotoxicosis," *The American Journal of Medicine*, vol. 80, no. 6, pp. 1245–1248, 1986.

[18] R. Wilson, J. H. McKlllop, G. T. Crocket et al., "The effect of lithium therapy on parameters thought to be involved in the development of autoimmune thyroid disease," *Clinical Endocrinology*, vol. 34, no. 5, pp. 357–361, 1991.

[19] F. Fairbrother, N. Petzl, J. G. Scott, and S. Kisely, "Lithium can cause hyperthyroidism as well as hypothyroidism: a systematic review of an under-recognised association," *Australian & New Zealand Journal of Psychiatry*, vol. 53, no. 5, pp. 384–402, 2019.

[20] O. K. Tuncel, F. Akdeniz, S. S. Ozbek, G. Kavukcu, and G. U. Kocabas, "Thyroid function and ultrasonography abnormalities in lithium-treated bipolar patients: a cross-

sectional study with healthy controls," *Noro Psikiyatri Arsivi*, vol. 54, no. 2, pp. 108–115, 2017.

[21] T. Kontozoglou and N. Mambo, "The histopathologic features of lithium-associated thyroiditis," *Human Pathology*, vol. 14, no. 8, pp. 737–739, 1983.

[22] D. H. Myers, R. A. Carter, B. H. Burns, A. Armond, S. B. Hussain, and V. K. Chengapa, "A prospective study of the effects of lithium on thyroid function and on the prevalence of antithyroid antibodies," *Psychological Medicine*, vol. 15, no. 1, pp. 55–61, 1985.

[23] J. R. Calabrese, A. D. Gulledge, K. Hahn, R. Skwerer, M. Kotz, and O. P. Schumacher, "Autoimmune thyroiditis in manic depressive patients treated with lithium," *American Journal of Psychiatry*, vol. 142, no. 11, pp. 1318–1321, 1985.

[24] A. H. Dang and J. M. Hershman, "Lithium-associated thyroiditis," *Endocrine Practice*, vol. 8, no. 3, pp. 232–236, 2002.

6

Can Met-PET/CT Predict Sporadic Multiglandular Hyperparathyroidism? Report of a Case and Review of the Literature

Andreas Hillenbrand,[1] Johannes Lemke,[1] Doris Henne-Bruns,[1] Ambros J. Beer,[2] and Vikas Prasad[2]

[1]*Department of General and Visceral Surgery, University Medical Center Ulm, Ulm, Germany*
[2]*Department of Nuclear Medicine, University Medical Center Ulm, Ulm, Germany*

Correspondence should be addressed to Andreas Hillenbrand; andreas.hillenbrand@uniklinik-ulm.de

Academic Editor: Carlo Capella

Background. Primary hyperparathyroidism (pHPT) is a common endocrine disorder of the parathyroid glands. In most cases pHPT is caused by single gland disease, but about 10% of patients suffer from sporadic multiglandular disease (MGD). Patients with MGD, especially with ectopic parathyroid adenomas, have an increased risk for persistence/recurrence after surgery. Normally, sporadic MGD cannot be diagnosed preoperatively by parathyroid scintigraphy. We analyzed the potential of positron emission tomography/computed tomography (Met-PET/CT) to predict MGD. *Methods and Case Presentation.* We reviewed the literature, if preoperative Met-PET/CT could predict MGD in patients with pHPT. Further, we present a 71-year-old female with ectopic MGD. Preoperative localization via Met-PET/CT showed MGD with two areas suspected to be enlarged parathyroid glands (left lateral to the thyroid lobe and posterior mediastinum). Both diagnostic findings were extirpated and parathormone dropped into normal levels. *Results.* We identified four additional manuscripts, referring to MGD and Met-PET/CT with divergent results. Preoperative localization diagnostics using Met-PET/CT may not necessarily identify MGD. In most cases, Met-PET/CT localized only one adenoma and localizes larger adenomas more reliably than smaller adenomas. *Conclusion.* Identifying patients at risk of MGD preoperatively remains challenging. We found MET-PET/CT seems to predict MGD in patients with large size and high weight PTH adenomas. For ectopic parathyroid adenomas, accurate preoperative localization is the key to successful surgical removal. Met-PET/CT appears to have great potential in soft-tissue analysis of complex anatomical regions and can predict ectopic parathyroid adenomas.

1. Introduction

Primary hyperparathyroidism (pHPT) is a common endocrine disorder caused by parathyroid gland adenomas secreting excess amounts of parathyroid hormone (PTH). As a result, the blood calcium increases, which in turn causes kidney stones, psychiatric abnormalities, and/or bone disease. Several imaging modalities have been proposed for the detection of parathyroid adenomas in patients with primary hyperparathyroidism. Ultrasound (US) examination and parathyroid scintigraphy usually performed as SPECT with low-dose CT with Tc-99m methoxy-isobutyl-isonitrile (MIBI) are the predominant imaging techniques used in the setting of pHPT [1].

In patients with negative US or MIBI scans, C-11 methionine positron emission tomography/computed tomography (Met-PET/CT) might identify hyperfunctioning parathyroid glands [2]. Met-PET/CT is a highly sensitive method to localize parathyroid adenomas, particularly for cases in which conventional imaging techniques, such as ultrasound or sestamibi scintigraphy, have failed [3].

Therapeutically, surgical resection of the hormone-releasing adenoma(s) remains standard therapy. Most patients with pHPT have a single gland adenoma. However, about 10% of patients suffer from sporadic multiglandular disease (MGD) [4]. Identifying patients at risk of MGD preoperatively remains challenging. Patients with MGD

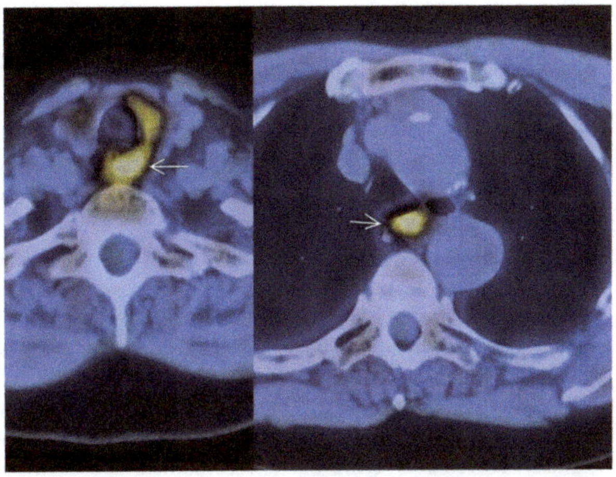

FIGURE 1: Preoperative localization via Met-PET/CT showed an intense uptake left lateral to the thyroid lobe and in the posterior mediastinum.

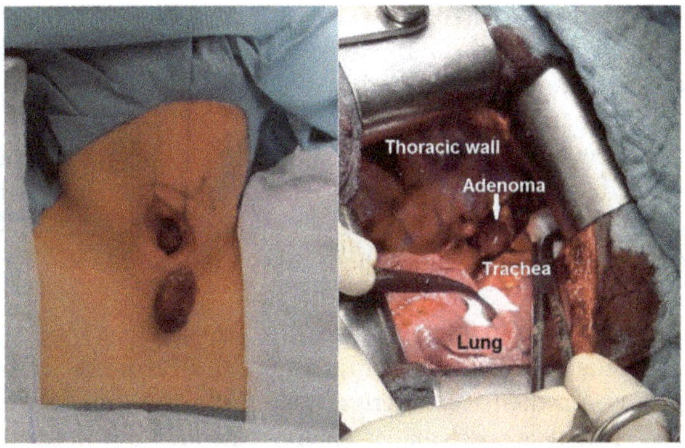

FIGURE 2: Extirpation of the left upper parathyroid gland and left thoracotomy with enlarged mediastinal parathyroid adenoma.

are considered to have higher risk of persistent disease. Therefore, a possible identification of patients with MGD could reduce the risk of a postoperative persistent hyperparathyroidism [5]. Further, ectopic parathyroid glands are found in about 1–3% of the population [6]. For ectopic parathyroid adenomas, accurate preoperative localization is the key to successful surgical removal. Met-PET/CT appears to have great potential in soft-tissue analysis of complex anatomical regions [7]. Aim of this study was to analyze if Met-PET/CT can predict MGD.

2. Case Report

Here, we report a case of a 71-year-old female diagnosed with MGD. The patient had no concurrent diseases and was not under any long-term medication. During a routine checkup, a hypercalcemia (3.7 mmol/l) with elevated parathyroid hormone (PTH: 233 pg/ml) was detected. Despite the very high serum calcium levels, the patient did not suffer from pHPT-specific symptoms such as kidney stones. A bone density measurement was not done. A preoperative neck and thyroid ultra-sonogram and a 99mTc-sestamibi SPECT/CT did not reveal an enlarged parathyroid adenoma in any location. An ultra-sonogram revealed a slightly enlarged multinodular thyroid and 99mTc-sestamibi SPECT/CT an uptake of radiotracers in the left lower thyroid, which intraoperatively turned out to be an inflammatory thyroid node.

Preoperative localization via Met-PET/CT showed a MGD with two areas suspected to be enlarged parathyroid glands (left lateral to the thyroid lobe and posterior mediastinum; Figure 1). Both diagnostic findings were extirpated in a two-stage procedure. First, a Kocher transverse collar incision was performed and the left thyroid area was explored. An enlarged left upper parathyroid gland (weight: 7.6 g, size: 4 × 2.5 × 1 cm) was extirpated, and a left caudal parathyroid gland was intraoperatively found to be normal in size (Figure 2). Further, a lower pole resection of the left thyroid (histology: inflammatory goiter node) and a left-sided thymus resection (histology: atrophic thymus with a cyst) was performed. Intraoperative PTH levels declined from 342 pg/ml to 197 pg/ml 10 minutes after extirpation. Three months later, a right thoracotomy was performed, and an enlarged parathyroid gland was extirpated from the posterior mediastinum (weight: 10.2 g size: 5 × 2.3 × 1.5 cm; Figure 2). Afterwards, intraoperative PTH levels declined from 189 pg/ml to 43 pg/ml at 10 minutes after extirpation. The postoperative course was uneventful and patient was discharged after one week with normal serum calcium levels (2.3 mmol/l; PTH: 51 pg/ml).

3. Discussion

The current imaging standard for patients with hyperparathyroidism is MIBI scintigraphy in combination with ultrasonography [1]. The sensitivity and specificity of these methods are high (approximately 90%) in patients with solitary parathyroid adenomas, but low if multiple gland pathology is encountered [8]. Normally, sporadic MGD cannot be diagnosed preoperatively by parathyroid scintigraphy due to low accuracy, sensitivity and specificity of any preoperative localization tests performed, although two cases of double parathyroid adenoma evidenced by 99mTc-MIBI SPECT/CT are reported [5, 9–11]. Moreover, negative preoperative localization studies are even highly predictive of MGD [4]. In our reported case, MGD was preoperatively diagnosed by Met-PET/CT.

To identify additional cases of double adenomas identified preoperatively by Met-PET/CT, a Medline search was performed using the terms "Met-PET/CT", "parathyroid adenoma", and "double adenoma". Publications were screened and manuscripts relevant for the current study were selected for further analysis. We identified four additional manuscripts, referring to MGD and Met-PET/CT. Interestingly, we found divergent results in these reports. In the first three case series, six patients with MGD and a preoperative Met-PET/CT were reported. In only one of these patients Met-PET/CT localized more than one hyperfunctioning parathyroid gland [12–14]. Weber et al. analyzed 2017 results of preoperative Met-PET/CT in patients with negative Tc-99 sestamibi (MIBI) scintigraphy. Three patients with double adenomas were reported and Met-PET/CT correctly located five of six parathyroids [2].

Review of the literature revealed that preoperative localization diagnostics using Met-PET/CT may not necessarily identify MGD. In the majority of cases, Met-PET/CT localized only one adenoma in these cases, comparable to MIBI scintigraphy.

It appears that Met-PET/CT localizes larger adenomas more reliably than smaller adenomas. Braeuning et al. reported in their case series that all lesions missed by PET/CT had a size smaller than 9 mm and a volume of less than 0.2 ml [12]. Moreover, Weber et al. reported a highly significant correlation between true-positive findings and size of parathyroid adenomas. Reported mean size of adenomas was 1.81 ± 0.84 cm and mean weight was 1.50 ± 2.56 g. Weight and size of the two parathyroid glands in our patient were comparably very high (7.6 and 10.2 g or $4 \times 2.5 \times 1$ cm and $5 \times 2.3 \times 1.5$ cm). The large size and high weight are potentially the reason why both adenomas in our case were detected in the preoperative Met-PET/CT. As mentioned before, some studies have suggested that MIBI scintigraphy also has the potential to identify MGD. However, whether Met-PET/CT identifies MGD more reliably than MIBI scintigraphy remains to be shown in future studies.

Therapy of patients with MGD is challenging since there is no reliable diagnostic tool to identify patients with MGD preoperatively. In particular, ectopic adenomas in patients with MGD are difficult to detect. Our observation suggests that the use of Met-PET/CT can help to identify MGD preoperatively or prior to second intervention. In patients with larger adenomas, Met-PET/CT is able to predict MGD.

Disclosure

We certify that no funding has been received.

Authors' Contributions

Andreas Hillenbrand and Doris Henne-Bruns performed the operative procedure, Vikas Prasad and Ambros J. Beer performed the preoperative diagnostic workup, and Johannes Lemke, Vikas Prasad, and Andreas Hillenbrand performed the research. Johannes Lemke and Andreas Hillenbrand wrote the manuscript. All authors read and approved the manuscript.

References

[1] E. Hindié, Ö. Ugur, D. Fuster et al., "2009 EANM parathyroid guidelines," *European Journal of Nuclear Medicine and Molecular Imaging*, vol. 36, no. 7, pp. 1201–1216, 2009.

[2] T. Weber, M. Gottstein, S. Schwenzer, A. Beer, and M. Luster, "Met-PET/CT was able to identify hyperfunctioning parathyroid glands in 74% of patients with pHPT and negative sestamibi scans," *World Journal of Surgery*, vol. 41, no. 4, pp. 980–985, 2017.

[3] C. Caldarella, G. Treglia, M. A. Isgrò, and A. Giordano, "Diagnostic performance of positron emission tomography using 11C-methionine in patients with suspected parathyroid adenoma: a meta-analysis," *Endocrine Journal*, vol. 43, no. 1, pp. 78–83, 2013.

[4] E. Kebebew, J. Hwang, E. Reiff et al., "Predictors of single-gland vs multigland parathyroid disease in primary hyperparathyroidism," *JAMA Surgery*, vol. 141, no. 8, p. 777, 2006.

[5] M. Barczyński, R. Bränström, G. Dionigi, and R. Mihai, "Sporadic multiple parathyroid gland disease—a consensus report of the European Society of Endocrine Surgeons (ESES)," *Langenbeck's Archives of Surgery*, vol. 400, no. 8, pp. 887–905, 2015.

[6] K. Cupisti, C. Dotzenrath, D. Simon, H. Röher, and P. E. Goretzki, "Therapy of suspected intrathoracic parathyroid adenomas. Experiences using open transthoracic approach and video-assisted thoracoscopic surgery," *Langenbeck's Archives of Surgery*, vol. 386, no. 7, pp. 488–493, 2002.

[7] S. Purz, R. Kluge, H. Barthel et al., "Visualization of ectopic parathyroid adenomas," *The New England Journal of Medicine*, vol. 369, no. 21, pp. 2067–2069, 2013.

[8] E. Hindié, D. Mellière, C. Jeanguillaume, P. Ureña, C. DeLabriolle-Vaylet, and L. Perlemuter, "Unilateral surgery for primary hyperparathyroidism on the basis of technetium Tc 99m sestamibi and iodine 123 subtraction scanning," *JAMA Surgery*, vol. 135, no. 12, pp. 1461–1468, 2000.

[9] L. De Gregorio, C. C. Lubitz, R. A. Hodin et al., "The Truth about double adenomas: incidence, localization, and intraoperative parathyroid hormone," *Journal of the American College of Surgeons*, vol. 222, no. 6, pp. 1044–1052, 2016.

[10] A. Krishnamurthy, U. Majhi, G. Rangarajan, V. Ramshankar, and R. Kumar, "The diagnostic and therapeutic challenges in the management of a double giant parathyroid adenoma," *Indian Journal of Nuclear Medicine*, vol. 31, no. 4, p. 301, 2016.

[11] M. Martínez-Valle Torres, E. Ramos Moreno, T. Amrani Raissouni, S. Sanz Viedma, A. Delgado Garcia, and J. Jiménez-Hoyuela Garcia, "A rare case of double parathyroid adenoma evidenced by 99mTc-sestaMIBI SPECT/CT," *Revista Española de Medicina Nuclear e Imagen Molecular*, vol. 36, no. 1, pp. 57-58, 2017.

[12] U. Braeuning, C. Pfannenberg, B. Gallwitz et al., "11C-methionine PET/CT after in conclusive 99mTc-MIBI-SPECT/CT for localisation of parathyroid adenomas in primary hyperparathyroidism," *Nuklearmedizin / Nuclear Medicine*, vol. 54, no. 01, pp. 26–30, 2017.

[13] T. Weber, G. Cammerer, C. Schick et al., "C-11 methionine positron emission tomography/computed tomography localizes parathyroid adenomas in primary hyperparathyroidism," *Hormone and Metabolic Research*, vol. 42, no. 03, pp. 209–214, 2010.

[14] T. Weber, C. Maier-Funk, D. Ohlhauser et al., "Accurate preoperative localization of parathyroid adenomas With C-11 methionine PET/CT," *Annals of Surgery*, vol. 257, no. 6, pp. 1124–1128, 2013.

7

A Case of Subacute Thyroiditis following COVID-19 Infection

Sameh Samir Elawady,[1] Diwakar Phuyal,[2] Rakesh Kumar Shah,[3] and Lubna Mirza[4]

[1]*Faculty of Medicine, Tanta University, Tanta, Egypt*
[2]*Kirtipur Hospital, PHECT Nepal, Kathmandu, Nepal*
[3]*Kathmandu Medical College, Kathmandu, Nepal*
[4]*Norman Endocrinology Associates, Norman, OK, USA*

Correspondence should be addressed to Sameh Samir Elawady; sameh.elawady1@gmail.com

Academic Editor: Wayne V. Moore

Background/Objective. Since the start of the pandemic, COVID-19 has been associated with several postinfection complications. Subacute thyroiditis (SAT) is an inflammatory disorder of the thyroid that has been reported in the literature following COVID-19 infection. We report a case of SAT following COVID-19 infection. *Case Report*. A 33-year-old female presented with neck pain two weeks after resolution of COVID-19 infection. Her thyroid function tests together with ultrasonographic pictures were consistent with SAT. She was treated with three rounds of medrol dose pack without relief. She then required oral prednisone 40 mg per day and ibuprofen 800 mg once daily for another several weeks that eventually resulted in improvement of her symptoms. *Discussion*. SAT most commonly occurs in females during or after viral infection. The usual course of the disease is hyperthyroidism then hypothyroidism followed by resolution. SAT is clinically diagnosed by lab findings of decreased TSH in the setting of negative thyroid-stimulating and thyroid peroxidase antibodies. All these data are consistent with our case. *Conclusion*. SAT following COVID-19 infection presents with a similar clinical presentation and course as the classic form of SAT, but we should consider the fact that a high-dose corticosteroid treatment might be necessary for such patients.

1. Introduction

Coronavirus disease 2019 (COVID-19) has been rapidly spreading world-wide with over 5 million infected individuals having died through November 26, 2021 [1]. COVID-19 has a clinical presentation varying from asymptomatic to mild upper respiratory tract infection, to severe complications including multiple organ failure especially lungs and kidneys. COVID-19 has been linked to many postinfection complications including subacute thyroiditis (SAT) [2]. Subacute thyroiditis (SAT), also known as de Quatrain thyroiditis, is a self-limiting thyroid disorder linked to some viral infections. It is reported that SAT is linked with several respiratory viruses such as coxsackievirus, mumps, Epstein–Barr virus, cytomegalovirus, and influenza virus [3]. SAT most commonly affects females in their 40s and 50s [4]. It typically presents with fever, myalgia, malaise, pain, and tenderness in the thyroid region, which may radiate to the jaw or neck [5, 6]. The usual course of action is hyperthyroidism, then hypothyroidism followed by resolution within weeks, but some cases may persist for months or may reoccur [7]. The diagnosis of SAT is a clinical diagnosis supported by lab findings of decreased TSH in the setting of negative thyroid-stimulating and thyroid peroxidase antibodies [5]. Here, we present a case of a 33-year-old female patient with post-COVID SAT.

2. Case Presentation

A 33-year-old female was referred to endocrinology due to anterior neck pain for four weeks. This pain developed two weeks after contracting COVID-19 infection, which presented with flu-like illness that was confirmed by PCR and resolved within 2 weeks. She initially noticed a swelling and pain in her neck radiating towards the right ear. She also had fever, malaise, and myalgia. She is a nonsmoker, not

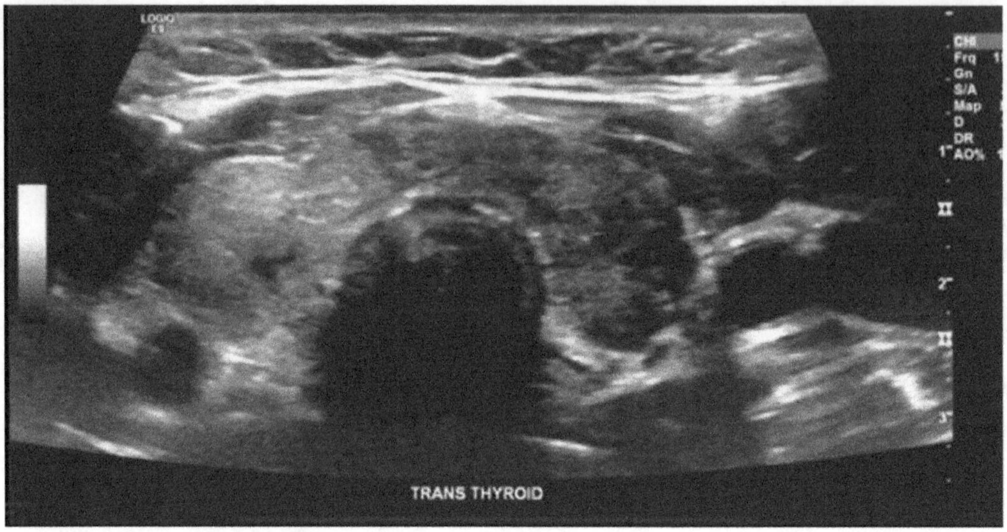

Figure 1: Ultrasound of the thyroid gland showing a heterogeneously enlarged thyroid gland with two small 4 mm solid hypoechoic solid nodules in the isthmus.

alcoholic, and is married with four children. Her past medical history included depression, abnormal pap smear, breast biopsies, and pregnancy-induced hypertension. Her medications included duloxetine HCl 30 mg capsule, delayed release particles once a day, and clonazepam 0.5 mg tablet as needed for severe anxiety. On general physical examination, she was alert, oriented, with intact cognitive function. She was cooperative, had good eye contact, judgment, and insight. She had a height of 157.5 cm, weight of 80.74 kg, and body mass index (BMI) of 32.55 kg/m^2. She had a temperature of 36.8°C, blood pressure of 118/84 mm hg, heart rate of 92 beats/min, and respiratory rate of 12 breaths/min. Head, neck, eye, and extremities examination revealed no abnormalities. Cardiac auscultation showed normal S1, S2, with no murmurs. Lung auscultation was clear. Abdomen was soft, nontender, and nondistended. Neurological examination showed a symmetrical deep tendon reflex of 2+ and good balance. Examination of the neck revealed thyromegaly with tenderness over the anterior neck. Laboratory investigations showed low TSH level (0.04 mU/L), normal free T4, normal free T3, negative thyroid peroxidase antibody (TPO) (0.9 IU/mL), and negative thyroid-stimulating immunoglobulin (TSI) (1.0). Ultrasound of the neck (Figure 1) revealed a heterogeneously enlarged thyroid gland with two small 4 mm solid hypoechoic solid nodules in the isthmus. Right thyroid lobe measured 1.64 ∗ 4.90 ∗ 1.69 cm. Left thyroid lobe measured 1.42 ∗ 4.03 ∗ 1.38 cm. Isthmus width was 0.49 cm. No abnormal lymph nodes were demonstrated. She was treated with medrol dosepack three times without relief. She continued to feel severe pain with swelling and compressive symptoms requiring oral prednisone 40 mg per day and ibuprofen 800 mg once daily for several weeks. Her symptoms, physical exam, and TSH level normalized within two weeks and steroids were tapered off gradually. An oral consent was obtained from the patient for research and publication, but no written consent has been obtained as there is no patient identifiable data included in this case report.

3. Discussion

Thyroiditis refers to heterogeneous groups of disorders that are characterized by some form of thyroid inflammation. SAT is a rare cause of thyroiditis which most commonly occurs two to eight weeks after viral infection. The most common viruses implicated include mumps, measles, influenza, enterovirus, cytomegalovirus, HIV, coxsackievirus, adenovirus, and EBV [3, 5]. SAT could either be due to direct injury by the virus or by the host's immunologic response to the virus [2]. SAT is associated with HLA-B ∗ 35, HLA-B ∗ 18.01, DRB1 ∗ 01, and C ∗ 04: 01, which confirms genetic predisposition in almost all patients [8].

The prevalence and association of subacute thyroiditis with SARS-CoV-2 varies in the literature. In a prospective study conducted by Bahçecioğlu et al. in Turkey, among 64 patients with SAT, 18.2% of those were associated with SARS-CoV-2. It also concluded that the rate of exposure of SARS-CoV-2 in SAT patients was increased, though the total number of SAT cases pre- and postpandemic period was comparable [9]. In an Italian case series, it was found that, of ten patients referred due to SAT, there were four patients who had evidence SARS-CoV-2 infection [10]. However, another one from Italy concluded that there was no increase in incidence of subacute thyroiditis during the pandemic period in the city of Brescia [11]. A systematic analysis conducted by Giovanella et al., including seven studies and 1237 COVID-19 patients, shows that thyroid dysfunction (defined as abnormal thyroid function tests) varies among the included studies between 13 and 64% [12].

The exact mechanism by which COVID-19 causes SAT is not known, but several explanations have been proposed including induction of an inflammatory response supported by inflammatory infiltration and apoptotic cells inside the thyroid gland [13]. This systemic immune and inflammatory response includes activation of coagulation and complement system, with elevation of many inflammatory cytokines such as IL-6, IL-1β, and TNF-α [14]. Another possible mechanism is the interaction with ACE2 receptors and transmembrane protease serine 2 (TMPRSS2) receptors, which are abundant in the thyroid tissue and at the same time coronavirus has a high affinity towards [15].

Our patient was diagnosed with SAT based on neck swelling, tenderness, low TSH, negative antibodies, ultrasonographic picture, and disease resolution after treatment with corticosteroids. Our patient have not undergone CRP or ESR testing, which is considered a limitation of our case report as it is considered as one of the main diagnostic criteria of SAT according to Stasiak and Lewiński [16].

A systematic review [2] including 19 articles which included 27 patients with SAT between May 21, 2020, and April 14, 2021, showed that about 83.3% SAT occurred after COVID-19 after a median of 30 days. 12.5% of patients had COVID-19 and SAT concurrently, and in one patient (4.2%), SAT preceded COVID-19 infection. Our patient had SAT after four weeks of COVID-19 and fitted in the group with the majority of the cases. In the study, overt thyrotoxicosis with a decrease in TSH was present in all cases with available reports, which was also the case with our patient who presented with low thyroid-stimulating hormone (TSH) of 0.04 mU/L. Thyroid ultrasound in our patient and most of the patients of the systematic review (20/27) had patchy hypoechogenic areas. Most of the patients in the systematic review had resolution after steroid treatment, with prednisone being the most commonly prescribed steroid at a median dose of 25 mg (IQR 25–35). In contrast to this, SAT in our patient relapsed even with three courses of medrol pack, and required treatment with high-dose prednisone 40 mg per day with ibuprofen 800 mg.

4. Conclusion

SAT after COVID-19 presents with a similar clinical presentation and similar course as the classic form of SAT, but we should consider the fact that high-dose corticosteroid treatment might be necessary for such patients.

References

[1] WHO, *WHO Coronavirus (COVID-19) Dashboard*, WHO, Geneva, Switzerland, 2021, https://covid19.who.int.

[2] P. Trimboli, C. Cappelli, L. Croce, L. Scappaticcio, L. Chiovato, and M. Rotondi, "COVID-19-Associated subacute thyroiditis: evidence-based data from a systematic review," *Frontiers in Endocrinology*, vol. 12, Article ID 707726, 2021.

[3] R. Desailloud and D. Hober, "Viruses and thyroiditis: an update," *Virology Journal*, vol. 6, p. 5, 2009.

[4] A. Bindra and G. D. Braunstein, "Thyroiditis," *American Family Physician*, vol. 73, no. 10, pp. 1769–1776, 2006.

[5] R. T. Shrestha and J. Hennessey, "Acute and subacute, and riedel's thyroiditis," in *Endotext. South Dartmouth (MA)*, K. R. Feingold, B. Anawalt, and A. Boyce, Eds., MDText.com, Inc, South Dartmouth, MA, USA, 2000.

[6] M. Stasiak and A. Lewiński, "New aspects in the pathogenesis and management of subacute thyroiditis," *Reviews in Endocrine & Metabolic Disorders*, vol. 22, 2021.

[7] V. Fatourechi, J. P. Aniszewski, G. Z. E. Fatourechi, E. J. Atkinson, and S. J. Jacobsen, "Clinical features and outcome of subacute thyroiditis in an incidence cohort: olmsted County, Minnesota, study," *Journal of Clinical Endocrinology & Metabolism*, vol. 88, no. 5, pp. 2100–2105, 2003.

[8] M. Stasiak, B. Tymoniuk, R. Michalak, B. Stasiak, M. L. Kowalski, and A. Lewiński, "Subacute thyroiditis is associated with HLA-B*18:01, -DRB1*01 and -C*04:01-The significance of the new molecular background," *Journal of Clinical Medicine*, vol. 9, no. 2, 2020.

[9] A. B. Bahçecioğlu, Z. C. Karahan, B. I. Aydoğan, I. A. Kalkan, A. Azap, and M. F. Erdoğan, "Subacute thyroiditis during the COVID-19 pandemic: a prospective study," *Journal of Endocrinological Investigation*, vol. 45, 2022.

[10] A. Brancatella, D. Ricci, D. Cappellani et al., "Is subacute thyroiditis an underestimated manifestation of SARS-CoV-2 infection? Insights from a case series," *Journal of Clinical Endocrinology & Metabolism*, vol. 105, no. 10, 2020.

[11] I. Pirola, E. Gandossi, M. Rotondi et al., "Incidence of De Quervain's thyroiditis during the COVID-19 pandemic in an area heavily affected by Sars-CoV-2 infection," *Endocrine*, vol. 74, no. 2, pp. 215–218, 2021.

[12] L. Giovanella, R. M. Ruggeri, P. P. Ovčariček, A. Campenni, G. Treglia, and D. Deandreis, "Prevalence of thyroid dysfunction in patients with COVID-19: a systematic review," *Clin Transl Imaging*, vol. 9, no. 3, pp. 233–240, 2021.

[13] X. H. Yao, T. Y. Li, Z. C. He et al., "[A pathological report of three COVID-19 cases by minimal invasive autopsies]," *Zhonghua Bing Li Xue Za Zhi*, vol. 49, no. 5, pp. 411–417, 2020.

[14] R. M. Ruggeri, A. Campennì, D. Deandreis et al., "SARS-COV-2-related immune-inflammatory thyroid disorders: facts and perspectives," *Expert Review of Clinical Immunology*, vol. 17, no. 7, pp. 737–759, 2021.

[15] M. Y. Li, L. Li, Y. Zhang, and X. S. Wang, "Expression of the SARS-CoV-2 cell receptor gene ACE2 in a wide variety of human tissues," *Infect Dis Poverty*, vol. 9, no. 1, 45 pages, 2020.

[16] M. Stasiak and A. Lewiński, "New aspects in the pathogenesis and management of subacute thyroiditis," *Reviews in Endocrine & Metabolic Disorders*, vol. 22, no. 4, pp. 1027–1039, 2021.

8

A Case of Gitelman Syndrome with Hypercalcemia Secondary to Primary Hyperparathyroidism

Zeinab Alnahas,[1] **Marko Markov**,[2] **and Mohamad H. Horani**[2]

[1]*Department of Internal Medicine, Cairo University, Cairo 11956, Egypt*
[2]*Chandler Regional Medical Center, Chandler 85224, Arizona, USA*

Correspondence should be addressed to Zeinab Alnahas; zeinab.elnahas@gmail.com

Academic Editor: Osamu Isozaki

Gitelman syndrome is a rare autosomal recessive salt-losing tubulopathy characterized by hypokalemia, hypomagnesemia, hypocalciuria, and secondary hyperaldosteronism. However, hypercalcemia secondary to hypocalciuria is extremely rare during the disease. A 36-year-old normotensive man who suffered a motor vehicle accident was presented with hypokalemia, hypomagnesemia, and mild hypercalcemia. He had a past medical history significant for bipolar depression disorder and a history of chronic atrial fibrillation. He was diagnosed with Gitelman syndrome. However, he was noncompliant with his medications. A laboratory workup revealed hypokalemia, hypomagnesemia, hypercalcemia, and a high parathyroid hormone level. Thorough investigations identified primary hyperparathyroidism as the primary cause of hypercalcemia. To our knowledge, Gitelman syndrome and primary hyperparathyroidism are an extremely rare association that is present in our case.

1. Background

Gitelman syndrome, also known as familial hypokalemia-hypomagnesemia, is a rare autosomal recessive hereditary disorder characterized by hypokalemic metabolic alkalosis, hypomagnesemia, hypocalciuria, and secondary hyperaldosteronism [1]. Gitelman syndrome tends to manifest during adolescence by various clinical presentations, including nonspecific symptoms such as fatigue, dizziness, nocturia, abdominal pain, muscle weakness, or muscle cramps and severe symptoms, such as tetany, paralysis, rhabdomyolysis, or fatal arrhythmia. However, individuals with Gitelman syndrome are usually asymptomatic and diagnosed by chance during routine blood testing [2]. The estimated prevalence of Gitelman syndrome is about 1 in 40,000 persons, with a significantly higher prevalence in the Asian population [3]. Although hypocalciuria is a distinctive characteristic of Gitelman syndrome caused by defective tubular reabsorption, it seldom can cause any change in the total plasma calcium level. Thus, the occurrence of hypercalcemia would require further investigation.

2. Case Presentation

We reported a 36-year-old normotensive man with a past medical history significant for bipolar depression disorder and gastroesophageal reflux disease and a history of atrial fibrillation. He was diagnosed with Gitelman syndrome based on the presence of hypokalemia, hypomagnesemia, and hypocalciuria. However, he was noncompliant with spironolactone, potassium, and magnesium supplementation. He suffered a motor vehicle accident, and on presentation to the emergency room, he was found with a serum potassium of 2.5 mmol/L (reference value 3.5–5.1 m·mol/L), serum magnesium of 0.8 mg/dL (reference value 1.7–2.2 mg/dL), total serum calcium of 11.3 mg/dL (reference value 8.4–10.2 mg/dL), serum phosphorus of 2.7 mg/dl (reference value 2.8–4.5 mg/dL), serum 25-dihydroxyvitamin D of 22.5 ng/mL (sufficient >25 ng/mL), random urine potassium of 122.1 mmol/L (reference value 20 mmol), 24-hour urinary calcium of 0.8 mg/kg/day (reference value < 4 mg/kg/day), and estimated fractional excretion of calcium of 0.004. He denied thiazide use, calcium, and vitamin D supplementation.

Further investigations were done to identify the potential causes of hypercalcemia and revealed a high intact parathyroid hormone of 144 pg/mL (reference value 10–65 pg/mL) consistent with primary hyperparathyroidism. His CT neck scan showed a 1.5 cm nodule inferior to the right thyroid lobe pole, consistent with an inferior parathyroid adenoma. However, a parathyroid radionuclide scan using technetium-99m MIBI showed no radiopharmaceutical localization for parathyroid adenoma within the neck or mediastinum. His abdominal CT scan excluded the presence of nephrolithiasis or nephrocalcinosis, and his echocardiography showed normal left ventricular function with no significant valvular pathology. Because the patient's serum calcium was higher than 1 mg/dL above the upper limits of the normal range, he underwent right inferior parathyroidectomy. The histological examination of the excised adenoma showed hypercellular parathyroid gland (678 milligrams) which confirmed the diagnosis of primary hyperparathyroidism. Shortly after the surgery, his serum calcium and parathyroid hormone levels were normalized, reaching 10 mg/dL and 56 pg/mL, respectively.

3. Discussion

Gitelman syndrome results from mutations at the SLC12A3 gene that encodes thiazide-sensitive sodium chloride cotransporter (NCCT) and magnesium channels in the renal distal convoluted tubule, causing salt-losing tubulopathy [4]. However, molecular genetic testing is not required for diagnosis, which can be established by the presence of the characteristic electrolyte imbalance [5]. Hypercalcemia is extremely rare in Gitelman syndrome, offset by the action of concomitant hypomagnesemia, which impairs the function of calciotropic hormones. This includes the function of parathyroid hormone (PTH) and 1,25-dihydroxyvitamin D [1,25 $(OH)_2D$], resulting in decreased intestinal absorption of calcium. Lack of magnesium hinders the activation of 1 alpha-hydroxylase by PTH, leading to a decreased level of 1,25 $(OH)_2D$. In addition, the negative relationship between circulating calcium levels and PTH is blunted in patients with Gitelman syndrome [6].

Therefore, the presence of hypercalcemia in patients with Gitelman syndrome requires further investigation to identify the potential causes of high calcium levels associated with elevated PTH levels, which may include primary hyperparathyroidism and familial hypocalciuric hypercalcemia. In primary hyperparathyroidism, there is a nonsuppressed secretion of PTH often from a single parathyroid adenoma, leading to high calcium levels. PTH stimulates osteoclast activity and suppresses osteoblast activity, resulting in bone breakdown and calcium release. Also, it increases renal calcium reabsorption and the formation of 1,25 $(OH)_2D$, which stimulates intestinal calcium absorption [7]. The most common presentation of primary hyperparathyroidism is asymptomatic hypercalcemia. Nevertheless, it can cause a broad spectrum of clinical presentations, including fatigue, depression, memory loss, muscle and bone pain, and gastroesophageal reflux disease, or the classical manifestations of bones, stones, abdominal moans, and psychic groans [8]. In comparison, familial hypocalciuric hypercalcemia is a rare genetic disorder resulting from mutations in the calcium-sensing receptor (CaSR) gene and less commonly due to autoantibodies blocking CaSR. It is clinically similar to primary hyperparathyroidism, resulting in abnormal urinary calcium levels and high levels of serum calcium and PTH [9].

The presence of low urinary calcium excretion is the most important parameter to distinguish familial hypocalciuric hypercalcemia from primary hyperparathyroidism. However, in a patient with Gitelman syndrome, the differentiation between the possible causes of hypercalcemia based on the urine excretion of calcium is not reasonable due to the presence of underlying hypocalcuria caused by enhanced renal tubular absorption of calcium [10]. In such cases, family history and genetic testing would be helpful in the differentiation. Also, renal imaging and measurement of bone mineral density using a DXA scan are interesting for evaluating primary hyperparathyroidism complications and are normal in familial hypocalciuric hypercalcemia [11]. In our case, the presence of a high level of PTH and low-normal phosphorus in conjugation with the imaging findings of inferior parathyroid adenoma on the CT neck scan supported the diagnosis of primary hyperparathyroidism which has been confirmed by the histological examination and the normalization of serum calcium level after the surgery. Moreover, our patient's gastrointestinal, psychological, and cardiac symptoms could be related to hypercalcemia and hyperparathyroidism, either directly or through activation of neurotransmitters and sodium/potassium pump [12–14]. Although primary hyperparathyroidism is diagnosed based on biochemical findings, imaging studies are used for preoperative localization and are not diagnostic tools. A radionuclide technetium-99m MIBI scan could localize approximately 75% of solitary parathyroid adenoma [15].

4. Conclusion

Hypercalcemia is extremely rare in Gitelman syndrome, offset by the action of concomitant hypomagnesemia. Our case shows the importance of investigating the potential causes of hypercalcemia, such as hyperparathyroidism, in individuals with Gitelman syndrome. To our knowledge, Gitelman syndrome and primary hyperparathyroidism are an extremely rare association that is present in our case.

References

[1] D. B. Simon, C. N. Williams, M. J. Bia et al., "Gitelman's variant of Barter's syndrome, inherited hypokalaemic alkalosis, is caused by mutations in the thiazide-sensitive Na–Cl cotransporter," *Nature Genetics*, vol. 12, no. 1, pp. 24–30, 1996.

[2] A. S. Balavoine, P. Bataille, P. Vanhille et al., "Phenotype-genotype correlation and follow-up in adult patients with hypokalaemia of renal origin suggesting Gitelman syndrome,"

European Journal of Endocrinology, vol. 165, no. 4, pp. 665–673, 2011.

[3] A. Kondo, C. Nagano, S. Ishiko et al., "Examination of the predicted prevalence of Gitelman syndrome by ethnicity based on genome databases," *Scientific Reports*, vol. 11, no. 1, Article ID 16099, 2021.

[4] I. Kurtz, J. J. Cohen, J. T. Harrington, N. E. Madias, and C. J. Zusman, "Molecular pathogenesis of Bartter's and Gitelman's syndromes," *Kidney International*, vol. 54, no. 4, pp. 1396–1410, 1998.

[5] National Organization for Rare Disorders, *Gitelman Syndrome*, National Organization for Rare Disorders, Danbury, CT, United States, 2018.

[6] M. G. Bianchetti, A. Bettinelli, J. P. Casez et al., "Evidence for disturbed regulation of calciotropic hormone metabolism in Gitelman syndrome," *Journal of Clinical Endocrinology and Metabolism*, vol. 80, no. 1, pp. 224–228, 1995.

[7] K. L. Insogna, "Primary hyperparathyroidism," *New England Journal of Medicine*, vol. 379, no. 11, pp. 1050–1059, 2018.

[8] T. Madkhali, A. Alhefdhi, H. Chen, and D. Elfenbein, "Primary hyperparathyroidism," *Turkish Journal of Surgery*, vol. 32, no. 1, pp. 58–66, 2016.

[9] M. C. Shinall, K. M. Dahir, and J. T. Broome, "Differentiating familial hypocalciuric hypercalcemia from primary hyperparathyroidism," *Endocrine Practice*, vol. 19, no. 4, pp. 697–702, 2013.

[10] C.-J. Cheng, J.-C. Shiang, Y.-J. Hsu, S.-S. Yang, and S.-H. Lin, "Hypocalciuria in patients with Gitelman syndrome: role of blood volume," *American Journal of Kidney Diseases*, vol. 49, no. 5, pp. 693–700, 2007.

[11] S. J. Silverberg, B. L. Clarke, M. Peacock et al., "Current issues in the presentation of asymptomatic primary hyperparathyroidism: proceedings of the Fourth International Workshop," *Journal of Clinical Endocrinology and Metabolism*, vol. 99, no. 10, pp. 3580–3594, 2014.

[12] B. Abboud, R. Daher, and J. Boujaoude, "Digestive manifestations of parathyroid disorders," *World Journal of Gastroenterology*, vol. 17, no. 36, p. 4063, 2011.

[13] R. Serdenes, M. Lewis, and S. Chandrasekhara, "A clinical review of the psychiatric sequelae of primary hyperparathyroidism," *Cureus*, vol. 13, no. 10, Article ID e19078, 2021.

[14] R. M. Kiewiet, H. H. Ponssen, E. N. W. Janssens, and P. W. Fels, "Ventricular fibrillation in hypercalcaemic crisis due to primary hyperparathyroidism," *The Netherlands Journal of Medicine*, vol. 62, no. 3, pp. 94–96, 2004.

[15] J. M. Ruda, C. S. Hollenbeak, and B. C. Stack, "A systematic review of the diagnosis and treatment of primary hyperparathyroidism from 1995 to 2003," *Otolaryngology-Head and Neck Surgery*, vol. 132, no. 3, pp. 359–372, 2005.

9

Delivery of Euthyroid Baby following Hyperthyroidism in Twin Gestation with Coexisting Complete Hydatidiform Mole

Rishi Raj, Edilfavia Mae Uy, Matthew Hager, and Kamyar Asadipooya

Department of Endocrinology, Diabetes and Metabolism, University of Kentucky, Lexington, KY, USA

Correspondence should be addressed to Rishi Raj; rishiraj91215@gmail.com

Academic Editor: John Broom

Context. Gestational trophoblastic disease (GTD) is a rare complication of pregnancy, ranging from molar pregnancy to choriocarcinoma. Twin pregnancies with GTD and coexisting normal fetus are extremely rare with an estimated incidence of 1 case per 22,000–100,000 pregnancies. Molecular mimicry between human chorionic gonadotrophin (hCG) and thyroid-stimulating hormone (TSH) leads to gestational trophoblastic hyperthyroidism (GTH) which is further associated with increased maternal and fetal complications. This is the first reported case in literature describing the delivery of a baby with biochemical euthyroid status following a twin pregnancy with hydatidiform mole (HM) associated with gestational trophoblastic hyperthyroidism (GTH). *Case Description.* A 24-year-old G4 P3 Caucasian female with twin gestation was admitted to hospital for gestation trophoblastic hyperthyroidism. She was later diagnosed to have twin pregnancy with complete mole and coexisting normal fetus complicated by gestational trophoblastic hyperthyroidism (GTH). Despite the risk associated with the continuation of molar pregnancy, per patient request, pregnancy was continued till viability of the fetus. The patient underwent cesarean section due to worsening preeclampsia and delivered a euthyroid baby at the 24th week of gestation. *Conclusions.* Twin pregnancy with gestational trophoblastic disease and coexisting normal fetus is associated with high risk of hyperthyroidism, and careful monitoring of the thyroid function test along with dose titration of thionamides is of utmost importance throughout the gestation. If normal thyroid hormone levels are maintained during the pregnancy, euthyroidism could be successfully achieved in the baby.

1. Case Presentation

A 24-year-old G4 P3 Caucasian female with a history of hypertension and type II diabetes mellitus presented to the emergency room with vaginal bleeding at 13 weeks of gestation. On presentation, she reported dizziness, diaphoresis, tremors, anxiety, palpitations, nausea, and leg swelling. Review of system was negative for headache or scotomas. Her vital signs showed blood pressure 141/80 mmHg, heart rate 97 beats per minute, respiratory rate 20 per minute, and temperature 98.4°F. Physical examination was significant for gravid uterus and bilateral lower extremity edema and had fine tremors of both hands. Thyroid gland was normal in size without any nodules. Laboratory studies (Tables 1 and 2) revealed suppressed TSH, elevated free T4, and absence of thyroid antibodies including thyrotropin-receptor antibodies (TRAb), thyroperoxidase antibodies (TPOAb), and thyroglobulin antibodies (TgAb). 24 hour urine protein was 200 mg/day and urine protein/creatinine ratio 0.2 in a random urine specimen. Pelvic ultrasound showed twin gestation with one complete HM and one coexisting normal fetus (Figures 1(a)–1(c)). Based on clinical and biochemical evidence of hyperthyroidism with elevated human chorionic gonadotrophin (hCG) levels in the absence of autoantibodies, a diagnosis of GTH was made.

After extensive discussion regarding risk of developing complications associated with molar pregnancy [1], she preferred to proceed with her current pregnancy until viability of fetus. As she was into her 2nd trimester of pregnancy, she was started on methimazole and the dose was titrated to achieve a goal free T4 in the upper range of normal (normal range = 0.8–1.7 ng/dL) to prevent fetal hypothyroidism. She was also on metoprolol 25 mg daily for chronic hypertension which was continued throughout the pregnancy. She also developed preeclampsia at 16 weeks of pregnancy with 24 hr urine protein of 3729 mg/day. She was

Table 1: Laboratory evaluation on admission.

Laboratory test	Result	Reference range
Anti-thyroid peroxidase Ab	<5	0–9 IU/mL
T3	405	87–187 ng/dL
Thyroglobulin antibody	<1.0	<4.0 IU/mL
TSH receptor antibody	<0.90	≤1.75
Urine protein creatinine ratio	0.2	<0.2 mg/mg
Total protein/day, urine	200	<150 mg/day if ambulatory <80 mg/day if bed rest
Platelet count	135	155–369 k/μL
Hemoglobin	9.1	11.2–15.7 g/dL
Hematocrit	27.9%	34–45%
WBC	4.9	3.7–10.3 k/μL
Glucose	83	74–99 mg/dL
Creatinine	0.35	0.60–1.10 mg/dL
Sodium	139	136–145 mmol/L
Potassium	3.9	3.7–4.8 mmol/L
Alkaline phosphatase	33	35–104 U/L
Alanine transaminase	9	8–33 U/L
Aspartate transaminase	8	11–32 U/L
Total bilirubin	0.3	0.2–1.1 mg/dL
LDH	171	116–250 U/L

Table 2: TSH, free T4, and hCG trends during and postpregnancy.

Laboratory Studies	TSH (range = 0.4–4.2 μIU/mL)	Free T4 (range = 0.8–1.7 ng/dL)	Methimazole dose (mg/day)	hCG, total beta (range <5 mIU/mL)
Weeks of gestation				
13th week	0.01	4.4	5	480, 579
15th week	0.01	2.6	30	746, 811
17th week	0.01	1.4	15	771, 692
18th week		1.2	10	706, 583
20th week		1.2	5	655, 027
22nd week		1.3	2.5	357, 387
24th week	0.02	1.3	2.5	415, 666
Postdelivery				
0.5th week	0.45	0.8		15, 942
2nd week				585
4th week				430
8th week				119
13th week				13
17th week				3
21st week				<1

again recommended termination of pregnancy, but she preferred to proceed with her pregnancy. At 24th weeks of gestation, pregnancy was complicated by worsening pre-eclampsia and she eventually underwent a lower segment cesarean section with delivery of a viable fetus and evacuation of molar pregnancy. The weight of the baby was 645 gram, and APGAR score was 1 at 1 minute, 2 at 5 minutes, and 3 at 10 minutes. Postoperatively, gross examination of the tissue revealed fragments of pink-red spongy soft tissue without any fetal parts or abnormal Z line, while microscopic examination revealed hydropic villi and trophoblastic proliferation confirming the diagnosis of a complete mole (Figures 1(d)–1(f)). Histopathology of placenta revealed a singleton placenta weighing 156 grams and measuring 13.8 × 11.3 × 2.6 cm. At the time of delivery, she was on very low dose of methimazole, and therefore, it was discontinued. She remained clinically and biochemically euthyroid in the postpartum period. Her hCG gradually trended to a normal range of 17 weeks after delivery, and she had spontaneous remission of molar pregnancy as supported by low hCG levels at 1-year follow-up (Figure 2). The preterm infant did not have any gross abnormalities, and screening for congenital hypothyroidism was negative both at birth with TSH < 2.91 μU/mL (normal range < 20 μU/mL) and free T4 8.2 μg/dL (normal range ≥ 5 μg/dL) and at two months postdelivery with TSH < 2.91 μU/mL (normal range < 20 μU/mL) and free T4 6.7 μg/dL (normal range ≥ 5°μg/dL). Unfortunately, the baby needed mechanical ventilation for respiratory distress syndrome and gradually developed bronchopulmonary dysplasia requiring need for prolonged mechanical ventilation and underwent tracheostomy. He was transferred to a long-term care facility.

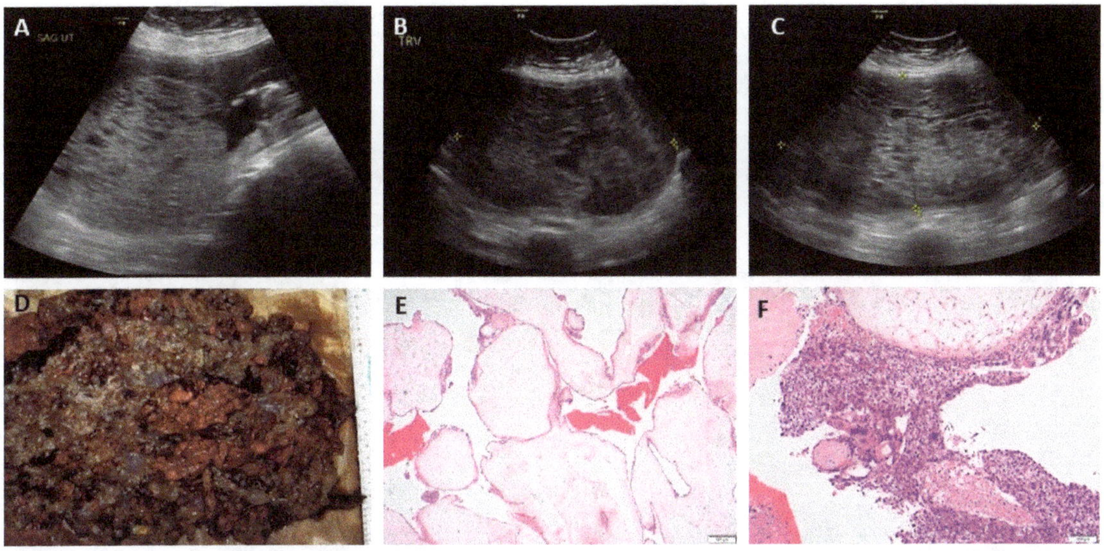

FIGURE 1: Ultrasound imaging of twin gestation (complete HM and coexisting normal fetus) at 14 weeks (a), 22 weeks (b), and 24 weeks (c). Histologic examination: (d) gross appearance with multiple tan-gray semitransparent vesicles of variable size admixed with solid fragments of tan-brown soft tissue and blood clot with no fetal parts; (e) diffuse villous enlargement with marked hydropic change; absent p57 immunostain (not shown) supporting the diagnosis of complete hydatidiform mole; (f) circumferential trophoblastic proliferation with focal necrosis and cytologic atypia, characteristics of complete HM.

2. Discussion

Gestational trophoblastic disease (GTD) is defined as a spectrum of proliferative disorders of trophoblastic cells and includes benign nonneoplastic placental site trophoblastic tumor, HM (complete or partial), gestational trophoblastic neoplasia, and choriocarcinoma [2]. HM is the most common form of GTD and results from errors of fertilization. It can be classified into complete or partial mole on the basis of karyotype, gross morphology of the specimen, histopathologic features, and clinical features [2]. Extreme maternal age (≤15 and >35 years) and previous history of molar pregnancy are considered to be risk factors [3]. In the US, HM occurs between 0.5 and 2.5 per 1000 pregnancies [3]. Twin gestation with HM is even rarer with an estimated incidence of 1 per 20,000 to 100,000 pregnancies [4] and is associated with severe maternal complications (massive vaginal bleeding, hyperemesis gravidarum, hyperthyroidism, preterm delivery, pregnancy-induced hypertension, preeclampsia, trophoblastic embolization, and gestational trophoblastic neoplasia) and fetal complications (fetal death) [1, 4–6]. A literature review by Lin et al. revealed a regional difference in clinical presentation of CHMCF with a higher rate of life-threatening conditions in South America compared to North America [1].

In our case, the patient chose to pursue her pregnancy until her fetus becomes viable for delivery knowing the possibility of severe complications of her pregnancy. If HM is associated with viable fetus as in our case, it is important to distinguish the specific type of mole as the normal cotwin of the complete mole has a better survival rate compared to the partial mole [7]. Cytogenetic analysis of complete HM reveals a diploid karyotype without fetal parts and has an androgenetic origin, while the partial mole has a triploid karyotype with fetal parts [7]. The fetus in the partial mole has triploidy without chance of life after delivery, and therefore, partial mole even with fetus alive should be interrupted [8]. P57 immunohistochemical staining helps in distinguishing between a complete and partial mole as seen in our case which is absent in complete HM and present in partial HM [9].

hCG is a glycoprotein hormone, made of a common alpha subunit encoded by a single gene on chromosome 6 and a hormone specific beta subunit encoded by a cluster of genes on chromosome 19 [10]. hCG shares the same alpha subunit as well as significant amino acid sequence in the beta subunit with TSH and hence is able to interact with the TSH receptor [11]. However, its potency for TSH receptor is significantly (~4000 times) less than TSH [12], and hence development of hyperthyroidism requires sustained elevation of hCG levels to >200,000 mIU/mL for several weeks [10]. In a normal pregnancy, secretion of hCG begins by the 3rd week and peaks to 200,000–300,000 mIU/mL between 9 and 11th weeks before gradual decline to 3,500–150,000 mIU/mL by the 20th week [10]. The peak hCG lasts for only few days and can occasionally lead to transient thyrotoxicosis with resultant elevation of T3 and T4 levels and suppression of TSH, bearing a mirror image of the hCG peak; however; treatment is rarely required beyond the 22nd week of pregnancy [12]. In contrast to normal pregnancy, HM secretes a large amount of hCG proportional to the tumor mass [12]. For every 10,000 mIU/ml increase in serum hCG, FT4 increases by 0.1 ng/dL and TSH decreases by 0.1 mIU/mL [13]. Furthermore, hCG produced from GTD is considered to have enhanced thyrotrophic activity compared to hCG in normal pregnancy as supported by increased cAMP production by GTD-associated hCG action on human TSH-R on Chinese hamster ovary cells [14]. This

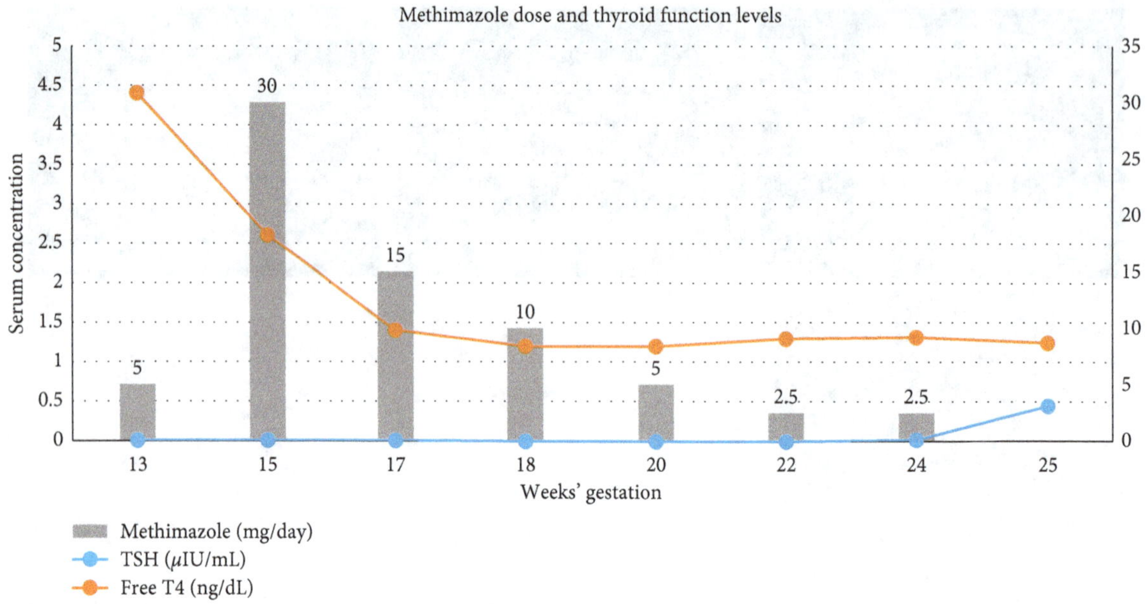

Figure 2

persistently elevated levels of hCG in molar pregnancy can lead hyperthyroidism and is defined as gestational trophoblastic hyperthyroidism.

Hyperthyroidism as a complication of HM was first described in 1955 [2]. The prevalence of biochemical hyperthyroidism with HM is relatively common and varies from 25 to 64% with 5% having clinical hyperthyroidism [10]. Clinically evident hyperthyroidism can manifest with weight loss, heat intolerance, palpitation, tremors, and diaphoresis with severity of symptoms being directly proportional to hCG levels [12]. In patients with uncontrolled hyperthyroidism, surgery and anesthesia may precipitate thyroid storm resulting in increased perioperative mortality [2].

Surgical evacuation of the molar pregnancy is the mainstay of management for HM and leads to prompt reduction in thyroid hormone levels secondary to decreased hCG concentrations [2]. In twin pregnancy with gestational trophoblastic disease and coexisting normal fetus, early termination of pregnancy had traditionally been advised but due to a better understanding of this condition, continuation of select pregnancy has been considered. Favorable obstetric outcome is seen among patients without antenatal maternal complications (pregnancy-induced hypertension, hyperthyroidism, and hyperemesis gravidarum) and initial serum hCG level less than 400,000°mIU/mL [4]. In those cases, continuation of twin pregnancy with gestational trophoblastic disease and coexisting normal fetus is an acceptable option with up to one-third chance of a live birth (7–37%) [7]. In our patient, although she developed preeclampsia and had significant hyperemesis gravidarum, she had successful fetal and maternal outcome which is extremely rare.

If pregnancy is desired, hyperthyroidism is mostly treated with beta blockers and thionamides while waiting for definitive management of the GTD [15]. The goal of thionamides is to reduce and maintain the mother's serum FT4 levels within a high normal range for nonpregnant females using the lowest dose to prevent fetal goiter and fetal hypothyroidism [15]. Transient central hypothyroidism may be seen in infants whose mother had poorly controlled hyperthyroidism during pregnancy, presumably due to suppression of the fetal-pituitary-thyroid-axis [15]. This is due to effect of uncontrolled maternal hyperthyroidism which leads to suppression of fetal TSH [16]. Both methimazole (MMI) and propylthiouracil (PTU) are equally effective in controlling hyperthyroidism. The choice of thionamide is based on consideration of their teratogenicity and risk of serious liver injury. The MMI embryopathy phenotype was described which includes scalp defects from aplasia cutis, choanal and esophageal atresia, trachea-esophageal fistula, abdominal wall defects like umbilicocele, developmental delay, athelia/hypothelia, hearing loss, and dysmorphic facie [10, 11]. American Thyroid Association (ATA) recommends use of PTU in the first trimester and MMI afterwards to reduce the risk of congenital malformations from MMI in the first trimester [15]. Beta adrenergic blocking agents (BBs) used for controlling hypermetabolic symptoms should be titrated based on clinical symptoms, as long-term use of BB has been associated with intrauterine growth restriction, fetal bradycardia, and neonatal hypoglycemia [15].

On extensive review of literature, we came across only one case of twin pregnancy with gestational trophoblastic disease and coexisting normal fetus where thyroid status of the newborn baby was discussed. In that case, the mother was treated with PTU and newborn delivered at 26 weeks had low FT4 and low normal TSH at birth but normalized at 5 weeks [11]. In our case, normal levels of FT4 were maintained during the course of pregnancy through a strict titration of MMI dose based on frequent monitoring of FT4 levels, and the baby was biochemically euthyroid on delivery as well as on follow-up, suggestive of importance of strict control of thyroid hormone levels. As the mother's hyperthyroidism was well controlled with antithyroid medication, this might have resulted in euthyroid status of the baby.

It is also important for postevacuation surveillance to detect persistence of molar tissue for potential development of gestational trophoblastic neoplasia (GTN) or choriocarcinoma [7]. Approximately, 3–5% of cases of HM can develop choriocarcinoma, whereas incidence of GTN following twin pregnancy with gestational trophoblastic disease and coexisting normal fetus is as high as 37% which is considerably higher compared to incidence of GTN with HM [4, 7, 10]. In our case, hCG levels started to trend down immediately postoperatively and was normal at 17 weeks postpartum. hCG levels are usually followed weekly until it reaches a normal range, which is usually within two to three months of evacuation of the molar pregnancy as seen in this case [17]. Once hCG levels are within the normal reference range, patients are followed every month for six months to look for any evidence of gestational trophoblastic neoplasia [2]. Intervention is not needed unless there is a rise of hCG levels [2, 17].

3. Conclusion

Twin pregnancy with gestational trophoblastic disease and coexisting normal fetus is an extremely rare condition, and there are limited data on safety outcome of mother and fetus. If pregnancy is desired until fetus becomes viable, careful monitoring of the mother for life-threatening complications could result in successful maternal and fetal outcome. As twin pregnancy with gestational trophoblastic disease and coexisting normal fetus is associated with high risk of hyperthyroidism, careful monitoring of the thyroid function test along with dose titration of thionamides is of utmost importance throughout the gestation, and if normal thyroid hormone levels are maintained during the pregnancy, euthyroidism could be safely achieved in the baby.

Abbreviations

HM: Hydatidiform mole
hCG: Human chorionic gonadotrophin
GTD: Gestational trophoblastic disease
GTN: Gestational trophoblastic neoplasia
MMI: Methimazole
PTU: Propylthiouracil
TSH: Thyroid-stimulating hormone
BB: Beta-blocker.

Authors' Contributions

Edilfavia Mae Uy, Rishi Raj, and Matthew Hager wrote the manuscript. Kamyar Asadipooya reviewed the manuscript and served as content expert. Katherine Vignes (Department of Obstetrics and Gynecology) and Autumn Vanover (Department of Pathology) contributed significantly in patient care and management.

References

[1] L. H. Lin, I. Maestá, A. Braga et al., "Multiple pregnancies with complete mole and coexisting normal fetus in North and South America: a retrospective multicenter cohort and literature review," *Gynecologic Oncology*, vol. 145, no. 1, pp. 88–95, 2017.

[2] S. Virmani, S. B. Srinivas, R. Bhat, R. Rao, and R. Kudva, "Transient thyrotoxicosis in molar pregnancy," *Journal of Clinical and Diagnostic Research*, vol. 11, no. 7, pp. QD01–QD02, 2017.

[3] A. Altieri, S. Franceschi, J. Ferlay, J. Smith, and C. L. Vecchia, "Epidemiology and aetiology of gestational trophoblastic diseases," *The Lancet Oncology*, vol. 4, no. 11, pp. 670–678, 2003.

[4] M. Suksai, C. Suwanrath, O. Kor-Anantakul et al., "Complete hydatidiform mole with co-existing fetus: predictors of live birth," *European Journal of Obstetrics & Gynecology and Reproductive Biology*, vol. 212, pp. 1–8, 2017.

[5] I. Nobuhara, N. Harada, N. Haruta et al., "Multiple metastatic gestational trophoblastic disease after a twin pregnancy with complete hydatidiform mole and coexisting fetus, following assisted reproductive technology: case report and literature review," *Taiwanese Journal of Obstetrics and Gynecology*, vol. 57, no. 4, pp. 588–593, 2018.

[6] N. J. Sebire, M. Foskett, F. J. Paradinas et al., "Outcome of twin pregnancies with complete hydatidiform mole and healthy co-twin," *The Lancet*, vol. 359, no. 9324, pp. 2165-2166, 2002.

[7] H. Imafuku, Y. Miyahara, Y. Ebina, and H. Yamada, "Ultrasound and MRI findings of twin pregnancies with complete hydatidiform mole and coexisting normal fetus: two case reports," *The Kobe Journal of Medical Sciences*, vol. 64, no. 1, pp. E1–E5, 2018.

[8] S. Y. Sun, D. P. Goldstein, M. R. Bernstein et al., "Maternal near miss according to world health organization classification among women with a hydatidiform mole: experience at the new england trophoblastic disease center, 1994–2013," *The Journal of Reproductive Medicine*, vol. 61, no. 5-6, pp. 210–214, 2016.

[9] H. Landolsi, N. Missaoui, S. Brahem, S. Hmissa, M. Gribaa, and M. T. Yacoubi, "The usefulness of p57KIP2 immunohistochemical staining and genotyping test in the diagnosis of the hydatidiform mole," *Pathology—Research and Practice*, vol. 207, no. 8, pp. 498–504, 2011.

[10] J. M. Hershman, "Physiological and pathological aspects of the effect of human chorionic gonadotropin on the thyroid," *Best Practice & Research Clinical Endocrinology & Metabolism*, vol. 18, no. 2, pp. 249–265, 2004.

[11] D. K. True, M. Thomsett, H. Liley et al., "Twin pregnancy with a coexisting hydatiform mole and liveborn infant: complicated by maternal hyperthyroidism and neonatal hypothyroidism," *Journal of Paediatrics and Child Health*, vol. 43, no. 9, pp. 646–648, 2007.

[12] L. Walkington, J. Webster, B. W. Hancock, J. Everard, and R. E. Coleman, "Hyperthyroidism and human chorionic gonadotrophin production in gestational trophoblastic disease," *British Journal of Cancer*, vol. 104, no. 11, pp. 1665–1669, 2011.

[13] D. Glinoer, "The regulation of thyroid function in pregnancy: pathways of endocrine adaptation from physiology to pathology," *Endocrine Reviews*, vol. 18, no. 3, pp. 404–433, 1997.

[14] K. Kato, M. Mostafa, K. Mann, A. Schindler, and R. Hoermann, "The human chorionic gonadotropin molecule from patients with trophoblastic diseases has a high thyrotropic activity but is less active in the ovary," *Gynecological Endocrinology*, vol. 18, no. 5, pp. 269–277, 2004.
[15] E. K. Alexander, E. N. Pearce, G. A. Brent et al., "2017 guidelines of the American thyroid association for the diagnosis and management of thyroid disease during pregnancy and the postpartum," *Thyroid*, vol. 27, no. 3, pp. 315–389, 2017.
[16] N. Bhavani, "Transient congenital hypothyroidism," *Indian Journal of Endocrinology and Metabolism*, vol. 15, no. 6, pp. S117–S120, 2011.
[17] R. Agarwal, S. Teoh, D. Short, R. Harvey, P. M. Savage, and M. J. Seckl, "Chemotherapy and human chorionic gonadotropin concentrations 6 months after uterine evacuation of molar pregnancy: a retrospective cohort study," *The Lancet*, vol. 379, no. 9811, pp. 130–135, 2012.

10

Thyroid Storm with Multiorgan Failure Treated with Plasmapheresis

Ann Miller and Kristi D. Silver

Division of Endocrinology, Diabetes, and Nutrition, Department of Medicine, University of Maryland School of Medicine, Baltimore, MD, USA

Correspondence should be addressed to Kristi D. Silver; ksilver@som.umaryland.edu

Academic Editor: Osamu Isozaki

Background. Thyroid storm is a severe manifestation of thyrotoxicosis and can present with multiorgan failure. First line treatment of thyroid storm is directed towards decreasing thyroid hormone production and peripheral conversion of T4 to T3, and treating adrenergic symptoms. When medical therapy fails, plasmapheresis is an alternative treatment option. Here we present a patient with thyroid storm and multiorgan failure who was treated with plasmapheresis. *Case.* A 50-year-old male with a history of hyperthyroidism, hypertension, and congestive heart failure presented to another hospital with fever and altered mentation. He was found to have pneumonia on imaging and was started on antibiotics. He developed shock complicated by atrial fibrillation with rapid ventricular rate which was treated with amiodarone. He was transferred to our hospital for further management. On arrival, TSH was <0.01 mIU/L, free T4 was >7 ng/dL and total T3 was 358 ng/dL. The endocrinology team determined he was in thyroid storm. His medical treatment of thyroid storm was aggressively titrated to maximal therapy. His hospital course was complicated by transaminitis, respiratory failure requiring intubation, shock requiring vasopressor support, kidney failure requiring continuous renal replacement therapy, and heart failure. Despite maximal anti-thyroid therapy, he had not improved clinically and T4 and T3 remained markedly elevated. A 4-day course of plasmapheresis was initiated resulting in marked lowering of T4 and T3 and clinical stability. *Conclusion.* While current guidelines for plasmapheresis for thyroid storm recommend individualized decision making, no further clarification is provided on who would be a good candidate for the procedure. We present a patient with thyroid storm and multiorgan failure who was treated with plasmapheresis after failing maximal medical therapy. Given the significant improvement seen with plasmapheresis, endocrinologists should consider this mode of treatment earlier in the course of thyroid storm when patients are not improving with medical therapy alone.

1. Background

Thyroid storm is a severe manifestation of thyrotoxicosis and can present with multiorgan failure. Thyroid storm has an estimated mortality rate of 20%–30% [1]. First line treatment of thyroid storm is directed at decreasing thyroid hormone production and peripheral conversion of thyroxine (T4) to triiodothyronine (T3), and treating adrenergic symptoms. When medical therapy fails, therapeutic plasma exchange (TPE), also called therapeutic plasmapheresis, is an alternative treatment option. Here we present a patient with thyroid storm and multiorgan failure who was successfully treated with TPE.

2. Case

A 50-year-old African American male with a history of hyperthyroidism, hypertension, and congestive heart failure presented to an outside hospital with fever and an altered mental status. He was diagnosed with hyperthyroidism about three months prior to hospitalization. He was started on methimazole (MMI), but compliance taking the medication was low. His primary care provider had recommended thyroidectomy; however, he was unable to have the procedure due to lack of health insurance. On presentation to the outside hospital, imaging revealed right lower lobe pneumonia with an effusion and he was started on antibiotics.

Table 1: Admission laboratory studies.

Lab	Result	Reference range
WBC	29.7	4.5–11.0 K/μL
Hemoglobin	10.3	12.6–17.4 g/dL
Platelets	149	153–367 K/μL
Creatinine	1.43	0.66–1.25 mg/dL
AST	177	17–59 units/L
ALT	44	21–72 units/L
Total bilirubin	3.8	0.3–1.2 mg/dL
Lactate	2.8	0.5–1.6 mmol/L
Troponin	7.05	≤0.06 ng/mL

His clinical status deteriorated, and he developed shock complicated by atrial fibrillation with rapid ventricular rate with documented rates in the 140–190 beats per minute. His arrhythmia was refractory to digoxin, diltiazem, and two attempts at cardioversion with 200 Joules. He was initiated on an amiodarone infusion which stabilized his arrhythmia. His TSH documented at the outside hospital was 0.01 mIU/L and free T4 was 8 ng/dL.

He was transferred to our hospital for further management. Prior to transfer, he was started on hydrocortisone 50 mg every 6 hours and MMI 10 mg three times daily. MMI was used instead of propylthiouracil (PTU) due to elevated liver function tests. On the day of arrival to our hospital, the inpatient endocrinology team was consulted for assistance with thyroid management. He was intubated for respiratory distress at the time of the endocrinology team's initial assessment. His blood pressure, supported by two pressors, was 90/63 mmHg. His temperature was 36.9°C and his pulse ranged from 88 to 134 beats per minute on the amiodarone infusion. Physical examination was significant for scleral icterus and left neck fullness. No thyroid bruit or discrete nodules were identified; however, the neck exam was limited due to multiple central lines. His heart beat was irregular consistent with atrial fibrillation and a cardiac murmur was also detected. Lower extremities were notable for edema and hyperreflexia. The endocrinology team was unable to assess his mental status due to the patient being sedated. Thyroid labs on admission to our hospital included TSH <0.01 mIU/L (0.47–4.68 mIU/L), total T3 358 ng/dL (97–169 ng/dL), free T4 > 7 ng/dL (0.6–2.5 ng/dL) and thyroid stimulating antibodies >500% (normal ≤122%). Additional laboratory studies (Table 1) showed acute kidney injury and elevated liver function tests, troponin, and white blood cell count. Thyroid ultrasound with doppler showed an enlarged, heterogeneous thyroid gland, more pronounced on the right than the left without any nodules, although the view of the left side was limited due to the endotracheal tube and central line.

His Burch–Wartofsky score [2] for hyperthyroid storm was 100 which was highly concerning for thyroid storm. As the Burch–Wartofsky score can sometimes be misleading with elevated scores in critically ill patients without thyroidal illness, the Japan Thyroid Association thyroid storm criteria, a diagnostic criterion less likely to incorrectly diagnose thyroid storm in critically ill patients, was also utilized to assess for thyroid storm in our patient [3]. Employing this second diagnostic criterion, our patient again met criteria for thyroid storm based on the family report of altered mental status, tachycardia with documented rates of 140–190 per minute, heart failure with an estimated ejection fraction of 30%, and thyrotoxicosis with suppressed TSH and elevated free T4 and total T3 levels.

The endocrine consult team recommended increasing MMI to 20 mg three times daily and starting cholestyramine 4 g three times daily. Over the ensuing days, his renal function worsened such that he required continuous renal replacement therapy. On day 2, saturated potassium iodide solution (SSKI) 250 mg three times daily was initiated and cholestyramine was increased to 4 g four times daily. Liver function tests improved by day 3; therefore, he was switched from MMI to PTU 200 mg three times daily to take advantage of the decreased conversion of T4 to T3 seen with PTU. On day 4, TSH remained undetectable and free T4 was unchanged at >7 ng/dL. Total T3 began to decrease, but remained >200 ng/dL. Despite maximal medical therapy for thyroid storm, his clinical status continued to worsen with evidence of multiorgan failure. The endocrinology team consulted the hematology physicians for initiation of TPE.

He was started on daily TPE on hospital day 4. Replacement fluid contained half fresh frozen plasma (FFP) and half 5% albumin and was equal in volume to his total plasma volume (about 4L). His TPE treatment lasted about two hours each day and he received plasmapheresis daily for four days. After the first day of TPE, his free T4 and total T3 decreased to 5.3 ng/dL and 139 ng/dL, respectively. After 4 sessions of daily TPE, his free T4 was 1.9 ng/dL and total T3 was 77 ng/dL (Figure 1). With TPE, his clinical course significantly improved to the point where he was weaned off of pressors and extubated. Over the following 2 weeks, he was safely titrated off of SSKI and hydrocortisone, and switched from PTU to MMI. For definitive treatment of hyperthyroidism, the endocrine surgery team was consulted to evaluate the patient for total thyroidectomy. At the time of their evaluation, the patient was clinically euthyroid. Given his recent critical illness, the surgeons considered him to be a high-risk surgical candidate. Therefore, they recommended performing an elective thyroidectomy once the patient was further out from his critical illness and had undergone outpatient cardiac optimization. He was discharged home three weeks later on MMI 30 mg twice daily and cholestyramine 4 g twice daily. At time of discharge, he did not require any supplemental oxygen and his left ventricular ejection fraction improved to 48% as measured on positron emission tomography myocardial perfusion scan. He was no longer in atrial fibrillation as he had converted back to sinus rhythm and amiodarone had been discontinued. With the exception of total bilirubin, his liver function tests had normalized before discharge. By 2 months post discharge, his total bilirubin had also normalized. He was discharged with intermittent dialysis needs, though two weeks after leaving the hospital, dialysis was discontinued because his kidney function recovered.

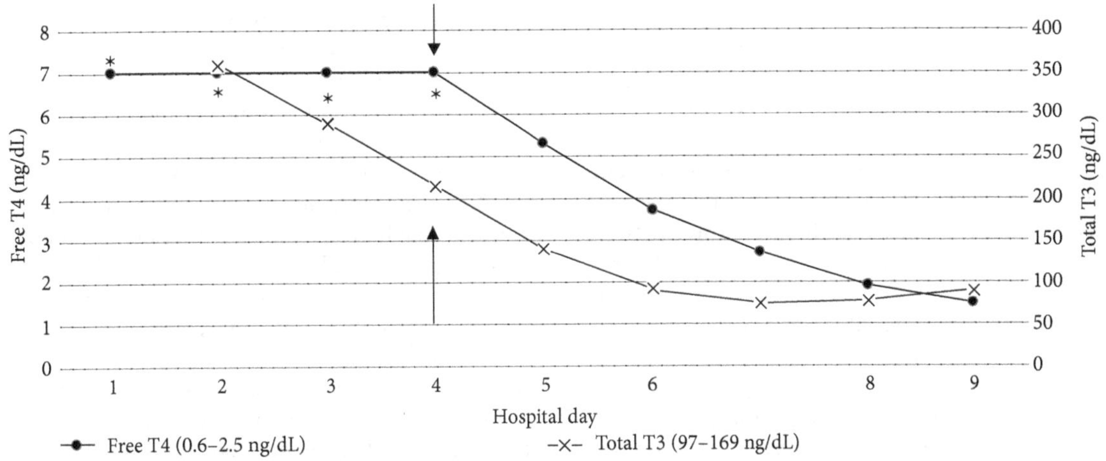

FIGURE 1: Free T4 and total T3 Levels during hospitalization. *Values were >7 ng/dL, → first day of plasmapheresis.

3. Discussion

Plasmapheresis is an extracorporeal blood purification technique that helps remove larger molecular weight substances from blood. Plasmapheresis is a general term that refers to removing plasma from blood. TPE is a type of plasmapheresis that involves removal of patient plasma and replacing it with something else (either donor plasma, colloid, or crystalloid). TPE is most often used to treat conditions, where a pathogenic substance or component is in the blood and needs to be rapidly removed. Examples of pathogenic substances include auto-antibodies, immunocomplexes, cryoglobulins, myeloma light chains, endotoxins, cholesterol containing lipoproteins, and as with our patient, plasma protein-bound thyroid hormones. The necessary tools for TPE include vascular access, either using large-bore needles in the limb veins or an implanted catheter in the large veins of the neck, chest, or groin, and a plasmapheresis machine. The machine separates the patient's plasma from the rest of the blood components and exchanges plasma with a replacement fluid. TPE is effective for treatment of thyroid storm as thyroid hormone is almost entirely bound to plasma proteins (99.97% of total serum T4 and 99.7% of total serum T3). The three main plasma proteins that bind T4 and T3 are thyroxine binding globulin (TBG), transthyretin, and albumin. TBG binds 75% of T4 and T3. Transthyretin binds 20% of T4 and <5% of T3. Albumin binds 5% of T4 and 20% of T3. TBG and transthyretin are relatively similar in size, 54 kDa and 55 kDa, respectively. Albumin is larger with a molecular mass of 66.5 kDa [4]. Because of the size of thyroid binding proteins, conventional dialysis cannot remove these proteins from blood. In contrast, TPE removes larger proteins, and thus can be used to reduce circulating thyroid hormone and treat refractory thyroid storm. TPE can also remove TSH receptor autoantibody (also referred to as thyroid stimulating immunoglobulin) and its removal has been predicted mathematically to result in rapid lowering of the free thyroxine levels [5].

Randomized placebo-controlled studies of TPE with medical management resistant thyroid storm have not been performed due to the rarity of the disorder. Therefore, guidelines for the use of TPE for thyroid storm are based on case reports, retrospective studies, and expert opinion. According to The American Society for Apheresis 2016 clinical practice guidelines, treatment of thyroid storm with plasmapheresis is a category III indication [6] meaning that the optimal role of TPE in thyroid storm is not established and the decision to use TPE for this indication should be individualized. Per these guidelines, when plasmapheresis is used to treat thyroid storm, FFP or albumin should be used as the replacement fluid. FFP has the benefit of increasing the concentration of TBG, which binds specifically to thyroxine and triiodothyronine, while albumin provides greater capacity for binding thyroid hormone. The recommended volume of replacement fluid is 1–1.5 times the total plasma volume. TPE treatment should be daily to every 3 days until clinical improvement is noted. TPE should be reserved for patients with severe symptoms of thyroid storm in whom first line medical therapies have failed or have had detrimental side effects that outweigh the benefits of treatment. These guidelines are similar to the guidelines set forth by The Japan Thyroid Association and Japan Endocrine Society in 2016 [7]. The Japanese guidelines recommend the use of TPE for treatment of thyroid storm if there is acute liver failure or no clinical improvement after 24–48 hours on optimized medical management. The Japanese guidelines recommend FFP over albumin as the replacement fluid due to its higher levels of TBG and specificity to bind thyroid hormone.

The effectiveness of TPE is dependent on multiple variables and is not a procedure without risk. The successful removal of pathogenic substances from blood through plasmapheresis depends on the volume of blood processed and plasma exchanged in each procedure, number of procedures performed, frequency of exchange, and rate of mobilization, stabilization, and re-synthesis of the cells or plasma components. Complications of plasmapheresis include bleeding, infection, disseminated intravascular coagulation (DIC), coagulation factor depletion leading to hypocoagulability, hypocalcemia, hypotension, and transfusion reactions such as transfusion associated infections, pulmonary edema, and pulmonary embolism. Despite these potential complications, the mortality rate of plasmapheresis is <1% [8].

Ashkar et al. first described thyrotoxicosis treated with plasmapheresis in 1970 in a case report of three thyrotoxic patients [9]. All three patients had deteriorating clinical status despite maximal medical treatment of thyrotoxicosis. The first patient underwent true TPE as his plasma was replaced with his red blood cells and lactate ringers. The other two patients were treated with plasmapheresis with removal of plasma with only their red blood cells returned to them. All three patients had significant clinical improvement. Since this initial description, case reports have described successful treatment with TPE in a variety of hyperthyroid scenarios ranging from post-operative thyroid storm complicated by pneumonia and septic shock [10] to MMI induced agranulocytosis [11] to amiodarone induced thyrotoxicosis [12]. While patients previously described as receiving plasmapheresis for thyroid storm were often critically ill, few have had multisystem organ failure similar to our patient. Of the few with multiorgan failure, one with a history of Graves' and medication noncompliance developed symptomatic thyrotoxicosis including palpitations, nausea, and vomiting. He was treated with medical therapy, but had to be switched from PTU to MMI due to liver dysfunction. He clinically decompensated despite medical therapy and developed DIC. He was treated with plasmapheresis and after two treatments, his free T4 and free T3 normalized. The same paper discusses a male with Graves' disease who also presented with thyrotoxicosis symptoms and medication noncompliance. This patient was started on oral medical therapy with MMI 20 mg daily and propranolol 40 mg twice daily. Shortly after admission, he became febrile with a temperature of 38.1°C and was found unresponsive and pulseless. He underwent cardiopulmonary resuscitation. He developed ventricular fibrillation and required electrical cardioversion. His clinical status further worsened with development of transaminitis and acute kidney injury with continued tachyarrhythmia. Neurologically, he was unresponsive off of sedation. After one day of plasmapheresis, his free T4 declined from 10.9 ng/dL to 8.57 ng/dL. He received two more treatments of plasmapheresis daily over the next two days. His free T4 continued to trend downwards as he continued to receive methimazole, SSKI, and steroids. While the paper does not talk about his neurological status after TPE, it did say that he became clinically and biochemically euthyroid and underwent definitive treatment with a total thyroidectomy [13]. Similarly, in a case reported by Baena et al., a 36-year-old woman with Graves' disease and multiorgan failure including acute liver and heart failure, acute kidney injury, cytopenia, rhabdomyolysis and coagulopathy improved with the use of medical management plus plasmapheresis [14].

Because of the infrequent use of TPE for treatment of thyroid storm/thyrotoxicosis, randomized controlled studies on its efficacy versus continuing with only maximal medical therapy have not yet been performed. Few retrospective reviews on TPE with thyroid storm involving more than one or two patients have been published. In a review by Ezer et al., 11 thyrotoxicosis patients successfully responded to pre-operative plasmapheresis treatment [15]. The etiologies of thyrotoxicosis (7-Graves' Disease, 3-toxic multinodular goiters, 1-iodine induced thyrotoxicosis) and the indications for plasmapheresis varied (7-poor response to medical therapy, 2-agranulocytosis, 1-iodine induced thyrotoxicosis and 1-urgent need for operation). All patients underwent plasmapheresis prior to surgery (10 patients underwent total thyroidectomy and 1 patient underwent an open reduction and internal fixation for femur fracture). The majority of patients required 1 to 3 plasmapheresis sessions to see clinical improvement and reductions in free T4 levels. Only one patient experienced a complication from plasmapheresis, a non-life threatening allergic reaction. Another patient had intraoperative bleeding from operative sites assumed to be secondary to the coagulopathy that can develop from TPE. Additionally, 50% of patients who underwent total thyroidectomy developed transient postoperative hypocalcemia. Hypocalcemia was presumed to be the result of long-term exposure to thyroid hormones with severe untreated hyperthyroidism, though postoperative hypocalcemia may have been due to parathyroid injury during surgery. Hyperthyroidism increases bone turnover which over time can lead to thyrotoxic osteodystrophy. After total thyroidectomy for hyperthyroidism, hypocalcemia can result from rapid recalcification of bones after loss of thyroid hormone stimulation [16].

In the largest retrospective study to date, 46 patients with thyrotoxicosis who were either unable to use anti-thyroid medications due to side effects, did not improve with standard thyrotoxicosis treatment or needed rapid improvement in thyroid function due to thyroid storm were treated with TPE [17]. Plasmapheresis was performed daily with sessions lasting 2.5–3 hours. The replacement fluid was FFP and the volume of replacement fluid was 1–1.5 times the calculated total plasma volume of the patient. The underlying etiology for the majority of the patients' thyrotoxicosis was Graves' disease with smaller numbers having amiodarone induced thyrotoxicosis or toxic nodular goiter. A significant improvement in free T4 levels from before to after plasmapheresis (free T4 2.9 ng/dL vs. 1.6 ng/dL, $P \leq 0.001$) was found in all patients. When stratified by hyperthyroid diagnosis, only the patients with Graves' disease had a statistically significant reduction in free T4 levels with TPE (free T4 2.9 ng/dL vs. 1.6 ng/dL, $P \leq 0.001$). While not statistically significant, possibly due to smaller numbers of subjects, the median free T4 did decrease after TPE in the patients with non-Graves' hyperthyroidism (free T4 3.1 ng/dL vs. 1.8 ng/dL, P = NS). In this study, complications related to TPE comprised of a deep vein thrombosis in a pregnant female and 2 catheter infections.

4. Conclusion

While current recommendations regarding TPE for treatment of thyroid storm recommend individualized decision making, little clarification regarding who would be a good candidate is available. In our case report, we present a patient with thyroid storm and multiorgan failure who was ineffectively treated with maximal medical anti-thyroid therapy alone, but was rapidly and successfully treated once plasmapheresis was added to medical anti-thyroid therapy. Our case is one of the first to show that a patient with severe critical multiorgan failure can benefit from TPE. Given our patient's extraordinary recovery and the remarkable improvements in other patients with thyroid storm treated with TPE, endocrinologists should have a lower threshold to pursue treatment of thyroid storm with plasmapheresis if patients are not improving with medical antithyroid therapy alone. Future research is needed to answer questions regarding optimal replacement fluid and volume, frequency, and duration at which TPE should proceed for thyroid storm.

Abbreviations

MMI: Methimazole
PTU: Propylthiouracil
SSKI: Saturated potassium iodide solution
TPE: Therapeutic plasma exchange
T4: Thyroxine
TBG: Thyroxine binding globulin
T3: Triiodothyronine.

References

[1] Tietgens, S. T. and M. C. Leinung, "Thyroid storm," *Medical Clinics of North America*, vol. 79, no. 1, pp. 169–184, 1995.

[2] H. B. Burch and L. Wartofsky, "Life-threatening thyrotoxicosis. thyroid storm," *Endocrinology and Metabolism Clinics of North America*, vol. 22, no. 2, pp. 263–277, 1993.

[3] T. Akamizu, T. Satoh, O. Isozaki et al., "Diagnostic criteria, clinical features, and incidence of thyroid storm based on nationwide surveys," *Thyroid*, vol. 22, no. 7, pp. 661–679, 2012.

[4] T. Pappa, A. M. Ferrara, and S. Refetoff, "Inherited defects of thyroxine-binding proteins," *Best Practice & Research Clinical Endocrinology & Metabolism*, vol. 29, no. 5, pp. 735–747, 2015.

[5] M. K.-S. Leow, "A mathematical model of pituitary–thyroid interaction to provide an insight into the nature of the thyrotropin–thyroid hormone relationship," *Journal of Theoretical Biology*, vol. 248, no. 2, pp. 275–287, 2007.

[6] J. Schwartz, A. Padmanabhan, N. Aqui et al., "Guidelines on the use of therapeutic apheresis in clinical practice-evidence-based approach from the writing committee of the american society for apheresis: the seventh special issue," *Journal of Clinical Apheresis*, vol. 31, no. 3, pp. 149–162, 2016.

[7] T. Satoh, O. Isozaki, A. Suzuki et al., "Guidelines for the management of thyroid storm from the Japan thyroid association and Japan endocrine society (first edition)," *Endocrine Journal*, vol. 63, no. 12, pp. 1025–1064, 2016.

[8] D. W. Huestis, "Mortality in therapeutic haemapheresis," *The Lancet*, vol. 321, no. 8332, p. 1043, 1983.

[9] F. S. Ashkar, R. B. Katims, and W. M. Smoak, "Thyroid storm treatment with blood exchange and plasmapheresis," *JAMA: The Journal of the American Medical Association*, vol. 214, no. 7, pp. 1275–1279, 1970.

[10] J Petry, P. E. Y. Van Schil, P. Abrams, and P. G. Jorens, "Plasmapheresis as effective treatment for thyrotoxic storm after sleeve pneumonectomy," *The Annals of Thoracic Surgery*, vol. 77, no. 5, pp. 1839–1841, 2004.

[11] A. A. Vyas, P. Vyas, N. L. Fillipon, R. Vijayakrishnan, and N. Trivedi, "Successful treatment of thyroid storm with plasmapheresis in a patient with methimazole-induced agranulocytosis," *Endocrine Practice*, vol. 16, no. 4, pp. 673–676, 2010.

[12] T. H. Diamond, R. Rajagopal, K. Ganda, A. Manoharan, and A. Luk, "Plasmapheresis as a potential treatment option for amiodarone-induced thyrotoxicosis," *Internal Medicine Journal*, vol. 34, no. 6, pp. 369–370, 2004.

[13] A. Carhill, A. Gutierrez, R. Lakhia, and R. Nalini, "Surviving the storm: two cases of thyroid storm successfully treated with plasmapheresis," *BMJ Case Reports*, vol. 2012, 2012.

[14] J. C. Baena, J. Padilla, and G. Guzman, "Thyroid storm associated with multiorganic dysfunction," *Medicina (B Aires)*, vol. 77, no. 4, pp. 337–440, 2017.

[15] A. Ezer, K. Caliskan, A. Parlakgumus, S. Belli, I. Kozanoglu, and S. Yildirim, "Preoperative therapeutic plasma exchange in patients with thyrotoxicosis," *Journal of Clinical Apheresis*, vol. 24, no. 3, pp. 111–114, 2009.

[16] P. Karunakaran, C. Maharajan, S. Ramalingam, and S. V. Rachmadugu, "Is hungry bone syndrome a cause of postoperative hypocalcemia after total thyroidectomy in thyrotoxicosis? a prospective study with bone mineral density correlation," *Surgery*, vol. 163, no. 2, pp. 367–372, 2018.

[17] I. Y. Simsir, M. Ozdemir, S. Duman, M. Erdogan, A. Donmez, and A. G. Ozgen, "Therapeutic plasmapheresis in thyrotoxic patients," *Endocrine*, vol. 62, no. 1, pp. 144–148, 2018.

11

Two Case Reports of Subacute Thyroiditis after Receiving Vaccine for COVID-19

Jan Adelmeyer,[1] Joachim Nils Goebel,[1] Alexander Kauka,[2] and Peter Herbert Kann[1]

[1]*Philipps-University Marburg, Endocrinology Baldingerstraße, 35043 Marburg, Germany*
[2]*General Practice Grossseelheim, Grossseelheim 35274, Germany*

Correspondence should be addressed to Jan Adelmeyer; adelmeye@med.uni-marburg.de

Academic Editor: J. Paul Frindik

The ongoing COVID-19 pandemic, caused by a coronavirus named SARS-CoV-2, has struck the planet with great force. As of December 2019, the virus has made its devasting route across all continents . In January 2022, the World Health Organization (WHO) registered over 5.5 million COVID-19 related deaths. Most of these people had suffered from pneumonia and acute respiratory distress syndrome , and in some cases, extensive damage to all organ systems. To get hold of this pandemic, it was vital to find effective vaccines against it. The two vaccine candidates BNT162b2 (BioNTech/Pfizer) and ChAdOx1 (University of Oxford and AstraZeneca) offer a high level of protection against COVID-19 by providing immunity due to antibody production against the spike protein of SARS-CoV-2. In addition to general side effects, immunological side effects such as subacute thyroiditis can follow the vaccination. This transient inflammatory condition of the thyroid gland is characterized with hyperthyroxinemia, inflammation, pain, and tenderness in the thyroid region, as well as an elevation of serum thyroglobulin concentration. There are only a few reports on the occurrence of this disease after receiving a COVID-19 vaccine. We present two cases of subacute thyroiditis after vaccination with the vaccines BNT162b2 and ChAdOx1 and try to enlighten the problem of immunological phenomena after vaccination. It must be discussed whether cross-reactivity of the spike protein and tissue proteins such as thyroid peroxidase (TPO), an "autoimmune/inflammatory syndrome by adjuvants" (ASIA), or the circulating spike protein itself after vaccination are responsible for the SAT.

1. Background

SAT, is an inflammatory disease of the thyroid gland [1-30], which primarily affects women and is manifested by pain and tenderness. Furthermore, patients mention fever, general malaise, myalgia, and arthralgia [10]. These typical clinical symptoms and the presence of elevated free thyroxine (fT4) and free triiodothyronine (fT3) with suppressed thyroid-stimulating hormone (TSH) as well as increased erythrocyte sedimentation rate (ESR) lead to the diagnosis of SAT. Symptoms of thyroid hormone excess may occur in the initial phase, and hypothyroidism affects about 5–10% of patients at annual follow-up [31].

The thyroid gland appears mostly focally hypoechogenic and of normal or enlarged size with no hypervascularity on ultrasound [32]. In addition, 99mTc-pertechnetate uptake is markedly reduced, indicating an inadequate metabolic pathway during inflammation [33].

To date, there is no known definitive cause for this disease. There are some studies that show an association between SAT and HLA-B35 in several ethnic groups, as well as a family-related occurrence [34]. Previous viral infections, such as influenza, coxsackie virus, and mumps virus, have been discussed as potential causes for a long time, but so far this has not been proven with absolute certainty [35]. This theory is partly supported by observing the seasonal occurrence of the SAT from summer to early autumn in some studies [36, 37]. The search for a viral infection is often useless unless there is a therapeutic consequence for the viral disease as such.

Recently, there have been several case reports that showed the occurrence of SAT after infection with SARS-

Table 1: A review of previously published cases of SAT associated with vaccination against SARS-CoV-2. Only SAT cases from each manuscript are listed in this table.

Reference	Gender	Age	Vaccine	Dose	Time from vaccination until onset of symptoms	Symptoms	History of thyroid disease	fT3	fT4	TSH	ESR (mm) (RR < 15)	TgAb	TRAb	TPO-ab
Our case 1	F	36	BNT162b2 (Comirnaty®)	2nd	1 day	Neck pain, restlessness, fatigue	None	↔	↔	↔	44	Neg	Neg	Neg
Our case 2	M	65	ChAdOx1 (Vaxzevria®)	1st	3 days	Malaise	None	↔	↔	↓	21	Pos	Neg	Neg
Iremli et al. [11]														
Case 1	F	35	PiCoVacc (CoronaVac®)	2nd	4 days	Left-side anterior neck pain, fever, fatigue, palpitations	None	↑	↔	↔	53	Neg	Neg	Neg
Case 2	F	34	PiCoVacc (CoronaVac®)	1st	4 days	Anterior neck pain, fever, fatigue, palpitations	None	↑	↓	↓	19	Neg	Neg	Neg
Case 3	F	37	PiCoVacc (CoronaVac®)	2nd	7 days	Mild anterior neck pain	None	↑	↔	↔	25	Neg	Neg	Neg
Reference	Gender	Age	Vaccine	Dose	Days until symptoms	Symptoms	History of thyroid disease	fT3	fT4	TSH	ESR (mm) (RR < 15)	TgAb	TRAb	TPO-Ab
Bornemann et al. [12]														
Case 1	F	26	ChAdOx1 (Vaxzevria®)	1st	14 days	Fever, cervical pain radiated in both ears	None	↑	↔	↔	ND	Neg	Neg	Neg
Case 2	F	49	mRNA-1273 (Spikevax®)	1st	14 days	Sore throat with radiation to the ear, headache	None	↔	↔	↔	ND	Neg	Neg	Neg
Patel et al. [13]														
	M	48	ND	2nd	7 days	Right neck swelling, throat discomfort, palpitations, fever, weight loss	ND	ND	3.6 ng/dl (no RR)	0.01 mIU/L (no RR)	ND	ND	ND	ND
Reference	Gender	Age	Vaccine	Dose	Days until symptoms	Symptoms	History of thyroid disease	fT3	fT4	TSH	ESR (mm) (RR < 15)	TgAb	TRAb	TPO-ab
Saygili et al. [14]														
	F	38	PiCoVacc (CoronaVac®)	2nd	14 days	Neck swelling, pain, fatigue, loss of appetite, sweating	None	↑	↔	↓	78	Neg	ND	Neg
	F	34	BBV152 (COVAXIN®)	1st	5–7 days	Fever, palpitation, anterior neck pain	None	↑	↑	↓	60	ND	ND	ND
Chatzi et al. [15]														
	F	35	BNT162b2 (Comirnaty®)	1st	12 days	Neck pain, fatigue, palpations	ND	ND	↑	↓	75	Neg	Neg	Neg
	F	32	BNT162b2 (Comirnaty®)	2nd	4 days	Neck pain, fatigue	ND	ND	↔	↓	40	Neg	Neg	Neg

Table 1: Continued.

Reference	Gender	Age	Vaccine	Dose	Time from vaccination until onset of symptoms	Symptoms	History of thyroid disease	fT3	fT4	TSH	ESR (mm) (RR < 15)	TgAb	TRAb	TPO-ab
Reference	Gender	Age	Vaccine	Dose	Days until symptoms	Symptoms	History of thyroid disease	fT3	fT4	TSH	ESR (mm) (RR < 15)	TgAb	TRAb	TPO-ab
Kyriacou et al. 10/21 [16]														
	F	40	BNT162b2 (Comirnaty ®)	2nd	12 hours	Malaise, anterior neck pain,	None	ND	↑	↓	67	Pos	Neg	Neg
Siolos et al. [17]														
	F	51	BNT162b2 (Corminaty®)	1st	4 days	Nausea, mild anterior neck pain, fever	None	↔	↑	↓	103	Neg	Neg	Neg
Reference	Gender	Age	Vaccine	Dose	Days until symptoms	Symptoms	History of thyroid disease	fT3	fT4	TSH	ESR (mm) (RR < 15)	TgAb	TRAb	TPO-ab
Jeeyavudeen et al. [18]														
	F	ND	BNT162b2 (Comirnaty®)	2nd	14 days	Painful swelling, poor sleep, night sweats, hyperdefecation, weight loss	None	↑	↑	↓	ND	Neg	ND	Neg
Plaza-Enriquez et al. [19]														
	F	42	mRNA-1273 (Spikevax®)	2nd	5–6 days	Earache radiating down to the neck and jaw,	None	↑	↔	↓	81	ND	ND	Neg
Reference	Gender	Age	Vaccine	Dose	Days until symptoms	Symptoms	History of thyroid disease	fT3	fT4	TSH	ESR (mm) (RR < 15)	TgAb	TRAb	TPO-ab
Khan et al. [20]														
	F	42	BNT162b2 (Comirnaty®)	2nd	4 days	Fever, palpitations, painful left-sided neck swelling	ND	ND	↑	↓	60	ND	Neg	Neg
Sözen et al. [21]														
	M	41	BNT162b2 (Comirnaty®)	2nd	8 days	Anterior neck pain, fatigue, palpitation	None	↑	↑	↓	32	Neg	Neg	Neg
	F	40	BNT162b2 (Comirnaty®)	1st	6 days	Neck pain, palpitation, sweating	None	↔	↔	↓	34	Pos	Neg	Neg
	M	40	BNT162b2 (Comirnaty®)	1st	4 days	Neck pain, nervousness, fatigue	None	↔	↔	↔	15	Neg	ND	Neg
Reference	Gender	Age	Vaccine	Dose	Days until symptoms	Symptoms	History of thyroid disease	fT3	fT4	TSH	ESR (mm) (RR < 15)	TgAb	TRAb	TPO-Ab
	F	26	BNT162b2 (Comirnaty®)	2nd	6 days	Neck pain	None	↑	↑	↓	34	Pos	Neg	Pos

Table 1: Continued.

Reference	Gender	Age	Vaccine	Dose	Time from vaccination until onset of symptoms	Symptoms	History of thyroid disease	fT3	fT4	TSH	ESR (mm) (RR < 15)	TgAb	TRAb	TPO-ab
	F	44	BNT162b2 (Comirnaty®)	2nd	9 days	Neck pain, headache, palpitation, sweating, tremor	Hashimoto thyroiditis	↔	↔	↓	44	Neg	Neg	Pos
Schimmel et al. [22]														
	F	57	BNT162b2 (Comirnaty®)	2nd	1 day	Anterior neck pain, swelling	None	↔	↔	↓	ND	Neg	Neg	Neg
Franquemont et al. [23]														
	F	42	BNT162b2 (Comirnaty®)	1st	5 days	Sore throat, palpitations	None	11.8 (no RR)	4.58 (no RR)	<0.01 (no RR)	62	Neg	Neg	Neg
Reference	Gender	Age	Vaccine	Dose	Days until symptoms	Symptoms	History of thyroid disease	fT3	fT4	TSH	ESR (mm) (RR < 15)	TgAb	TRAb	TPO-ab
Oyibo et al. [24]														
	F	55	ChAdOx1 (Vaxzevria®)	1st	21 days	Headache, sore throat, generalized aches, palpitations	None	ND	↑	↓	51	ND	ND	Neg
Sahin Tekin et al. [25]														
	M	67	PiCoVacc (CoronaVac®)	2nd	19 days	Fever, mild neck pain,	None	↑	↑	↓	67	Neg	Neg	Neg
Reference	Gender	Age	Vaccine	Dose	Days until symptoms	Symptoms	History of thyroid disease	fT3	fT4	TSH	ESR (mm) (RR < 15)	TgAb	TRAb	TPO-ab
Pla Peris et al. [26]														
	M	67	mRNA-1273 (Spikevax®)	1st	10–14 days	Neck pain radiating to the ears, asthenia, mild fever, tachykardia	None	ND	↑	↓	60	Neg	Neg	Pos
	M	47	BNT162b2 (Comirnaty®)	1st	10–14 days	Neck pain radiating to the ears, asthenia, mild fever, tachykardia	None	ND	↔	↓	70	Neg	Neg	Neg

Note: the pathological values are printed in bold. fT3: free triiodothyronine; fT4: free thyroxine; TSH: thyroid-stimulating hormone; ESR: erythrocyte sedimentation rate; TgAb: antithyroglobulin antibody; TRAb, TSH receptor antibodies; TPO-Ab: thyroid peroxidase antibody; pos: positive; neg: negative; ND: no data; RR : reference range; ↔: normal; ↑: increased; ↓: decreased.

CoV-2 [38]. However, not only could the infection itself trigger SAT, but also the new vaccines are suspected of causing this thyroidal dysfunction [11–26].

We present two additional cases of SAT following vaccination with BNT162b2 (BioNTech/Pfizer) and ChAdOx1 (University of Oxford and AstraZeneca).

2. Case Presentation I

A 36-year old woman presented to our endocrinology outpatient clinic in April 2021, four weeks after receiving her second vaccine dose against COVID-19 with BNT162b2 (BioNTech/Pfizer, Comirnaty®). She reported that she had developed neck pain one day after receiving this second dose.

Following symptom onset, she had presented to an ear, nose, and throat doctor. After a laryngoscopy, which found no pathological findings, the doctor performed an ultrasound examination of the thyroid gland, which was assessed to be abnormal. In addition, there was an increased C-reactive protein (CRP), leukocytosis, and an increased thyroglobulin in the external blood tests, so the colleague began a three-day therapy with prednisolone 60 mg/d to treat his suspected diagnosis of SAT. A few hours after starting this treatment the pain disappeared but returned shortly after prednisolone was discontinued. The symptoms worsened over the following weeks, so the woman presented herself in our endocrinology outpatient clinic for further examination and treatment advice. At that time, the patient complained about neck pain, restlessness, as well as fatigue.

She did not have any known preexisting diseases, especially no previous history or family history of thyroid disease or COVID-19. The patient was a cigarette smoker.

2.1. Investigation. At examination, she was 170 cm tall and weighed approximately 55 kilograms (body mass index, 19 kg/m^2). There were no pathological findings regarding heart rate, blood pressure, and temperature. The neck pain could be induced by palpating the thyroid gland. Our initial biochemical blood tests showed a slight leukocytosis as well as moderately increased CRP and significantly increased ESR. In addition, there was a markedly elevated thyroglobulin level with normal fT4, fT3, and TSH indicating an euthyroid state, most likely due to the fact that the patient presented four weeks after the onset of symptoms. No thyroid peroxidase autoantibodies (TPO-Ab), TSH receptor stimulating antibodies (TRAb), or antithyroglobulin antibodies (TgAb) were detected (Table 1).

Ultrasound examination of the thyroid gland showed a hypoechogenic texture with pseudonodular lesions (Figure 1). The volume was about 18 ml, and some enlarged nonsuspicious lymph nodes were seen. The appearance was typical for SAT, and the pain could be induced by pressure with the ultrasound probe right above the thyroid gland. There was no evidence of a current corona infection in the rapid antigen test.

2.2. Treatment. Based on strong evidence suggesting SAT with normal thyroidal function at presentation, we discussed the treatment options with our patient. We offered her therapy with nonsteroidal anti-inflammatory drugs (NSAIDs) or a longer course of prednisolone therapy. She decided on the former, and we advised her to begin a prednisolone therapy if there was no improvement on NSAID with a starting dose of 30 mg/d with tapering the daily dosage by 5 mg every 5–7 days.

2.3. Outcome and Follow-Up. During a telephone call two weeks later, the patient reported that the neck pain had worsened while she was taking ibuprofen and that she had developed subfebrile temperatures. Therefore, as recommended, she started prednisolone therapy, which promptly resulted in improvement. She took prednisolone in a tapering scheme over six weeks. The symptoms did not return after stopping the prednisolone, and she has been fine. An intermittent unintentional weight loss of five kilograms was also resolved. The ultrasound examination showed an almost complete recovery. Thyroglobulin decreased by about 75%, and the CRP was normal. Mild leukocytosis may have been explained by smoking. Her thyroid function tests still showed an euthyroid state.

3. Case Presentation II

A 65-year old man visited his family doctor in June 2021 because of malaise after receiving his first vaccine against COVID-19 with ChAdOx1 (University of Oxford and AstraZeneca, Vaxzevria®) three days before. Due to an increase in CRP and an increased ESR, the doctor suspected another sigmoid diverticulitis because of several episodes since 2018. The patient also complained of pain in the thyroid region and hoarseness; in secondary findings, a decreased TSH was detected. Therefore, a referral to our endocrinology outpatient clinic was arranged. At the time of the appointment, the local symptoms were decreasing and the patient was fine. There was no history of thyroid disease, neither in the patient nor in their family.

3.1. Investigation. The man was in good condition. Blood pressure was normal, and the heart rate was moderately elevated (100 bpm). Due to decreased appetite, he had lost eight kilograms. The thyroid gland was slightly enlarged and palpable without tenderness. Blood examination revealed moderately elevated CRP, normal white blood cell count, mild normochromic normocytic anemia, and elevated ESR. In addition, there was a reduced TSH with normal fT3 and fT4 and increased TgAb, which we assessed as unspecific (Table 1). Other antibodies related to the thyroid gland were negative (TRAb and TPO-Ab).

Ultrasound examination of the thyroid showed a hypoechogenic texture and a diffusely hypoperfused parenchyma. The volume was slightly enlarged (36 ml) and there were some enlarged nonsuspicious lymph nodes (Figure 2). A COVID-19 rapid antigen test was negative.

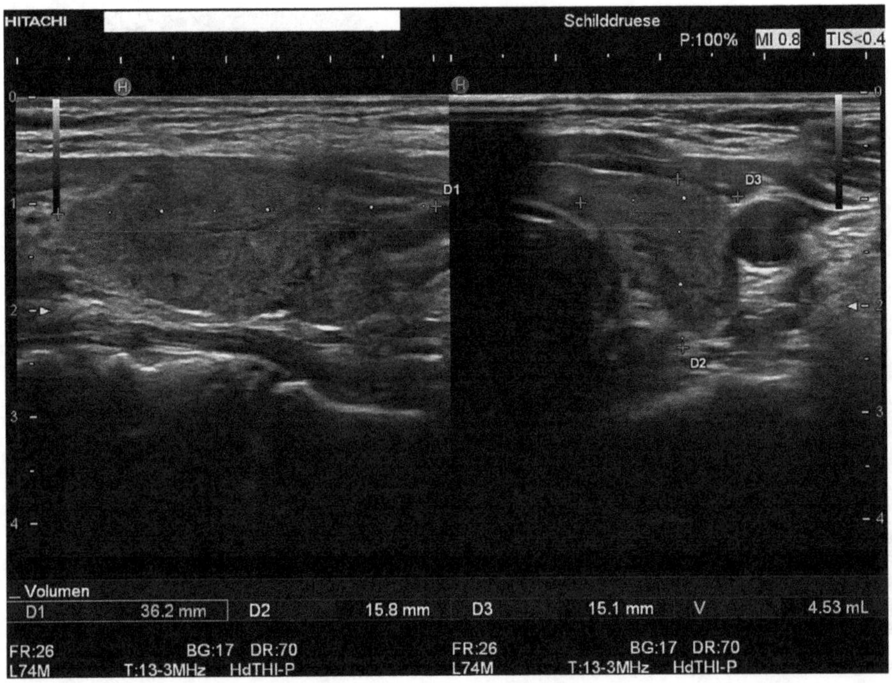

Figure 1: This ultrasound picture shows a hypoechogenic texture with pseudonodular lesions typical for SAT.

3.2. Treatment. No special treatment was required because of the regressive symptoms.

3.3. Outcome and Follow-Up. At the recommended appointment three months later, the patient felt well. Blood tests showed mild anemia but no more signs of inflammation, and the TSH was normalized. Sonographic examination of the thyroid gland showed a reduced volume. There was no tenderness or pressure on the thyroid region.

4. Discussion

The current COVID-19 pandemic is causing various medical problems. In addition to the main infections, e.g., lung infection, the infection affects the entire body system. Initial studies by Somasundaram et al. in June 2020 suggested possible damage to the endocrine system by SARS-CoV-2 [39]. Only a few months later, the first reports underscored this suspicion [40]. The thyroid gland could be affected by several mechanisms.

First of all, the virus enters human tissues using the angiotensin-converting enzyme 2 (ACE2) as a cell receptor, which is strongly expressed in thyroid cells and can probably damage the thyroid gland by direct viral cytopathic effects [41, 42]. Early research had shown that there are some homologies between amino acid sequences of, e.g., the spike glycoprotein subunits S1 and S2 from the virus and tissue proteins such as thyroid peroxidase (TPO). This can cause autoimmunity against thyroid cells or exacerbate an existing autoimmunity [43].

In addition, uncontrolled immune responses to the virus in severe cases of COVID-19 should be discussed. This leads to an extensive inflammatory state and an enhanced Th1/Th17 immune response, which results in the release of inflammatory cytokines that are also seen in autoimmune thyroid diseases [44].

Furthermore, the exact pathomechanism of SAT in general is unknown. It is hypothesized that autoreactive T-cells generated by molecular mimicry on thyroid cells promote an autoimmune response against the thyroid gland. Another explanation is that a virus infection results in the presentation of viral products or virus antigens by host cells. As a result, the thyroid cells are recognized as foreign and destroyed by the immune system [45].

But the infection by the virus itself is not only discussed as a cause of SAT. The occurrence of this disease has also been detected after the injection of the new vaccines [11–26]. Recent studies show that the spike protein could be detected in subjects after administration of the mRNA vaccine [30] because both vaccines lead to endogenous production of these spike proteins through different mechanisms to induce immunity against SARS-CoV-2 [6, 7].

In addition, animal experiments have shown that this protein alone can cause cell damage [29]. Since the thyroid cells, as already described, show a high level of expression of the ACE2 receptor, which serves as a cell receptor, direct damage by the protein could be an explanation. However, this theory should be explored in more detail in further studies, and of course, the idea cannot be applied to other vaccinations (e.g., influenza) and the occurrence of SAT.

Another explanation that should be mentioned is the "autoimmune/inflammatory syndrome by adjuvants" known as ASIA. Bragazzi et al. summarized 50 cases of SAT after vaccination that were attributed to this syndrome [28]. Adjuvants are substances that can increase the effectiveness of vaccines and, in some cases, can cause relevant damage by triggering immunological phenomena through activation of

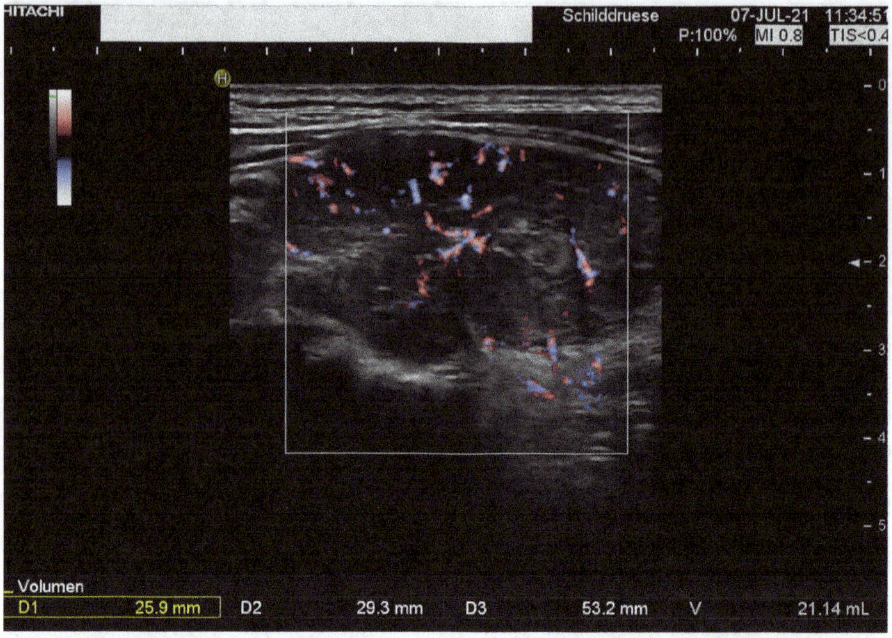

FIGURE 2: The right lobe of the thyroid gland with a hypoechogenic texture and a diffusely hypoperfused parenchyma.

B lymphocytes or molecular mimicry [46]. In the case of the vaccine BNT162b2 (BioNTech/Pfizer), lipid nanoparticles (e.g., ALC-0159) have an adjuvant effect in terms of stabilizing the mRNA and transporting it to the target site [47, 48]. In contrast, the vaccine ChAdOx1 (the University of Oxford and AstraZeneca) does not contain any relevant adjuvant substances in the true sense [49] but processed polysorbate 80 (E 433), which is part of AS03, an adjuvant of influenza vaccines [50].

So, ASIA could also be a possible cause of the development of SAT after vaccination against COVID-19. However, ASIA cannot explain the association of SAT with the infection itself.

To our knowledge, there have been publications of 26 cases of SAT following vaccination against SARS-CoV-2 [11–26].

Our cases are in line with the published cases of SAT after COVID-19 vaccination so far (Table 1). The typical clinical presentation with neck pain and malaise, as well as the ultrasound of the thyroid gland and the time since administration (1–3 days), confirm the diagnosis of vaccination-associated SAT. In contrast to most of the cases reported in the literature, our first patient had completely normal thyroid function due to a longer history since the onset of symptoms. Among the 26 cases, there are three others who were euthyroid, and only 62% of the patients had hyperthyroidism. The positive TgAb in our second case was interpreted as unspecific. Nishihara et al. 2019 examined 40 patients in the early phase of SAT and were able to show that 52.5% had positive TgAb, which decreased over time [37]. Three of the 26 cases of vaccine-associated SAT also had positive TgAb.

We must note that although we ruled out corona infection by antigen testing, we did not arrange for further virologic testing for other pathogens. However, there was no evidence of infection.

We would like to point out that, based on the accumulation of case reports, SAT appears to be a possible but rare sequelae of SARS-CoV-2 vaccination that should be considered by practicing physicians. The course of SAT is often mild and disproportionate to the harmfulness of COVID-19 but may be important because of the substantial increase in the global vaccination rate, with more than 9.5 billion doses of vaccine administered [4].

Nevertheless, temporal findings can be no proof of a causal relationship. To date, there have been many reports of SAT following SARS-CoV-2 infection. But a study from a region in northern Italy heavily affected by SARS-CoV-2 could not document a rise in cases of SAT in their outpatient emergency clinic during the pandemic [51]. Likewise, the temporal association of the reported cases of SAT after vaccination against SARS-CoV-2 could still be a coincidence.

Because case reports can only raise suspicion of a causal relationship, studies should compare the incidence of SAT in the weeks after vaccination with an unvaccinated group or with the incidence of SAT before vaccination. In addition, when SAT is diagnosed in temporal association with vaccine use, physicians should make a report to the appropriate pharmacovigilance institution.

Data Availability

The data used to support the findings of this study are included within the article.

Additional Points

Subacute thyroiditis (SAT) is a temporary inflammatory disease of the thyroid gland that is probably triggered by multiple viral infections with a genetic predisposition to HLA-B35. In the past, the occurrence of SAT has been described, for example, after influenza vaccination. Recently, several reports have described the appearance of SAT as being associated with the injection of the new COVID-19 vaccines. Cross-reactivity between the spike protein and tissue proteins of the thyroid gland, ASIA, or the circulating spike protein as a cause for SAT after vaccination should be discussed.

Consent

Written informed consent has been obtained from the patient (or patient's guardian) for publication of the submitted article and accompanying images.

Authors' Contributions

The patients described were medically advised by Dr. Kauka, Goebel, and Prof. Kann, who gave full approval. The cases were presented by Dr. Adelmeyer.

References

[1] N. Zhu, D. Zhang, W. Wang et al., "A novel coronavirus from patients with pneumonia in China, 2019," *New England Journal of Medicine*, vol. 382, no. 8, pp. 727–733, 2020.

[2] S. K. Mishra and T. Tripathi, "One year update on the COVID-19 pandemic: where are we now?" *Acta Tropica*, vol. 214, Article ID 105778, 2021.

[3] C. R. Triggle, D. Bansal, H. Ding et al., "A comprehensive review of viral characteristics, transmission, pathophysiology, immune response, and management of SARS-CoV-2 and COVID-19 as a basis for controlling the pandemic," *Frontiers in Immunology*, vol. 12, Article ID 631139, 2021.

[4] W. H. Organisation, *WHO Coronavirus (COVID-19) Dashboard*, https://covid19.who.int22, 2022.

[5] P. Zhou, X.-L. Yang, X.-G. Wang et al., "A pneumonia outbreak associated with a new coronavirus of probable bat origin," *Nature*, vol. 579, no. 7798, pp. 270–273, 2020.

[6] F. P. Polack, S. J. Thomas, N. Kitchin et al., "Safety and efficacy of the BNT16 2b2 mRNA covid-19 vaccine," *New England Journal of Medicine*, vol. 383, no. 27, pp. 2603–2615, 2020.

[7] M. Voysey, S. A. C. Clemens, S. A. Madhi et al., "Safety and efficacy of the ChAdOx1 nCoV-19 vaccine (AZD1222) against SARS-CoV-2: an interim analysis of four randomised controlled trials in Brazil, South Africa, and the UK," *Lancet (London, England)*, vol. 397, no. 10269, pp. 99–111, 2021.

[8] C. M. Girgis, R. R. Russo, and K. Benson, "Subacute thyroiditis following the H1N1 vaccine," *Journal of Endocrinological Investigation*, vol. 33, no. 7, Article ID 506, 2010.

[9] F. A. Altay, G. Güz, and M. Altay, "Subacute thyroiditis following seasonal influenza vaccination," *Human Vaccines & Immunotherapeutics*, vol. 12, no. 4, pp. 1033-1034, 2016.

[10] K. R. Feingold, B. Anawalt, A. Boyce, G. Chrousos, W. W. de Herder, and K. Dhatariya, Endotext Review, 2000.

[11] B. G. İremli, S. N. Şendur, and U. Ünlütürk, "Three cases of subacute thyroiditis following SARS-CoV-2 vaccine: post-vaccination ASIA syndrome," *The J ournal o f C inical Endocrinology and Metabolism*, vol. 106, no. 9, 2021.

[12] C. Bornemann, K. Woyk, and C. Bouter, "Case report: two cases of subacute thyroiditis following SARS-CoV-2 vaccination," *Frontiers of Medicine*, vol. 8, Article ID 737142, 2021.

[13] K. R. Patel, M. E. Cunnane, and D. G. Deschler, "SARS-CoV-2 vaccine-induced subacute thyroiditis," *American Journal of Otolaryngology*, vol. 43, no. 1, Article ID 103211, 2022.

[14] E. S. Saygılı and E. Karakilic, "Subacute thyroiditis after inactive SARS-CoV-2 vaccine," *BMJ Case Reports*, vol. 14, no. 10, 2021.

[15] S. Chatzi, A. Karampela, C. Spiliopoulou, and G. Boutzios, "Subacute thyroiditis after SARS-CoV-2 vaccination: a report of two sisters and summary of the literature," *Hormones*, vol. 21, no. 1, pp. 177–179, 2022.

[16] A. Kyriacou, S. Ioakim, and A. A. Syed, "COVID-19 vaccination and a severe pain in the neck," *European Journal of Internal Medicine*, vol. 94, pp. 95-96, 2021.

[17] A. Siolos, K. Gartzonika, and S. Tigas, "Thyroiditis following vaccination against COVID-19: report of two cases and review of the literature," *Metabolism Open*, vol. 12, Article ID 100136, 2021.

[18] M. S. Jeeyavudeen, A. W. Patrick, F. W. Gibb, and A. R. Dover, "COVID-19 vaccine-associated subacute thyroiditis: an unusual suspect for de Quervain's thyroiditis," *BMJ Case Reports*, vol. 14, no. 11, 2021.

[19] L. Plaza-Enriquez, P. Khatiwada, M. Sanchez-Valenzuela, and A. Sikha, "A case report of subacute thyroiditis following mRNA COVID-19 vaccine," *Case Rep Endocrinol*, vol. 2021, Article ID 8952048, 2021.

[20] F. Khan and M. J. Brassill, "Subacute thyroiditis post-Pfizer-BioNTech mRNA vaccination for COVID-19," *Endocrinol Diabetes Metab Case Rep*, vol. 2021, 2021.

[21] M. Sözen, Ö Topaloğlu, B. Çetinarslan et al., "COVID-19 mRNA vaccine may trigger subacute thyroiditis," *Human Vaccines & Immunotherapeutics*, vol. 17, no. 12, pp. 5120–5125, 2021.

[22] J. Schimmel, E. L. Alba, A. Chen, M. Russell, and R. Srinath, "Letter to the editor: thyroiditis and thyrotoxicosis after the SARS-CoV-2 mRNA vaccine," *Thyroid*, vol. 31, no. 9, Article ID 1440, 2021.

[23] S. Franquemont and J. Gálvez, "Subacute thyroiditis after mRNA vaccine for covid-19," *J Endocrine Society*, vol. 2021, no. 1, Article ID A956, 2021.

[24] S. O. Oyibo, "Subacute thyroiditis after receiving the adenovirus-vectored vaccine for coronavirus disease (COVID-19)," *Cureus*, vol. 13, no. 6, Article ID e16045, 2021.

[25] M. Şahin Tekin, S. Şaylısoy, and G. Yorulmaz, "Subacute thyroiditis following COVID-19 vaccination in a 67-year-old male patient: a case report," *Human Vaccines & Immunotherapeutics*, vol. 2021, pp. 1–3, 2021.

[26] B. Pla Peris, A. Merchante Alfaro, F. J. Maravall Royo, P. Abellán Galiana, S. Pérez Naranjo, and M. González Boillos, "Thyrotoxicosis following SARS-COV-2 vaccination: a case series and discussion," *Journal of Endocrinological Investigation*, vol. 1-7, 2022.

[27] S. Benvenga and F. Guarneri, "Molecular mimicry and autoimmune thyroid disease," *Reviews in Endocrine & Metabolic Disorders*, vol. 17, no. 4, pp. 485–498, 2016.

[28] N. L. Bragazzi, A. Hejly, A. Watad, M. Adawi, H. Amital, and Y. Shoenfeld, "ASIA syndrome and endocrine autoimmune disorders," *Best Practice & Research Clinical Endocrinology & Metabolism*, vol. 34, no. 1, Article ID 101412, 2020.

[29] Y. Lei, J. Zhang, C. R. Schiavon et al., "SARS-CoV-2 spike protein impairs endothelial function via downregulation of ACE 2," *Circulation Research*, vol. 128, no. 9, pp. 1323–1326, 2021.

[30] A. F. Ogata, C. A. Cheng, M. Desjardins, Y. Senussi, A. C. Sherman, and M. Powell, "Circulating SARS-CoV-2 vaccine antigen detected in the plasma of mRNA-1273 vaccine recipients," *Clinical Infectious Diseases*, vol. 2021, 2021.

[31] V. Fatourechi, J. P. Aniszewski, G. Z. E. Fatourechi, E. J. Atkinson, and S. J. Jacobsen, "Clinical features and outcome of subacute thyroiditis in an incidence cohort: olmsted County, Minnesota, study," *Journal of Clinical Endocrinology & Metabolism*, vol. 88, no. 5, pp. 2100–2105, 2003.

[32] S. Y. Park, E.-K. Kim, M. J. Kim et al., "Ultrasonographic characteristics of subacute granulomatous thyroiditis," *Korean Journal of Radiology*, vol. 7, no. 4, pp. 229–234, 2006.

[33] Y. Hiromatsu, M. Ishibashi, I. Miyake, and K. Nonaka, "Technetium-99m tetrofosmin imaging in patients with subacute thyroiditis," *European Journal of Nuclear Medicine and Molecular Imaging*, vol. 25, no. 10, pp. 1448–1452, 1998.

[34] A. B. Kramer, C. Roozendaal, and R. P. F. Dullaart, "Familial occurrence of subacute thyroiditis associated with human leukocyte antigen-B35," *Thyroid*, vol. 14, no. 7, pp. 544–547, 2004.

[35] R. Volpé, V. V. Row, and C. Ezrin, "Circulating viral and thyroid antibodies in subacute thyroiditis," *Journal of Clinical Endocrinology & Metabolism*, vol. 27, no. 9, pp. 1275–1284, 1967.

[36] E. Martino, L. Buratti, L. Bartalena et al., "High prevalence of subacute thyroiditis during summer season in Italy," *Journal of Endocrinological Investigation*, vol. 10, no. 3, pp. 321–323, 1987.

[37] E. Nishihara, H. Ohye, N. Amino et al., "Clinical characteristics of 852 patients with subacute thyroiditis before treatment," *Internal Medicine*, vol. 47, no. 8, pp. 725–729, 2008.

[38] J. Christensen, K. O'Callaghan, H. Sinclair, K. Hawke, A. Love, and K. Hajkowicz, "Risk factors, treatment and outcomes of subacute thyroiditis secondary to COVID-19: a systematic review," *Internal Medicine Journal*, vol. 2021, 2021.

[39] N. P. Somasundaram, I. Ranathunga, V. Ratnasamy et al., "The impact of SARS-cov-2 virus infection on the endocrine system," *Journal of the Endocrine Society*, vol. 4, no. 8, Article ID bvaa082, 2020.

[40] N. Kothandaraman, A. Rengaraj, B. Xue et al., "COVID-19 endocrinopathy with hindsight from SARS," *American Journal of Physiology - Endocrinology And Metabolism*, vol. 320, no. 1, pp. E139–E150, 2021.

[41] L. Scappaticcio, F. Pitoia, K. Esposito, A. Piccardo, and P. Trimboli, "Impact of COVID-19 on the thyroid gland: an update," *Reviews in Endocrine & Metabolic Disorders*, vol. 22, no. 4, 2020.

[42] M. Rotondi, F. Coperchini, G. Ricci et al., "Detection of SARS-COV-2 receptor ACE-2 mRNA in thyroid cells: a clue for COVID-19-related subacute thyroiditis," *Journal of Endocrinological Investigation*, vol. 44, no. 5, pp. 1085–1090, 2021.

[43] A. Vojdani, E. Vojdani, and D. Kharrazian, "Reaction of human monoclonal antibodies to SARS-CoV-2 proteins with tissue antigens: implications for autoimmune diseases," *Frontiers in Immunology*, vol. 11, Article ID 617089, 2020.

[44] R. M. Ruggeri, A. Campennì, D. Deandreis et al., "SARS-COV-2-related immune-inflammatory thyroid disorders: facts and perspectives," *Expert Review of Clinical Immunology*, vol. 17, no. 7, pp. 737–759, 2021.

[45] R. Domin, E. Szczepanek-Parulska, D. Dadej, and M. Ruchala, "Subacute Thyroiditis - literature overview and COVID-19," *JMS (Interent)*, vol. 89, no. 4, 2020.

[46] A. Watad, N. L. Bragazzi, H. Amital, and Y. Shoenfeld, "Hyperstimulation of adaptive immunity as the common pathway for silicone breast implants, autoimmunity, and lymphoma of the breast," *The Israel Medical Association Journal : The Israel Medical Association Journal*, vol. 21, no. 8, pp. 517–519, 2019.

[47] A. Khurana, P. Allawadhi, I. Khurana et al., "Role of nanotechnology behind the success of mRNA vaccines for COVID-19," *Nano Today*, vol. 38, Article ID 101142, 2021.

[48] A. Pujol, L. A. Gómez, C. Gallegos, J. Nicolau, P. Sanchís, and M. González-Freire, "Thyroid as a target of adjuvant autoimmunity/inflammatory syndrome due to mRNA-based SARS-CoV2 vaccination: from Graves' disease to silent thyroiditis," *Journal of Endocrinological Investigation*, vol. 45, no. 4, 2021.

[49] A. F. Hernández, D. Calina, K. Poulas, A. O. Docea, and A. M. Tsatsakis, "Safety of COVID-19 vaccines administered in the EU: should we be concerned?" *Toxicol Rep*, vol. 8, pp. 871–879, 2021.

[50] C. Cohet, R. van der Most, V. Bauchau et al., "Safety of AS03-adjuvanted influenza vaccines: a review of the evidence," *Vaccine*, vol. 37, no. 23, pp. 3006–3021, 2019.

[51] I. Pirola, E. Gandossi, M. Rotondi, F. Marini, A. Cristiano, and L. Chiovato, "Incidence of De Quervain's thyroiditis during the COVID-19 pandemic in an area heavily affected by Sars-CoV-2 infection," *Endocrine*, vol. 74, no. 2, 2021.

Hypokalemic Periodic Paralysis Precipitated by Thyrotoxicosis and Renal Tubular Acidosis

Ian Jackson,[1] **Yazan Addasi**,[1] **Moeed Ahmed**,[1] **Bashar Ramadan**,[1] **Karson Kalian**,[1] **Noor Addasi**,[2] **Ali Nayfeh**,[3] **Jocelyn Taylor**,[1] **Khalid Bashir**,[4] **and Bryan Krajicek**[3]

[1]*Department of Medicine, Creighton University School of Medicine, Omaha, NE, USA*
[2]*Department of Endocrinology, University of Nebraska Medical Center, Omaha, NE, USA*
[3]*Department of Pulmonary and Critical Care, Creighton University School of Medicine, Omaha, NE, USA*
[4]*Department of Nephrology, Creighton University School of Medicine, Omaha, NE, USA*

Correspondence should be addressed to Ian Jackson; ianjackson@creighton.edu

Academic Editor: Lucy Mastrandrea

Background. Hypokalemic periodic paralysis is a rare neuromuscular disorder characterized by transient episodes of flaccid paralysis due to a defect in muscle ion channels. Most cases are hereditary, but it can be acquired. We present a case of acquired hypokalemic periodic paralysis associated with hyperthyroidism and renal tubular acidosis. *Clinical Case.* A 38-year-old female with a history of Graves' disease presented to the emergency department with generalized weakness and associated nausea, vomiting, and weight loss. Examination was significant for diffuse weakness in all extremities. Labs showed hypokalemia, hyperthyroidism, and nonanion gap metabolic acidosis with a positive urine anion gap. She was treated for hypokalemic periodic paralysis and renal tubular acidosis. Potassium replacement, propranolol, methimazole, and sodium bicarbonate were initiated. Her potassium gradually corrected with resolution of her symptoms. Further investigation revealed a history of dry eyes, dry mouth, and recurrent dental carries. She had positive ANA, SS-A, and SS-B antibodies. She was diagnosed with Sjögren's syndrome, which may have been associated with her Graves' disease and thus contributed to both her RTA and hyperthyroidism. *Conclusion.* Early recognition and treatment of thyrotoxic periodic paralysis are important to prevent cardiac complications. Management includes potassium replacement with careful monitoring to prevent rebound hyperkalemia. The definitive treatment is to achieve euthyroid status.

1. Introduction

Periodic paralysis is a rare neuromuscular disorder caused by a defect in muscle ion channels. It is characterized by episodes of painless muscle weakness. Hypokalemic periodic paralysis (HPP) is a subset of periodic paralysis that occurs in the presence of low serum potassium. HPP may be inherited or occur sporadically in the setting of hyperthyroidism. We are presenting a rare case of HPP associated with hyperthyroidism and renal tubular acidosis. We discuss the pathophysiology, clinical manifestations, assessment, and management of HPP.

2. Case Presentation

A 38-year-old female with a medical history of Graves' thyrotoxicosis presented to the emergency department (ED) complaining of generalized weakness that started several days prior to her presentation. It was associated with nausea, vomiting, and weight loss. She denied diarrhea, pain, or shortness of breath. Her only medication was methimazole 10 milligrams twice daily which she had been taking for three years with intermittent compliance. She was alert and oriented to person, place, and time. Her vitals on presentation were blood pressure of 127/80 mmHg, heart rate of 80, respiratory rate of 22, and temperature of 98.4°F. Neurological exam yielded intact cranial nerves with no sensory deficit. However, she had diffuse weakness in all extremities with strength of 2/5 in the lower extremities and 2/5 in the upper extremities. The rest of the physical examination showed no abnormalities.

Workup in the ED revealed multiple lab abnormalities including hypokalemia, a nonanion gap metabolic acidosis, and hyperthyroidism (Table 1). Her EKG showed changes consistent with hypokalemia including a QTc interval of 686 milliseconds (Figure 1). A chest X-ray and computed tomography of the head without contrast showed no acute abnormalities. Renal ultrasound and abdominal X-ray were negative for hydronephrosis or kidney stones.

The patient was given intravenous potassium in the ED and transferred to the intensive care unit (ICU) with continuous cardiac monitoring. The endocrinology team recommended starting propranolol and increasing her dose of methimazole. She was treated with additional intravenous and oral potassium supplementation in the ICU. The potassium level was checked frequently due to concern for rebound hyperkalemia. Based on the patient's acute onset of diffuse weakness without cranial nerve dysfunction or pain, hypokalemia, elevated free T4, and low TSH, a presumptive diagnosis of thyrotoxic periodic paralysis was made.

The patient's potassium was gradually corrected with subsequent resolution of her paralysis and decrease of her QTc interval. However, she continued to have a nonanion gap acidosis. Urine studies showed a urine pH of 8 (normal range 4.5–8), urine chloride of 105 mmol/L (normal range 55–125 mmol/L), urine potassium of 39.8 mmol/L (normal range 12–62 mmol/L), and urine sodium of 90 mmol/L (normal range 20–110 mmol/L) resulting in a positive urine anion gap of 24.8. This was attributed to renal tubular acidosis (RTA) type 1. The patient was started on sodium bicarbonate in addition to her oral potassium supplementation. These medications were gradually titrated and later discontinued as her labs normalized (Figure 2).

Further history revealed intermittent dry eyes, dry mouth, and recurrent dental carries. This prompted additional workup which was significant for positive ANA, SS-A, and SS-B. The patient was eventually referred to rheumatology for further evaluation and management of Sjögren's syndrome. She was started on hydroxychloroquine. With this treatment, her RTA completely resolved, and she no longer required potassium or bicarbonate supplementation. The patient maintained follow-up with endocrinology, and she preferred to continue antithyroid medications rather than pursue radioactive iodine ablation.

Table 1: Initial laboratory values.

Lab	Result	Normal range
Sodium	142 mmol/L	135–144 mmol/L
Potassium	1.6 mmol/L	3.7–5.1 mmol/L
Chloride	114 mmol/L	96–110 mmol/L
CO_2	16 mmol/L	22–32 mmol/L
Creatinine	0.92 mg/dL	0.5–1.6 mg/dL
Magnesium	2.3 mg/dL	1.8–2.6 mg/dL
Phosphorus	1.4 mg/dL	2.5–4.9 mg/dL
pH	7.25	7.35–7.45
pCO_2	34 mmol/L	35–45 mmol/L
TSH	<0.005 UIU/mL	0.4–3.8 UIU/mL
T4, free	1.6 ng/dL	0.7–1.4 ng/dL

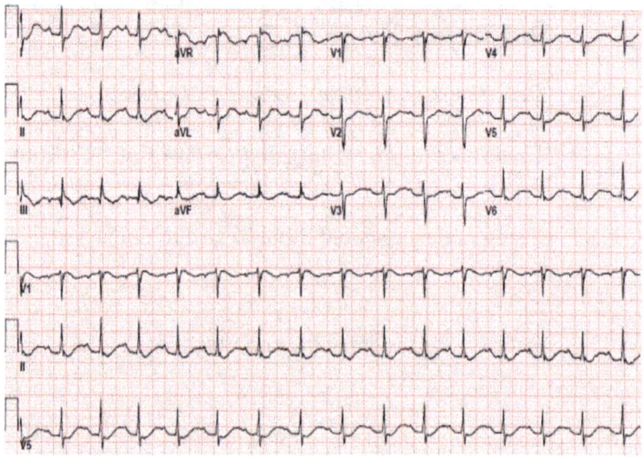

Figure 1: EKG with changes indicative of hypokalemia.

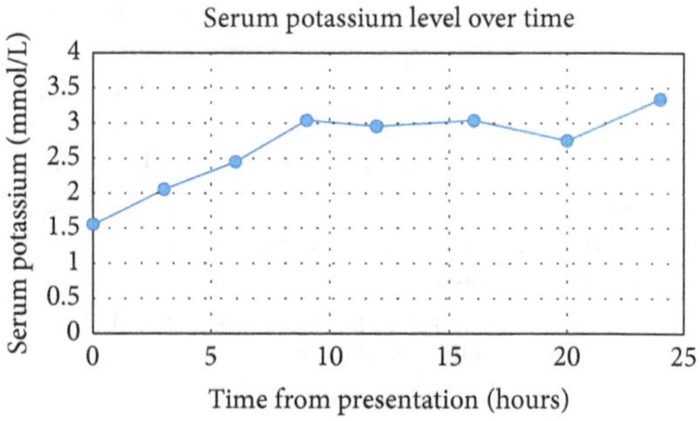

Figure 2: Serum potassium level over time.

3. Discussion

Periodic paralysis is a neuromuscular disorder associated with defective muscle ion channels and characterized by episodes of painless muscle weakness. It is classified as hypokalemic or hyperkalemic based on the serum potassium level. The majority of cases are familial and inherited in an autosomal dominant pattern. Less commonly, hypokalemic periodic paralysis (HPP) can also be acquired in patients with thyrotoxicosis. Thyrotoxic periodic paralysis (TPP) can be caused by any form of thyrotoxicosis but is most common in Graves' disease. Unlike other forms of thyroid disease, TPP is more common in males. It is also more frequent in Asian populations with an incidence of approximately 2% in patients with thyrotoxicosis [1].

Although the exact pathogenesis is unclear, it is hypothesized that patient's with TPP have an underlying defect in muscle ion channels that remains asymptomatic in patients with normal thyroid function. However, when thyroid hormone levels are elevated, it increases tissue responsiveness to beta-adrenergic stimulation. This in turn increases sodium-potassium ATPase activity and drives potassium into cells. The intracellular shift of potassium causes hyperpolarization of the muscle membrane, resulting in inexcitability of the muscle. It is not caused by a deficiency in total body potassium [2]. Furthermore, obese patients are more susceptible to episodes of TPP because high levels of insulin also stimulate a shift of potassium into cells [3, 4].

TPP manifests as transient episodes of painless muscle weakness with preserved consciousness. The episodes typically last for hours to days. The weakness is generalized, but often more pronounced in proximal muscles. Episodes can be exacerbated by high carbohydrate foods, exercise, stress, infection, anesthesia, or exposure to extreme temperatures [5]. Our patient reported having a large fast-food meal the night prior to onset of her symptoms. Other less common symptoms include myalgia, hyporeflexia or areflexia, and associated hyperthyroid symptoms such as tachycardia. TPP can rarely cause potentially fatal arrhythmias.

Diagnosis of TPP should be suspected when a patient presents with paralysis associated with hypokalemia and hyperthyroidism. TPP must be distinguished from other causes of acute paralysis including myasthenic crisis, botulism, Guillain–Barre syndrome, acute myelopathy, and acute thyrotoxic myopathy. In our case, the patient had normal cranial nerve function, making myasthenic crisis or botulism unlikely. Her weakness was present diffusely without an ascending pattern that would indicate Guillain–Barre syndrome. Her lack of pain, normal creatine kinase level, and nondermatomal distribution were also inconsistent with acute thyrotoxic myopathy or acute myelopathy. Paralysis in TPP usually occurs when the potassium level is less than 3 mmol/L. In one study of 78 patients with TPP, the mean serum potassium level was 2.1 mmol/L [6]. EKG changes often include tachycardia and changes consistent with hypokalemia.

Acute treatment of TPP primarily involves potassium supplementation. Oral potassium chloride is the preferred method, but intravenous potassium may be necessary in patients with impaired swallowing. One protocol suggests a dose of 30 milliequivalents orally every 15–30 minutes until serum potassium is normalized [7]. Rebound hyperkalemia is common, so close monitoring of serum potassium and cardiac telemetry should be used. In cases refractory to potassium replacement, intravenous propranolol may help to reverse the excess beta-adrenergic stimulation causing potassium to shift into the cells. Long-term preventative treatment of TPP is through restoration of euthyroid state, which can be accomplished through antithyroid medications, radioactive iodine ablation, or thyroidectomy.

RTA secondary to Sjögren's syndrome may have also contributed to HPP in this case. Approximately 5% of patients with primary Sjögren's syndrome have clinically significant renal involvement, with distal RTA being the most common manifestation. The resulting hypokalemia and metabolic acidosis can contribute to muscle weakness and periodic paralysis [8]. Corticosteroids are the most widely used therapy. The efficacy of steroid-sparing agents, such as hydroxychloroquine used for our patient, remains unknown [9].

Our patient had several atypical features for HPP. First, acquired cases of HPP are far more common in Asian males, while our patient was a Caucasian female. Second, the presence of both thyrotoxicosis and renal tubular acidosis as underlying causes of HPP is very rare. The combination of these two mechanisms in our patient is likely due to her diagnosis of Sjögren's syndrome, which can not only cause distal RTA but has also been associated with autoimmune thyroid disorders. The coexistence of Sjögren's syndrome and autoimmune thyroid disorders, such as Graves' disease in our patient, is potentially due to common pathogenetic mechanisms shared by the two conditions [10].

4. Conclusion

Early diagnosis and treatment of TPP are important to prevent serious cardiac complications. Potassium replacement should be gradual, with serial monitoring of potassium to avoid rebound hyperkalemia. The definitive treatment is to achieve euthyroid status to prevent recurrent attacks.

Disclosure

The details of this study were presented in "Fellows Critical Care Posters" as part of the annual CHEST conference in Glenview, IL, on October 18–21, 2020.

References

[1] A. Vijayakumar, G. Ashwath, and D. Thimmappa, "Thyrotoxic periodic paralysis: clinical challenges," *Journal of Thyroid Research*, vol. 2014, Article ID 649502, 6 pages, 2014.

[2] A. Pompeo, A. Nepa, M. Maddestra, V. Feliziani, and N. Genovesi, "Thyrotoxic hypokalemic periodic paralysis: an overlooked pathology in western countries," *European Journal of Internal Medicine*, vol. 18, no. 5, pp. 380–390, 2007.

[3] S.-H. Lin and C.-L. Huang, "Mechanism of thyrotoxic periodic paralysis," *Journal of the American Society of Nephrology*, vol. 23, no. 6, pp. 985–988, 2012.

[4] A. W. C. Kung, "Thyrotoxic periodic paralysis: a diagnostic challenge," *The Journal of Clinical Endocrinology & Metabolism*, vol. 91, no. 7, pp. 2490–2495, 2006.

[5] J. Finsterer, "Primary periodic paralyses," *Acta Neurologica Scandinavica*, vol. 117, no. 3, pp. 145–158, 2008.

[6] J. C. Shiang, C. J. Cheng, M. K. Tsai et al., "Therapeutic analysis in Chinese patients with thyrotoxic periodic paralysis over 6 years," *European Journal of Endocrinology*, vol. 161, no. 6, pp. 911-916, 2009.

[7] S. L. Venance, S. C. Cannon, D. Fialho et al., "The primary periodic paralyses: diagnosis, pathogenesis and treatment," *Brain*, vol. 129, no. 1, pp. 8-17, 2006.

[8] S. Maripuri, J. Grande, T. Osborn et al., "Renal involvement in primary Sjogren's syndrome: a clinicopathologic study," *Clinical Journal of the American Society of Nephrology*, vol. 4, no. 9, p. 1423, 2009.

13

TIO Associated with Hyperparathyroidism: A Rarity, a Rule, or a Novel HPT-PMT Syndrome—A Case Study with Literature Review

Michael Salim,[1] **Mohannad Samy Behairy**,[2] **and Elena Barengolts**[3]

[1]*Department of Internal Medicine, Mount Sinai Hospital, Chicago, IL 60608, USA*
[2]*Ross University School of Medicine, Bridgetown, Barbados*
[3]*Department of Medicine, University of Illinois Medical Center and Department of Medicine, Jesse Brown VA Medical Center, Chicago, IL 60612, USA*

Correspondence should be addressed to Michael Salim; michael.salim91@gmail.com

Academic Editor: Michaël R. Laurent

Objective. Association of primary hyperparathyroidism (pHPT) with phosphaturic mesenchymal tumors (PMT) is rarely reported. This report entertains the hypothesis of the causal association of HPT with tumor-induced osteomalacia (TIO) and of the existence of HPT-PMT syndrome. *Case Presentation.* A 49-year-old man presented with fragility rib fractures, generalized bone pain, and muscle weakness worsening over the past 3 years. Initial tests demonstrated hypophosphatemia and high PTH. The diagnosis of pHPT was entertained, but parathyroid scan was negative. During a 2-year follow-up, the patient reported minimal improvement of symptoms after intermittent treatment with calcitriol and phosphate. Biochemical evaluation showed persistent hypophosphatemia with renal phosphate wasting, elevated FGF23, and osteopenia on DXA scan. TIO was suspected. Multiple MRIs and whole-body FDG-PET scans were inconclusive. The patient subsequently underwent ^{68}Ga-DOTATATE PET-CT, which revealed a somatostatin receptor-positive lesion in the lung. The resected mass was confirmed as PMT. The patient had dramatically improved symptoms, normal phosphate, calcium, and FGF23. During follow-up over 3 years postsurgery, the patient had slowly rising calcium and persistently elevated PTH. *Conclusion.* The debate whether the patient had pHPT or tertiary HPT prompted literature review showing that aberrant genes including FGFR1, FGF1, fibronectin 1, and Klotho were mechanistically involved in the HPT-PMT association. This case highlights the pitfalls contributing to delayed diagnosis and treatment of TIO and hypothesizes the association between pHPT and PMT.

1. Introduction

Tumor-induced osteomalacia (TIO) is a rare paraneoplastic syndrome caused by phosphaturic mesenchymal tumors (PMT) secreting fibroblast growth factor 23 (FGF23) [1]. Physiologically produced predominantly by osteocytes and osteogenic cells, FGF23, a peptide hormone, is the primary regulator of serum phosphate (phosphatonin) through its effects on the parathyroid glands, kidneys, and vitamin D metabolism. Clinically, TIO presents with myalgia, bone pain, osteomalacia, and fragility fractures; the laboratory hallmarks of TIO are renal phosphate wasting, hypophosphatemia, low or inappropriately normal vitamin D, and normal serum calcium and parathyroid hormone (PTH) [1]. Definitive treatment of TIO is surgical resection of the offending tumor followed by biochemical and clinical resolution of the disease state. The rarity of the disorder, difficulty in tumor localization, and potential comorbidities often make TIO diagnosis and treatment challenging and delayed [1]. Increased or inappropriately normal (for the degree of hypophosphatemia) PTH is rarely diagnosed as hyperparathyroidism (HPT) [2]. We report a case of a patient with PMT and primary hyperparathyroidism (pHPT) and possible existence of HPT-PMT syndrome.

2. Case Presentation

A 49-year-old man was seen in the endocrinology clinic with a 3-year history of fragility rib fractures, muscle weakness, and generalized bone pain unrelieved with high-dose opioids. Rheumatologic workup was negative. Initial tests showed elevated circulating PTH 114.1 pg/mL (14–72 pg/mL) and alkaline phosphatase (ALP) 283 IU/L (44–174 IU/L), reduced phosphate 1.6 mg/dL (2.5–4.9 mg/dL), 25(OH)D 16 ng/mL (30–100 ng/mL), 1,25(OH)$_2$D 9 pg/mL (18–72 pg/mL), and eGFR 58 mL/min/1.73 m^2, and normal calcium level 9.2 mg/dL (8.5–10.1 mg/dL) (Table 1). The diagnosis of primary normocalcemic HPT or secondary HPT (sHPT, due to vitamin D deficiency) was entertained. A sestamibi scan showed normal parathyroid uptake.

During a 2-year follow-up, the patient was intermittently taking vitamin D, calcitriol, and phosphate (phosphate in low dose and with poor adherence due to side effects) and reported some improvement of symptoms. Further investigations showed persistent hypophosphatemia with renal phosphate wasting (elevated urinary fractional phosphate excretion 44%, ref. <20%), high FGF23 291 RU/mL (0–180 RU/mL), and osteopenia on DXA. TIO due to PMT (TIO-PMT) was suspected. Over the next few years, investigations included three whole-body FDG PET-CT scans revealing several suspicious areas, yet no tumor was seen on multiple MRIs. Follow-up laboratory tests showed persistent hypophosphatemia, increasing FGF23 (up to 1330 RU/mL) and PTH (up to 274.4 pg/mL), and normal calcium, 25(OH)D, and 1,25(OH)$_2$D (Table 1). The ^{68}Ga-DOTATATE PET-CT revealed a somatostatin receptor-positive lesion involving the left upper lobe of the lung (Figure 1).

The lung mass was resected with histopathology confirming PMT (Figure 2). At a 6-month postoperative follow-up, the patient reported dramatically improved symptoms, and tests showed normal phosphate, calcium, ALP, and FGF23 (160 RU/mL) (Table 1) and improved DXA. Phosphorus supplementation was discontinued. At follow-up 3 years postsurgery, the patient was asymptomatic, and tests showed normal phosphate, 25(OH)D, and FGF23 (174 RU/mL) but high calcium (10.6 mg/dL) and PTH (126.3 pg/mL) (Table 1). A diagnosis of tertiary HPT (tHPT) was suspected, but the patient did not meet the criteria for surgical treatment, so no investigations were done. The nature of HPT, whether pHPT (since PTH was high at the initial presentation) or tHPT (due to long-standing hypovitaminosis D), was debated and prompted literature review.

3. Discussion

The patient was initially diagnosed as pHPT with a normal parathyroid scan, similar to previous reports in TIO-PMT [3]. Hyperparathyroidism was uncommonly acknowledged in TIO-PMT cases [1, 2], and predominantly, HPT was diagnosed as sHPT [1] or tHPT [1, 4]. Tertiary HPT would not apply to our case since PTH was high at the initial presentation. Secondary HPT was described in TIO-PMT and explained by the suppressive action of FGF23 on renal 25(OH)D-1-α-hydroxylase [5], similar to FGF23-induced TIO in animal models, showing HPT and parathyroid hyperplasia [6]. Vitamin D and specifically calcitriol usually normalized PTH in sHPT [5]. In our patient, two years of vitamin D and calcitriol treatment normalized 25(OH)D and 1,25(OH)$_2$D, but PTH remained high, suggesting factors other than or in addition to vitamin D deficiency contributed to HPT. Primary HPT was rarely diagnosed in patients presenting with TIO. In our case, there is the possibility that the patient had primary normocalcemic hyperparathyroidism at the beginning evolving into primary hypercalcemic hyperparathyroidism. In a published case diagnosed as pHPT and TIO due to unlocalizable PMT, the patient was treated with total (four glands) parathyroidectomy [3]. Particularly, insightful was a case of a young patient with a de novo germline translocation involving α-Klotho gene resulting in high circulating α-Klotho, FGF23, and PTH [7]. The patient was diagnosed and treated for hypophosphatemic rickets. There was no localizable PMT, yet, 30 years later, the patient developed two PMT in the mastoid bone [8]. The published reports and our case could imply that the association of PMT and HPT was not accidental, and perhaps, FGF23 per se or FGF23 pathway (including FGFR1-Klotho receptor) was the primary inducer of hyperparathyroidism.

Accumulating research has provided new insights showing that FGF23 is an important ligand for the FGFR1-Klotho receptor pathway playing a pivotal role in FGF23 hypersecretion phenotype and pathogenesis of PMT [8, 9]. FGFR1, a cell surface receptor with tyrosine kinase activity, works in union with its obligatory coreceptor Klotho, a transmembrane protein with a β-glucuronidase activity. Both FGF23 and Klotho can be cleaved and shed and act as circulating hormones. The binding of FGF23 to FGFR1-Klotho activates downstream events regulating mineral metabolism, cell differentiation, and aging [8, 9]. Specifically, fusion of fibronectin 1 (FN1) with FGFR1 or FGF1 creates aberrant fusion genes FN1-FGFR1 and FN1-FGF1, which are overexpressed in 42% and 6% of PMT, respectively [9], while aberrant α-Klotho (or less commonly β-Klotho) genes are overexpressed in 8 of 10 fusion-negative PMT [8]. These aberrant genes activate the FGF1-FGFR signaling pathway resulting in paracrine positive feedback with upregulation of FGF23 gene and uncontrolled secretion of FGF23 by PMT [8, 9].

There are no published studies exploring mechanisms of the association between PMT and HPT. In clinical cases, pHPT has been reported as rare and accidental [3]. Alternatively, however, the coexistence of HPT and PMT may not be accidental but related to common factors contributing to the development of HPT-PMT syndrome similar to HPT-jaw tumor syndrome [10]. Review of literature reveals that several genes can be implicated as potential candidates for inducing PMT and HPT. Aberrant genes overexpressed in PMT can also initiate changes in parathyroid glands resulting in hyperplasia and autonomous secretion of PTH. Consistent with this hypothesis, published data show that parathyroid glands had an abundant expression of FGF1-α-Klotho receptors [10, 11]. Correspondingly, in clinical HPT due to parathyroid tumors, frequent upregulation of FGF1 and FGFR1 genes has been reported [10]. In experimental models of HPT, FGF23–FGFR1-Klotho signaling upregulates PTH gene expression, PTH secretion, and parathyroid cell proliferation [11].

Table 1: Laboratory evaluation.

Measure	Ref	2011[a]	2012[a]	2013[a]	2014[a]	2015[a]	2016[a]	2017[a]	2018[b]	2019[b]	2020[b]
PTH, pg/mL	14–72	114.1	—	110.6	247.6	220.4	—	274.4	—	—	126.3
Ca, mg/dL	8.5–10.1	9.2	8.9	9.2	9.5	9.0	8.3	9.8	10.1	9.9	10.6
PO_4, mg/dL	2.5–4.9	1.6	1.6	1.0	1.7	0.9	2.3	1.7	3.0	3.0	2.6
Vit D 25(OH)D, ng/mL	30–100	16	—	46	31	32	—	30	30	24	37
Vit D $1,25(OH)_2$, pg/mL	18–72	9	—	27	-	29	—	27	70	37	-
ALP, IU/L	44–174	283	—	252	243	262	—	103	71	71	71
FGF23, RU/mL	0–180	—	—	291	-	-	—	1330	160	174	174
eGFR, mL/min/1.73 m^2	>60	58	—	85	90	75	66	64	66	66	61
FeP	<20%	—	—	44%	—	—	—	—	—	—	—

ALP, alkaline phosphatase; Ca, calcium; eGFR, estimated glomerular filtration rate; FeP, fractional excretion of phosphate; FGF, fibroblast growth factor; PO_4, phosphate; PTH, parathyroid hormone; Ref, reference. [a]Prior to tumor resection. [b]Following tumor resection.

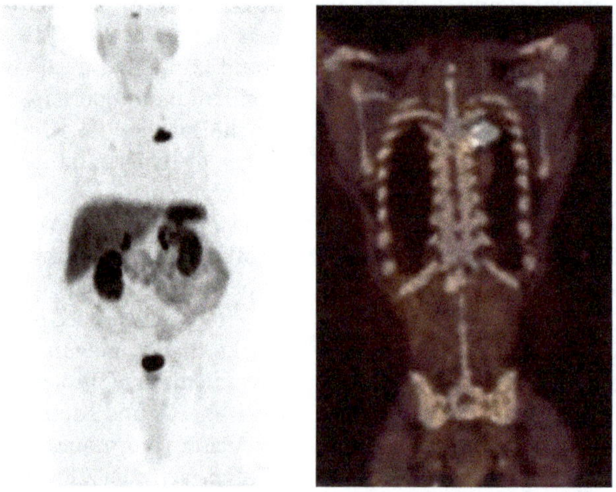

(a) (b)

Figure 1: ^{68}Ga-DOTATATE PET-CT maximum intensity projection coronal (a) and representative-fused PET/CT coronal (b) views demonstrating somatostatin receptor-positive lesion involving the posteromedially located pleural-based 3.5 cm mass in the left upper lobe.

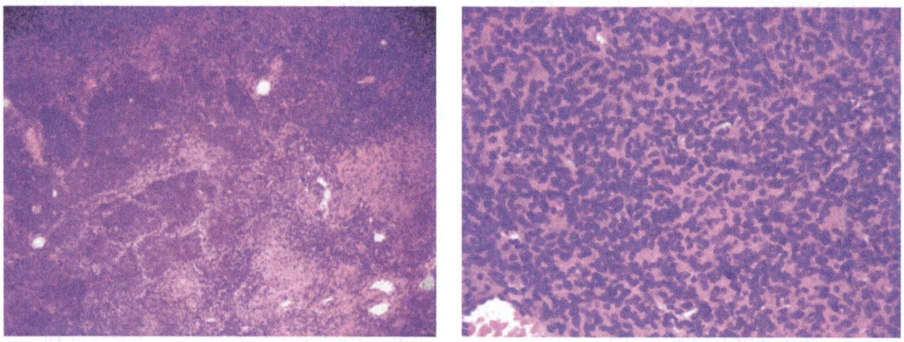

(a) (b)

Figure 2: Histopathologic images showing hemangiopericytoma-like vasculature and calcified chondroid-like matrix in intermediate power (a) and cellular spindle cell lesion in high power (b) consistent with mesenchymal tumor.

In addition to aberrant expression of FGF-related genes, mutations of some other genes, e.g., MEN1 and EEF2K, may be associated with the development of PMT and HPT. The multiple endocrine neoplasia type 1 (MEN1) gene encodes menin, a transcription factor expressed in many tissues and involved in the development of endocrine and nonendocrine tumors [12]. Since the cloning of the MEN1 gene, more than 1,500 germline and somatic mutations have been reported, including those found in 35–50% of parathyroid adenomas [12], parathyroid hyperplasia [13], and some mesenchymal tumors [14]. Of relevance, MEN1 mutation has been found in a patient with HPT and TIO due to benign chondroblastoma [13]. The patient has presented with generalized bone pain, difficulties walking, hypophosphatemia, osteomalacia, and high

PTH and diagnosed as HPT. He has been treated with a subtotal (three and a half glands) parathyroidectomy and pathology-confirmed hyperplastic lesions in all parathyroid glands [13]. Due to persistent hypophosphatemia, further investigations have been performed and have shown high circulating FGF23 prompting the diagnosis of TIO, while genetic testing has shown somatic mutation of the MEN1 gene in hyperplastic parathyroid lesions. On follow-up, a benign chondroblastoma of the femur has been found and presumed to be the cause of TIO [13].

The EEF2K gene encoding for eukaryotic elongation factor 2 kinase (eEF2K) is suggested to be involved in tumorigenesis [15]. EEF2K is differentially expressed in parathyroid adenomas compared to normal parathyroid tissue and can contribute to the development of parathyroid hyperplasia and HPT [16]. In addition, EEF2K is shown to be important in epithelial-mesenchymal transition (EMT) [15]. The EMT is a highly regulated and reversible process that allows a polarized epithelial cell to undergo multiple biochemical changes resulting in a mesenchymal cell phenotype. The EMT is suggested to play an important role in the development and progression of multiple tumors, including mesenchymal tumors [17]. Of interest, a nonclassical vitamin D pathway is important in promoting epithelial differentiation while diminishing the expression of several EMT inducers and suppressing the EMT process [17]. The available published data can imply that long-standing vitamin D deficiency via its influence on EMT and PTH may contribute to the simultaneous development of PMT and hyperparathyroidism.

In conclusion, the mechanism of PMT tumorigenesis remains elusive, and the hypothesis for the existence of HPT-PMT syndrome remains a hypothesis. Further molecular and experimental studies can improve our understanding and help to discover novel genes and/or pathways to answer the question of whether the association between hyperparathyroidism and PMT is a rarity or a rule.

Acknowledgments

The authors acknowledge Dr. Terry Unterman for following up with the patient in the clinic and Dr. Liza Escuadro for the pathology expertise.

References

[1] S. Minisola, M. Peacock, S. Fukumoto et al., "Tumour-induced osteomalacia," *Nature Reviews Disease Primers*, vol. 3, no. 1, Article ID 17044, 2017.

[2] J. Feng, Y. Jiang, O. Wang et al., "The diagnostic dilemma of tumor induced osteomalacia: a retrospective analysis of 144 cases," *Endocrine Journal*, vol. 64, no. 7, pp. 675–683, 2017.

[3] S. K. Bhadada, S. Palnitkar, S. Qiu, N. Parikh, G. B. Talpos, and S. D. Rao, "Deliberate total parathyroidectomy: A potentially novel therapy for tumor-induced hypophosphatemic osteomalacia," *The Journal of Clinical Endocrinology & Metabolism*, vol. 98, no. 11, pp. 4273–4278, 2013.

[4] S. Tournis, V. Samdanis, D. Economopoulos, P. Giannikou, and G. P. Lyritis, "Autonomous hyperparathyroidism following long-term phosphate treatment for tumor-induced osteomalacia," *The Endocrinologist*, vol. 17, no. 5, pp. 263–266, 2007.

[5] S. S. Harris, E. Soteriades, J. A. S. Coolidge, S. Mudgal, and B. Dawson-Hughes, "Vitamin D insufficiency and hyperparathyroidism in a low income, multiracial, elderly Population," *The Journal of Clinical Endocrinology & Metabolism*, vol. 85, no. 11, pp. 4125–4130, 2000.

[6] X. Bai, D. Miao, J. Li, D. Goltzman, and A. C. Karaplis, "Transgenic mice overexpressing human fibroblast growth factor 23 (R176Q) delineate a putative role for parathyroid hormone in renal phosphate wasting disorders," *Endocrinology*, vol. 145, no. 11, pp. 5269–5279, 2004.

[7] C. A. Brownstein, F. Adler, C. Nelson-Williams et al., "A translocation causing increased -Klotho level results in hypophosphatemic rickets and hyperparathyroidism," *Proceedings of the National Academy of Sciences*, vol. 105, no. 9, pp. 3455–3460, 2008.

[8] C.-H. Lee, S.-Y. Su, K. Sittampalam et al., "Frequent overexpression of klotho in fusion-negative phosphaturic mesenchymal tumors with tumorigenic implications," *Modern Pathology*, vol. 33, no. 5, pp. 858–870, 2020.

[9] J.-C. Lee, S.-Y. Su, C. A. Changou et al., "Characterization of FN1-FGFR1 and novel FN1-FGF1 fusion genes in a large series of phosphaturic mesenchymal tumors," *Modern Pathology*, vol. 29, no. 11, pp. 1335–1346, 2016.

[10] J.-Y. Lee, S. Y. Kim, E.-Y. Mo et al., "Upregulation of FGFR1 expression is associated with parathyroid carcinogenesis in HPT-JT syndrome due to an HRPT2 splicing mutation," *International Journal of Oncology*, vol. 45, no. 2, pp. 641–650, 2014.

[11] Y. Fan, W. Liu, R. Bi et al., "Interrelated role of Klotho and calcium-sensing receptor in parathyroid hormone synthesis and parathyroid hyperplasia," *Proceedings of the National Academy of Sciences*, vol. 115, no. 16, pp. E3749–E3758, 2018.

[12] G. Westin, "Molecular genetics and epigenetics of nonfamilial (sporadic) parathyroid tumours," *Journal of Internal Medicine*, vol. 280, no. 6, pp. 551–558, 2016.

[13] K. Sato, T. Obara, K. Yamazaki et al., "Somatic mutations of theMEN1Gene and microsatellite instability in a case of tertiary hyperparathyroidism occurring during high phosphate therapy for acquired, hypophosphatemic osteomalacia," *The Journal of Clinical Endocrinology & Metabolism*, vol. 86, no. 11, pp. 5564–5571, 2001.

[14] V. Nuzzo, L. Tauchmanová, A. Falchetti et al., "MEN1 family with a novel frameshift mutation," *Journal of Endocrinological Investigation*, vol. 29, no. 5, pp. 450–456, 2006.

[15] R. Liu and C. G. Proud, "Eukaryotic elongation factor 2 kinase as a drug target in cancer, and in cardiovascular and neurodegenerative diseases," *Acta Pharmacologica Sinica*, vol. 37, no. 3, pp. 285–294, 2016.

[16] M. Lu, H. Kjellin, O. Fotouhi et al., "Molecular profiles of oxyphilic and chief cell parathyroid adenoma," *Molecular and Cellular Endocrinology*, vol. 470, pp. 84–95, 2018.

[17] M. J. Larriba, A. García de Herreros, and A. Muñoz, "Vitamin D and the epithelial to mesenchymal transition," *Stem Cells International*, vol. 2016, Article ID 6213872, 11 pages, 2016.

14

Intravenous Iodinated Contrast Induced Thyrotoxic Periodic Paralysis: A Case Report

S. Alrushaid[1] **and T. Alessa**[2,3]

[1]*Kuwait University, Kuwait City, Kuwait*
[2]*Division of Endocrinology, Diabetes and Metabolism, Jaber Al-Ahmad Hospital, Kuwait City, Kuwait*
[3]*Dasman Diabetes Institute, Kuwait City, Kuwait*

Correspondence should be addressed to T. Alessa; thamermd@gmail.com

Academic Editor: Wei Wu

Thyrotoxic periodic paralysis (TPP) is an entity that has been described in the literature as a transient, symmetrical, flaccid paralysis, mainly affecting the lower limbs of patients with a current or previous history of hyperthyroidism. In most cases, Graves' disease is the cause of hyperthyroidism. Contrast and iodine-induced TPP have been described in the literature, but only one case of intravenous contrast induced TPP has been reported. We report a case of TPP following administration of intravenous contrast for a computed tomography scan of the neck prior to lymph node excision. A 35-year-old Kuwaiti male with known Graves' disease in remission until two months of his presentation, reported to the emergency room one early morning in December 2020. He sustained a fall from the stairs due to bilateral lower limb weakness, mostly proximal. The upper limbs were spared, and the patient did not experience any numbness or headache. His potassium was found to be 2.1 mmol/L and an electrocardiogram showed U waves and ST segment changes. He was initiated on 20 mEq of intravenous potassium chloride in 500 mL sodium chloride over one hour, following which his potassium approached normal and his weakness resolved. He was last known to be euthyroid in November 2019 but noted in October 2020 to be in the hyperthyroid state when thyroid function testing showed a thyroid-stimulating hormone of <0.005 (0.27–4.2 uIu/mL) and free thyroxine (T4) of 27.6 (7.8– pmol/L). In patients with known hyperthyroidism, more caution is required when iodine-containing substances are administered without proper evaluation of thyroid function.

1. Case Report

A 35-year-old Kuwaiti man with known Graves' disease, brought by ambulance to the emergency room (ER) in Mubarak Al-Kabeer Hospital early morning in December 2020 with an acute episode of bilateral lower limb weakness. The weakness was of a sudden onset, first noticed as the patient was getting up from a seated position late at night. On walking, the patient noticed his legs felt heavy. Upon attempting to go up the stairs, his legs were weak and gave away, causing him to fall and sustain some minor injuries. There was no associated numbness or paresthesia, blurry vision, or speech disturbances. His upper limbs were completely free from any symptoms. He denied any symptoms of hyperthyroidism.

Before the event, he denied consuming a high carbohydrate meal, but mentioned drinking a small cup of milk with tea 2–4 hours before his symptoms began. He also denied exercise or alcohol consumption prior to the incident. However, he did receive 80 mL of low osmolality iodinated intravenous (IV) contrast (Visipaque) in the morning of the incident for contrast computed tomography (CT) imaging of the neck at Al-Sabah Hospital, as a surgery for excising an enlarged isolated cervical lymph node was planned. Visipaque is available in concentrations of 270 and 320 mg of organically bound iodine per mL (550 and 652 mg of iodixanol per mL, respectively). No discussion of his hyperthyroidism condition was performed by the radiology department before the CT procedure.

In the ER, his temperature was 36.8 degrees C, heart rate 86 bpm, and oxygen saturation 99%. The initial basic blood chemistry test was done showing low potassium (2.1 mmol/L). Electrocardiogram (ECG) was performed twice, initially showing *U* waves and later ST segment abnormalities.

Two months prior in October 2020, the patient was admitted to a local hospital for the diagnosis of acute gastroenteritis. He presented with symptoms of abdominal pain, vomiting, and diarrhea. He was managed conservatively with intravenous fluids. During admission, several laboratory tests were done, including a thyroid function test showing thyroid-stimulating hormone (TSH) < 0.005 (0.27–4.2 uIu/mL) and free thyroxine (FT4) 27.6 (7.8–16 pmol/L). The caring medical team decided not to use antithyroid medications as it was believed to be a transient hyperthyroidism related to his acute illness.

The patient was diagnosed with hyperthyroidism due to Graves' disease in 2016 after presenting with palpitations, sweating, anxiety, and agitation. At the time, his TSH was 0.12 (0.27–4.2 uIu/mL), FT4 of 14.1 (7.8–16 pmol/L), and free T3 of 8.0 (3.5–6.7 pmol/L). Thyroid uptake scan showed homogenously increased radiotracer distribution in both lobes, with no discrete areas showing decreased or increased uptake. Four-hour and 24-hour radio-iodine uptakes were 33.6% and 62%, respectively. These findings were consistent with a diffuse, toxic thyroid gland, diagnosed as Graves' disease. Medical therapy with carbimazole was initiated. He was maintained euthyroid and kept on medical therapy. The patient and his caring endocrinologist have not planned an alternative therapy for the management of his hyperthyroidism. In 2018, thyroid ultrasound showed normal sized thyroid lobes but coarse echotexture and geographic hypoechoic areas with increased vascularity, suggesting thyroiditis. He was taken off carbimazole therapy in early 2019, and his thyroid function test was within the reference range since then. During the patient's last visit to his endocrinologist in November 2019, he did not report any symptoms of hyperthyroidism nor ophthalmic symptoms. His thyroid function test done during that visit showed a TSH of 0.95 (0.27–4.2 uIu/mL) and free T4 of 11.6 (7.8–16 pmol/L). His thyroid gland was mildly diffusely enlarged, nontender with no audible bruit or nodularity.

The patient also has hypertension and hyperlipidemia, both reported to be controlled on medical therapy with telmisartan 40 mg once daily and rosuvastatin 20 mg once daily. He does not use any illicit drugs or consume alcohol. He smokes an electric cigarette for two years. The patient had no previous surgeries except for laser-assisted in situ keratomileusis (LASIK) for a refractive error of his both eyes. He is married with two children and works at the Ministry of Education.

Both patient's parents have hypothyroidism diagnosed during adulthood, with no history of thyroid surgery. His mother had nephrectomy for a malignant renal tumor. There is no reported family history of other renal conditions or potassium abnormalities. His father is 74 years old and became bed-ridden after a stroke. The patient reported no family history of similar presentation of temporary paralysis.

2. Investigations

Initial basic blood chemistry performed in the ER (Table 1) was significant for hypokalemia (2.3 mmol/L). Elevated random serum glucose (8.9 mmol/L) and low phosphate (0.73 mmol/L) were also noted. The anion gap was elevated (20), although serum bicarbonate was normal (26 mmol/L). A few hours later, laboratory results showed elevated magnesium (1.37 mmol/L), low albumin (34 g/L), and normal corrected serum calcium (2.27 mmol/L). Electrocardiography (ECG) showed *U* waves and ST segment abnormalities.

3. Outcome and Follow-Up

In the ER, the patient was administered 20 mEq potassium chloride (KCl) in 500 mL sodium chloride (NaCl) intravenously over one hour and 2 g magnesium sulfate (MgSO4) over half an hour soon after the initial test result, which allowed gradual improvement of his weakness until resolution with improvement of his serum potassium (Table 1) in less than four hours. Serum magnesium levels noted to be elevated (1.37 mmol/L) possibly due to MgSO4 infusion but no baseline level was available. Patient was connected to continuous cardiac monitoring during treatment of hypokalemia and no cardiac arrythmias or abnormal findings were detected during the potassium replacement therapy. Beta-blocker were not administered during his ER stay. The patient was discharged home from the ER on paracetamol and advised to follow a high potassium diet. No potassium supplements were given. He did, however, sustain superficial bruises with pain in his lower extremities that lasted for 48 hours afterwards.

Two weeks following the event, he was evaluated by another endocrinologist, and a new thyroid function test performed showing TSH <0.005 (0.27–4.2 uIu/mL) and FT4 of 13 (7.8–16 /L) indicating most likely a resolving hyperthyroidism. He was not started on any antithyroid therapy. His TSH values improved over the next eight months reaching 1.32 (0.27–4.2 uIu/mL) with normal FT4 in August 2021.

4. Discussion

Thyrotoxic periodic paralysis (TPP) is an entity that has been described in the literature as a transient, symmetrical, flaccid paralysis, mainly affecting the lower limbs of patients with a current or previous history of hyperthyroidism [1, 2]. In most cases, Graves' disease is the cause of hyperthyroidism [3]. Other causes include toxic multinodular goiter, thyroiditis, or iodine-induced thyrotoxicosis [4]. It is more common in people of Asian descent and following a carbohydrate-rich meal, which results in an increase in the insulin level [5, 6]. Patients tend to present during early morning hours, as a catecholamine peak occurs during this time [3]. Both insulin and catecholamines are known to inhibit the Kir channel in the skeletal muscle, a channel that allows potassium to move extracellularly, which could explain why a rise in either could precipitate hypokalemia in

Table 1: Serum laboratory findings in the emergency room.

Tests	6:48 AM	7:25 AM	10:16 AM	11:05 AM	Reference range
Glucose		8.9			4.1–5.9 mmol/L
Urea		4.8			2.8–7.2 mmol/L
Creatinine		84			64–104 μmol/L
Sodium		141			136–146 mmol/L
Potassium	2.10	2.31	3.50		3.5–5.1 mmol/L
Chloride		104			101–109 mmol/L
Phosphate		0.73			0.81–1.45 mmol/L
Calcium				2.15	2.2–2.65 mmol/L
Magnesium				1.37	0.73–1.06 mmol/L
Corrected calcium				2.27	2.2–2.6 mmol/L
Albumin				34	35–52 g/L
CO2		28			21–31 mmol/L
Anion gap		11.3			

susceptible people [3]. The cardinal finding is hypokalemia and the culprit in this case is thought to be a rise in thyroid hormone levels [7, 8]. The severity of the weakness correlates with the degree of hypokalemia [5, 7]. During thyrotoxicosis, there is an increase in transcription of Na/K ATPase pumps as well as increased activity through two mechanisms: directly by thyroid hormones and via the resulting increased B2-adrenergic receptor sensitivity [4, 7, 9]. The influx of potassium into the intracellular compartment results lowered the levels of plasma potassium, leading to periodic paralysis [1]. The increased Na/K ATPase activity allows for more intracellular displacement of potassium, causing lower plasma potassium levels which leads to periodic paralysis [1, 3, 4, 7]. Genetic changes have been identified in TPP, involving the Na/K ATPase pump and Kir channel [3, 4, 7]. The Kir channel normally allows potassium to flow out of the cell, so loss of function mutations involving the Kir channel gene predispose to TPP [3, 4, 7]. This condition has a male predominance which makes these genetic alterations possibly X-linked, or that sex hormones play a role in the pathophysiology. In fact, androgens are known to increase the activity of the Na/K ATPase pump, while estrogen and progesterone inhibit it [3, 9, 10]. Furthermore, androgens induce muscle growth and hypertrophy, which increases the amount of Na/K ATPase pumps available for stimulation [10].

TPP is often confused with familial periodic paralysis (FPP) [11]. FPP occurs due to autosomal dominantly inherited mutations in skeletal muscle sodium, potassium, or calcium receptors [11, 12]. It may be hypokalemic, hyperkalemic, or normokalemic [11, 12]. The associated transient paralysis lasts anywhere from minutes to days [12]. Family history of thyroid conditions, rather than of transient paralysis may be helpful in distinguishing the two entities, especially since familial periodic paralysis has an autosomal dominant inheritance pattern [1, 7, 11]. History or findings of hyperthyroidism is also useful [7, 11]. Both patient's parents have hypothyroidism, both had it as a primary condition and not proceeded by hyperthyroidism. No reported transient paralysis was noted in the patient's family history. In addition, hypomagnesemia and hypophosphatemia tend to occur in TPP only due to intracellular shift from a catecholamine increase [4, 5]. The initial laboratory findings for our patient did not include magnesium test but his phosphate was low. Patients with TPP also tend to have a preserved acid-base balance as well as low creatinine [5, 7]. In our patient, the anion gap was elevated while the bicarbonate level was normal. This observation could not be explained due to lack of further clinical and laboratory data.

During the attack, patients may present with signs and symptoms of hyperthyroidism, such as palpitations, tremors, and tachycardia [11, 13]. Our patient, however, did not experience any symptoms of hyperthyroidism during the attack apart from systolic hypertension in the emergency room, which made the diagnosis challenging. Most patients with TPP have only mild or subclinical hyperthyroidism but our patient had a significant hyperthyroidism thyroid profile with suppressed TSH and FT4 double the upper normal range detected two months before his presentation [5, 14]. This could have facilitated the development of TPP in our patient. With correction of the hypokalemia, affected patients classically regain complete motor function in their lower limbs within hours, sometimes up to days [3].

There are multiple reported cases of iodine-induced TPP after ingestion of amiodarone and other iodine-containing substances, such as radioactive iodine and kelp [1, 14–18]. However, only one case of TPP following administration of intravenous iodine-containing contrast has been reported which was also managed urgently with potassium replacement [19]. In that case, proximal weakness of both his upper and lower limbs with inability to stand independently one day after cardiac catheterization with iodinated contrast was reported [19]. Our patient's presentation spared the upper limbs. Other reports of TPP mentioned using beta-blockers, which was not used in our Case [1]. Beta-blockers are given to cause intracellular shifting of potassium and counteract the increased B-adrenergic receptor sensitivity [1].

The Jod–Basedow phenomenon can be used to explain the pathophysiology of iodine-induced TPP [20]. Normally, those exposed to large amounts of exogenous iodine will experience a transient reduction in thyroid hormone synthesis [20]. This inhibition is independent of TSH and is called the Wolff–Chaikoff effect [20]. Patients with hyperthyroidism could escape this effect as thyroid hormone synthesis is not controlled by pituitary TSH, and comparatively large quantities of iodine or iodide when ingested can lead to iodine-induced hyperthyroidism (Jod–Basedow effect) [19]. Our patient had significant hyperthyroidism before receiving the intravenous iodine contrast, escaping the Wolff–Chaikoff effect would be likely and optimal precontrast preparation was required.

Intravenous potassium replacement is the main element in the management of TPP and needs to be done as soon as possible; however, as these patients' total body potassium is normal, rebound hyperkalemia may result from potassium replacement along with eventual extracellular shifting [3]. Inhibitors of thyroid hormone synthesis are given to treat the underlying cause [3]. It is unclear whether potassium supplementation is helpful prophylactically; however, beta-blockers and antithyroid medication are beneficial in the long-term [3, 10, 19]. Our patient was only advised to maintain a potassium-rich diet after the episode. Furthermore, in those with contrast or iodine-induced TPP, this should be noted for more precautions to be taken in the future. Our patient showed laboratory features of improving hyperthyroidism in the months following the event, it is not clear whether his relapse was transient and remitted spontaneously.

TPP is a challenging diagnosis, especially in the emergency setting. Intravenous contrast-induced TPP is even more challenging. Increasing the awareness of patients and their physicians is crucial in allowing timely diagnosis and management. As most patients will not have overt hyperthyroidism, this must be sought out using a high index of suspicion based on previous history of thyroid disease in a patient with acute weakness or paralysis. Proper investigations to differentiate between thyrotoxic and familial forms of periodic paralysis are helpful and should be carried out. As the paralysis is transient, patients must be reassured and educated following the episode. In patients with documented hyperthyroidism, more caution is required when iodine-containing substances are administered without proper control of thyroid function.

Consent

Written informed consent was obtained from the patient.

Authors' Contributions

Alrushaid S. wrote the article. Alessa T. contributed to the writing and discussion of the article and was the named physician involved in the care of the patient. All authors read and approved the manuscript.

References

[1] M. Haider, A. Z. Khan Chachar, and A. Munir, "Thyrotoxic periodic paralysis," *Journal of Ayub Medical College, Abbottabad*, vol. 31, no. 4, pp. 619–621, 2019.

[2] S. Chandran, R. Balakrishnan, G. Thirumalnesan, and N. Doraisamy, "Thyrotoxic periodic paralysis," *Indian Journal of Endocrinology and Metabolism*, vol. 15, no. 6, pp. S147–S149, 2011.

[3] Q. Z. Iqbal, M. Niazi, Z. Zia, and S. B. A. Sattar, "A literature review on thyrotoxic periodic paralysis," *Cureus*, vol. 12, no. 8, Article ID e10108, 2020.

[4] S. Siddamreddy and V. H. Dandu, *Thyrotoxic Periodic Paralysis*, StatPearls, Treasure Island (FL), 2022.

[5] M. Alziadat and M. Ismail, "Thyrotoxic periodic paralysis after urethral dilatation," *Avicenna Journal of Medicine*, vol. 10, no. 4, pp. 249–251, 2020.

[6] M. Patel and K. Ladak, "Thyrotoxic periodic paralysis: a case report and literature review," *Clinical Medicine Research*, vol. 19, no. 3, pp. 148–151, 2021.

[7] S. H. Lin and C. L. Huang, "Mechanism of thyrotoxic periodic paralysis," *Journal of the American Society of Nephrology*, vol. 23, no. 6, pp. 985–988, 2012.

[8] L. Lam, R. J. Nair, and L. Tingle, "Thyrotoxic periodic paralysis," *Baylor University Medical Center Proceedings*, vol. 19, no. 2, pp. 126–129, 2006.

[9] P. Dunne, N. Kaimal, J. MacDonald, and A. A. Syed, "Iodinated contrast-induced thyrotoxicosis," *Canadian Medical Association Journal*, vol. 185, no. 2, pp. 144–147, 2013.

[10] J. T. Batch, M. U. Jahngir, and I. Rodriguez, "Thyrotoxic periodic paralysis: an incidental diagnosis!" *Cureus*, vol. 12, no. 2, Article ID e7041, 2020.

[11] C. H. Hsieh, S. W. Kuo, D. Pei et al., "Thyrotoxic periodic paralysis: an overview," *Annals of Saudi Medicine*, vol. 24, no. 6, pp. 418–422, 2004.

[12] J. M. Statland, B. Fontaine, M. G. Hanna et al., "Review of the diagnosis and treatment of periodic paralysis," *Muscle & Nerve*, vol. 57, no. 4, pp. 522–530, 2018.

[13] J. Gilbert, "Thyrotoxicosis - investigation and management," *Clinical Medicine*, vol. 17, no. 3, pp. 274–277, 2017.

[14] S. E. Yun, Y. Kang, E. J. Bae et al., "Iodine-induced thyrotoxic hypokalemic paralysis after ingestion of Salicornia herbace," *Renal Failure*, vol. 36, no. 3, pp. 461–463, 2014.

[15] H. A. Tran, "Inadvertent iodine excess causing thyrotoxic hypokalemic periodic paralysis," *Archives of Internal Medicine*, vol. 165, no. 21, p. 2536, 2005.

[16] S. Akar, A. Comlekci, M. Birlik et al., "Thyrotoxic periodic paralysis in a Turkish male; the recurrence of the attack after radioiodine treatment," *Endocrine Journal*, vol. 52, no. 1, pp. 149–151, 2005.

[17] S. T. Laroia, K. M. Zaw, A. K. Ganti, W. Newman, and A. O. Akinwande, "Amiodarone-induced thyrotoxicosis presenting as hypokalemic periodic paralysis," *Southern Medical Journal*, vol. 95, no. 11, pp. 1326–1328, 2002.

[18] K. P. Ober and J. F. Hennessy, "Jodbasedow and thyrotoxic periodic paralysis," *Archives of Internal Medicine*, vol. 141, no. 9, pp. 1225–1227, 1981.

[19] M. P. Kane and R. S. Busch, "Drug-induced thyrotoxic periodic paralysis," *The Annals of Pharmacotherapy*, vol. 40, no. 4, pp. 778–781, 2006.

[20] M. Higgs, E. Hull, and E. Lujan, "A case report of post-operative jod-basedow phenomennon following oral and IV iodine contrast administration," *Case Reports in Endocrinology*, vol. 2014, Article ID 980283, 3 pages, 2014.

15

The Use of ^{99m}Tc-Methoxy-isobutyl-isonitrile (sestaMIBI) Uptake on Scintigraphy (^{99m}-STS) in Amiodarone-Induced Thyrotoxicosis: Case Series and Review of the Literature

Ghada Elshimy,[1,2,3] Mahmoud Alsayed,[2] Jerome Targovnik,[2,3] Gamal Sidarous,[4] and Kresimira M. Milas[5]

[1]*Endocrinology, Diabetes and Metabolism Division, Medical College of Georgia, Augusta University, Augusta, GA, USA*
[2]*Endocrinology Division, University of Arizona College of Medicine, Phoenix, AZ, USA*
[3]*Endocrinology Division, Phoenix VA Health Care System, Phoenix, AZ, USA*
[4]*Nuclear Medicine Department, University of Arizona College of Medicine, Phoenix, AZ, USA*
[5]*Endocrine Surgery Department, University of Arizona College of Medicine, Phoenix, AZ, USA*

Correspondence should be addressed to Ghada Elshimy; ghadaelchimi87@gmail.com

Academic Editor: Toshihiro Kita

Amiodarone is a class III antiarrhythmic drug, used by cardiologists to treat arrhythmia including atrial fibrillation (A fib) and ventricular fibrillation. However, amiodarone is associated with endocrine dysfunction including both hypo- and hyperthyroidism. In the literature, two types of amiodarone-induced thyrotoxicosis (AIT) were described: AIT-1 and AIT-2. Mixed AIT also called AIT type 3 (AIT-3) has been described in the literature when the cases do not have a typical presentation. In order to differentiate different types of AIT, various clinical, biochemical, and radiological tools have been proposed. The use of ^{99m}Tc-methoxy-isobutyl-isonitrile (sestaMIBI) uptake on scintigraphy (^{99m}-STS) has been suggested in the literature in only few studies (no large retrospective or prospective studies have been established in the United States). We present a case series describing 5 patients presenting to the University of Arizona with AIT where we used ^{99m}-STS to assess in diagnosis and treatment of different types of AIT followed by a review of the literature.

1. Introduction

Amiodarone is a class III antiarrhythmic drug, used by cardiologists to treat arrhythmia including atrial fibrillation (A fib) and ventricular fibrillation. However, amiodarone is associated with endocrine dysfunction including both hypo- and hyperthyroidism. This dysfunction is explained by the high iodine content (containing 75 mg of iodine per 200 mg tablet) and its direct toxic effect on the thyroid [1]. Amiodarone principle metabolite is desethylamiodarone (DEA), which accumulates in different tissues including the lung, the adipose tissues, and the thyroid. Given the very long elimination half-lives of amiodarone and DEA (40 ± 10 days and 57 ± 27 days, respectively), the drug and its metabolites remain available for a long time after withdrawal of the medication [2].

The intrinsic properties of the drug explain the effect of amiodarone on thyroid hormone. It inhibits the outer ring 5'-monodeiodination of thyroxine (T4). Additionally, it inhibits the intracellular T4 transport and pituitary type 2 idothyronine deiodinase (D2), thus leading to a decrease in the triiodothyronine (T3) production with an increase in the reverse T3 level. Furthermore, DEA blocks T3-receptor binding to nuclear receptors and decreases the expression of some thyroid hormone-related genes. In addition, there is a direct toxic effect on the thyroid follicular cells, resulting in a destructive thyroiditis referred to amiodarone-induced thyrotoxicosis type 2 (AIT-2). The iodine content in amiodarone mediates amiodarone-induced thyrotoxicosis type 1 (AIT-1) and amiodarone-induced hypothyroidism (AIH). AIT-1 has underlying abnormal thyroid gland (nodular goiter and latent Graves' disease) with positive antibody testing which explains the pathophysiology of the disease [3–6].

Amiodarone can have additional effects on the thyroid function tests. There is a transient increase in thyroid-stimulating hormone (TSH) in the first months of treatment in nearly all patients treated with amiodarone given the Wolff-Chaikoff effect explained by the adaptation of the thyroid gland to iodine overload with inhibition of iodine organification and reduction of the thyroid hormones production rate [3–6].

In the literature, two types of amiodarone-induced thyrotoxicosis (AIT) were described: AIT-1 and AIT-2. Mixed AIT also called AIT type 3 (AIT-3) has been described in the literature when the cases do not have a typical presentation. Some authors further divided the mixed AIT-3 form into mixed AIT/type 1 and mixed AIT/type 2 [7, 8]. In order to differentiate different types of AIT, various clinical, biochemical, and radiological tools have been proposed. On clinical examination, the presence of Graves' disease or Graves' ophthalmopathy or goiter points toward AIT-1. Laboratory testing as measurement of the inflammatory mediators has been suggested. Erythrocyte sedimentation rate (ESR) and C-reactive protein (CRP) can be elevated in AIT-2 in the context of thyroiditis, while interleukin-6 (IL-6) is considered a better marker for the destructive process. Unfortunately, sometimes, it can be falsely low, which limits its usefulness. In addition, coexisting illness such as heart failure or preexisting thyroid disease like Graves' disease can produce high IL-6 making it an unreliable marker in differentiating between AIT types [4, 9–11]. Multiple imaging modalities have been suggested including color flow Doppler sonography (CFDS) and radioactive iodine uptake scan (RAIU). Absent vascularity on CFDS is seen in patients with AIT-2, while uneven patchy parenchymal flow to markedly diffuse increase in the flow is seen in AIT-1. Studies comparing both modalities showed that CFDS is more accurate, but combined modalities have been suggested for more accurate results [12–14]. Moreover, differences in populations' iodine supply have often been mentioned as one of the main reasons for the poor reproducibility of CFDS and RAIU [15, 16].

In the past couple of years, the use of ^{99m}Tc-methoxy-isobutyl-isonitrile (sestaMIBI) uptake on scintigraphy (^{99m}-STS) has been suggested in the literature in only few studies to differentiate between different types of AIT (no large retrospective or prospective studies have been established in the United States). The rationale behind using ^{99m}-STS is that given the short half-life of the pure gamma emitter tracer Tc-99m, it has ability to accumulate in the mitochondrial rich cells, and it can differentiate between AIT-1 and AIT-2. There is positive uptake in hyperfunctioning thyroid in AIT-1, and no uptake is observed in AIT-2. The duration of the test is shorter in comparison to RAIU, and the results are not influenced by the iodine supply in the population making it a more promising diagnostic tool. In 2008, Piga et al. used it to distinguish AIT-1 from AIT-2 in Italy and stated that it is an effective tool superior to CFDS and RAIU [17]. In 2015, Pattison et al. described 15 patients in Australia, and in 2017, Wang and Zhang described 15 patients in China where they used ^{99m}-STS [18, 19]. In 2018, Censi et al. used ^{99m}-STS with target to background ratio (TBR) on 30 patients with AIT in Italy and suggested that ^{99m}-STS has 100% specificity and 91.7% sensitivity in differentiating different types of AIT [8]. We present a case series describing 5 patients presenting to the University of Arizona with AIT where we used ^{99m}-STS to assess in diagnosis and treatment of different types of AIT followed by a review of the literature.

2. Materials and Methods

In the case series, ^{99m}-STS was performed in our facility at the University of Arizona for all the described patients. It is a dual-head gamma camera equipped with pinhole collimators (Siemens, Symbia Evos). Images were acquired after intravenous injection of about 10–25 mCi of sestaMIBI. Early images were acquired at 10–15 minutes, and the late images were acquired at 60–180 minutes in different patients. Most of the prior reports acquired late images at 60 minutes; however, since this is a new modality used for AIT, the nuclear medicine department suggested extending the duration up to 180 minutes to assess if it will have an effect on the diagnosis, to ensure the complete washout of the tracer without any residuals and to rule out any mixed AIT pattern.

A qualitative assessment was based on the pattern of tracer uptake: diffuse tracer retention in the early images and a complete washout of the radiopharmaceutical in the late images prompted the patient to be classified as a case of AIT-1; if there was no significant tracer uptake in the early images, the patient was diagnosed as having AIT-2. This is similar to Piga et al. in 2008 and Censi et al. in 2018 description for the use of 99m-STS in AIT patients. Regarding the mixed AIT (AIT-3) pattern, it was suggested to use the description of Censi et al., which further classified AIT-3 into mixed/AIT-1 and mixed/AIT-2. Mixed/AIT-1 was diagnosed if the scan had a normal or slightly lower uptake than in AIT-1 in the early images and only a partial washout in the late images. Mixed/AIT-2 was diagnosed if the scan showed a slightly higher uptake than in AIT-2 in the early images and partial or complete washout in the late ones [8, 17]. However, none of our patients had a mixed pattern.

The laboratory reference ranges throughout the manuscript were as follow: TSH: 0.45–5 mIU/L; free T4: 0.8–1.7 ng/dl; free T3: 2–4.8 pg/ml; thyroid-stimulating immunoglobulin (TSI): <140%; TSH receptor antibodies (TRAb): <OR = 16%, microsomal thyroid peroxidase (TPO) antibody: ≤34 IU/ml; and 24 hours urine iodine: 70–500 mcg/24 h.

3. Cases Description

3.1. Patient 1. A 69-year-old male with a history of type 2 diabetes, hypertension, multinodular goiter (MNG) without compressive symptoms, and A fib was referred to our endocrine clinic given abnormal thyroid function tests. He had an automatic implantable cardioverter-defibrillator (AICD) implant, and he has been on amiodarone for almost 12 months to control his A fib. He denied any symptoms of hyperthyroidism. He was following with his cardiologist, and laboratory tests showed suppressed TSH <0.01 mU/l with high normal free T4 1.7 ng/dl, 6 months after starting the amiodarone. There was no documented baseline TSH prior to the amiodarone use. Repeat laboratory workup showed normal free T4 1.3 ng/dl and normal free T3 3.1 pg/ml with TSH <0.01 mU/l. Antibodies testing showed TSI <89%, TRAb 7%, and TPO antibody 31 IU/mL. A 24-hour urine iodine was ordered and came back elevated >1000 mcg/L, so ^{99m}-STS was ordered instead of RAIU to assess for AIT. The ^{99m}-STS showed intense initial intense uptake of the tracer activity within the thyroid parenchyma followed by a near complete washout in the 3-hour delayed images suggestive of AIT-1 (Figure 1). Thyroid ultrasound (US) showed diffusely enlarged (left more than right) thyroid gland with relatively isoechoic, predominantly solid nodules replacing the entire gland. Right lobe has dominant mid-upper pole nodule 3.7 × 1.9 × 2.2 cm. Two lower pole nodules measure 2.6 × 1.2 × 1.3 cm and 1.9 × 1.3 × 1.9 cm. Left lobe contains a dominant nodule measuring 7.1 × 5.1 × 5.7 cm. There was mild diffuse internal blood flow on CFDS. The patient was started on methimazole 10 mg tablets orally (PO) daily, and he was referred to endocrine surgery for total thyroidectomy given the large-size goiter and the worsening underlying cardiac condition. Pathology revealed multinodular colloid goiter with no evidence of malignancy. Afterward, thyroid function tests normalized. Amiodarone was continued to control his A fib.

3.2. Patient 2. A 62-year-old male with a history of non-ischemic cardiomyopathy and recurrent ventricular tachycardia (VT) status post-AICD implant 2 years before was admitted to an outside hospital with recurrent persistent VT. The patient was on amiodarone 200 mg PO daily for 1 year and then he was switched to sotalol around 10 months prior to the presentation. Baseline TSH was normal prior to the start of amiodarone. Laboratory workup showed free T4 2.83 ng/dl and TSH <0.005 mU/L. Thyroid US showed mild diffuse enlargement with no nodules. Methimazole 20 mg 4 times PO daily with metoprolol tartrate 100 mg twice PO daily were started without any further workup with a presumptive diagnosis of AIT-1. The patient presented to our hospital 3 months later with recurrent VT. Repeat laboratory workup showed free T4 5.06 ng/dl, TSH <0.01 mU/L, free T3 6 pg/ml with negative antibodies testing, TSI 113%, and TRAb 2%. The patient stated that he was compliant to his medications. Given the persistent hyperthyroidism despite high-dose methimazole, ^{99m}-STS was ordered. The ^{99m}-STS showed similar results to patient 1, suggesting AIT-1 (Figure 2). Methimazole was discontinued, and propylthiouracil 200 mg every 6 hours was started. After 10 days, repeat free T4 showed significant improvement (2.2 ng/dl) with normalization of free T3 at 3 pg/ml.

3.3. Patient 3. A 55-year-old female with a history of end-stage renal disease secondary to Goodpasture syndrome, secondary hyperparathyroidism, osteoporosis, MNG with multiple benign fine-needle aspiration (FNA) of different nodules, and amiodarone use for VT 100 mg daily for 1 year was referred to the endocrine clinic given symptoms of hyperthyroidism including weight loss, recurrent palpitations, tremors, and heat intolerance. Laboratory workup showed suppressed TSH 0.06 mU/L, high free T4 2.3 ng/dl, and normal free T3 2.6 pg/ml. Negative antibodies testing showed the following values: microsomal TPO antibody <10, TSI <89%, and TRAb <1%. Thyroid US showed enlarged multinodular goiter with normal vascularity of the thyroid gland on CFDS. The ^{99m}-STS showed intense initial intense uptake of the tracer activity within both thyroid lobes followed by a complete washout in the 2-hour delayed images suggestive of AIT-1 as observed in patients 1 and 2 (Figure 3). Methimazole 10 mg PO daily was started, and metoprolol 50 mg PO twice daily previously prescribed by the cardiologist was continued. Repeat thyroid function tests 2 months later showed normalization of free T4 and TSH. The patient continued to be on amiodarone to control the VT.

3.4. Patient 4. A 75-year-old female with a past medical history of persistent A Fib on amiodarone for 2 years that was stopped 5 months earlier presented to the emergency department with recurrent A fib and underwent ablation. She complained of recurrent palpitation with weight loss around 10 pounds in the last month despite having a very large appetite. She had a family history of Hashimoto's hypothyroidism in her father. Laboratory workup showed suppressed TSH 0.01 mU/L, slightly elevated free T4 1.75 ng/dl, normal free T3 3.2 pg/ml, mildly positive TSI 159% and negative TRAb <9 IU/l. Two months prior to the presentation, TSH was normal (1.85 mU/l). The patient had a computerized tomography angiogram with contrast 1 month prior to this presentation ordered by the cardiologist. Decision was to order ^{99m}-STS to assess for AIT. It showed no evidence of tracer labeling within the thyroid lobes at the initial 15 minutes' images and the 1-hour follow-up image confirming AIT-2 (Figure 4). Prednisone 40 mg PO daily was started leading to a significant improvement in the patient's symptoms. Prednisone was tapered off over a couple of months with a complete normalization of the thyroid function tests.

3.5. Patient 5. A 69-year-old male with a past medical history of A fib, type 2 diabetes, hypertension, and heart failure was admitted for recurrent A fib with rapid ventricular rate. Endocrinology service was consulted for suppressed TSH. He has been on amiodarone for 18 months prior to this admission. He complained of tremors and palpitations but no other symptoms related to hyperthyroidism. Physical examination was significant for resting tremors with a palpable mild goiter, but without discrete thyroid nodule or bruit. Laboratory testing showed TSH <0.004 uIU/mL, free T4 3.4 ng/dL, free T3 5.72 pg/mL, negative antibodies with TSI <89%, and TRAb <0.9 IU/L. Thyroid US showed mildly homogenously enlarged thyroid gland. CFDS showed absent vascularity. Based on the lack of underlying thyroid pathology and the absence of vascularity on US, prednisone 40 mg PO daily was started with a presumptive diagnosis of AIT-2.

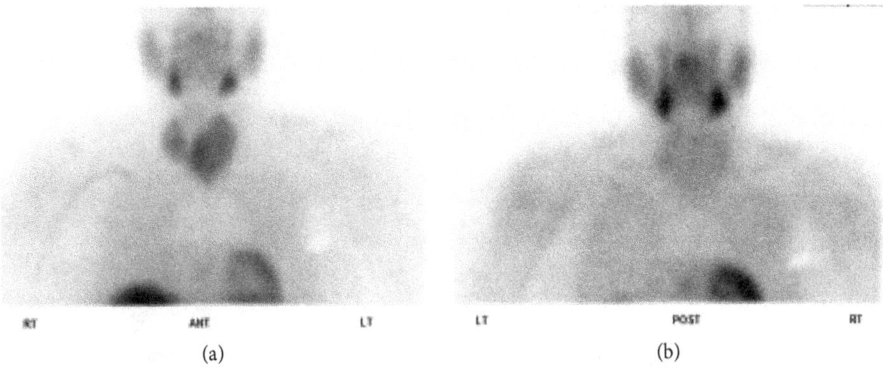

Figure 1: The ^{99m}-STS with a dose of 21.8 mCi showed intense initial uptake of the tracer activity within the thyroid parenchyma followed by a near complete washout in the 3-hour delayed images suggestive of AIT-1. In addition, there is diffuse enlargement of the thyroid gland (left more than right) and physiologic pattern of tracer distribution observed in the nasopharyngeal mucosa, salivary glands, and imaged parts of the liver and myocardium. A photopenic area in the left chest region correlates with the pacemaker. (a) 10 min postinjection; (b) 3 hr postinjection.

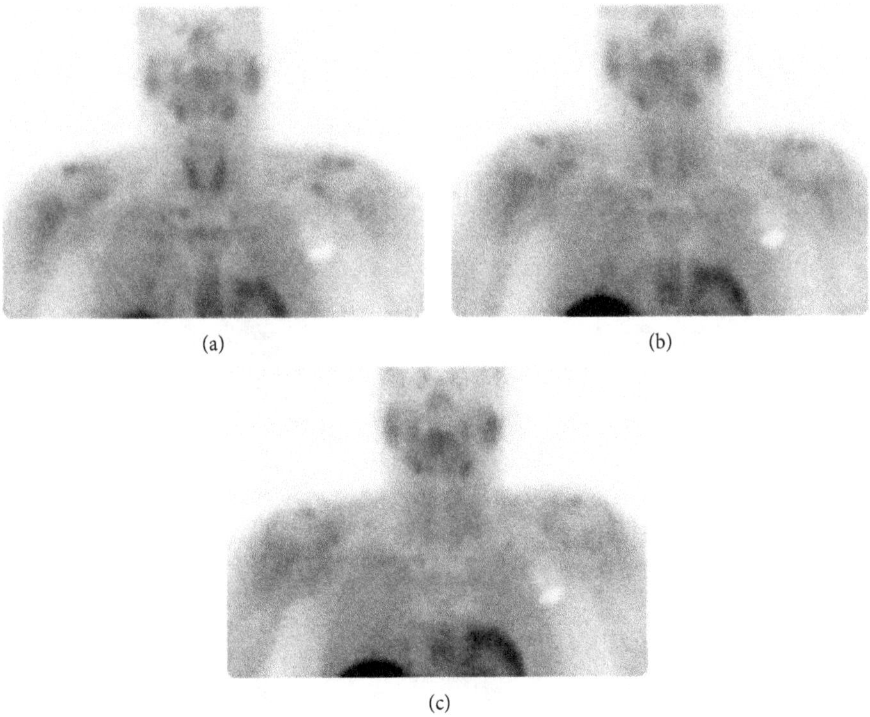

Figure 2: The ^{99m}-STS with a dose of 19.4 mCi showed intense initial intense uptake of the tracer activity within the thyroid parenchyma followed by bilateral symmetrical gradual washout of tracer activity in the 1-hour and 2-hour delayed images suggestive of AIT-1. (a) 15 min delay; (b) 1 hr delay; (c) 2 hr delay.

Given no improvement in the patient's clinical condition, repeated thyroid function tests were ordered, and it showed persistent hyperthyroid status with TSH <0.004, free T4 2.18, free T3 2.1, and 24 hours' urine iodine 2905 μg (100–460 ug/24 hours). ^{99m}-STS showed persistent activity in the right and left lobes of the slightly enlarged thyroid gland at 10 minutes, unchanged from the 2-minute image and declining at 60 minutes' compatible with AIT-1 (Figure 5). Prednisone dose was tapered, and methimazole 20 mg daily was initiated. Over the 4-month period, he was on methimazole, and the patient was demonstrating clinical and biochemical improvement with normalization of thyroid function tests. Amiodarone was continued as per cardiology recommendation. Table 1 summarize the 5 cases.

4. Discussion

Amiodarone is an iodine-rich antiarrhythmic agent used by cardiologists in the treatment of multiple conditions. Treated patients invariably have underlying heart diseases, which can

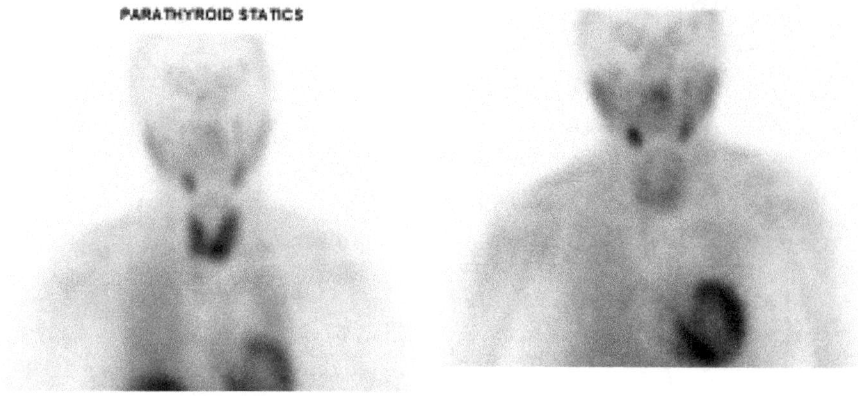

(a) (b)

Figure 3: ^{99m}-STS with a dose of 19.43 mCi showed an intense initial intense uptake of the tracer activity within both thyroid lobes (a) followed by a complete washout in the 2-hour delayed images (b) suggestive of AIT-1.

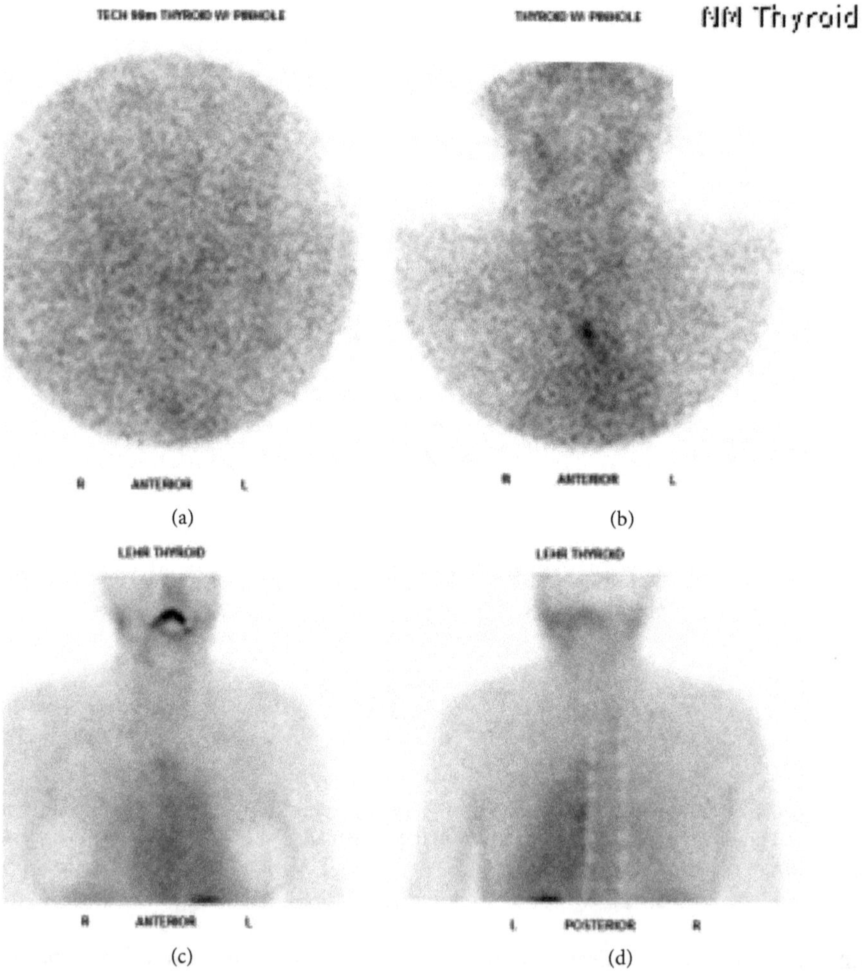

Figure 4: ^{99m}-STS showed failure of localization of the tracer within the thyroid gland, by imaging criteria suggesting destructive effect of amiodarone to the function of the gland and confirming AIT-2 (a, b) 15 minutes delay high- and low-resolution images. (c, d) 1 hour delayed anterior and posterior images.

deteriorate in the setting of hyperthyroidism secondary to AIT raising a concern of an increase in these patient's morbidity and mortality. Given the pharmacological drug composition, around 15–20% of the patients on amiodarone will develop thyroid dysfunction including either AIT or AIH. The iodine intake plays a key role in developing amiodarone-induced thyroid dysfunction. This explains the increased prevalence of AIH in iodine-replete and AIT in iodine-

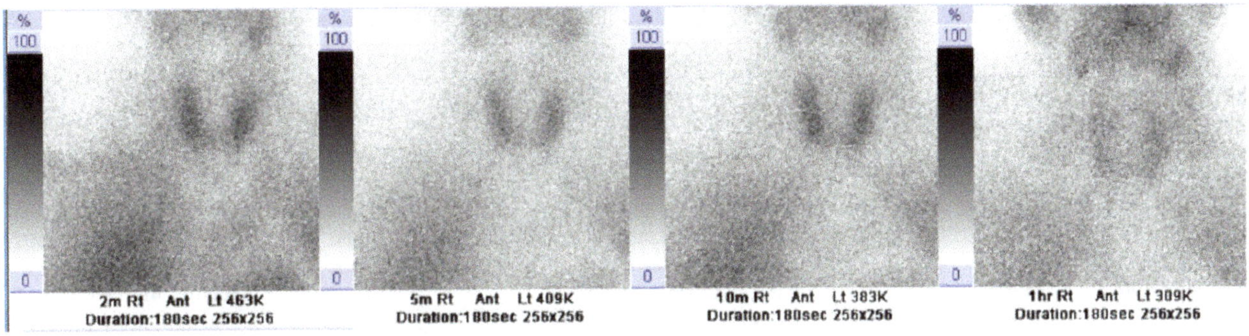

FIGURE 5: ^{99m}-STS with a dose of 24.9 mCi demonstrating persistent activity in the right and left lobes of the slightly enlarged thyroid gland at 10 minutes, declining at 60 minutes' image confirming diagnosis of AIT-1.

TABLE 1: Summary of the patient's duration of amiodarone use and biochemical and radiological workup.

Patient	TSH	Free T4	Free T3	TRAb	TSI	Thyroid US	^{99m}-STS	Duration of amiodarone use prior to presentation
Patient 1	<0.001	1.3	3.1	Negative	Negative	MNG	AIT-1	1 year
Patient 2	<0.01	5.06	6	Negative	Negative	Mild diffuse enlargement	AIT-1	1 year
Patient 3	0.06	2.3	2.6	Negative	Negative	MNG (multiple benign FNA)	AIT-1	1 year
Patient 4	0.01	1.75	3.2	Negative	Mildly positive	Not done	AIT-2	2 years
Patient 5	<0.004	3.4	5.72	Negative	Negative	Mild diffuse enlargement	AIT-1	18 months

deficient geographical area [1, 15]. The pathophysiology of AIT-1 is explained by an excessive thyroidal hormone synthesis and release induced by the iodine load in patients with underlying thyroid autonomy (nodular or diffuse goiter or latent Graves' disease). This iodide-induced thyrotoxicosis is an example of the Jod–Basedow phenomenon seen in patients with endemic iodine-deficient goiter who are given iodide replacement, thus explaining why thyrotoxicosis is more common in iodine depleted areas. However, AIT-2 is a consequence of a destructive process in patients with normal thyroid gland [3–6]. The differentiation between AIT-1 and AIT-2 is an important prerequisite for the correct therapeutic choice to avoid unnecessary use of combined medications; thus, different modalities have been used including clinical, biochemical, and radiological imaging (Table 2).

The presence of thyroid antibodies can be misleading. Positive TRAb, TPO, or thyroglobulin antibodies usually point toward AIT-1 as they indicate underlying thyroid autoimmune disease. However, the presence of positive titers does not rule out AIT-2. Therefore, further imaging studies are required for the complete workup of AIT in these patients [15, 16, 19, 20]. This has occurred in patient 4 who had a mildly positive TSI 159% (reference 140%) in the setting of positive family history of Hashimotos' hypothyroidism in his father; however, the ^{99m}-STS showed AIT-2 with a good response to prednisone 40 mg. We should keep in consideration that these antibodies can be positive in patients with a family history of autoimmune disease, and these patients need a close follow-up. Regarding the other 4 patients, all of them had negative antibody titers which was not helpful in the diagnosis. Thyroid US in patients 1 and 3 showed multinodular goiter, while patients 2 and 5 showed only mild diffuse enlargement of the thyroid. As explained before, the patients with MNG have a higher risk for AIT-1. CFDS can also be misleading sometimes as in patient 5. It showed absent vascularity which led to the diagnosis of AIT-2. Given no response to the treatment, ^{99m}-STS was ordered which was able to give an accurate diagnosis. To sum up, the ^{99m}-STS was a helpful tool in confirming the diagnosis in all of these patients.

Upon review of the literature, initially, in 2008, ^{99m}-STS was described by Piga et al. in a series of 20 patients as being superior to all other diagnostic tests for differentiating AIT subtypes and, in particular, is the only test capable of prospectively identifying AIT [17]. The rationale behind the use of ^{99m}-STS lies in that sestaMIBI is accumulated by mitochondria-rich cells, whereas necrotic and apoptotic tissues are unable to take up the sestaMIBI tracer because their mitochondrial membrane potential has collapsed. Hence, this explained the increased retention in hyperfunctioning thyroid tissue as a result of increased mitochondrial numbers in hypermetabolic cells in AIT-1 and the absent of tracer uptake in AIT-2. When a qualitative assessment of the ^{99m}-STS image is clearly compatible with AIT-1 or AIT-2, the diagnosis is extremely accurate, and patients can be treated accordingly. Pattison et al. in 2015 reported that the use of quantitative TBR improves the interobserver reliability of reporting ^{99m}-STS for investigation of different types of AIT [19]. When the qualitative assessment suggests a mixed form, Censi et al. in 2018

Table 2: Summary of clinical, biochemical, and radiological imaging differentiation between AIT-1 and AIT-2 [1–19].

Modalities	AIT-1	AIT-2
Underlying thyroid disease	Yes (Graves' disease or MNG)	No
Time after starting amiodarone	Short (median 3 months)	Long (median 30 months)
Thyroid antibodies including TSI, TRAb, microsomal TPO antibodies	May be positive	Usually absent
RAIU	Low/normal/increased (uptake can be inhibited in high intrathyroidal iodine concentration and increased in iodine-deficient regions)	Low/absent
Circulating IL-6	Normal to high	Frequently marked elevated
T4/T3 ratio	Usually <4	Usually >4
Thyroid US	Diffuse or nodular goiter	Normal or small thyroid
CFDS	Increased	Absent
^{99m}-STS	Increased uptake in the thyroid in the initial images followed by washout in the delayed images	Absent uptake in the thyroid in the initial and delayed images

Table 3: Summary of the different literature using ^{99m}-STS in AIT.

Study	Type of the study	Number of patients	Country	Results
Piga et al. [17]	Prospective	20 patients	Italy	^{99m}-STS can be proposed as an easy and highly effective diagnostic tool for the differential diagnosis of AIT, with positive persistent scans in AIT-1 and negligible uptake in AIT-2. It appears also to give some insights into indeterminate forms of AI. ^{99m}-STS is superior to all other diagnostic tools including CFDS and RAIU.
Oki et al. [24]	Prospective	23 patients on amiodarone for more than 4 months (4 out of 23 patients had AIT)	Brazil	^{99m}-STS may be an alternative tracer for thyroid scintigraphy and uptake measurement of patients on chronic use of amiodarone. ^{99m}-STS seems to be better than Tc-99m pertechnetate for the scintigraphic evaluation of the thyroid in euthyroid and hyperthyroid patients.
Souto et al. [22]	Case report	1 patient	Portugal	^{99m}-STS used to diagnosis undetermined AIT.
Pattison et al. [19]	Retrospective	15 patients	Australia	Use of quantitative TBR improves the interobserver reliability of reporting ^{99m}-STS for investigation of different types of AIT.
Patel et al. [21]	Case report	1 patient	Houston	^{99m}-STS used to diagnosis AIT-1 in addition to the RAIU.
Victor et al. [23]	Case report	1 patient	Portugal	^{99m}-STS used to diagnosis undetermined AIT.
Wang and Zhang [18]	Prospective	15 patients	China	^{99m}-STS imaging alone can accurately distinguish types I and II and mixed-type AIT.
Censi et al. [8]	Retrospective	30 patients	Italy	^{99m}-STS combined with the TBR proved a very useful approach to the classification of AIT, enabling patients to be offered appropriate treatment as soon as they are diagnosed. It has 100% specificity and 91.7% sensitivity in differentiating different types of AIT.

recommended applying the TBR: a value below the cut-off of 0.482 is indicative of AIT-2, while a higher value suggests a genuine mixed type of thyrotoxicosis [8]. Few case reports and studies have been documented in the literature regarding the utility of ^{99m}-STS in AIT, but no large prospective studies have been established yet [21–24] (Table 3).

There are some advantages of ^{99m}-STS in comparison to CFDS and RAIU. Differences in populations' iodine supply have often been mentioned as one of the main reasons for the poor reproducibility of CFDS and RAIU [15, 16]. However, prior studies showed that ^{99m}-STS results were not affected by different geographical distributions in either iodine-deficient areas (like Censi et al. in north east Italy) or iodine sufficient areas (like Piga et al. in Sardinia Italy and Wang et al. in China) [8, 17, 18]. The short duration of the test (1 hour in comparison to 24 hours needed in RAIU) and the short half-life of the pure gamma emitter tracer Tc-99m (6 hours) make ^{99m}-STS a superior diagnostic study in comparison to the conventional methods used for the diagnosis of AIT. Additionally, Tc-99m is much safer than the gamma and beta emitter I 131 used in RAIU scintigraphy [8].

AIT-2 is usually a self-limited disease, and patients become euthyroid in 3–5 months. However, given the underlying cardiac disease and the fear of the deterioration of the clinical condition especially in elder population and in patients with left ventricular dysfunction, early treatment to achieve euthyroidism is usually required. Prednisone is considered the most effective treatment in AIT-2 given the anti-inflammatory and membrane stabilization effect. However, thionamides, with or without potassium or sodium perchlorate, are used in AIT-1 in addition to beta-blockers for heart rate and adrenergic symptoms control. The mechanism of action of these medications is to block the thyroid hormones production and deplete the intrathyroidal iodine stores in patients with underlying thyroid diseases. These medications are ineffective in AIT-2; however, they can be used in combination with steroids in AIT-3 (mixed AIT) when the diagnosis is inconclusive [2, 7]. We described different patients with different scenarios. Interestingly, patient 2 was resistant to methimazole treatment, so switching to propylthiouracil after confirming the diagnosis of AIT-1 with ^{99m}-STS was the appropriate approach. There was significant improvement in his clinical condition afterward. This implies the importance of making the correct diagnosis in these patients to avoid unnecessary and potentially dangerous combined overtreatment. According to the European Thyroid Association 2018 guidelines, total thyroidectomy without delay is recommended in AIT patients with deterioration of the cardiac function or when they are unresponsive to the medical therapy [7]. Patient 1 had large MNG in the setting of deterioration of his medical condition, and he underwent total thyroidectomy. Improvement in the patient's clinical condition was noticed afterward.

5. Conclusion

^{99m}-STS imaging is a valuable method for the diagnosis and classification of AIT. It can distinguish different types of AITs especially the mixed-types which are usually difficult to cure. ^{99m}-STS has shown great advantages over the conventional methods. Further large prospective studies are required.

Abbreviation

AIH: Amiodarone-induced hypothyroidism
AIT: Amiodarone-induced thyrotoxicosis
AIT-1: Amiodarone-induced thyrotoxicosis type 1
AIT-2: Amiodarone-induced thyrotoxicosis type 2
AIT-3: AIT type 3
A fib: Atrial fibrillation
CRP: C-reactive protein
CFDS: Color flow Doppler sonography
DEA: Desethylamiodarone
ESR: Erythrocyte sedimentation rate
FNA: Fine-needle aspiration
IL-6: Interleukin-6
MNG: Multinodular goiter
PO: Orally
RAIU: Radioactive iodine uptake scan
TBR: Target to background ratio
TSH: Thyroid-stimulating hormone
T4: Thyroxine
T3: Triiodothyronine
TSI: Thyroid-stimulating immunoglobulin
TRAb: TSH receptor antibodies
TPO: Thyroid peroxidase
US: Ultrasound
VT: Ventricular tachycardia
^{99m}-STS: ^{99m}Tc-Methoxy-isobutyl-isonitrile (sestaMIBI) uptake on scintigraphy.

Authors' Contributions

All authors read and approved the manuscript before submission.

References

[1] T. A. lomp, J. M. van Rossum, E. O. Robles de Medina et al., "Pharmacokinetics and body distribution of amiodarone in man," *Arzneimittelforschung*, vol. 34, pp. 513–520, 1984.

[2] S. A. Eskes and W. M. Wiersinga, "Amiodarone and thyroid," *Best Practice & Research Clinical Endocrinology & Metabolism*, vol. 23, no. 6, pp. 735–751, 2009.

[3] R. H. Rao, V. R. McCready, and G. S. Spathis, "Iodine kinetic studies during amiodarone treatment," *The Journal of Clinical Endocrinology & Metabolism*, vol. 62, no. 3, pp. 563–568, 1986.

[4] J. A. Franklyn, J. R. Davis, M. D. Gammage, W. A. Littler, D. B. Ramsden, and M. C. Sheppard, "Amiodarone and thyroid hormone action jayne a," *Clinical Endocrinology*, vol. 22, no. 3, pp. 257–264, 1985.

[5] H. C. Van Beeren, O. Bakker, and W. M. Wiersinga, "Structure-function relationship of the inhibition of the 3,5,3′-triiodothyronine binding to the alpha1- and beta1-thyroid hormone receptor by amiodarone analogs," *Endocrinology*, vol. 137, no. 7, pp. 2807–2814, 1996.

[6] E. Roti, R. Minelli, E. Gardini et al., "Thyrotoxicosis followed by hypothyroidism in patients treated with amiodarone. A possible consequence of a destructive process in the thyroid," *Archives of Internal Medicine*, vol. 153, no. 7, pp. 886–892, 1993.

[7] L. Bartalena, F. Bogazzi, L. Chiovato, A. Hubalewska-Dydejczyk, T. P. Links, and M. Vanderpump, "2018 European thyroid association (ETA) guidelines for the management of amiodarone-associated thyroid dysfunction," *European Thyroid Journal*, vol. 7, no. 2, pp. 55–66, 2018.

[8] S. Censi, V. Bodanza, J. Manso et al., "Amiodarone-induced thyrotoxicosis," *Clinical Nuclear Medicine*, vol. 43, no. 9, pp. 655–662, 2018.

[9] C. M. Newman, A. Price, D. W. Davies, T. A. Gray, and A. P. Weetman, "Amiodarone and the thyroid: a practical guide to the management of thyroid dysfunction induced by

amiodarone therapy," *Heart*, vol. 79, no. 2, pp. 121–127, 1998 Feb.

[10] L. Bartalena, L. Grasso, S. Brogioni, F. Aghini-Lombardi, L. E. Braverman, and E. Martino, "Serum interleukin-6 in amiodarone-induced thyrotoxicosis," *The Journal of Clinical Endocrinology & Metabolism*, vol. 78, no. 2, pp. 423–427, 1994.

[11] G. H. Daniels, "Amiodarone-induced thyrotoxicosis," *The Journal of Clinical Endocrinology & Metabolism*, vol. 86, no. 1, pp. 3–8, 2001.

[12] W. Tsang and R. L. Houlden, "Amiodarone-induced thyrotoxicosis: a review," *Canadian Journal of Cardiology*, vol. 25, no. 7, pp. 421–424, 2009.

[13] F. Bogazzi, E. Martino, E. Dell'Unto et al., "Thyroid color flow Doppler sonography and radioiodine uptake in 55 consecutive patients with amiodarone-induced thyrotoxicosis," *Journal of Endocrinological Investigation*, vol. 26, no. 7, pp. 635–640, 2003.

[14] S. E. M. Eaton, H. A. Euinton, C. M. Newman, A. P. Weetman, and W. M. Bennet, "Clinical experience of amiodarone-induced thyrotoxicosis over a 3-year period: role of colour-flow Doppler sonography," *Clinical Endocrinology*, vol. 56, no. 1, pp. 33–38, 2002.

[15] E. Martino, L. Bartalena, F. Bogazzi, and L. E. Braverman, "The effects of amiodarone on the thyroid," *Endocrine Reviews*, vol. 22, no. 2, pp. 240–254, 2001.

[16] F. Bogazzi, L. Bartalena, and E. Martino, "Approach to the patient with amiodarone-induced thyrotoxicosis," *The Journal of Clinical Endocrinology & Metabolism*, vol. 95, no. 6, pp. 2529–2535, 2010.

[17] M. Piga, M. C. Cocco, A. Serra, F. Boi, M. Loy, and S. Mariotti, "The usefulness of ^{99m}Tc-sestaMIBI thyroid scan in the differential diagnosis and management of amiodarone-induced thyrotoxicosis," *European Journal of Endocrinology*, vol. 159, no. 4, pp. 423–429, 2008.

[18] J. Wang and R. Zhang, "Evaluation of ^{99m}Tc-MIBI in thyroid gland imaging for the diagnosis of amiodarone-induced thyrotoxicosis," *The British Journal of Radiology*, vol. 90, no. 1071, Article ID 20160836, 2017.

[19] D. A. Pattison, J. Westcott, M. Lichtenstein et al., "Quantitative assessment of thyroid-to-background ratio improves the interobserver reliability of technetium-^{99m} sestamibi thyroid scintigraphy for investigation of amiodarone-induced thyrotoxicosis," *Nuclear Medicine Communications*, vol. 36, no. 4, pp. 356–362, 2015.

[20] L. Bartalena, W. M. Wiersinga, M. L. Tanda et al., "Diagnosis and management of amiodarone-induced thyrotoxicosis in Europe: results of an international survey among members of the European Thyroid Association," *Clinical Endocrinology*, vol. 61, no. 4, pp. 494–502, 2004.

[21] N. R. Patel, L. A. Tamara, and H. Lee, "^{99m}Tc sestamibi thyroid scan in amiodarone-induced thyrotoxicosis type I," *Clinical Nuclear Medicine*, vol. 41, no. 7, pp. 566-567, 2016.

[22] S. B. Souto, H. Fernandes, M. J. Matos, D. C. Braga, J. Pereira, and D. Carvalho, "Importance of ^{99m}Tc-sestaMIBI thyroid scan in a case of amiodarone-induced thyrotoxicosis," *Arquivos Brasileiros de Endocrinologia & Metabologia*, vol. 55, no. 7, pp. 486–489, 2011.

[23] M. Victor, A. G. Ferreira, S. Carmona et al., "The role of ^{99m}Tc-sestamibi in amiodarone-induced thyrotoxicosis—case report," *Endocrine Abstracts*, vol. 49, Article ID EP1298, 2017.

[24] G. C. R. Oki, D. E. Zantut-Wittmann, A. de Oliveira Santos et al., "Tc-^{99m} sestamibi thyroid imaging in patients on chronic amiodarone treatment," *Clinical Nuclear Medicine*, vol. 35, no. 4, pp. 223–227, 2010.

16

Hereditary Hypercalcemia Caused by a Homozygous Pathogenic Variant in the *CYP24A1* Gene: A Case Report and Review of the Literature

Daniele Cappellani,[1] Alessandro Brancatella,[1] Martin Kaufmann,[2] Angelo Minucci,[3] Edda Vignali,[1] Domenico Canale,[1] Elisa De Paolis,[3] Ettore Capoluongo,[3,4] Filomena Cetani,[1] Glenville Jones,[2] and Claudio Marcocci[1]

[1]*Department of Clinical and Experimental Medicine, Unit of Endocrinology, University of Pisa, Pisa, Italy*
[2]*Department of Biomedical and Molecular Sciences, Queen's University, Kingston, ON, Canada*
[3]*Fondazione Policlinico Universitario A. Gemelli IRCCS, Roma, Italy*
[4]*Università Cattolica del Sacro Cuore, Roma, Italy*

Correspondence should be addressed to Claudio Marcocci; claudio.marcocci@med.unipi.it

Academic Editor: Mihail A. Boyanov

Introduction. Loss of function mutations of CYP24A1 gene, which is involved in vitamin D catabolism, cause vitamin D-mediated PTH-independent hypercalcemia. The phenotype varies from life-threatening forms in the infancy to milder forms in the adulthood. *Case Presentation.* We report a case of a 17-year-old woman with a history of nephrolithiasis, mild PTH-independent hypercalcemia (10,5mg/dL), and high serum 1,25$(OH)_2$D concentrations (107pg/mL). Other causes of hypercalcemia associated with the above biochemical signature were excluded. Family history revealed nephrolithiasis in the sister. Blood testing in first-degree relatives showed serum PTH in the low-normal range and 1,25$(OH)_2$D at the upper normal limit or slightly elevated. The CYP24A1 gene analysis revealed a known homozygous loss-of-function pathogenic variant (c.428_430delAAG, rs777676129, p.Glu143del). The panel of vitamin D metabolites evaluated by liquid chromatography showed the typical profile of CYP24A1 mutations, namely, low 24,25$(OH)_2D_3$, elevated 25$(OH)D_3$:24,25$(OH)_2D_3$ ratio, and undetectable 1,24,25$(OH)_3D_3$. The parents and both the siblings harbored the same variant in heterozygosis. We decided for a watchful waiting approach and the patient remained clinically and biochemically stable over a 24-month followup. *Conclusion. CYP24A1* gene mutations should be considered in cases of PTH-independent hypercalcemia, once that more common causes (hypercalcemia of malignancy, granulomatous diseases, and vitamin D intoxication) have been ruled out.

1. Introduction

Pathogenic variants (PVs) in the human cytochrome P450 24 subfamily A member 1 (*CYP24A1*) gene are associated with Idiopathic Infantile Hypercalcemia (IIH, OMIM 143880), a rare disease recently related to vitamin D catabolism impairment [1]. The *CYP24A1* gene encodes a 24-hydroxylase enzyme, which catalyzes the degradation of the active form of vitamin D, 1,25-dihydroxyvitamin D [1,25$(OH)_2$D] by multiple pathways [2]. *CYP24A1* loss of function leads to an increase in serum 1,25$(OH)_2$D concentration, which may be associated with various degrees of hypercalcemia and hypercalciuria and low-or-undetectable plasma parathyroid hormone (PTH) levels. The phenotype of IIH embraces a wide range of clinical scenarios [3], from severe forms diagnosed early in the infancy (severe hypercalcemia associated with dehydration, vomiting, nephrocalcinosis, and sometimes death) [4] to milder forms, often diagnosed in the adulthood during workout for recurrent nephrolithiasis [5]. Since the recognition in 2011[1] that PVs in *CYP24A1* are responsible for IIH, a large number of cases have been reported, leading to an increased insight into the diagnostic and therapeutic management of this disease [6, 7].

Table 1: Clinical and biochemical data at admission to our clinic.

Analyte	Result	Normal adult reference range
Total calcium (mg/dL)	10.5	8.6-10.2
Ionized calcium (mmol/L)	1.35-1.36-1.45*	1.13-1.32
Phospate (mg/dL)	3.1	2.7-4.5
Magnesium (mg/dL)	2.02	1.7-2.2
Albumin (g/dL)	4.6	3.6-5.2
PTH (pg/mL)	< 4-7*	8-40
Calcitonin (pg/mL)	< 2	< 11.5
25-hydroxy vitamin D (ng/mL) §	30.3	
1,25-dihydroxyvitamin D (pg/mL) ∫	107	20-67
Osteocalcin (ng/mL)	61.6	6.8-34
Bone-specific alcaline phophatase (mcg/L)	23	2-20
Carboxy-terminal collagen crosslinks (ng/mL)	1.042	0.112-0.738
Urine calcium (mg/24h)	150-410-455*	100-321
Urine phosphates (mg/24h)	697-875*	400-1300
Urine magnesium (mg/24h)	140-164*	60-120
Creatinine (mg/dL)	0.69-0.72*	0.5-0.9
Urine creatinine (mg/24h)	1050-1085-1148*	740-1570
Angiotensin converting enzyme (U/L)	80	65.8-114.4

*When available, repeated measures are reported

§: 25(OH)D was assayed at University of Pisa laboratory as total 25(OH)D (i.e. the sum of $25(OH)D_2 + 25(OH)D_3$) using a chemiluminescence immunoassay (IDS-iSYS, Immunodiagnostic systems, Boldon, Tyne and Wear, UK)

∫: $1,25(OH)_2D$ was assayed at University of Pisa laboratory as total $1,25(OH)_2D$ (i.e. the sum of $1,25(OH)_2D_2 + 1,25(OH)_2D_3$) using a radioimmunoassay (IDS, Immunodiagnostic systems, Boldon, Tyne and Wear, UK)

Herein we describe a case of recurrent nephrolithiasis and moderate PTH-independent hypercalcemia of undetermined origin referred to our outpatient clinic for further investigation. The familial nature of hypercalcemia prompted us to search for genetic causes and we identified a loss of function variant in the *CYP24A1* gene.

2. Case Presentation

A 17-year-old woman was referred to the Endocrine Unit of the University Hospital of Pisa for further evaluation of hypercalcemia associated with undetectable/low PTH levels.

Her clinical history was unremarkable except for a previous admission to the local Emergency Unit for renal colic 3 years before; an abdominal ultrasound revealed unilateral kidney stones. On that occasion, the patient was treated with analgesics and hydration and no further investigations were performed. One year later she underwent extracorporeal shockwave lithotripsy for the recurrence of renal colics. At that time, routine blood tests revealed hypercalcemia [12.4 mg/dL; (reference range 8.4-10.2)], hypercalciuria [390 mg/24h, (100-300)], and undetectable PTH (< 4 pg/mL; NV 8-40) and a 25-hydroxyvitamin D [25(OH)D] level of 37.4 ng/mL. The family history was unremarkable with the exception of nephrolithiasis in the sister.

At admission, physical examination was normal, with no evidence of major bone abnormalities. Lab tests confirmed hypercalcemia, hypercalciuria, and low/undetectable PTH levels; bone turnover markers were slightly above the upper limit of adult reference range (Table 1). Routine biochemistry was normal. Chest X-ray and abdominal and neck ultrasound were unremarkable. The long lasting hypercalcemia, the negative medical history beyond nephrolithiasis, and the normal imaging studies made unlikely the hypothesis of paraneoplastic hypercalcemia. Further evaluation revealed elevated serum levels of $1,25(OH)_2D$ suggesting vitamin D-dependent hypercalcemia. A granulomatous disease could be ruled out on the basis of normal serum concentration of angiotensin converting enzyme and the absence of specific signs at chest X-rays.

Because of the young age of the patient and the family history of nephrolithiasis, biochemical tests were performed in first-degree relatives. Total and ionized serum calcium, phosphate, PTH, and $1,25(OH)_2D$ levels were in the normal range in both parents, who had a low vitamin D status. Interestingly, in the siblings PTH concentration was in the low-normal range and $1,25(OH)_2D$ at the upper normal limit or slightly elevated (Table 2). The latter findings, together with the biochemical profile of the patient, suggested that hypercalcemia might be due to an impairment of the CYP24A1 catabolic pathway. The genetic analysis in the proband was made using High Resolution Melting Analysis (HRMA) [8] and further confirmed using gene amplification and sequencing [9], revealing a known homozygous PV (c.428_430delAAG, rs777676129, p.Glu143del) in the *CYP24A1* gene (Figure 1(a)). The same heterozygous variant was detected in the parents

TABLE 2: Clinical and biochemical findings in the patient's first degree family members.

	I.1	I.2	II.1	II.2
Age (years)	52	53	26	20
History of nephrolithiasis	No	No	Yes	No
Total calcium (mg/dL)	10	9.8	9.9	9.8
Ionized calcium (mmol/L)	1.28	1.23	1.29	1.26
Phosphate (mg/dL)	3.6	2.9	3.9	3.1
PTH (pg/mL)	17	18	11	8
25 hydroxyvitamin D (ng/mL)	7.8	17.3	28.4	22.5
1,25- dihydroxyvitamin D (pg/mL)	39	37	72	66

The reported values are the mean of two independent samples collected in two consecutive days. For family member identification see Figure 1(b). See Table 1 for the normal adult reference range at our laboratory and details about 25(OH)D and $1,25(OH)_2D$ assays.

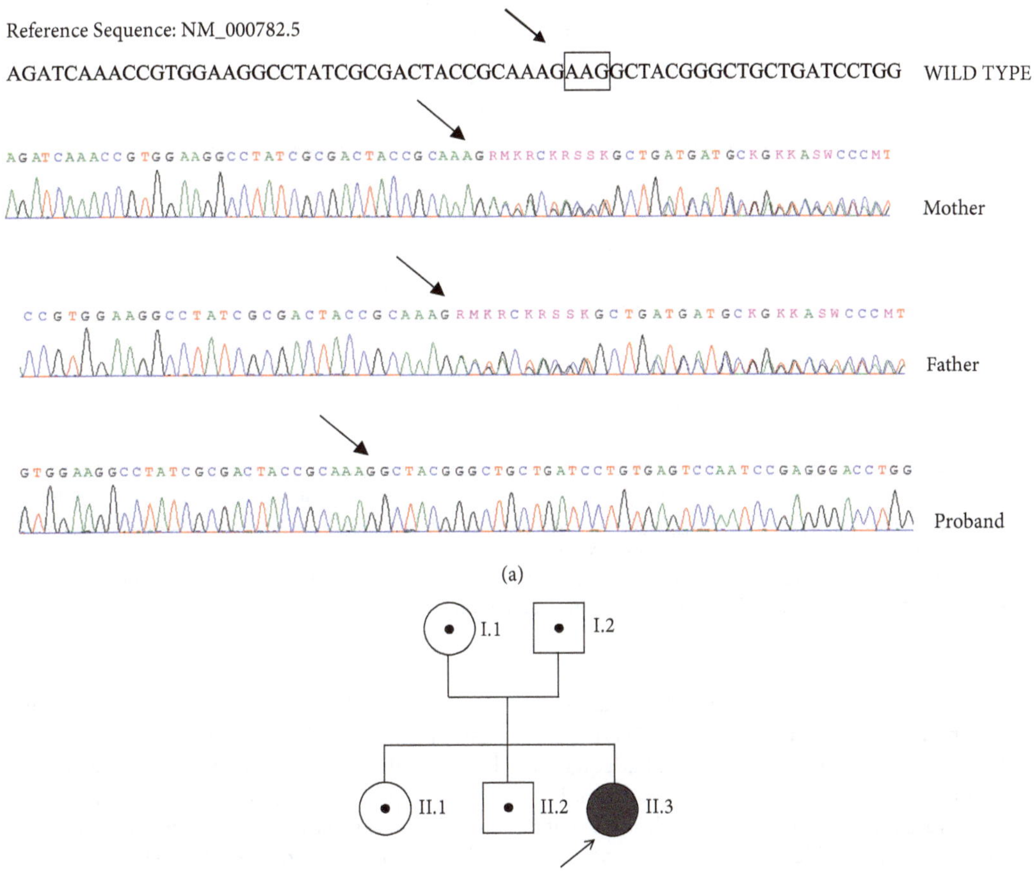

(a)

(b)

FIGURE 1: (a) Sequences of the *CYP24A1* exon 2 obtained by proband and her parents. *CYP24A1* gene amplification and sequencing were performed as reported. Sequences of the exon 2 obtained by proband and her parents were shown. Arrows indicate the position of *c.428_430delAAG* heterozygous and homozygous variant in the parents and the proband, respectively. (b) Family tree.

and the siblings (Figure 1(b)). The parents excluded consanguinity, even though they came from the same small village.

To complete the biochemical profile of vitamin D metabolites, liquid chromatography tandem mass spectrometry (LC-MS/MS) was run on stored serum samples of all the family members. Serum samples were prepared by immunoextraction and derivatized with 4-[2-(6,7-dimethoxy-4-methyl-3,4-dihydroquinoxalinyl)ehtyl]-1,2,4-triazoline-3,5-dione (DMEQ-TAD), as reported [10]. We observed that the proband exhibited low $24,25(OH)_2D_3$ (0.42 ng/mL) and elevated $25(OH)D_3$:$24,25(OH)_2D_3$ ratio (118; cutoff >80) which confirmed the diagnosis of impaired CYP24A1 function. A more rigorous chromatographic method[11] was also used to assay the same sample ($25(OH)D_3$:$24,25(OH)_2D_3$ ratio = 3117; cutoff>140), which also indicated inappropriately low levels of $24,25(OH)_2D_3$ in the proband. The other family members, who present as heterozygous variants, exhibited essentially normal serum $24,25(OH)_2D_3$ concentrations and $25(OH)D_3$:$24,25(OH)_2D_3$ ratios (Table 3 and Figure 2).

Table 3: Liquid chromatography tandem mass spectrometry analysis results.

	I.1	I.2	II.1	II.2	II.3
$25(OH)D_3$ (ng/mL)	13.16	28.88	38.03	28.25	49.87
$24,25(OH)_2D_3$ (ng/mL)	0.44	1.14	1.94	1.66	0.02
$25(OH)D_3:24,25(OH)_2D_3$ ratio	30.1	25.4	19.6	17.1	3117
$1,25(OH)_2D_3$ (pg/mL)	41.1	37.4	66.9	66.6	118.4
$1,24,25(OH)_3D_3$ (pg/mL)	6.5	7.7	16.9	21.4	< 2

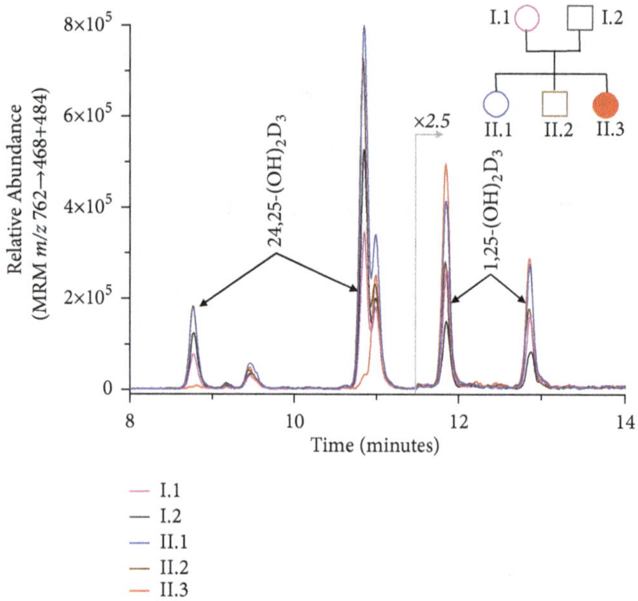

Figure 2: LC-MS/MS chromatogram of dihydroxylated vitamin D metabolites. Serum samples were prepared by immunoextraction and derivatized with DMEQ-TAD. Peaks corresponding to 6S and 6R isomers of DMEQ-TAD adducts of $24,25(OH)_2D_3$ and $1,25(OH)_2D_3$ were observed using the multiple reaction monitoring (MRM) transition of mass/charge (m/z) 762.3-->468.1+484.1, from which serum concentrations of these metabolites were determined. The figure reveals the dramatically reduced concentration of $24,25(OH)_2D_3$ in the proband II.3 as well as elevated $1,25(OH)_2D_3$, in comparison to unaffected family members.

Because of the mild hypercalcemia, we did not advise pharmacologic treatments aimed at modulating $1,25(OH)_2D$ metabolism and we recommended maintenance of adequate hydration and avoidance of unprotected excessive sunlight exposure. Followup evaluation up to 24 months showed that the patient was in an overall stable condition, with serum calcium concentration slightly above the upper normal limit and renal ultrasound showing no recurrent nephrolithiasis.

The patient and the family gave written informed consent for the genetic analysis and the use of their clinical data for scientific purposes, including publication.

3. Discussion

Hypercalcemia is a common disorder, with a prevalence of 1/500 patient in the outpatient setting[12]. Primary hyperparathyroidism is the most common cause of hypercalcemia [13]. Vitamin D-induced hypercalcemia is a heterogeneous group of diseases that includes vitamin D intoxication, granulomatous diseases, and abnormalities of vitamin D metabolism. Hypercalcemia due to loss of function variants in the *CYP24A1* gene is a genetic disorder recently described in patients with IIH [1]. Nowadays the name "idiopathic infantile hypercalcemia" is considered a misnomer [6], because in most patients a genetic cause can be identified (namely, a loss-of-function mutation in the *CYP24A1* or in the *SCL34A1* or large deletions on chromosome 7 causing the Williams-Beuren syndrome), and the clinical phenotype is no longer confined to infancy.

Vitamin D is mainly produced in the skin or supplied by dietary sources. It undergoes an initial activation by 25-hydroxylation in the liver, catalyzed by CYP2R1, thus generating 25(OH)D. A second hydroxylation by 1α-hydroxylase (CYP27B1) takes place mainly in the kidney, but also in several extrarenal tissues, and converts 25(OH)D to $1,25(OH)_2D$, the active form of vitamin D [14]. The *CYP24A1* gene, located at 20q13.2, encodes the cytochrome P450 component of the mitochondrial 24-hydroxylase enzyme, which catalyzes the degradation of 25(OH)D and $1,25(OH)_2D$ into the multistep 24-oxidation pathway to calcitroic acid [15, 16]. The *CYP24A1* gene has been cloned in animals [17, 18] and humans [19]. Its expression is induced by vitamin D receptor agonists [20] by interacting with a vitamin D response element in the promoter of the gene [18]. Furthermore, many hormones involved in bone mineral metabolism regulate the CYP24A1 enzyme. PTH attenuates the $1,25(OH)_2D$-mediated induction of the *CYP24A1* gene, through a direct effect on the transcription of the gene [21]. Fibroblast growth factor 23 (FGF23) decreases $1,25(OH)_2D$ levels by inhibiting *CYP27B1* expression and inducing *CYP24A1* in the kidney [22].

CYP24A1 loss-of-function variants are recognized as a cause of vitamin D-mediated hypercalcemia [23]. As a matter of fact, defective 24-hydroxylase activity results in high $1,25(OH)_2D$ concentrations and, as a consequence, PTH-independent hypercalcemia with hypercalciuria, in the absence of hypophosphatemia. Twenty-one PVs of *CYP24A1* have so far been described in literature [6]. The disease is inherited as a recessive trait and a genotype-phenotype correlation has been postulated [3].

Biallelic variants, independently of whether in homozygosis or compound heterozygosis, result in a significant phenotype [1, 24], which may range from severe to mild and misrecognized forms [1, 3]. The majority of cases diagnosed in early infancy presents the classic manifestations of IIH, namely, severe hypercalcemia, dehydration, polyuria, vomiting, failure to thrive, nephrocalcinosis, muscular hypotonia, and lethargy, occasionally leading to death [1, 4, 23]. Conversely, cases with biallelic mutations diagnosed in the adulthood commonly present mild to moderate hypercalcemia [23] and recurrent nephrolithiasis [5, 25].

It is still not clear whether different PVs may be associated with different phenotypes. As a matter of fact, the specific PV may influence the extent of the variation in the enzyme activity, thus contributing to the severity of the clinical picture [26]. Specifically, most patients harboring p.Glu143del biallelic mutation present a late-onset clinical picture, which mainly consists in urological manifestations, such as nephrolithiasis and/or nephrocalcinosis [26–29]. Until now, the small number of patients so far reported does not allow drawing significant genotype-phenotype correlations both for the p.Glu143del and for other rarer PVs.

Data about heterozygote carriers are mainly derived from studies involving relatives of index cases carrying biallelic variants. Whether the presence of monoallelic mutation can lead to an overt clinical phenotype is still a matter of debate [24]. Heterozygote carriers usually have a milder biochemical phenotype compared to patients affected by biallelic variants [7, 25, 30, 31], with mild hypercalcemia and less frequently nephrolithiasis [25]. Moreover, others suggest that these patients are mainly asymptomatic and that incidental nephrolithiasis may be due to other causes [7]. This is in keeping with the finding in our kindred, where the clinical and biochemical picture in heterozygous mutation carriers was heterogeneous, thus suggesting that other factors might contribute to the phenotype (see below). Conversely, a study reported two children with monoallelic *CYP24A1* intron-exon splice junction mutations (IVS5+1G>A and IVS6-2A>G) with severe hypercalcemia and the classical phenotype of IIH, commonly due to biallelic mutation [31]. The authors postulated that the symptomatic picture could be due to an autosomal dominant inheritance pattern. Additional environmental factors or predisposing conditions, including vitamin D administration [1, 32], sunlight exposure [33], and pregnancy [34], may contribute to the development of a clinically relevant phenotype in patients with either biallelic or monoallelic mutations.

In clinical practice loss-of-function mutations in *CYP24A1* should be searched in patients with hypercalcemia and hypercalciuria, associated with low serum PTH concentrations and $1,25(OH)_2D$ levels in the upper normal range or slightly above. Serum 25(OH)D concentrations can be low, normal, or mildly elevated. The finding of markedly elevated 25(OH)D levels raises the suspicion of vitamin D intoxication. An additional diagnostic clue is the measurement of $24,25(OH)_2D_3$, the main product of CYP24A1 [10], that is expected to be decreased. Unfortunately, the assay of this metabolite is not routinely available. Moreover, measurement of absolute $24,25(OH)_2D_3$ concentration alone has limited diagnostic value, because low $24,25(OH)_2D_3$ can also occur due to low $25(OH)D_3$ in addition to CYP24A1 mutation. We observed in patient I.1 (hetorozygote carrier) a $24,25\text{-}(OH)_2D_3$ concentration of 0.56 ng/mL, similar to patient II.3 (proband). Calculation of a $25(OH)D_3$:$24,25(OH)_2D_3$ ratio indicates when 24,25-$(OH)_2D_3$ concentration is inappropriately low for a given $25(OH)D_3$ level. In unaffected individuals serum levels of $24,25(OH)_2D$ are proportional to those of 25(OH)D and the ratio ranges between 5 and 25. In the patients affected by *CYP24A1* loss-of-function mutations, the ratio is markedly increased, up to more than 80 [10, 25, 31] by short method and over 140 by the long method, reported here. Currently, the measurement of the 25(OH)D:$24,25(OH)_2D$ is considered the most accurate screening tool for the identification of patients to be submitted to genetic testing.

Treatment of patient with *CYP24A1* PVs is directed towards the control of hypercalcemia. In severe cases, treatment starts with vigorous fluids administration eventually followed by a loop diuretic as furosemide when the patient is adequately hydrated. Other options include calcitonin and bisphosphonates. The use of corticosteroid to reduce intestinal calcium absorption is not advised in the setting of hypercalcemia related to *CYP24A1* PVs [35] because its therapeutic benefit requires a functioning CYP24A1 enzyme [36]. Another therapeutic approach aims to modulate the metabolism of $1,25(OH)_2D$. Ketoconazole reduces the synthesis of $1,25(OH)_2D$ by inhibiting the CYP27B1 enzyme and has been effective in patients affected by *CYP24A1* loss-of-function mutations in the acute and in the chronic setting [31, 37]. Fluconazole has been proposed as a valid alternative to ketoconazole, especially for the less pronounced long-term toxicity [38].

Rifampin, given its capacity to induce CYP3A4 enzyme, catalyzes a nonspecific hydroxylation of $1,25(OH)_2D$ to an inactive metabolite, $1,23,25(OH)_3D$, and has been used with overall good results [39].

Independently of the pharmacologic approaches, it seems reasonable to avoid exogenous vitamin D supplementation, implement a low-calcium diet, and avoid unprotected excessive sunlight exposure, even though the benefit of these approaches remains to be clarified [6].

In the case of females of child-bearing age with biallelic CYP24A1 mutations, it should be noted that the advent of pregnancy constitutes an added risk for hypercalcemia, as the placenta is a known site of additional $1,25(OH)_2D_3$ synthesis. Several cases have been described in which the patient's hypercalcemia is exacerbated during recurrent pregnancies, a condition which dissipates during nonpregnant periods[28, 34].

4. Conclusion

The patient reported herein represents a typical case of homozygous *CYP24A1* loss-of-function mutation discovered in the early adulthood with recurrent nephrolithiasis.

About 2 years passed from the initial episode of renal colic to the first measurement of serum calcium and the discovery of hypercalcemia. This is a common finding in many adult patients presenting with nephrolithiasis and hypercalcemia due to PV of the CYP24A1 enzyme [1, 5, 38] and reflects the common attitude to approach the treatment of kidney stones rather than investigating the causes.

The differential diagnosis of hypercalcemia encompasses many different conditions. The possibility of mutation of the *CYP24A1* gene as a cause of hypercalcemia should be considered in cases of PTH-independent hypercalcemia, once that more common causes, namely, hypercalcemia of malignancy, granulomatous diseases, activated vitamin D intoxication, have been ruled out.

The clinical expression of the *CYP24A1* mutation is heterogeneous both in biallelic (age at diagnosis and severity) and monoallelic members of the same kindred (as in our family). Treatment should be individually tailored, taking into account the risk-benefit ratio. The severity of the clinical manifestations, the patient's age, the expected side effects of the medication proposed (which should be taken possibly for a lifetime), and the patient's preference should be taken into account.

Acknowledgments

This research was partially supported by University of Pisa funds to Professor Claudio Marcocci. Aspects of this work were supported by a grant from the European Rare Diseases Consortium (E-Rare 2) & the Canadian Institutes for Health Research (#ERA-132931) to G. Jones. Waters Corporation (Milford, MA, USA) generously provided the LC-MS/MS instrumentation used in these studies through a Queen's University/Waters Corporation Agreement. We are grateful to the patients for their effort to help out with this research.

References

[1] K. P. Schlingmann, M. Kaufmann, S. Weber et al., "Mutations in CYP24A1 and idiopathic infantile hypercalcemia," *The New England Journal of Medicine*, vol. 365, no. 5, pp. 410–421, 2011.

[2] G. Jones, D. E. Prosser, and M. Kaufmann, "Cytochrome P450-mediated metabolism of vitamin D," *Journal of Lipid Research*, vol. 55, no. 1, pp. 13–31, 2014.

[3] D. T. O'Keeffe, P. J. Tebben, R. Kumar, R. J. Singh, Y. Wu, and R. A. Wermers, "Clinical and biochemical phenotypes of adults with monoallelic and biallelic CYP24A1 mutations: evidence of gene dose effect," *Osteoporosis International*, vol. 27, no. 10, pp. 3121–3125, 2016.

[4] R. Lightwood and T. Stapleton, "Idiopathic hypercalcaemia in infants," *The Lancet*, vol. 262, no. 6779, pp. 255-256, 1953.

[5] T. P. Jacobs, M. Kaufman, G. Jones et al., "A lifetime of hypercalcemia and hypercalciuria, finally explained," *The Journal of Clinical Endocrinology & Metabolism*, vol. 99, no. 3, pp. 708–712, 2014.

[6] G. Jones, M. L. Kottler, and K. P. Schlingmann, "Genetic diseases of vitamin D metabolizing enzymes," *Endocrinology and Metabolism Clinics of North America*, vol. 46, no. 4, pp. 1095–1117, 2017.

[7] A. Molin, R. Baudoin, M. Kaufmann et al., "CYP24A1 mutations in a cohort of hypercalcemic patients: Evidence for a recessive trait," *The Journal of Clinical Endocrinology & Metabolism*, vol. 100, no. 10, pp. E1343–E1352, 2015.

[8] E. De Paolis, A. Minucci, M. De Bonis et al., "A rapid screening of a recurrent CYP24A1 pathogenic variant opens the way to molecular testing for Idiopathic Infantile Hypercalcemia (IIH)," *Clinica Chimica Acta*, vol. 482, pp. 8–13, 2018.

[9] P. M. Ferraro, A. Minucci, A. Primiano et al., "A novel CYP24A1 genotype associated to a clinical picture of hypercalcemia, nephrolithiasis and low bone mass," *Urolithiasis*, vol. 45, no. 3, pp. 291–294, 2017.

[10] M. Kaufmann, J. C. Gallagher, M. Peacock et al., "Clinical utility of simultaneous quantitation of 25-hydroxyvitamin D and 24,25-dihydroxyvitamin D by LC-MS/MS involving derivatization with DMEQ-TAD," *The Journal of Clinical Endocrinology & Metabolism*, vol. 99, no. 7, pp. 2567–2574, 2014.

[11] M. Kaufmann, N. Morse, B. J. Molloy et al., "Improved screening test for idiopathic infantile hypercalcemia confirms residual levels of serum 24,25-(OH)2 D3 in affected patients," *Journal of Bone and Mineral Research*, vol. 32, no. 7, pp. 1589–1596, 2017.

[12] M. W. Yeh, P. H. G. Ituarte, H. C. Zhou et al., "Incidence and prevalence of primary hyperparathyroidism in a racially mixed population," *The Journal of Clinical Endocrinology & Metabolism*, vol. 98, no. 3, pp. 1122–1129, 2013.

[13] C. Marcocci and F. Cetani, "Primary hyperparathyroidism," *The New England Journal of Medicine*, vol. 365, no. 25, pp. 2389–2397, 2011.

[14] H. F. DeLuca, "Vitamin D: the vitamin and the hormone," *Fed Proc*, vol. 33, no. 11, pp. 2221-2219, 1974.

[15] G. Jones, D. E. Prosser, and M. Kaufmann, "25-Hydroxyvitamin D-24-hydroxylase (CYP24A1): Its important role in the degradation of vitamin D," *Archives of Biochemistry and Biophysics*, vol. 523, no. 1, pp. 9–18, 2012.

[16] G. S. Reddy and K.-Y. Tserng, "Calcitroic acid, end product of renal metabolism of 1,25-dihydroxyvitamin D3 through C-24 oxidation pathway," *Biochemistry*, vol. 28, no. 4, pp. 1763–1769, 1989.

[17] Y. Ohyama and K. Okuda, "Isolation and characterization of a cytochrome P-450 from rat kidney mitochondria that catalyzes the 24-hydroxylation of 25-hydroxyvitamin D3," *The Journal of Biological Chemistry*, vol. 266, no. 14, pp. 8690–8695, 1991.

[18] Y. Ohyama, M. Noshiro, Y. Kato et al., "Structural Characterization of the Gene Encoding Rat 25-Hydroxyvitamin D3 24-Hydroxylase," *Biochemistry*, vol. 32, no. 1, pp. 76–82, 1993.

[19] K.-S. Chen, J. M. Prahl, and H. F. Deluca, "Isolation and expression of human 1,25-dihydroxyvitamin D3 24-hydroxylase cDNA," *Proceedings of the National Acadamy of Sciences of the United States of America*, vol. 90, no. 10, pp. 4543–4547, 1993.

[20] G. Jones, S. A. Strugnell, and H. F. DeLuca, "Current understanding of the molecular actions of vitamin D," *Physiological Reviews*, vol. 78, no. 4, pp. 1193–1231, 1998.

[21] M. Kaufmann, S. M. Lee, J. W. Pike, and G. Jones, "A high-calcium and phosphate rescue diet and VDR-expressing transgenes normalize serum Vitamin D metabolite profiles and renal Cyp27b1 and Cyp24a1 expression in VDR null mice," *Endocrinology*, vol. 156, no. 12, pp. 4388–4397, 2015.

[22] T. Shimada, H. Hasegawa, Y. Yamazaki et al., "FGF-23 is a potent regulator of vitamin D metabolism and phosphate homeostasis," *Journal of Bone and Mineral Research*, vol. 19, no. 3, pp. 429–435, 2004.

[23] P. J. Tebben, R. J. Singh, and R. Kumar, "Vitamin D-mediated hypercalcemia: Mechanisms, diagnosis, and treatment," *Endocrine Reviews*, vol. 37, no. 5, pp. 521–547, 2016.

[24] T. O. Carpenter, "CYP24A1 loss of function: Clinical phenotype of monoallelic and biallelic mutations," *The Journal of Steroid Biochemistry and Molecular Biology*, vol. 173, pp. 337–340, 2017.

[25] M. Cools, S. Goemaere, D. Baetens et al., "Calcium and bone homeostasis in heterozygous carriers of CYP24A1 mutations: A cross-sectional study," *Bone*, vol. 81, pp. 89–96, 2015.

[26] T. Jobst-Schwan, A. Pannes, K. P. Schlingmann, K.-U. Eckardt, B. B. Beck, and M. S. Wiesener, "Discordant clinical course of vitamin-D-hydroxylase (CYP24A1) associated Hypercalcemia in Two Adult Brothers with Nephrocalcinosis," *Kidney and Blood Pressure Research*, vol. 40, no. 5, pp. 443–451, 2015.

[27] H.-F. Ji and L. Shen, "CYP24A1 mutations in idiopathic infantile hypercalcemia," *The New England Journal of Medicine*, vol. 365, no. 18, pp. 1741–1743, 2011.

[28] D. Dinour, M. Davidovits, S. Aviner et al., "Maternal and infantile hypercalcemia caused by vitamin-D-hydroxylase mutations and vitamin D intake," *Pediatric Nephrology*, vol. 30, no. 1, pp. 145–152, 2015.

[29] D. Dinour, P. Beckerman, L. Ganon, K. Tordjman, Z. Eisenstein, and E. J. Holtzman, "Loss-of-function mutations of CYP24A1, the vitamin D 24-hydroxylase gene, cause long-standing hypercalciuric nephrolithiasis and nephrocalcinosis," *The Journal of Urology*, vol. 190, no. 2, pp. 552–557, 2013.

[30] A. Dauber, T. T. Nguyen, E. Sochett et al., "Genetic defect in CYP24A1, the vitamin D 24-hydroxylase gene, in a patient with severe infantile hypercalcemia," *The Journal of Clinical Endocrinology & Metabolism*, vol. 97, no. 2, pp. E268–E274, 2012.

[31] P. J. Tebben, D. S. Milliner, R. L. Horst et al., "Hypercalcemia, hypercalciuria, and elevated calcitriol concentrations with autosomal dominant transmission due to CYP24A1 mutations: Effects of ketoconazole therapy," *The Journal of Clinical Endocrinology & Metabolism*, vol. 97, no. 3, pp. E423–E427, 2012.

[32] M. Castanet, E. Mallet, and M.-L. Kottler, "Lightwood syndrome revisited with a novel mutation in CYP24 and vitamin D supplement recommendations," *Journal of Pediatrics*, vol. 163, no. 4, pp. 1208–1210, 2013.

[33] M.-L. Figueres, A. Linglart, F. Bienaime et al., "Kidney function and influence of sunlight exposure in patients with impaired 24-hydroxylation of vitamin D due to cyp24a1 mutations," *American Journal of Kidney Diseases*, vol. 65, no. 1, pp. 122–126, 2014.

[34] A. D. Shah, E. C. Hsiao, B. O'Donnell et al., "Maternal hypercalcemia due to failure of 1,25-dihydroxyvitamin-D3 catabolism in a patient With CYP24A1 mutations," *The Journal of Clinical Endocrinology & Metabolism*, vol. 100, no. 8, pp. 2832–2836, 2015.

[35] G. Colussi, L. Ganon, S. Penco et al., "Chronic hypercalcaemia from inactivating mutations of vitamin D 24-hydroxylase (CYP24A1): Implications for mineral metabolism changes in chronic renal failure," *Nephrology Dialysis Transplantation* , vol. 29, no. 3, pp. 636–643, 2014.

[36] R. St-Arnaud, "CYP24A1-deficient mice as a tool to uncover a biological activity for vitamin D metabolites hydroxylated at position 24," *The Journal of Steroid Biochemistry and Molecular Biology*, vol. 121, no. 1-2, pp. 254–256, 2010.

[37] M. Nguyen, H. Boutignon, E. Mallet et al., "Infantile hypercalcemia and hypercalciuria: New insights into a vitamin D-dependent mechanism and response to ketoconazole treatment," *Journal of Pediatrics*, vol. 157, no. 2, pp. 296–302, 2010.

[38] J. Sayers, A. M. Hynes, S. Srivastava et al., "Successful treatment of hypercalcaemia associated with a CYP24A1 mutation with fluconazole," *Clinical Kidney Journal*, vol. 8, no. 4, pp. 453–455, 2015.

[39] C. P. Hawkes, D. Li, H. Hakonarson, K. E. Meyers, K. E. Thumme, and M. A. Levine, "CYP3A4 Induction by Rifampin: An alternative pathway for Vitamin D inactivation in patients with CYP24A1 mutations," *The Journal of Clinical Endocrinology & Metabolism*, vol. 102, no. 5, pp. 1440–1446, 2017.

17

Reidel's Thyroiditis, a Diagnostic and Management Challenge: A Case Report and Review of the Literature

Yassine Er-Rahali,[1] Mohammed Massine El Hammoumi,[2] Jad Issouani,[1] Colna Antonio Nfad,[1] Souad El Moussaoui,[1] El Hassane Kabiri,[2] and Ahmed Anass Guerboub[1]

[1]*Endocrinology Department, Mohammed V Military Academic Hospital, Faculty of Medicine and Pharmacy, Mohammed V-Souissi University, Rabat, Morocco*
[2]*Thoracic Surgery Department, Mohammed V Military Academic Hospital, Faculty of Medicine and Pharmacy, Mohammed V-Souissi University, Rabat, Morocco*

Correspondence should be addressed to Yassine Er-Rahali; yassine0388@gmail.com

Academic Editor: Mihail A. Boyanov

Riedel's thyroiditis is a very rare inflammatory condition. It affects not only the thyroid gland but also the adjacent vital structures. It may also be associated with different forms of systemic fibrotic disorders. The exact etiology is unknown, but currently, the most favorable opinion is that it is a localized form of the systemic fibrotic process. We report the case of a 38-year-old woman, presented with a 10-month history of progressive hypothyroidism, dysphonia, and dysphagia. A Doppler ultrasound study revealed massive thyroid enlargement with multiple Eu TIRADS 3 and 4 nodules. Fine needle aspiration was noncontributive on two occasions. A hard subtotal thyroidectomy was performed. Pathological study confirmed Riedel's thyroiditis with the presence of IgG4 antibodies in immunohistochemistry. The patient was successfully treated with levothyroxine replacement and corticosteroid therapy with rapid resolution of obstructive symptoms. The case descriptions highlight the diagnostic challenge of this disease, describe the response to surgical management and corticosteroid therapy, and give a short review of the subject.

1. Introduction

Riedel's thyroiditis (RT) is a rare fibrosclerotic condition affecting the thyroid gland. It is characterized by thyroid parenchyma replacement with fibrous tissue. It was first described by Bernhard Riedel in 1896 [1]. Until now, there have been almost 200 cases reported in the literature. This sclerotic process may not only be limited to only the thyroid but also invades the surrounding vital structures such as vessels, nerves, trachea, esophagus, and parathyroid that leads to compressive symptoms and endocrine abnormalities [2]. It is a rare condition, with a prevalence of 1 per 100,000 inhabitants, which affects more frequently women between 30 and 50 years of age. RT accounts for less than 0.06% of patients undergoing thyroidectomies [3]. The precise etiology of this disorder is still unclear. An association with systemic fibrotic processes, autoimmune diseases, and more recently with diseases from the spectrum of excessive immunoglobulin G type 4 (IgG4) has been described [4]. We report the case of a 38-year-old woman presented with clinical features initially suggestive of malignant goiter, which turned out to be Riedel's thyroiditis.

2. Case Report

We report the case of a 38-year-old woman who came to the endocrinology department with a 10-month history of progressive hypothyroidism and an enlargement at the base of her neck. She had noted dysphonia, dyspnea, and progressive difficulty in swallowing solid food. Thyroid-stimulating hormone was normal under on L-thyroxin replacement therapy. Antithyroglobulin and antiperoxidase

Table 1: Patient's laboratory results.

Laboratory tests		Patient values	Normal range
TSH		0.89 μU/ml	0.40–4.00
Free T4		1.35 ng/dl	0.70–1.48
TPO ab		10.2 U/l	<34
Tg ab		1.57 U/ml	0.20–4.11
Calcium	Before surgery	91 mg/l	80–105
	Follow-up	77 mg/l	
PTH	Before surgery	66 pg/ml	15–68
	Follow-up	21 pg/ml	
Serum-IgG4		0.071 g/L	0.039–0.864

TSH: thyroid stimulating hormone; TPO ab: thyroid peroxidase antibodies; Tg ab: thyroglobulin antibodies; PTH: parathyroid hormone; IgG4: subclass 4 of immunoglobin G.

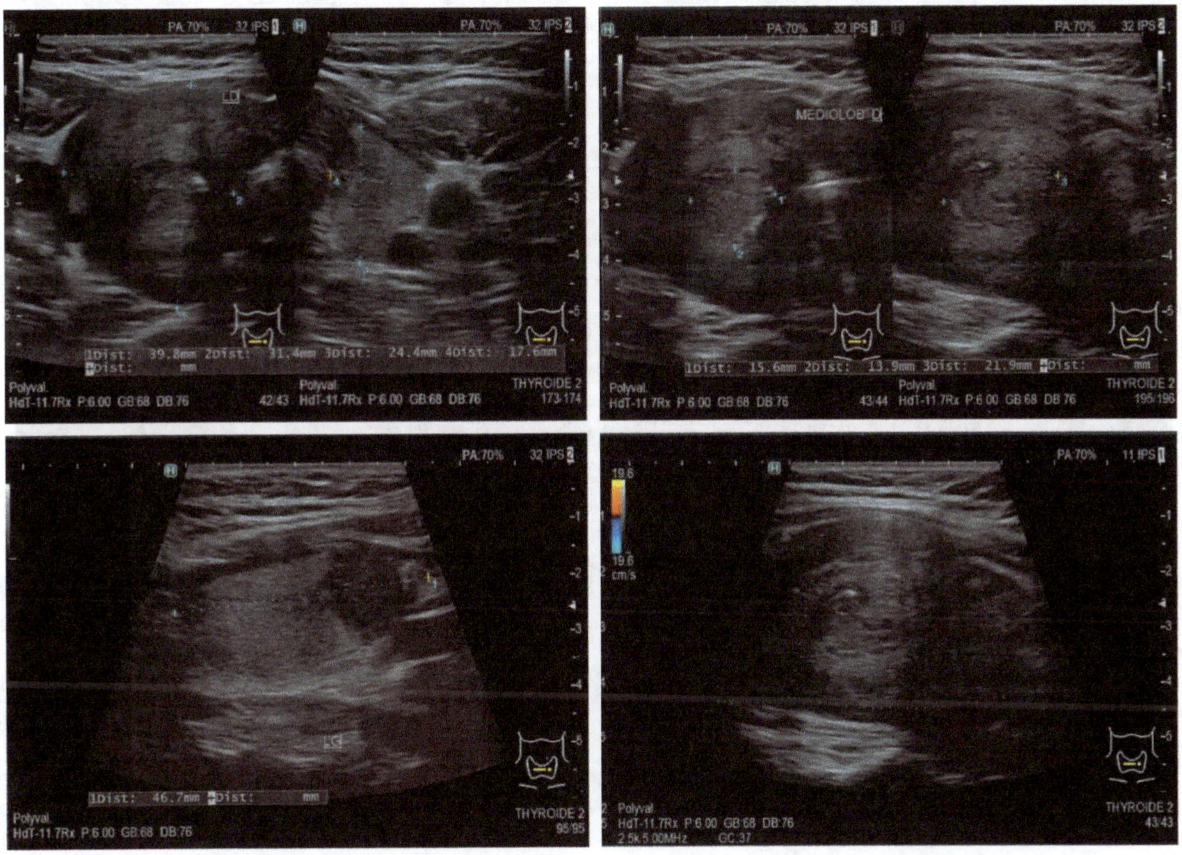

Figure 1: Patient's cervical ultrasound showing a hypovascularized nodular goiter.

antibodies were negative. Parathormone and calcemia levels were normal before surgery (Table 1). A Doppler ultrasound study of the woman's neck revealed a massive thyroid enlargement with multiple Eu TIRADS 3 and 4 nodules (Figure 1). CT scan showed a large nodular goiter with tracheal deviation and stenosis (Figure 2). Fine needle aspiration was noncontributive on two separate occasions (Bethesda I).

The patient was referred to surgery for thyroidectomy. Intraoperative findings revealed a goiter with a hard stony consistency, adhesive to the visceral planes suggestive of huge malignancy. Peroperative pathological examination of a specimen suspected malignant thyroid disease. The surgical team performed despite a subtotal thyroidectomy with placement of a temporary tracheostomy. The definitive pathological study confirmed surprising diagnosis of Riedel's thyroiditis with the presence of IgG4 antibodies in immunohistochemistry.

Evolution was marked by progressive dyspnea. The patient was put on short courses of corticosteroids with a transitory symptom improvement. The patient was admitted to our department 5 months after surgery because of COVID-19 pandemic. On physical examination, the patient presented signs of hypocalcemia with dyspnea. Laboratory tests confirmed hypoparathyroidism treated by substitutive therapy (alfacalcidol + calcium). A cervico-thoraco-

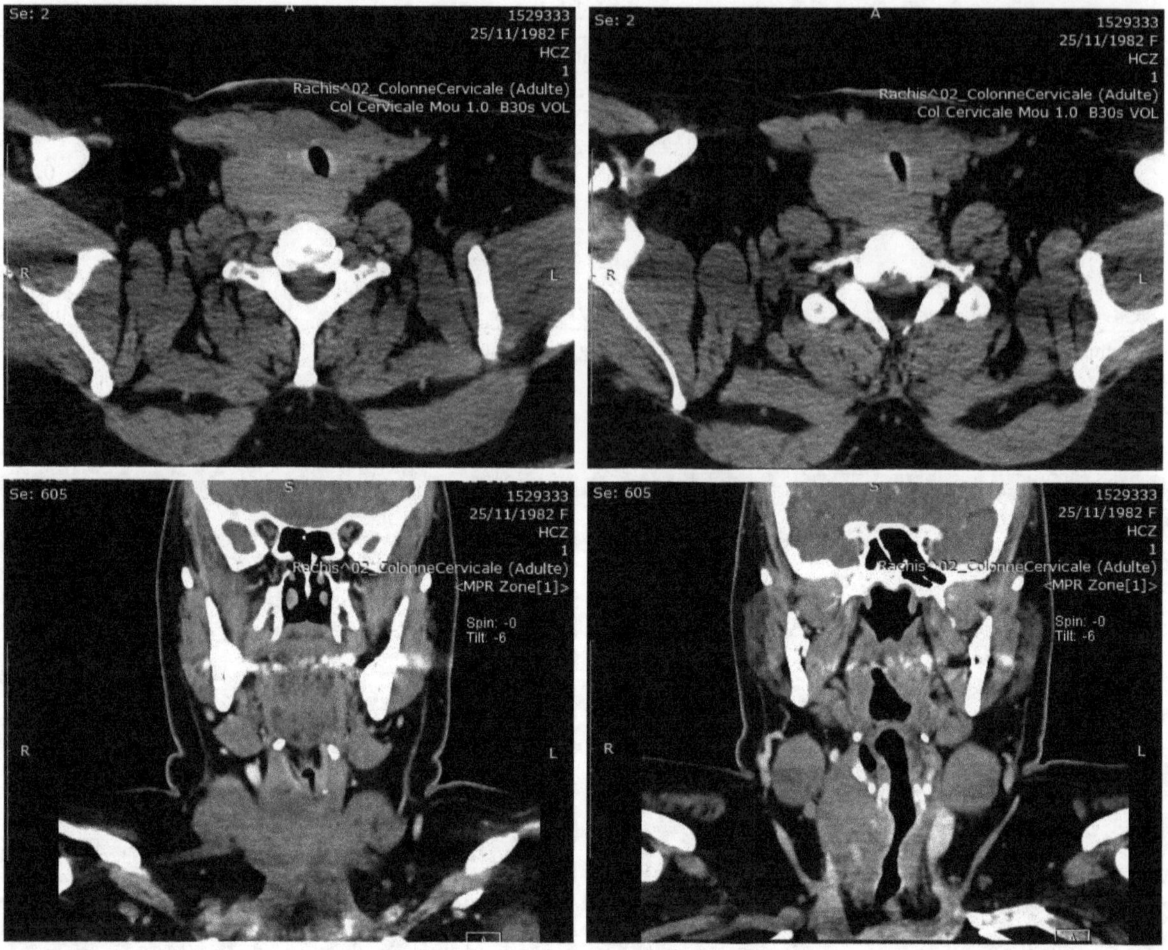

FIGURE 2: CT image in transverse and coronal sections showing a large goiter with tracheal deviation and stenosis.

abdominal CT scan revealed a right thyroid infiltrating process and plunging into the upper mediastinum. This process encases the right primary carotid artery up to its bifurcation. A partial thrombosis of the right internal jugular vein was noted. No fibrous lesion elsewhere. The orbital CT scan was normal. The serum level for immunoglobulin G4 (IgG4) subclass had been normal.

The patient was successfully treated with oral levothyroxine replacement (100 μg per day) high-dose corticosteroid therapy (60 mg/day) for 1 month. Internal jugular vein thrombosis was treated successfully with the 3-month use of enoxaparin.

On follow-up, dyspnea had resolved. A gradual reduction of corticosteroid doses was performed. Currently, the patient is on 7.5 mg/d of prednisolone. The cervical ultrasound shows a stable right thyroid residue.

3. Discussion

Riedel's thyroiditis is extremely rare. The incidence is now estimated to be 1 in 100,000, with higher incidence in women. It is most frequent in middle age adults (30–50 years) [2, 3]. There are multiple hypotheses regarding its pathogenesis, but its exact etiology remains uncertain. Autoimmune etiology is the most likely hypothesis. Some authors consider Riedel's thyroiditis as a part of multifocal fibrosclerosis, relating to the group of IgG4 sclerosing diseases. [5].

Patients with RT usually present compressive symptoms related to fibrosis, such as hoarseness, aphonia, dysphagia, and/or dyspnea. Physical exam often finds a firm, fixed thyroid, which suspects a malignant tumor. If neck surgery is pursued, like in our case, surgeons will find a large fibrotic mass involving the thyroid and perithyroid tissue without an obvious tissue plane [6]. As the fibroinflammatory process progresses, it can affect the thyroid and parathyroid glands, leading to hypothyroidism and/or hypoparathyroidism. Evidence collected over time shows that RT-associated hypothyroidism occurs in 25–80% of patients [7].

The thyroid ultrasound typically finds a diffuse hypoechogenous thyroid that seems to be hypovascular on color Doppler. A thyroid mass or node may also be found, as in our patient's case. Additional imaging techniques have also been performed: ultrasound elastography revealed increased gland stiffness. 18-Fluoro-deoxyglucose PET/CT showed increased uptake by the lesion, inconstantly decreased by corticoids, and 99mTc thyroid scintigraphy showed poor radioactive uptake. MRI results vary widely among authors. Although numerous imaging techniques have been used, clinicians remain unable to differentiate Riedel's thyroiditis from other thyroid pathologies, including neoplasms [8]. Cytology is not always diagnostic in RT and may fail to prove the invasive nature of fibrosis [9]. The diagnosis of RT is most commonly suggested after pathologic evaluation of resected thyroid tissue. Findings like storiform fibrosis and occlusive phlebitis argue for RT, and, in the case of IgG4 involvement, elevation of IgG4 positive plasma cells with an IgG-4 ratio >40% [10].

Because of its low incidence, no guidelines or large clinical studies exist for the optimal management of Riedel's thyroiditis. Most authors agree that therapy must focus on treating hypothyroidism and managing fibrosclerotic manifestations [11]. Systemic steroids are the first-line therapy, decreasing the size and hardness of the goiter in only a few patients. Prolonged treatment is often required due to the risk of losing the improvement achieved once the doses are reduced. Tamoxifen is another agent used successfully, at doses of 10–20 mg twice a day. Significant reduction in goiter size has been reported in patients who have not responded to steroids previously [12].

Other potential therapies exist, but may be less well studied. There are a few reports of the use of low-dose radiation for the treatment of RT, but no systematic evaluation of this therapy exists to date. Mycophenolic acid, the active metabolite of mycophenolate, induces inhibition of T- and B-cell production, thus reducing the spread of antibody levels [13]. Rituximab has been reported to have favorable effects in IgG4-related systemic disorders and in some cases of RT [14]. As far as surgical management is considered, the indications are essentially two: sample for histopathological diagnostic confirmation and relieving compression or obstruction in the trachea or esophagus. The complete resection of the gland is not recommended due to the high risk of damaging nearby structures such as neck vessels, the parathyroid, and recurrent laryngeal nerves because of the lack of resection margins [11].

4. Conclusion

Reidel's thyroiditis is a very rare form of fibrous destruction of thyroid parenchyma, which leads to thyroid dysfunction and progressive airway and digestive tract obstruction. Glucocorticoids are still the mainstay of therapy. The need of consensual guidelines to better manage this rare disease becomes mandatory to prevent associated complications.

References

[1] S. A. Ng, I. Corcuera-Solano, V. V. Gurudutt, and P. M. Som, "A rare case of Reidel thyroiditis with associated vocal cord paralysis: CT and MR imaging features," *American Journal of Neuroradiology*, vol. 32, no. 11, pp. E201–E202, 2011.

[2] A. A. Shafi, N. B. Saad, and B. AlHarthi, "Riedel's thyroiditis as a diagnostic dilemma - a case report and review of the literature," *Annals of Medicine and Surgery*, vol. 52, pp. 5–9, 2020.

[3] V. Navarro-Sánchez, L. A. Marín-Castañeda, C. A. Gallegos, O. Quiroz, and M. Ahumada-Ayala, "IgG4-Related fibrous thyroiditis (Riedel's Thyroiditis): a Case Report," *American Journal of Case Reports*, vol. 21, Article ID e928046, 2020.

[4] V. M. Blanco, C. A. Páez, A. M. Victoria et al., "Riedel's Thyroiditis: Report of Two Cases and Literature Review," *Case Reports in Endocrinology*, vol. 2019, pp. 1–4, Article ID 5130106, 2019.

[5] M. Darouichi and P. E. Constanthin, "Riedel's thyroiditis," *Radiology Case Reports*, vol. 11, no. 3, pp. 175–177, 2016.

[6] J. V. Hennessey, "Riedel's Thyroiditis: A Clinical Review," *Journal of Clinical Endocrinology & Metabolism*, vol. 96, no. 10, pp. 3031–3041, 2011.

[7] M. M. Fatourechi, I. D. Hay, B. McIver, T. J. Sebo, and V. Fatourechi, "Invasive Fibrous Thyroiditis (Riedel Thyroiditis): The Mayo Clinic Experience, 1976-2008," *Thyroid*, vol. 21, no. 7, pp. 765–772, 2011.

[8] R. Slman, H. Monpeyssen, S. Desarnaud et al., "Ultrasound, Elastography, and Fluorodeoxyglucose Positron Emission Tomography/Computed Tomography Imaging in Riedel's Thyroiditis: Report of Two Cases," *Thyroid*, vol. 21, no. 7, pp. 799–804, 2011.

[9] N. Kumar, R. Gupta, S. Sayed, Z. Moloo, S. Vinayak, and M. Ahmed, "Difficulties in diagnosis of Riedel's thyroiditis on aspiration cytology: A case report and brief review of the literature," *Diagnostic Cytopathology*, vol. 47, no. 5, pp. 512–516, 2019.

[10] V. Deshpande, Y. Zen, J. K. Chan et al., "Consensus statement on the pathology of IgG4-related disease," *Modern Pathology*, vol. 25, no. 9, pp. 1181–1192, 2012.

[11] H. Falhammar, C. C. Juhlin, C. Barner, S.-B. Catrina, C. Karefylakis, and J. Calissendorff, "Riedel's thyroiditis: clinical presentation, treatment and outcomes," *Endocrine*, vol. 60, no. 1, pp. 185–192, 2018.

[12] S. K. Y. Gosi, M. Nguyen, and V. V. Garla, *Riedel Thyroiditis*StatPearls Publishing, Treasure Island, FL, USA, 2021, http://www.ncbi.nlm.nih.gov/books/NBK537303/.

[13] J. M. Levy, C. P. Hasney, P. L. Friedlander, E. Kandil, E. A. Occhipinti, and M. J. Kahn, "Combined Mycophenolate Mofetil and Prednisone Therapy in Tamoxifen- and Prednisone-Resistant Reidel's Thyroiditis," *Thyroid*, vol. 20, no. 1, pp. 105–107, 2010.

[14] S. V. Mammen and M. B. Gordon, "Successful Use of Rituximab in a Case of Riedel Thyroiditis Resistant to Treatment with Prednisone and Tamoxifen," *AACE Clinical Case Reports*, vol. 5, no. 3, pp. e218–e221, 2019.

18

Rhabdomyolysis in a Young Patient due to Hypothyroidism without Any Precipitating Factor

Dhineshreddy Gurala ,[1] Kartikeya Rajdev ,[1] Roshan Acharya,[1] Pretty Sara Idiculla,[2] Saad Habib,[1] and Michael Krzyzak[3]

[1]*Resident, Internal Medicine, Staten Island University Hospital, Northwell Health, Staten Island, NY, USA*
[2]*Foreign Medical Graduate, Sree Gokulam Medical College and Research Foundation, Alamthara, India*
[3]*Hospitalist, Internal Medicine, Staten Island University Hospital, Northwell Health, Staten Island, NY, USA*

Correspondence should be addressed to Dhineshreddy Gurala; dineshgurala@gmail.com

Academic Editor: Osamu Isozaki

Hypothyroidism is characterized by decreased hormone production, which results in various clinical manifestations in different organ systems. Muscular symptoms are common in patents with clinical hypothyroidism which includes muscle cramps, myalgia, and mild to moderate elevation of creatinine kinase less than five times the upper limit of normal. However, rhabdomyolysis due to hypothyroidism is rare and in most of the reported cases a precipitating factor has been found. We report a unique case of a 35-year-old male with no past medical history who presented with rhabdomyolysis due to newly diagnosed hypothyroidism without any precipitating factors and was treated successfully with intravenous fluids and levothyroxine.

1. Introduction

Hypothyroidism is found in 4.6% of the U.S. population, with 0.3% presenting clinically and 4.3% being subclinical [1]. Muscle involvement in hypothyroidism is common, involving 79% of patients [2]. Muscular manifestations range from muscle weakness, myalgia, muscle cramps with mild to moderate elevation of creatinine kinase to more severe such as Hoffman's syndrome or rhabdomyolysis [3, 4]. Rhabdomyolysis due to skeletal muscle necrosis in hypothyroidism is rare [5, 6] and usually associated with precipitating factor such as statin medication or severe exercise, illicit drugs. However, without any obvious precipitating factors, the incidence of rhabdomyolysis is infrequent [3]. Here in we report a unique case of rhabdomyolysis in young male due to hypothyroidism without any associated precipitating factors.

2. Case Presentation

A 35-year-old male with no significant medical history presented to the emergency department with diffuse muscle pain for one week prior to presentation. It initially started in his neck which progressed to his shoulder, trunk, and bilateral lower extremities and was associated with excessive fatigue and recent weight gain of 4.54 kg over two weeks. Review of systems was negative for dry skin, thinning of hair, fever, chills, upper respiratory tract infection, weakness in upper or lower extremities, double vision, changes in memory, or puffy skin. He denied the use of illicit drugs, alcohol abuse, herbal medications, trauma or prolonged immobilization, and did not report any family history of thyroid disease. His vitals were stable with a heart rate of 70 beats per minute, and blood pressure was 130/80 mm Hg. Physical examination was positive for diffuse mild muscle tenderness with normal 5/5 motor strength in upper and lower extremities. Electrocardiography showed normal sinus rhythm. Laboratory examination revealed normal hemogram and serum electrolytes including phosphate and calcium levels as shown in the Table 1. His serum creatinine was 1.2 mg/dl (baseline creatinine is 1.0–1.2). He had elevated serum creatinine kinase (CK) of 11760 U/L and elevated lactate dehydrogenase (LDH) of 544 U/L. His lipid profile was deranged with total cholesterol of 240 mg/dl, triglyceride of 284 mg/dl, and LDL-cholesterol of 138 mg/dl.

Table 1: Laboratory results.

Variable	Reference range	Day 1	Day 2	Day 3
Hemoglobin (mg/dl)	14–18	15.6		
WBC count (K/μl)	4.8–10.8	7.84		
Platelets (K/μl)	130–400	206		
Glucose random (mg/dl)	70–99	94		
Serum sodium (mmol/litre)	135–146	137	138	141
Serum potassium (mmol/litre)	3.5–5.0	4.3	3.8	3.8
Serum chloride (mmol/litre)	98–110	96	97	101
Anion gap	7–14	15	13	14
BUN (mg/dl)	10–20	14	11	9
Serum creatinine (mg/dl)	0.7–1.5	1.2	1.3	1.2
Calcium (mg/dl)	8.5–10.1	9.3	8.7	8.6
Magnesium (mg/dl)	1.8–2.4			1.9
TSH (μIU/ml)	0.27–4.2	111	100	
T4 (μg/dl)	4.6–12		0.5	
LDH (U/l)	50–242	544		
CK (U/l)	0–225	9553	11760	7600
CRP (mg/dl)	0–0.4		0.27	
RF (IU/ml)	0–13		<10	
CCP (units)	0–19		<8	
Ds DNA (IU/ml)	≤29		<12	
ESR (mm/hr)	0–10		3	
TG (mg/dl)	40–150	284		
HDL-cholesterol (mg/dl)	40–60	29		
LDL-cholesterol (mg/dl)	50–100	138		
Total-cholesterol (mg/dl)	100–200	240		

His urine was bloody in appearance, and urine analysis was negative for erythrocytes but was positive for urine myoglobin.

The patient was admitted to the hospital for rhabdomyolysis and was started on intravenous fluids. He was found to have an TSH (Thyroid Stimulating Hormone) of 100 micro IU/ml with a low free T4 level of 0.5 micro g/dl (Table 1). He was diagnosed with hypothyroidism and treatment with levothyroxine was initiated. Further work-up including Rheumatoid Factor (RF), Cyclic Citrullinated Peptide (CCP) Antibody, Antinuclear Antibody (ANA), Erythrocyte Sedimentation Rate (ESR), C-Reactive Protein (CRP), ds DNA, Coombs test, HIV, and urine drug screen was normal. Our patient showed significant improvement in his symptoms and the CK levels went down to 7600 μ/l with hydration by the third day of hospitalization. He was eventually discharged home on the fourth day of hospitalization and followed up as an out-patient.

3. Discussion

Hypothyroidism causes a broad spectrum of clinical manifestations such as generalized fatigue, dry skin, constipation, bradycardia, hypothermia, diastolic hypertension, and pericardial effusion. Muscular symptoms range from muscle weakness, stiffness, myalgia, muscle cramps to severe rhabdomyolysis, and pseudohypertrophy of the muscles (Hoffman's syndrome) [3, 4].

Rhabdomyolysis is defined by skeletal muscle necrosis and release of intracellular muscle contents into the circulation. Common causes of rhabdomyolysis include seizure, trauma, medications such as a statin, illicit drugs (methadone), alcohol, strenuous exercise, inflammatory myopathies (polymyositis), electrolyte abnormalities (hyponatremia, hypokalemia, hypocalcemia), and some of the glycogen storage disorders [7]. Rarely, it may also develop in patients with hypothyroidism [8, 9]. The pathophysiology of rhabdomyolysis in hypothyroidism is still unclear. Myolysis is attributable to changes in muscle fibers from fast twitching to slow twitching muscle fibers, deposition of glycosaminoglycans, poor contractility of actin-myosin units, low myosin ATPase activity, or low ATP turn over in the skeletal muscles [10]. Some of the possible explanations for these are inhibition of mitochondrial oxidative phosphorylation results in reduced ATP production and dysregulation of metabolic pathways such as the Kreb's cycle, fatty acid catabolism, and glycolytic energy production [11].

Diagnosis of rhabdomyolysis is based on the elevation of creatinine kinase up to five times the standard limit. Our patient had 50 times the usual limit of CK, had clinical symptoms of hypothyroidism such as weight gain, extreme fatigue, and laboratory examination showed high TSH, low T4 and dyslipidemia. Our patient did not have any other risk factors for the development of rhabdomyolysis and his work-up was negative for infectious, inflammatory, or autoimmune etiology. These findings led to the diagnosis of hypothyroidism induced rhabdomyolysis.

Initial management of rhabdomyolysis consists of intravenous fluids administration and to correct electrolyte abnormalities such as hyperkalemia, hyperphosphatemia, hypocalcemia, hyperuricemia, and metabolic acidosis. Acute kidney injury (AKI) is one of the most common complications with the reported frequency of AKI ranges from 15 to over 50% [12, 13]. Early and aggressive fluid resuscitation is necessary to prevent acute kidney injury [12]. The type of fluid and rate of repletion are unclear, however, initial fluid resuscitation with isotonic saline at the rate of 100 to 200 ml/hour is suggested to maintain or enhance renal perfusion, thereby minimizing ischemic injury. Sequential monitoring of CK levels, volume status of the patient, and urine output are needed to monitor response to the treatment and to adjust the rate of intravenous fluids. Fluid repletion should be continued until CK levels decreases to <5000 U/l and continue to fall. Measurement of TSH and free T4 every 4–6 weeks is necessary to assess the response. If TSH remains above the reference range, the dose can be increased by 25 to 50 μg/day until therapeutic goal has been achieved.

We suggest to keep hypothyroidism in one of the differential diagnosis in patients with rhabdomyolysis. According to the American Thyroid Association clinical guidelines, an increase in serum concentration of either CK or LDH for at least two weeks is enough to screen patients for hypothyroidism [13]. Our case illustrates the importance of screening for hypothyroidism in patients with rhabdomyolysis, and symptoms of hypothyroidism in the absence of other etiologies [14, 15].

4. Conclusion

Rhabdomyolysis is a rare but potentially severe complication of hypothyroidism. Clinicians should be aware of this unique possibility and be cautious in patients presenting with symptoms of hypothyroidism and muscular manifestations. It is necessary to screen patients with elevated muscle enzymes for hypothyroidism, as recommended by the American Thyroid Association. Early diagnosis and prompt treatment of hypothyroidism induced rhabdomyolysis are essential in preventing grave consequences.

References

[1] J. G. Hollowell, N. W. Staehling, W. D. Flanders et al., "Serum TSH, T4, and thyroid antibodies in the United States population (1988 to 1994): National Health and Nutrition Examination Survey (NHANES III)," *The Journal of Clinical Endocrinology & Metabolism*, vol. 87, no. 2, pp. 489–499, 2002.

[2] R. F. Duyff, J. Van den Bosch, D. M. Laman, B. J. van Loon, and W. H. Linssen, "Neuromuscular findings in thyroid dysfunction: a prospective clinical and electrodiagnostic study," *Journal of Neurology, Neurosurgery & Psychiatry*, vol. 68, no. 6, pp. 750–755, 2000.

[3] A. A. Khaleeli, D. G. Griffith, and R. H. T. Edwards, "The clinical presentation of hypothyroid myopathy and its relationship to abnormalities in structure and function of skeletal muscle," *Clinical Endocrinology*, vol. 19, no. 3, pp. 365–376, 1983.

[4] F. H. Norris Jr and B. J. Panner, "Hypothyroid myopathy. Clinical, electromyographical, and ultrastructural observations," *Archives of Neurology*, vol. 14, no. 6, pp. 574–589, 1966.

[5] A. Sindoni, C. Rodolico, M. A. Pappalardo, S. Portaro, and S. Benvenga, "Hypothyroid myopathy: a peculiar clinical presentation of thyroid failure. Review of the literature," *Reviews in Endocrine and Metabolic Disorders*, vol. 17, no. 4, pp. 499–519, 2016.

[6] M. N. Chowta and N. K. Chowta, "Hypothyroidism-associated rhabdomyolysis," *Indian Journal of Medical Sciences*, vol. 62, no. 12, p. 496, 2008.

[7] M. J. Barahona, A. Mauri, N. Sucunza, R. Paredes, and A. M. Wägner, "Hypothyroidism as a cause of rhabdomyolysis," *Endocrine Journal*, vol. 49, no. 6, pp. 621–623, 2002.

[8] B. Katipoglu, I. Ates, F. Acehan, A. Meteris, and N. Yılmaz, "Rhabdomyolysis case based on hypothyroidism," *Endocrinology, Diabetes & Metabolism Case Reports*, vol. 2016, no. 1, 2016.

[9] N. Salehi, E. Agoston, I. Munir, and G. J. Thompson, "Rhabdomyolysis in a patient with severe hypothyroidism," *The American Journal of Case Reports*, vol. 18, pp. 912–918, 2017.

[10] C. M. Wiles, A. Young, D. A. Jones, and R. H. Edwards, "Muscle relaxation rate, fibretype composition and energy turnover in hyper- and hypo-thyroid patients," *Clinical Science*, vol. 57, no. 4, pp. 375–384, 1979.

[11] P. D. Thompson, P. Clarkson, and R. H. Karas, "Statin-associated myopathy," *JAMA*, vol. 289, no. 13, pp. 1681–1690, 2003.

[12] P. A. Gabow, W. D. Kaehny, and S. P. Kelleher, "The spectrum of rhabdomyolysis," *Medicine*, vol. 61, no. 3, pp. 141–152, 1982.

[13] G. Melli, V. Chaudhry, and D. R. Cornblath, "Rhabdomyolysis: an evaluation of 475 hospitalized patients," *Medicine*, vol. 84, no. 6, pp. 377–385, 2005.

[14] J. L. Zimmerman and M. C. Shen, "Rhabdomyolysis," *Chest*, vol. 144, no. 3, pp. 1058–1065, 2013.

[15] P. W. Ladenson, P. A. Singer, K. B. Ain et al., "American Thyroid Association guidelines for detection of thyroid dysfunction," *Archives of Internal Medicine*, vol. 160, no. 11, pp. 1573–1575, 2000.

19

Is it T3 Thyrotoxicosis? A Case of Falsely Elevated Tri-Iodothyronine (T3) Levels Leading to a Diagnosis of Multiple Myeloma

Nanik Ram,[1] Saira Furqan,[1] and Sibtain Ahmed[2]

[1]*Department of Medicine, Aga Khan University, Stadium Road, P.O. Box 3500, Karachi 74800, Pakistan*
[2]*Department of Pathology and Laboratory Medicine, Aga Khan University, Stadium Road, P.O. Box 3500, Karachi 74800, Pakistan*

Correspondence should be addressed to Sibtain Ahmed; sibtain.ahmed@aku.edu

Academic Editor: Wayne V. Moore

We are presenting a case of falsely elevated T3 levels in a patient due to interference from monoclonal immunoglobulins. A 56-year-old, clinically euthyroid man referred to the endocrinology clinic of the Aga Khan university, Karachi Pakistan, for possible T3 thyrotoxicosis after thyroid function tests revealed total T3 >12.32 nmol/L (reference range 0.6–2.79), normal TSH, and total T4 level. There was a mismatch in clinical and laboratory parameters and preliminary laboratory results were suggestive of thyroid binding globulin abnormalities. Further evaluation in this context unmasked multiple myeloma. The presence of monoclonal immunoglobulins can lead to assay interference and spurious results. To the best of our knowledge, this is the second case defining the cause of falsely elevated T3 levels, due to assay interferences with binding of T3 only to monoclonal immunoglobulins.

1. Introduction

As stated in the text book of clinical chemistry, "the clinical chemist confronted with an immunoassay result which does not appear to fit the clinical picture and perhaps also confronted with an alarmed physician should consider the possibility of a phantom in the immunoassay" [1]. The above statement refers to the spurious results which may be caused by interferences.

For the routine evaluation of thyroid function, analysis of thyrotropin (TSH), thyroxine (T4), and triiodothyronine (T3) are widely used diagnostic methods. However, they are subjected to nonspecific bindings that can interfere with the measurement of these hormones. Literature review revealed only one case till date that descripted the presence of a monoclonal immunoglobulin in the serum or urine, which may exhibit binding to T3 only and lead to falsely elevated results [2].

2. Case Presentation

Our patient is a 56-year-old man, who was referred from primary care physician for elevated T3 and possible T3 thyrotoxicosis. For the past few weeks, he had been complaining of fatigue, lethargy, and weight loss. On further evaluation, he had no diarrhea, heat intolerance, skin or hair changes, tremors, visual changes, and palpitations. Furthermore, there was no known personal or family history of thyroid disease. Physical exam was unremarkable except for palpable nodular goiter, and the patient was clinically euthyroid.

In context of fatigue, his primary care physician ordered thyroid function tests, which showed TSH 1.67 μIU/mL (reference range 0.5–8.9), total T3 > 12.32 nmol/L (reference range 0.6–2.79), total T4 4.5 μg/dL (4.6–10.5), free T4 1.08 ng/dL (reference range 0.89–1.76), and free T3 of 2.4 ng/mL (reference range 2.1–4.4). The patient was referred to the endocrinologist clinic for further evaluation The thyroid function test performed on the Siemens Advia centaur analyzer were rechecked, but similar results were obtained. The Siemens Advia centaur T3 assay is a two-site Sandwich/competitive immunoassay using direct chemiluminescent technology. T3 in the patient sample competes with a T3 analog, which is covalently coupled to paramagnetic particles in the solid phase for a limited amount of acridinium ester-labeled monoclonal mouse anti-T3 antibody in the reagent. Furthermore, the same sample was assayed using Abbot Architect Total T3 assay, and results were >8.0 nmol/L. The Architect total T3 assay is a two-step immunoassay to determine the presence of total T3 in human serum and plasma using chemiluminescent microparticle immunoassay technology. This raised the suspicion of a possible endogenous interferent in the sample.

Additional laboratory studies revealed normal liver and renal function tests, negative hepatitis panel. The biochemical parameters are enlisted in Table 1.

As the TSH levels were not suppressed, only raised total T3 level raised the suspicion for thyroid binding protein abnormality. To eliminate the possible interference generated by endogenous antibodies from multiple myeloma, serum of the patient was mixed with an equal proportion of polyethylene glycol (PEG) 6000, i.e., 200 μl. Alongside, a normal control serum was also precipitated with the PEG to ensure that the T3 was not precipitated. The solution was incubated at 37°C during 10 min and then centrifuged for 10 minutes at 5000 rpm. Total T3 activity was reassessed within the supernatant, and result was 0.82 nmol/L (reference range 0.6–2.79), i.e., within the normal reference range. Furthermore, the IgG levels which were 113.45 g/L (normal range: 6.5–16 g/L) at baseline declined to 0.74 g/L (normal range: 6.5–16 g/L) posttreatment with PEG.

However, the anti-mouse antibody blocking analysis and the linearity study with dilution to confirm the interference could not be carried out because we did not have enough baseline serum of the patient to carry out the analysis. However, the patient stated that he had no previous exposure to mice.

Serum protein electrophoresis (SPE) was undertaken which showed gamma globulin of 7.78 g/dL (0.5–1.6) with an M-spike, consistent with diagnosis of multiple myeloma and serum immunofixation (IFE) revealed IgG lambda monoclonal gammopathy as shown in (Figure 1).

Bone marrow examination showed cellular areas with diffuse infiltration with plasma cells (90–95%). Plasma cells positive for CD138 and CD56. Skeletal survey was positive for multiple lytic lesions. All findings were consistent with diagnosis of multiple myeloma.

As the patient was clinically and biochemically euthyroid, total T3 was falsely elevated which was determined to be due to the excess gamma globulins interference in serum with T3 only, and the case was further referred to hematologist for appropriate management. The patient underwent treatment for multiple myeloma as per the recommended protocol based on cyclophosphamide, bortezomib, and dexamethasone. The IgG levels which were 113.45 g/L (normal range: 6.5–16 g/L) at baseline normalized to 11.35 g/L (normal range: 6.5–16 g/L) posttreatment. Furthermore, the total T3 levels posttreatment were 1.25 nmol/L (reference range 0.6–2.79).

3. Discussion

Nearly, more than 99% of both total T3 and T4 are bound to either the thyroxine-binding globulin (TBG), transthyretin (TTR), or albumin. The remnant fraction is the hormonally active free hormone [3]. The routinely used total T3 and T4 immunoassays quantitate both the free and bound forms. Keeping this fact in mind, any degree of change in these binding proteins will result in change in the serum concentration of total T3 and T4, generating spurious results creating a dilemma for diagnosticians in the presence of normal TSH levels.

TBG abnormalities are usually suspected the cause when an endocrinologist encounters a patient with elevated T4 or T3 with normal TSH and the free forms of the hormone. TBG excess is primarily hereditary or it can be secondary to excess estrogens, hepatitis and certain medications 5-fluorouracil, opiates. [4, 5]. In our case, the history does not comprise any medication known to alter TBG levels alongside a negative hepatitis panel. Furthermore, hereditary excess TBG production was ruled out as the patient had previously normal thyroid function tests. Additionally, autoantibodies to T3 or T4 have also serve as thyroid hormone binding proteins and can falsely alter the levels of T3 and T4 [6]. However, as the prevalence of anti-T3 or anti-T4 antibodies among healthy individuals is very rare, it was not further evaluated.

In the 90s, a case of factitious hyperthyroxinemia, due to a monoclonal IgA kappa multiple myeloma was reported with falsely elevated total T3 and T4 not correlating with a normal TSH and free form of both the hormones [7]. In our case, there was absence of any clinical evidence suggesting abnormal TBG, so the high total T3 is most likely justified by the monoclonal immunoglobulin identified on serum protein electrophoresis and immunofixation, binding T3 with high affinity but not T4, as T4 levels were within normal limits. Furthermore, as the Advia Centaur immunoassay is a competitive binding assay, the tracer total T3 binding to the assay antibody follows an inverse relationship with the patient's total T3 levels, i.e., it will eventually decline as the patient's serum T3 levels go up (Figure 2). In the scenario of the monoclonal antibody interfering with the tracer binding, a significantly elevated total T3 would be expected. This is based on the fact that the T3 including the tracer T3 would bind more poorly. Based on this phenomenon, an erroneously elevated T3 was evident in this case. Since the concentration on the architect was also elevated, but other immunoassays based on different working principle were not explored and the possibility of interference with the other assays cannot be ruled out.

To the best of our knowledge, till date, only one similar case with interference with only T3 has been reported by Antonopoulou et al. with euthyroid hyper-tri-iodothyronemia. In

Table 1: Biochemical workup.

Hemoglobin	9.1 g/dl (normal range: 12.3–16.6 g/dl)
Hematocrit	28.9% (normal range: 38.4–50.7%)
White blood cell count	7.8×10^9/L (normal range: 4.8–11.3 $\times 10^9$/L)
Platelets	296×10^9/L (normal range: 154–433 $\times 10^9$/L)
IgG	113.45 g/L (normal range: 6.5–16 g/L)
Serum creatinine	0.9 mg/dl (normal range: 0.9–1.3 mg/dl)
Beta-2-microglobulin	6020 ng/ml (1210–2700 ng/ml)
Serum calcium	9.9 mg/dl (8.6–10.2 mg/dl)

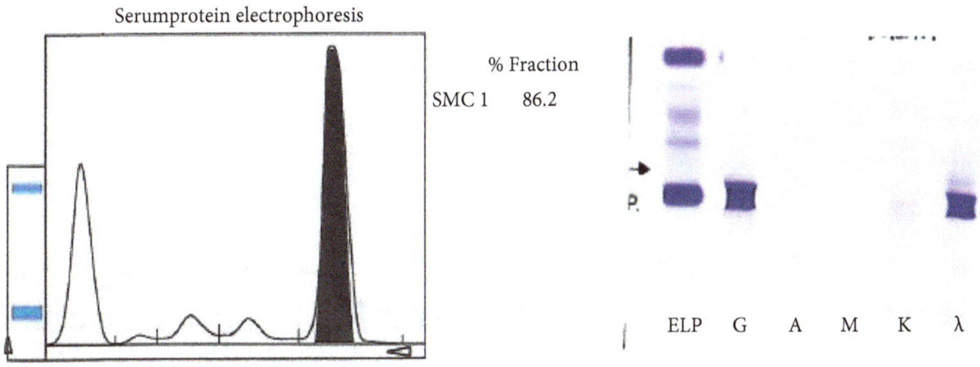

Fractions	%		(g/dl)	(g/dl) Normal
Albumin	29.5		4.20	3.20–5.50
Alpha 1	1.9		0.26	0.10–0.40
Alpha 2	7.0		0.99	0.40–1.20
Beta	6.8		0.97	0.50–1.10
Gamma	54.8		7.78$\uparrow$	0.50–1.60
A/G ratio 0.42		Tot. prot. (g/dl)	14.20$\uparrow$	6.40–8.30

Figure 1: Serum protein electrophoresis showing the M-spike and serum immunofixation (IFE) results consistent with IgG lambda monoclonal gammopathy.

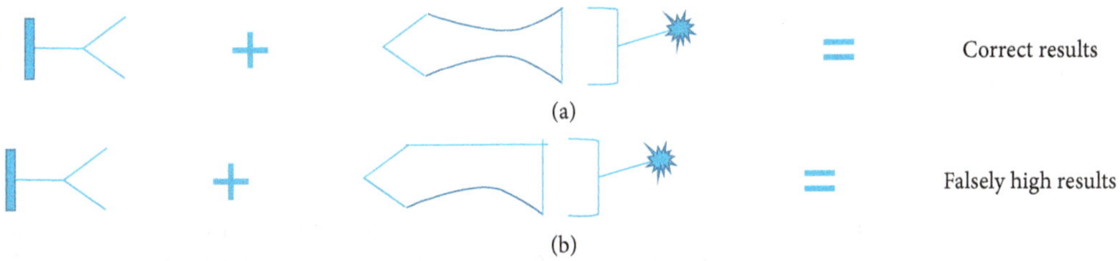

Figure 2: Crossreactions by interferents in two-site immunoassay. (a) Antibodies bind to specific analyte: correct result obtained; (b) cross-reactant sharing two epitopes in common with analyte: falsely high results obtained.

this case, the high total T3 was revealed to be due to the high monoclonal immunoglobulin level, binding T3 with high affinity but not T4, as evident by normal T4 levels revealing a diagnosis of multiple myeloma [2].

4. Conclusion

Our case report is only the second till date suggesting that monoclonal immunoglobulins from multiple myeloma may exhibit binding with higher affinity to T3 only leading to falsely elevated T3 levels in euthyroid patients. It is noteworthy to recognize that spurious results of total thyroid hormones in presence of normal TSH could be due to interferences and requires thorough evaluation based on appropriate clinical history and laboratory workup.

References

[1] M. H. Nahm and J. W. Hoffmann, "Heteroantibody: phantom of the immunoassay," *Clinical Chemistry*, vol. 36, no. 6, p. 829, 1990.

[2] M. Antonopoulou and A. Silverberg, "Spurious t3 thyrotoxicosis unmasking multiple myeloma," *Case Reports in Endocrinology*, vol. 2013, Article ID 739302, 3 pages, 2013.

[3] Y. Pirahanchi and I. Jialal, "Physiology, thyroid, stimulating hormone (TSH)," in *StatPearls*, StatPearls Publishing, Petersburg, FL, USA, 2018.

[4] T. Pappa, A. M. Ferrara, and S. Refetoff, "Inherited defects of thyroxine-binding proteins," *Best Practice & Research Clinical Endocrinology & Metabolism*, vol. 29, no. 5, pp. 735–747, 2015.

[5] A. O. Cheek, K. Kow, J. Chen, and J. A. McLachlan, "Potential mechanisms of thyroid disruption in humans: interaction of organochlorine compounds with thyroid receptor, transthyretin, and thyroid-binding globulin," *Environmental Health Perspectives*, vol. 107, no. 4, pp. 273–278, 1999.

[6] E. Fröhlich and R. Wahl, "Thyroid autoimmunity: role of anti-thyroid antibodies in thyroid and extra-thyroidal diseases," *Frontiers in Immunology*, vol. 8, p. 521, 2017.

[7] K. Cissewski, J. D. Faix, D. Reinwein, and A. C. Moses, "Factitious hyperthyroxinemia due to a monoclonal IgA in a case of multiple myeloma," *Clinical Chemistry*, vol. 39, no. 8, pp. 1739–1742, 1993.

An Unusual Amyloid Goiter in a 48-Year-Old Woman with Rheumatoid Arthritis, Secondary Amyloidosis and Renal Failure

B. López-Muñoz [1] L. Greco Bermúdez,[2] D. Marín-Jiménez [3] M. F. Sánchez de la Fuente,[2] A. Franca Capparelli,[4] I. Mascarell Martínez,[4] and S. Serrano Corredor [1]

[1]*Sección de Endocrinología y Nutrición, Hospital General Universitario de Alicante, ISABIAL-FISABIO, Valencia, Spain*
[2]*Sección de Anatomía Patológica, Hospital General Universitario de Alicante, ISABIAL-FISABIO, Valencia, Spain*
[3]*Sección de Anestesiología y Reanimación, Hospital General Universitario de Alicante, Alicante, Spain*
[4]*Sección de Endocrinología y Nutrición, Hospital Vega Baja de Orihuela, Alicante, Spain*

Correspondence should be addressed to S. Serrano Corredor; sol.serrcorr@gmail.com

Academic Editor: Eli Hershkovitz

Amyloid goiter (AG) is characterized by the presence of deposits of amyloid protein in the thyroid tissue in sufficient amounts to produce enlargement of the gland, accompanied by fat deposition or thyrolipomatosis. It can be seen in long-standing inflammatory disorders, with the common characteristic of amyloidotic renal failure. In daily practice, practitioners should pay attention to the differential diagnosis in patients with suggestive co-morbidities for amyloidosis. The clinic is a progressive increase of the thyroid gland with compressive symptomatology (dyspnea, dysphagia, and changes in the voice). The main imaging finding is diffuse fatty infiltration of the thyroid. The amyloid goitre was most probably in the general context of amyloidosis, regardless of the other complications. We present a case of a 48-years-old female with amyloid goiter secondary to rheumatoid arthritis and renal failure.

1. Introduction

Amyloid goiter (AG) is characterized by the presence of deposits of amyloid protein in the thyroid tissue, accompanied by a diffuse accumulation of adipose tissue, capable of producing a significant enlargement of the gland [1]. Although the normal thyroid gland may have adipocytes in peri and subcapsular areas and near the vessels, and, sometimes, focal microscopic deposition of amyloid might be seen in both primary and secondary amyloidosis, amyloid goiter is a very rare entity with only a few cases described in the literature [1–3]. The main finding of this entity is the diffuse infiltration of fat from the thyroid gland, which is also known as thyroid lipomatosis or thyrolipomatosis (TL), a confusion factor in the terminology of this pathology.

2. Aim

We describe the case of a 48-years-old female with a very extensive diffuse fatty infiltration of the thyroid gland in an AG in the context of secondary amyloidosis.

3. Case Report

In July 2018, a 48-year-old woman was submitted in Endocrinology for goiter grade 2. She reported progressive dysphagia, with a feeling of "stop" the food bolus in the middle sternal area for 2-3 years.

She had a medical history of rheumatoid arthritis, diagnosed when she was 20 years old, in treatment with prednisone for 17 years continuously (current dose of 10 mg daily) and biological treatments (including rituximab and tocilizumab) at different times; secondary amyloidosis, diagnosed in 2010, by a rectal biopsy in a colonoscopy during the study of abdominal pain; colonic diverticula; and terminal renal failure, secondary to amyloidosis, in dialysis for 6 years and a half.

The patient was diagnosed of subclinical hyperthyroidism (TSH 0.21 mU/L (0.38–4.84), FT4 2.27 ng/dL (0.8–2.0) and FT3 2.38 μg/ml (1.8–4.6)), without symptoms of thyroid hyperfunction and negative antithyroid antibodies. She was under treatment with Tiamazol 5 mg daily.

Thyroid ultrasound showed an enlargement thyroid gland, isoechoic and without nodules. Cervical computed tomography revealed an increase in size of thyroid gland, with a right

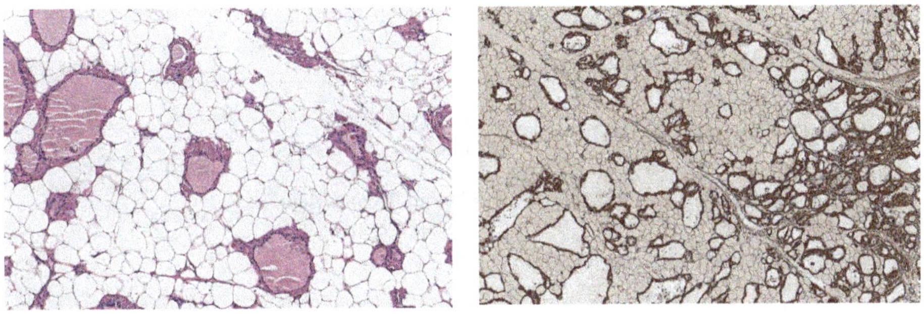

(a) (b)

FIGURE 1: (a) (Hematosilin-Eosin) thyroid tissue replaced by adipocytes, preserving only the thyroid follicles, surrounded by eosinophilic, hyaline, and amorphous aggregates, (b) (amyloid A staining) are positive in immunohistochemistry to amyloid AA antibody.

thyroid lobe (LTD) of 5×4.7×8.8 cm, a left thyroid lobe (LTI) of 4×3.5×6.5 cm and an isthmus of 2.5 cm, with polylobulated contours. It displaced the carotid artery and the internal jugular vein laterally, without causing stenosis or displacement of the trachea. The thyroid parenchyma showed a marked decrease in density, similar to fat density. On T1- and T2-weighted images, hyperintense lobulated areas that corresponded to fatty attenuation areas on CT were noted. Core needle biopsy reported an intense adipose replacement of normal tissue and interstitial deposits of positive eosinophilic substance for Congo Red staining, with green birefringence in polarized light and positivity for Thioflavin with UV light, compatible with amyloid deposits.

With the diagnosis of amyloid goiter, total thyroidectomy was performed. During the surgery, a large thyroid mass was found. It seemed to be like a big, friable, lipoma, completely different from a normal thyroid gland. Three fragments of tissue with dimensions of 13.5×4.5, 6.5×3.5 and 3.5×2.5 cm, respectively, were referred to pathological anatomy. The appearance of the fragment was like adipose tissue, surrounded by a reddish margin that seemed to be the thyroid parenchyma. Histologically, a diffuse adipose metaplasia of the thyroid stroma was observed, associated with the deposition of amyloid material in the vascular walls and in the thyroid interstitium (Figure 1). The postoperative coursed without incidences.

4. Discussion

Amyloid goiter is defined by the presence of amyloid protein in the thyroid in sufficient amounts to produce enlargement of the gland accompanied by fat deposition of varying extents [1, 4]. It has been described associated in both primary and secondary amyloidosis with long-standing inflammatory disorders (familiar Mediterranean fever, rheumatoid arthritis, ankylopoietic espodilitis, chronic osteomyelitis, tuberculosis, bronchiectasis and other connective tissue diseases), and, more rarely, with neoplastic processes (medullary carcinoma of the thyroid), with the common characteristic of amyloidotic renal failure [2].

Its current incidence and prevalence are unknown. It has been described associated with as a primary amyloidosis in 0.04% and a familial Mediterranean fever in 0.27% [1].

References in literature on AG are limited. Until 2000, García-Villanueva et al. referred 200–250 published cases [5]. In our review, we have only found 9 cases published in the last 10 years, all of them were associated with kidney disease (CKD), with or without kidney transplant: 3 of them were associated with familial Mediterranean fever [1, 6], 2 cases were associated with rheumatoid arthritis [3, 7], 1 case was associated with bronchiectasis [2], another case with bronchiectasis and ankylosing spondylitis [1], and other 2 cases were associated with Crohn's disease [4] and multiple myeloma [8] (Table 1). Hijazi et al. [9] reviewed four more cases of thyrolipomatosis until 2018, publishing a new case in a 53-year-old woman with renal failure secondary to diabetic nephropathy, without anatomopathological study for amyloid.

The pathophysiology of diffuse proliferation of mature adipose tissue in the thyroid gland is unclear. Fat accumulation in amyloid goiters can be explained by tissue hypoxia secondary to progressive capillary and thyroid follicle destruction due to amyloid deposition. Tissue hypoxia may result in metaplasia of stromal fibroblasts to become adipose cells, which accumulate adipose tissue in the gland, increasing its size [1, 6–8].

Thyroid lipomatosis is clinically apparent due to a progressive enlargement of the thyroid that can involve the airway and/or upper gastrointestinal tract, producing dyspnea, dysphagia, and changes in the voice [7]. They tend to show rapid progression, which means that differential diagnosis must be made with malignant processes such as lymphoma or anaplastic cancer [6, 7].

Physical examination usually shows a soft, nontender goiter that is nodular or diffuse. In most cases, tests show normal thyroid function, but both hyperthyroidism and hypothyroidism have been described in a few patients, usually mild, like our case [7].

Imaging patterns in amyloid goiters may vary depending on the amount of fat and amyloid deposition. By ultrasonography, amyloid deposition has a hypoechoic pattern, with or without nodules. In our case, as fatty infiltration predominated, sonography pattern was isoechoic and diffuse. CT scan show an enlarged thyroid with well-defined limits and low density, in the range of adipose tissue (−10 to −50 Hounsfield Units). On MRI, fatty infiltration causes increased signal intensity both on T1- and T2-weighted images, with suppression on fat-saturated sequences. Cases with diffused fatty infiltration can be difficult to differentiate from thyrolipomatosis [7].

TABLE 1: Amyloid goiter cases published since 2010.

Reference	Age (years old), sex	Associated pathology	Clinical features	Thyroid function	Thyroid autoantibodies
[1]	47, male	Ankylosing spondylitis Bronchiectasia AA	Incidental enlarged thyroid gland in thoracic TC	—	—
[1]	43, male	Familiar Mediterranean fever AA	Enlarged thyroid gland in physical examination	Normal	—
[1]	34, female	Familiar Mediterranean fever AA	—	—	—
[2]	30, male	Bronchiectasia Primary adrenal insufficiency due to amyloidosis	Dysphagia for solids	Normal	AntiTPO - AntiTG -
[3]	52, female	Rheumatoid arthritis AA	Dyspnea Neck swelling	Normal	AntiTPO - AntiTG -
[4]	55, male	Crohn's disease AA Kidney transplant	Neck swelling	Normal	—
[6]	31, female	Familiar Mediterranean fever AA	Enlarged thyroid gland in physical examination	Normal	—
[7]	36, female	Rheumatoid arthritis AA Kidney transplant	Dyspnea Enlarged thyroid gland in physical examination	Normal	—
[8]	45, male	Multiple mieloma AA	Dysphagia Dyspnea	Normal	—

AA: secondary amyloidosis, TC: computer tomography, antiTPO: antimicrosomal antibodies, antiTG: antithyroglobulin antibodies.

In a pathological examination, the thyroid reveals a loss of normal architecture with diffuse infiltration of mature adipose tissue without atypias. The number of follicles decreases and tends to be distorted and surrounded by an eosinophilic acellular amorphous material. There deposits are positive for Congo Red stained and for amyloid AA antibody in immunohistochemistry, showing green birefringence with polarized light. Some of the published cases have reported massively enlarged thyroids with masses of 500–700 g [7].

The usual treatment is total thyroidectomy [3], performed in our case and in the 9 cases mentioned, necessary both to relieve symptoms and to establish the definitive diagnosis. Preoperatory suspicion is important if there are long-standing co-morbidities, including confirmed amyloidiosis, because it is useful to guide the surgeon, due to the risk of local extension and differential diagnosis with a thyroid carcinoma.

5. Conclusion

Amyloid goiter is a rare entity, which should be suspected in the presence of a goiter, in the context of a systemic disease associated with renal failure with/without transplantation. Systemic amyloidosis is usually accompanied by fatty deposits in the thyroid, but enlargement of the gland due to a thyrolipomatosis is infrequent. We believe that in literature there is not a good differentiation between the concepts of AG vs TL, with an overlap in the diagnostic criteria between both entities. It remains to be clarified if it is a single entity or, on the contrary, they are two pathologies with shared characteristics.

References

[1] S. Bakan, S. G. Kandemirli, S. Akbas et al., "Amyloid goiter: a diagnosis to consider in diffuse fatty infiltration of the thyroid," *Journal of Ultrasound in Medicine*, vol. 36, no. 5, pp. 1045–1049, 2017.

[2] I. Oueslati, K. Khiari, H. Kaaroud et al., "Amyloid goiter as the first manifestation of systemic amyloidosis," *La Tunisie Médicale*, vol. 94, no. 1, p. 82, 2016.

[3] G. Uzum, F. O. Kaya, A. K. Uzum et al., "Amyloid goiter associated with amyloidosis secondary to rheumatoid arthritis," *Case Reports in Medicine*, vol. 2013, Article ID 792413, 3 pages, 2013.

[4] T. A. Jacques and M. P. Stearns, "Diffuse lipomatosis of the thyroid with amyloid deposition," *Journal of Laryngology & Otology*, vol. 127, no. 4, pp. 426–428, 2013.

[5] A. García Villanueva, M. J. García Villanueva, M. García Villanueva et al., "Surgical considerations about amyloid goiter," *Endocrinology and Nutrition*, vol. 60, no. 5, pp. 254–259, 2013.

[6] A. O. Aksu, M. N. Ozmen, K. K. Oguz, D. Akinci, U. Yasavun, and P. Firat, "Diffuse fatty infiltration of the thyroid gland in amyloidosis: sonographic, computed tomographic, and magnetic resonance imaging findings," *Journal of Ultrasound in Medicine*, vol. 29, no. 8, pp. 1251–1255, 2010.

[7] S. Bell, G. A. Sosa, A. Del Valle Jaen, and M. F. Russo Picasso, "Thyroid lipomatosis in a 36-year-old patient with rheumatoid arthritis and a kidney transplant," *Endocrinology, Diabetes & Metabolism Case Reports*, vol. 2016, p. 160007, 2016.

[8] M. A. Cannizzaro, S. L. Bianco, W. Saliba et al., "A rare case of primary thyroid amyloidosis," *International Journal of Surgery Case Reports*, vol. 53, pp. 179–181, 2018.

[9] D. M. Hijazi, F. A. Addas, N. M. Alghanmi, H. Z. Marzouki, and M. A. Merdad, "An Enlarged goiter presenting with a rare diffuse lipomatosis of the thyroid gland," *American Journal of Case Reports*, vol. 19, pp. 808–811, 2018.

21

Riedel's Thyroiditis: Report of Two Cases and Literature Review

Victor Manuel Blanco,[1] Camilo Andrés Páez,[1] Angela María Victoria,[2] Luis Guillermo Arango,[3] Ana María Arrunategui,[4] Juliana Escobar,[4] Veline Martínez,[1] and Guillermo Edinson Guzmán[3]

[1]*Internal Medicine Unit, Fundación Valle del Lili, Cra 98 #18-49, Cali 760032, Colombia*
[2]*Health Sciences Faculty, Universidad Icesi, Fundación Valle del Lili, Cra 98 #18-49, Cali 760032, Colombia*
[3]*Internal Medicine Unit - Department of Endocrinology, Fundación Valle del Lili, Cra 98 #18-49, Cali 760032, Colombia*
[4]*Pathology Surgery Unit, Fundación Valle del Lili, Cra 98 #18-49, Cali 760032, Colombia*

Correspondence should be addressed to Angela María Victoria; angelamav7@hotmail.com

Academic Editor: Eli Hershkovitz

Riedel's thyroiditis is a rare entity consisting of a fibrotic process of the thyroid which can generate gland destruction, infiltration of cervical structures and even airway obstruction. It has been associated with systemic fibrotic disorders, autoimmune diseases, and more recently with spectrum of diseases related to excess of Immunoglobulin G type 4 (IgG4). Two cases of Riedel's thyroiditis by IgG4, confirmed by immunohistochemistry and was managed surgically with favorable results during the follow-up time, are presented. These case descriptions highlight the diagnostic challenge of this disease, describe the response with surgical management, and make a brief update on the subject.

1. Introduction

Riedel's thyroiditis is a fibrotic process of the thyroid gland which characteristically extends through adjacent tissues generating gland destruction, infiltration in cervical structures and even air way obstruction. It is a rare condition, with a prevalence of one per 100.000 inhabitants, which affects more frequently women between 30 and 50 years of age. The precise etiology of this disorder is not still clear. It has been described an association with systemic fibrotic processes, autoimmune diseases, and more recently with diseases from the spectrum of excessive immunoglobulin G type 4 (IgG4).

Regarding the treatment for this condition there is no international consensus, but it has been described the surgical approach, use of systemic steroids and inmunosupressants like tamoxifen, rituximab, and mycophenolate mofetil, among others with varying rates of success. We describe two cases, in which diagnosis was confirmed by immunohistochemistry and additionally managed with surgical intervention, with satisfactory results until the follow-up date.

2. Case Presentation

2.1. Case 1. A 38-year-old female from Palmira, Colombia, without past medical history presented with a nonpainful mass in the anterior neck region of nine months of evolution associated to dysphagia, hoarseness, and dyspnea of night predominance. Physical examination revealed good general condition, no areas of swelling or local inflammation, and vital signs in normal ranges. A grade III goiter was palpable mainly in the right thyroid lobe, its diameter was about five centimeters and had a hard consistency without pulsatility or murmurs. Thyroid-stimulating hormone (TSH) test was reported as 0.153 μIU/mL (normal range 0.4–4.5), free T4 1.19 ng/dL (normal range 0.8–1.7), and negative antithyroid peroxidase (anti-TPO) antibodies. In addition, serological immunoglobulins were tested resulting in IgG 905 mg/dL (normal range 767–1590), IgM 150 mg/dL (normal range 37–286), and IgA 200 mg/dL (normal range 61–356). The patient had no signs or symptoms of hyperthyroidism; therefore, this condition was interpreted as subclinical hyperthyroidism. Fine-needle aspiration biopsy (FNAB) was

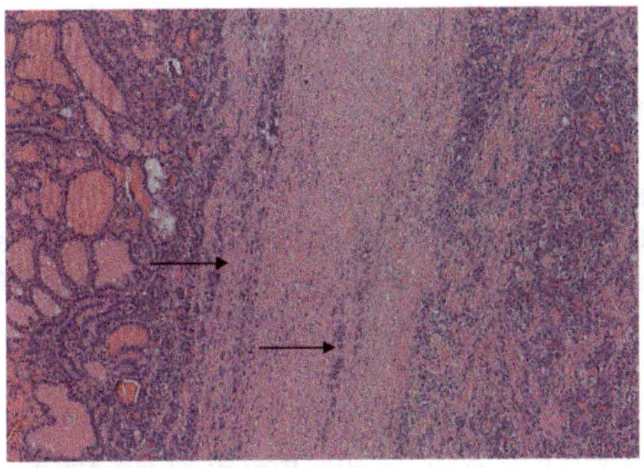

FIGURE 1: Thyroid gland pathology. Hematoxylin and eosin stain of histological sample from case 1, showing fibrosis and tissue distortion. Original magnification ×20.

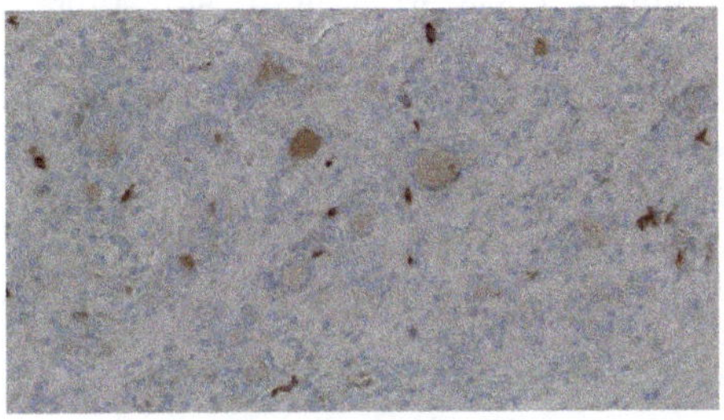

FIGURE 2: Thyroid gland pathology. Staining for IgG4. Multiple IgG4-positive cells were observed (brown color). Original magnification ×40.

taken from the right thyroid nodule with unsatisfactory results (Bethesda I). The patient was taken to total thyroidectomy; surgical findings depicted a five centimeters complex mass with hard consistency, whitish appearance and a thick capsule that compressed and deformed the trachea. Its histological study identified thyroid gland with follicles of different sizes, without oxyphilic changes, full of colloid material surrounded by abundant dense fibro-connective tissue with interspersed collagen and abundant lymphoplasmacytic inflammatory infiltrate with some eosinophils (Figure 1). The fibrous area constituted the majority of the nodular lesion, without evidence of malignancy, findings that corresponded to Riedel's thyroiditis. Immunohistochemistry tests were performed, which were positive for IgG4 (Figure 2). A favorable postsurgical evolution was obtained, achieving an euthyroid state with levothyroxine substitution.

2.2. Case 2. A 56-year-old male patient with medical history of hypertension, chronic obstructive pulmonary disease, and chronic kidney disease on renal replacement therapy, presented with a right cervical mass with progressive growth associated to dyspnea and dysphagia to solid foods. At physical examination the patient had vital signs in normal ranges; also, presented a large thyroid mass of right predominance with continuity up to the thoracic operculum, of approximately 12 cm in diameter and hard consistency without associated adenopathies. Initial TSH value was 269 μIU/mL and substitution with levothyroxine was started. Thyroid ultrasound showed enlarged thyroid lobes, with multiple nodular hypoechoic and hyperechoic images with irregular edges up

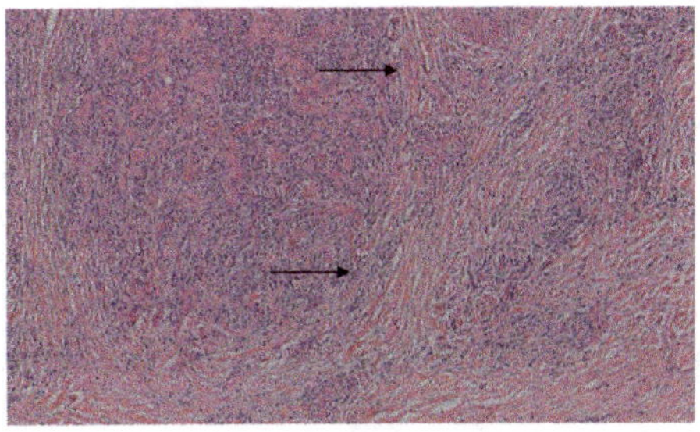

FIGURE 3: Thyroid gland pathology. Hematoxylin and eosin stain of histological sample from case 2, showing fibrosis and tissue distortion. Original magnification ×20.

to 2.5 cm. Through fibrobronchoscopy, extrinsic compression of the trachea was documented at three centimeters from the glottis, with occlusion of 20% of the luminal space, for which thyroidectomy was decided. During surgery, a large thyroid gland was visualized with an inflammatory, fibrotic, and multinodular aspect. The pathology report described a gland of 177.5 grams, of a dark-brown color, and a smooth surface, to which cuts were made, finding that the entire gland had fibrotic and multinodular aspect. Microscopic visualization showed tissue with architectural distortion due to the presence of extensive fibrosis, with severe atrophy of the follicles, evident dense inflammatory infiltrate and abundant plasma cells (Figure 3). Immunohistochemical study helped to confirm the diagnosis of Riedel's thyroiditis, with more than 10 IgG4-positive plasma cells per high-power field (HPF), with an IgG4/IgG ratio greater than 40%.

3. Discussion

Riedel's thyroiditis is a fibrotic process associated with infiltration by mononuclear inflammatory cells that compromise thyroid gland but usually extends beyond it invading the adjacent soft tissue. Fibrous involvement can extend to the recurrent laryngeal nerves causing dysphonia, towards the trachea causing compression or stenosis, towards the parathyroids causing hypoparathyroidism, or other tissues such as the mediastinum and chest wall. This invasive capacity differentiates Riedel's thyroiditis from other forms of infiltration of the thyroid gland. Epidemiologically, it is a rare disorder that affects more women than men, with an incidence of approximately one case per 100.000 patients, most frequently seen between the fourth and sixth decades of life [1].

To date, the etiology of Riedel's thyroiditis remains unknown, in some cases it has been considered as the thyroid manifestation of multifocal fibrosclerosis, which is partly supported by its association with other fibrotic disorders (retroperitoneal fibrosis, fibrosing mediastinitis, sclerosing cholangitis, among others); however, evidence for this association is scarce [2, 3]. The autoimmune etiology has also been suggested due to the histopathological findings of mononuclear infiltrate, vasculitis, and high prevalence of antithyroid antibodies in affected patients, in addition to the association with disorders such as Hashimoto's thyroiditis, Addison's disease, type I diabetes, Graves' disease, and pernicious anemia [4].

It is known that Riedel's thyroiditis can occur as part of systemic diseases associated with IgG4, being characteristic in these cases the tissue infiltration by IgG4 positive plasma cells, as well as elevated serum levels of this immunoglobulin, although normal serum levels can be seen in up to 30% of patients [5–7]. In none of our cases the presence of extra thyroid fibrosis was documented.

From the clinical point of view, there are no pathognomonic findings in Riedel's thyroiditis [8, 9]. Regarding the clinical manifestations of this disorder, goiter is usually found, which can vary in size but typically has a stony consistency and equally affects both thyroid lobes, it is usually slow-growing and in most cases is asymptomatic, although some patients may report dyspnea, dysphagia, dysphonia, or symptoms and signs of superior vena cava syndrome or lower respiratory infection (obstructive pneumonia secondary to compression created by the growing mass) [10]. The adjacent involvement can extend to cervical lymph nodes and can be accompanied by adenopathies attached to deep planes that may suggest a diagnosis of neoplastic etiology. In terms of symptomatic presentation, Fatourechi et al. found pain (24%), dysphagia (33%), vocal cord paralysis (29%), and tracheal narrowing (48%) [11]. In our experience, the cardinal symptoms were mainly respiratory due to extrinsic compromise of the airway.

Regarding diagnostic imaging strategies, scintigraphy usually shows a heterogeneous uptake, while computer tomography (CT) and nuclear magnetic resonance (NMR) show the extensive fibrosis of the thyroid parenchyma. The advantage of CT and NMR is that they can assess the extent of compromise to other structures of the neck, including the possibility of vascular invasion. Thyroid and neck ultrasound can also be helpful, showing multiple hypoechoic focal lesions, which lack blood flow when evaluated by color doppler mode [12]. Other imaging modalities that have been described include positron emission tomography with the use of fluorodeoxyglucose (PET-Scan), which shows areas of increased metabolism, modality that can be used for monitoring the disease activity [13].

Most patients have normal thyroid function, both TSH and Free T4 are normal in the vast majority of those affected, although it is reported that up to 30% have hypothyroidism [8]. In a 30-year retrospective analysis, Fatourechi et al. reported at the Mayo Clinic 17 hypothyroid patients and only one with hyperthyroidism out of the 22 total studied patients [11]. On the other hand, it is useful to perform the measurement of thyroid autoantibodies due to more than 50% of patients have high levels [8, 9]. In our case, the first patient had subclinical hyperthyroidism and negative anti-TPO antibodies and the second one exhibited hypothyroidism and did not have a report of antithyroid antibodies.

As to the histopathological findings, the sample can be obtained by both open surgery plus biopsy or FNAB, being the latter less helpful in Riedel's thyroiditis compared to other pathologies of the gland, since in many patients the sample is inconclusive evidencing only fibrosis and mononuclear infiltrate with few cells of thyroid epithelium, which is difficult to differentiate from other disorders with similar presentation like subacute thyroiditis, the fibrous variant of Hashimoto thyroiditis (where non-producing IgA plasma cells predominate), or the paucicellular variant of anaplastic thyroid carcinoma [14]. It is precisely due to the foregoing that many of the diagnostic confirmations require surgical removal, in which hard, whitish, and avascular tissue can be evidenced macroscopically.

In advanced stages, the predominant findings under the microscope are tissue fibrosis, absence of thyroid follicles and poor lymphocyte-predominant cellularity, being also characteristic the perithyroid infiltration of adipose tissue, vessels (even with associated thrombosis), nerves, and even the trachea and muscles. In up to one fourth of the patients, it can also be seen hemorrhagic cysts within the affected parenchyma. Deep tissues can be so compromised that in several cases complete removal of the gland becomes impossible. Thus, the trained eye of the pathologist will search for clues that suggest the diagnosis while, at the same time, could discard other probable etiologies such as malignancy or granulomatous entities, being of special interest the differential diagnosis with anaplastic paucicellular thyroid carcinoma, that may have a similar pattern of fibrosis and invasion to adjacent planes, in addition to characteristic tapered cells that can be detected by using immunohistochemistry for specific makers of the thyroid line [15].

Due to the low incidence of Riedel's thyroiditis, there are no guidelines or large clinical studies that refer to the optimal management of the condition, in addition, although most cases are progressive, there are reports of patients in whom the disease stabilizes or even reverses. Most authors agree that the therapy should be aimed at treating hypothyroidism in those who exhibit it and at managing the fibrosclerotic manifestations that can put the patient's life at risk (e.g., compression of the airway that may lead to recurrent pneumonias).

There are multiple approaches for the treatment of fibrosis, being systemic steroids, the first line of treatment given to the majority of patients, which decreases the size and hardness of the goiter in only a few of the patients, usually, being necessary prolonged therapy since it is not uncommon to lose the improvement achieved once the doses are titrated downwards [16]. Tamoxifen is another agent used with successful reports, at doses of 10–20 mg every 12 hours. There are descriptions with significant decrease in goiter size in patients who previously did not respond to steroids; the exact mechanism by which this improvement is achieved is not known in detail, but it would seem to be associated with reduction in fibroblast proliferation mediated by transforming growth factor beta (TGF-B) [17].

Regarding surgical management, the indications are basically two: sampling for histopathological diagnostic confirmation, as previously described, and compression or stenosis relief at the level of trachea or esophagus. It has to be considered that the management in these cases should be limited to the resection of the segment that is generating obstruction. The complete resection of the gland is inadvisable due to the high possibility of damaging nearby structures such as the parathyroid and recurrent laryngeal nerves because of the lack of margins of resection. In totally refractory cases, low-dose radiation therapy has been used as a final management, but there is not concrete information about its efficacy [18, 19].

4. Conclusion

As it has been depicted in this review, Riedel's thyroiditis is a rare entity, scarcely described, with characteristics that suggest association with systemic fibrosis and other disorders triggered by IgG4. Diagnosis can be challenging due to the unknown etiology, and the unspecific symptoms that overlap with other disorders. As to the treatment, there are no guidelines or general consensus, and the proposed treatments do not go beyond case reports or small case series. The aim of our publication was to describe the cases that occurred in the institution Fundación Valle del Lili in Cali, Colombia; diagnosed by histopathology and managed with surgical intervention, where good clinical evolution was achieved.

Acknowledgments

The authors hereby express their gratitude to the health staff, the Department of Endocrinology and the Clinical Research Center of Fundación Valle del Lili. The present investigation has not received any specific scholarship from public or commercial agencies, or nonprofit sectors.

References

[1] J. C. Lo, K. C. Loh, A. L. Rubin, I. Cha, and F. S. Greenspan, "Riedel's thyroiditis presenting with hypothyroidism and hypoparathyroidism: dramatic response to glucocorticoid and thyroxine therapy," *Clinical Endocrinology*, vol. 48, no. 6, pp. 815–818, 1998.

[2] M. F. Erdoğan, C. Anil, N. Türkçapar, D. Ozkaramanli, S. D. Sak, and G. Erdoğan, "A case of Riedel's thyroiditis with pleural and pericardial effusions," *Endocrine*, vol. 35, no. 3, pp. 297–301, 2009.

[3] J. V. Hennessey, "Riedel's thyroiditis: a clinical review," *The Journal of Clinical Endocrinology & Metabolism*, vol. 96, no. 10, pp. 3031–3041, 2011.

[4] T. Zimmermann-Belsing and U. Feldt-Rasmussen, "Riedel's thyroiditis: an autoimmune or primary fibrotic disease?" *Journal of Internal Medicine*, vol. 235, no. 3, pp. 271–274, 1994.

[5] M. Dahlgren, A. Khosroshahi, G. P. Nielsen, V. Deshpande, and J. H. Stone, "Riedel's thyroiditis and multifocal fibrosclerosis are part of the IgG4-related systemic disease spectrum," *Arthritis Care & Research*, vol. 62, no. 9, pp. 1312–1318, 2010.

[6] T. Kamisawa, Y. Zen, S. Pillai, and J. H. Stone, "IgG4-related disease," *The Lancet*, vol. 385, no. 9976, pp. 1460–1471, 2015.

[7] J. H. Stone, Y. Zen, and V. Deshpande, "IgG4-related disease," *New England Journal of Medicine*, vol. 366, no. 6, pp. 539–551, 2012.

[8] M. H. Cho, C. S. Kim, J. S. Park et al., "Riedel's thyroiditis in a patient with recurrent subacute thyroiditis: a case report and review of the literature," *Endocrine Journal*, vol. 54, no. 4, pp. 559–562, 2007.

[9] S. M. Schwaegerle, T. W. Bauer, and C. B. Esselstyn Jr, "Riedel's thyroiditis," *American Journal of Clinical Pathology*, vol. 90, pp. 715–722, 1988.

[10] T. Yasmeen, S. Khan, S. G. Patel et al., "Clinical case seminar: Riedel's thyroiditis: report of a case complicated by spontaneous hypoparathyroidism, recurrent laryngeal nerve injury, and Horner's syndrome," *The Journal of Clinical Endocrinology and Metabolism*, vol. 87, no. 8, pp. 3543–3547, 2002.

[11] M. M. Fatourechi, I. D. Hay, B. Mclver, T. J. Sebo, and V. Fatourechi, "Invasive fibrous thyroiditis (Riedel thyroiditis): the mayo clinic experience, 1976–2008," *Thyroid*, vol. 21, no. 7, pp. 765–72, 2011.

[12] G. Papi, S. Corrado, A. M. Cesinaro, L. Novelli, A. Smerieri, and C. Carapezzi, "Riedel's thyroiditis: clinical, pathological and imaging features," *International Journal of Clinical Practice*, vol. 56, no. 1, pp. 65–67, 2002.

[13] J. Lauwyck, Y. Piette, L. Van Walleghem, and F. De Geeter, "IgG4-related disease: the utility of (18) F-FDG PET/CT in diagnosis and treatment," *Hellenic Journal of Nuclear Medicine*, vol. 18, no. 1, pp. 155–159, 2015.

[14] M. Harigopal, S. Sahoo, W. M. Recant, and R. M. DeMay, "Fine-needle aspiration of Riedel's disease: report of a case and review of the literature," *Diagnostic Cytopathology*, vol. 30, no. 3, pp. 193–197, 2004.

[15] S. K. Wan, J. K. Chan, and S. K. Tang, "Paucicellular variant of anaplastic thyroid carcinoma. a mimic of Reidel's thyroiditis," *American Journal of Clinical Pathology*, vol. 105, no. 4, pp. 388–393, 1996.

[16] B. Vaidya, P. E. Harris, P. Barrett, and P. Kendall-Taylor, "Corticosteroid therapy in Riedel's thyroiditis," *Postgraduate Medical Journal*, vol. 73, no. 866, pp. 817–819, 1997.

[17] J. Few, N. W. Thompson, P. Angelos, D. Simeone, T. Giordano, and T. Reeve, "Riedel's thyroiditis: treatment with tamoxifen," *Surgery*, vol. 120, no. 6, pp. 993–999, 1996.

[18] J. V. Hennessey, "Riedels thyroiditis: a clinical review," *The Journal of Clinical Endocrinology & Metabolism*, vol. 96, no. 10, pp. 3031–3041, 2011.

[19] H. Falhammar, C. C. Juhlin, C. Barner, S.-B. Catrina, C. Karefylakis, and J. Calissendorff, "Riedel's thyroiditis: clinical presentation, treatment and outcomes," *Endocrine*, vol. 60, no. 1, pp. 185–192, 2018.

22

First Case Report of Arrhythmogenic Right Ventricular Cardiomyopathy Showing Refractory Ventricular Tachycardia Induced by Thyroid Storm due to Graves' Disease

Masaki Matsubara[1] **Tomohiro Tanaka,**[2] **Akinori Wakamiya,**[2] **Tamiko Tamanaha,**[1] **Hisashi Makino,**[1] **Tomonori Tanei,**[3] **Takeshi Aiba,**[2] **Kengo Kusano,**[2] **and Kiminori Hosoda**[1]

[1]*Division of Diabetes and Lipid Metabolism, National Cerebral and Cardiovascular Center, 6-1 Kishibe-Shimmachi, Suita, Osaka 564-8565, Japan*
[2]*Department of Cardiovascular Medicine, National Cerebral and Cardiovascular Center, 6-1 Kishibe-Shimmachi, Suita, Osaka 564-8565, Japan*
[3]*Department of Breast and Endocrine Surgery, Osaka University Graduate School of Medicine, 2-2-E10 Yamadaoka, Suita, Osaka 565-0871, Japan*

Correspondence should be addressed to Masaki Matsubara; matsubara.m@ncvc.go.jp

Academic Editor: Toshihiro Kita

A 48-year-old man who was diagnosed with arrhythmogenic right ventricular cardiomyopathy (ARVC) due to a plakophilin 2 gene mutation developed acute both-sided heart failure with rapid atrial fibrillation and was hospitalized. After admission, sustained ventricular tachycardia, which was refractory to antiarrhythmic agents, occurred repeatedly, and required electrical cardioversion. He was diagnosed with thyroid storm due to Graves' disease, and treatment for hyperthyroidism was initiated. After the treatment, lethal arrhythmia did not reoccur, and biventricular heart failure ameliorated. To our best knowledge, this is the first report in English of a patient with ARVC showing refractory arrhythmia induced by thyroid storm due to Graves' disease.

1. Introduction

Arrhythmogenic right ventricular cardiomyopathy (ARVC) is characterized by an enlargement and hypofunction of the right ventricle and arrhythmia of the right ventricular origin and can cause sudden death due to arrhythmia in juveniles [1]. Thus, early diagnosis and appropriate treatment are important. ARVC is caused by genetic factors, one of which is a plakophilin 2 gene (*PKP2*) mutation, which is mainly expressed in the epidermis and cardiomyocytes, including Purkinje fibers and constituted desmosomes. Moreover, the connections between cardiomyocytes are impaired by mutations of this protein, leading to weakened myocardial structure [1, 2].

Graves' disease is a common disease, and it can induce a life-threatening condition, namely, thyroid storm (TS) [3]. Regarding the cardiovascular system affected by thyrotoxicosis, high-output heart failure with decreased systemic vascular resistance is expected [4]. However, low-output heart failure related to dilated cardiomyopathy has been reported as an unusual type of cardiac complication, which is usually reversible with hyperthyroidism treatment [5].

We herein report the first case of a patient with ARVC showing refractory ventricular tachycardia (VT) induced by TS due to Graves' disease. Moreover, the patient suffered from biventricular heart failure. Hyperthyroidism treatment was initiated, and it proved to be really effective. No lethal arrhythmia recurred after the treatment, and both-sided heart failure improved as well.

2. Case Presentation

The patient was a 48-year-old man diagnosed with ARVC due to PKP2 mutation [2] and constitutional jaundice. At the age of 35 years, catheter ablation of the right ventricular apical septum was performed for sustained VT with left bundle branch block-type and superior QRS axis. The thyroid function was euthyroid at the time; the thyroid-stimulating hormone (TSH) level was 1.53 (normal range, 0.5–5.5) μU/mL, the free triiodothyronine (T3) level was 3.6 (normal range, 2.6–4.6) pg/mL, and the free thyroxine (T4) level was 1.5 (normal range, 1.1–1.8) ng/dL. Thereafter, under daily metoprolol intake of 80 mg, VT did not recur. He complained of palpitation six months before admission, and 80 mg/day sotalol was started. His laboratory data are shown in Table 1. Although palpitation was reduced, he had general fatigue and discontinued taking sotalol one month before consultation. He presented to our emergency department with worsening dyspnea, bilateral lower leg edema, a 5 kg weight gain, and watery diarrhea. As for vital signs, he was alert, his blood pressure was 123/87 mmHg, his heart rate was 150/min and irregular, his blood oxygen saturation was 95% (room air), and his body temperature was 37.7°C. Physical examination revealed jugular venous distention, coarse crackles in both lungs, pitting edema in the legs, and tremors of the upper limbs. Exophthalmos and ocular motility disturbances were not observed. A chest radiograph and electrocardiogram showed cardiac dilation, bilateral pleural effusion, and a rapid atrial fibrillation (AF) rhythm (Figures 1(a) and 2). Transthoracic echocardiography clarified dilation of the intravenous cava, right atrium, and right ventricle (RVDd = 57 mm), decreased right ventricular contractile function (TAPSE = 8 mm), compression of the left ventricle by the dilated right ventricle, and tricuspid regurgitation (peak pressure gradient = 15 mmHg) at the right side. LVDd and LVDs were 46 mm and 33 mm, respectively; however, they might have been underestimated owing to compression. Furthermore, a decreased ejection fraction (visual 30%) and absence of vegetation at the valves were observed. The plasma brain natriuretic peptide (BNP) and serum total bilirubin levels were elevated (Table 1). He was diagnosed with both-sided acute heart failure with rapid AF and admitted to the coronary care unit (CCU). The SOFA and APACHE II scores at admission were 2 and 8, respectively. He was given 80 mg/day intravenous furosemide and 0.25 mg intravenous digoxin, and heparinization was started. After admission, sustained VT occurred, so an electrical cardioversion was performed and intravenous amiodarone was administered (Figure 2). Moreover, atrial tachycardia, for which both 50 mg intravenous lidocaine and 20 milliequivalent magnesium sulfate were ineffective, occurred and required electrical cardioversion again, and 1 μg/kg/min intravenous landiolol was initiated (Figure 2). Thereafter, VT reoccurred; thus, electrical cardioversion was reperformed, and intravenous landiolol was increased to 3 μg/kg/min. Blood chemistry revealed suppressed TSH level (<0.01 μU/mL) and elevated free T3 (16.4 pg/mL) and free T4 levels (>7.7 ng/dL), and the patient was referred for hyperthyroidism. Thyrotropin receptor antibody (TRAb) measured using the electrochemiluminescence assay method was 24.7 (normal range, <2.0) IU/L, and goiter with increased blood flow was confirmed by ultrasonography (Figure 1(b)). Hence, the patient was diagnosed with Graves' disease. The total bilirubin level increased to 5.6 mg/dL at that time. Thus, he fulfilled the following diagnostic criteria for TS proposed by the Japan Thyroid Association [3]: thyrotoxicosis, tachycardia, and gastrointestinal/hepatic manifestations, and the findings in this case correspond to TS2 (suspected TS). The Burch–Wartofsky Point Scale (BWPS) score, which was proposed in 1993 and had been widely used for the diagnosis of TS, of 45 and >45 is suggestive of TS [6]. Although the total bilirubin level of this patient could not be appropriately evaluated due to constitutional jaundice, BWPS was 60 even when the heading of "gastrointestinal-hepatic dysfunction" among the diagnostic criteria was underscored as "moderate" (if a patient showed jaundice, it was scored as "severe"). Therefore, he was diagnosed with TS, and treatment with 150 mg/day intravenous hydrocortisone, 30 mg/day oral methimazole (MMI), and 200 mg/day potassium iodide (KI) was initiated. After initial treatment of the TS, lethal arrhythmia including VT did not reoccur, and he returned to a normal sinus rhythm several days later (Figure 2). As thyroid function gradually decreased, intravenous hydrocortisone was tapered off and altered to oral prednisolone (PSL), and KI was decreased to 100 mg/day. Regarding his cardiac function, when he was referred for hyperthyroidism, the central venous pressure (CVP) decreased from 25 mmHg at admission to 17 mmHg, and compression of the left ventricle was substantially reduced. However, EF did not improve after the abovementioned therapy. Treatment for TS was started at this time, and the echocardiography performed 6 days after the hyperthyroid treatment showed improvement in contractile function and dilation of the left ventricle. The EF was 60%–65%, and the LVDds and LVDs were 42 mm and 28 mm, respectively. In addition, right ventricular dilation and function improved (RVDd = 52 mm; TAPSE = 11.7 mm). The thyroid function test results 6 days after the initiation of TS therapy were as follows: free T3 = 3.4 pg/mL and free T4 = 3.7 ng/dL (Figure 3). The free T4 level remained high, but the free T3 level returned to normal. Consequently, furosemide and landiolol were also tapered off and discontinued, and amiodarone was adjusted according to the serum concentration and shifted to oral administration. Although an implantable cardioverter-defibrillator placement was recommended for possibly recurrent VT [7], the patient declined. Finally, symptoms such as dyspnea, leg edema, and watery diarrhea improved, and his body weight reduced approximately 10 kg compared with admission data, so he was discharged on day 28. When he left the hospital, his medications were 2.5 mg PSL on alternate days, 30 mg/day MMI and 100 mg/day KI for hyperthyroidism, 10 mg/day apixaban for anticoagulation, 2.5 mg/day bisoprolol and 150 mg/day amiodarone for the prevention of arrhythmia, and 2.5 mg/day enalapril for heart failure. His blood test results at the time of discharge are shown in Table 1.

Table 1: Laboratory data at 6 months before the first admission, on admission, and at the time of discharge for thyroid storm.

Laboratory data	Six months before first admission	First admission for TS	Discharge for TS	Normal range
TP	6.7	6.6	6.0	6.7–8.3 g/dL
Alb	3.9	3.8	3.4	4.0–5.0 g/dL
T-bil	3.1	4.8	2.3	0.3–1.2 mg/dL
AST	31	37	18	13–33 U/L
ALT	35	25	27	8–42 U/L
LDH	209	250	160	119–229 U/L
γ-GTP	59	93	219	10–47 U/L
ALP	413	483	342	115–359 U/L
CPK	71	277	42	62–287 U/L
CPK-MB		7		≤25 U/L
Troponin T		0.015		≤0.014 ng/mL
BUN	12	21	13	8.0–22.0 mg/dL
Cre	0.80	0.80	0.83	0.60–1.10 mg/dL
Na	145	142	140	138–146 mEq/L
K	3.9	4.4	3.8	3.6–4.9 mEq/L
Cl	107	107	102	99–109 mEq/L
BNP	197.3	305.3	286.6	<18.4 pg/ml
WBC	6280	5800	5990	4000–9000/μL
PLT	25.0	19.3	19.7	15–35 × $10^4/\mu$L
CRP		0.21		<0.3 mg/dL
PT-INR		1.47		0.90–1.47
Antithrombin		75.0		80–120%
Fibrinogen		273		150–340 mg/dL
FDP		4		<5 μg/ml
D-dimer		1.2		<1.0 μg/ml
T-CHO	111	77	132	128–219 mg/dL
Triglyceride	105	41	66	30–149 mg/dL
HDL-C		26	46	40–96 mg/dL
LDL-C		39	70	<140 mg/dL

TS: thyroid storm; TP: total protein; Alb: albumin; T-bil: total bilirubin; AST: aspartate aminotransferase; ALT: alanine aminotransferase; LDH: lactate dehydrogenase; γ-GTP: gamma-glutamyl transpeptidase; ALP: alkaline phosphatase; CPK: creatine phosphokinase; BUN: blood urea nitrogen; Cre: creatinine; Na: sodium; K: potassium; Cl: chloride; BNP: brain natriuretic peptide; WBC: white blood cell; PLT: platelet count; CRP: C-reactive protein; PT-INR: prothrombin time international normalized ratio; FDP: fibrin/fibrinogen degradation products; T-CHO: total cholesterol; HDL-C: high-density lipoprotein cholesterol; and LDL-C: low-density lipoprotein cholesterol.

He became febrile and was transported to our hospital 22 days after discharge. His neutrophils decreased to 6/μL and he was diagnosed with agranulocytosis due to MMI. He recovered after the initiation of empirical broad-spectrum antibiotics, granulocyte colony-stimulating factor (G-CSF), and acetaminophen treated in a clean room. Thyroid function was maintained by 100 mg/day KI and arrhythmia did not occur during the second admission. Additionally, some medications were changed because of drug-induced liver injury. The clinical course of second admission is shown in Figure 4. Total thyroidectomy was performed 48 days after the second discharge, and there were no complications, such as arrhythmia. Pathological observation showed that the resected thyroid was swelling slightly, and nodules were not detected. Hyperplasia of the large and small follicles and vacuolization where the epithelium contacted the colloid was observed. These findings were compatible with those of Graves' disease. After the operation, levothyroxine was initiated and adjusted according to the thyroid function. The total clinical course of the patient is shown in Figure 3.

3. Discussion

We herein report the first case of a patient with ARVC who presented with lethal arrhythmia, which was refractory to medication and electrical cardioversion induced by TS due to Graves' disease. Palpitation and decreased serum total cholesterol level were observed 6 months before the first hospitalization, and it is likely that he had already developed Graves' disease around this period. We considered that the cessation of sotalol might have triggered TS, which induced arrhythmia and led to the onset of biventricular heart failure. The treatment of TS was effective, succeeded to suppress refractory arrhythmias, and ameliorated both-sided heart failure. Thereafter, he developed agranulocytosis incidentally due to MMI. Finally, total thyroidectomy was performed without any complications and his thyroid function was controlled within the normal range by administering levothyroxine.

No previous English report describing a case complicated with ARVC and Graves' disease or the relationships between them has been published. Two cases of ARVC

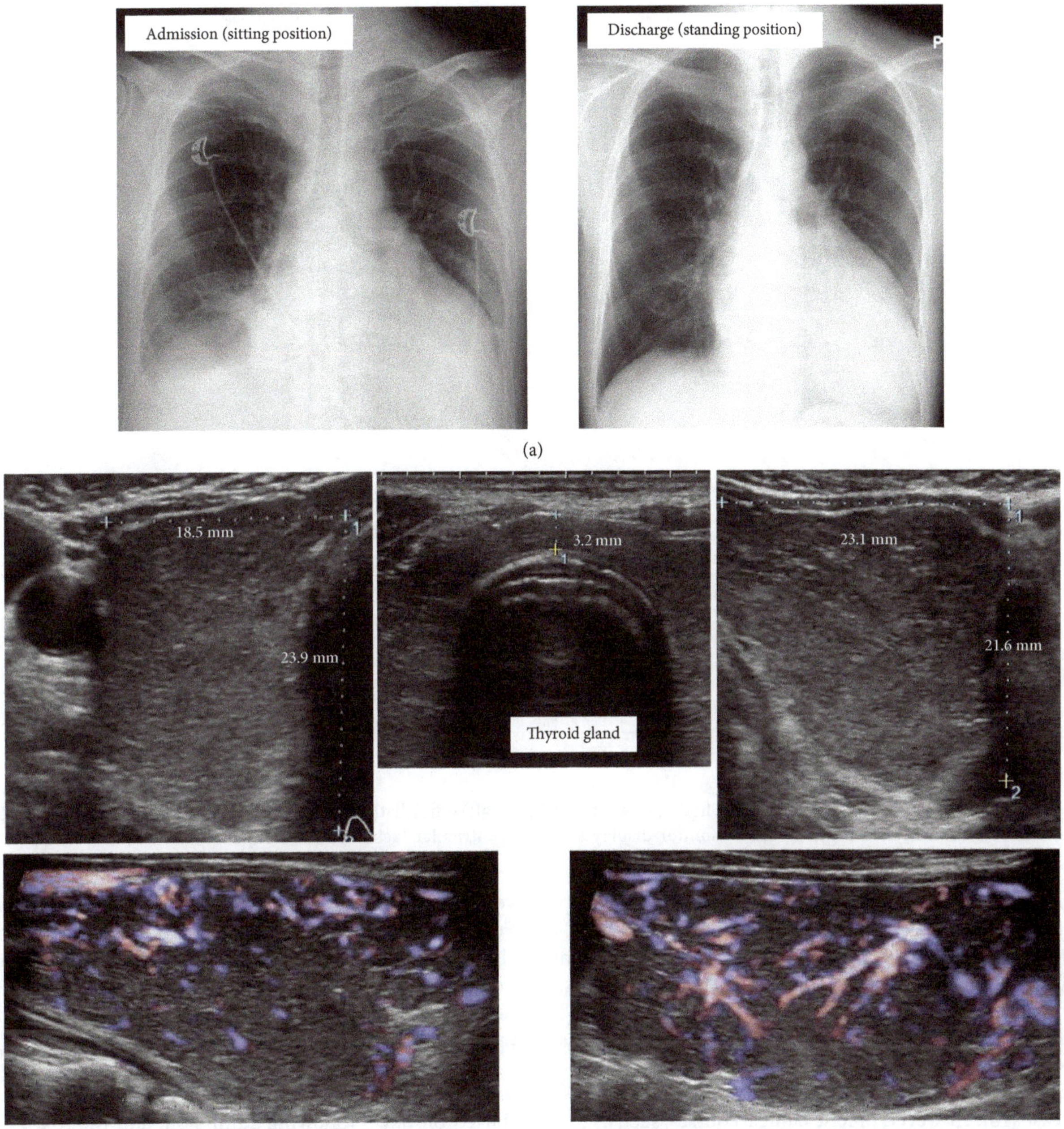

Figure 1: Imaging findings at first admission. (a) Chest X-ray on admission and discharge. (b) An ultrasonogram showing enlargement and increased blood flow of the thyroid gland.

complicated with hyperthyroidism have been reported in Japanese. Although the cause of hyperthyroidism was not noted in both cases [8, 9], we considered they were complicated with Graves' disease since MMI was used for treatment. One case with ARVC complicated with hyperthyroidism repeated VT and required catheter ablation [8]. The other case was diagnosed with ARVC during treatment of hyperthyroidism and atrial tachycardia occurred when serum thyroid hormone levels elevated [9]. However, their clinical courses were not described in detail. Since PKP2 is rarely expressed in the thyroid gland [10], it is speculated that patients with ARVC harboring PKP2 mutation are not likely to develop thyroid diseases. As for Graves' disease, it is one of the autoimmune diseases induced by the production of autoantibodies to TSH receptors. Though mechanism of autoimmunity, namely, myocarditis, has been also implied in some ARVC patients [11], the association of Graves' disease and ARVC is unclear. Arrhythmia, especially AF, is a common complication of Graves' disease induced by activating the arrhythmogenic activity of the pulmonary veins [12]. Thus, when patients with ARVC are incidentally complicated with Graves' disease, hyperthyroidism can easily trigger arrhythmia. As for hyperthyroidism other than Graves' disease, amiodarone, which is often initiated for

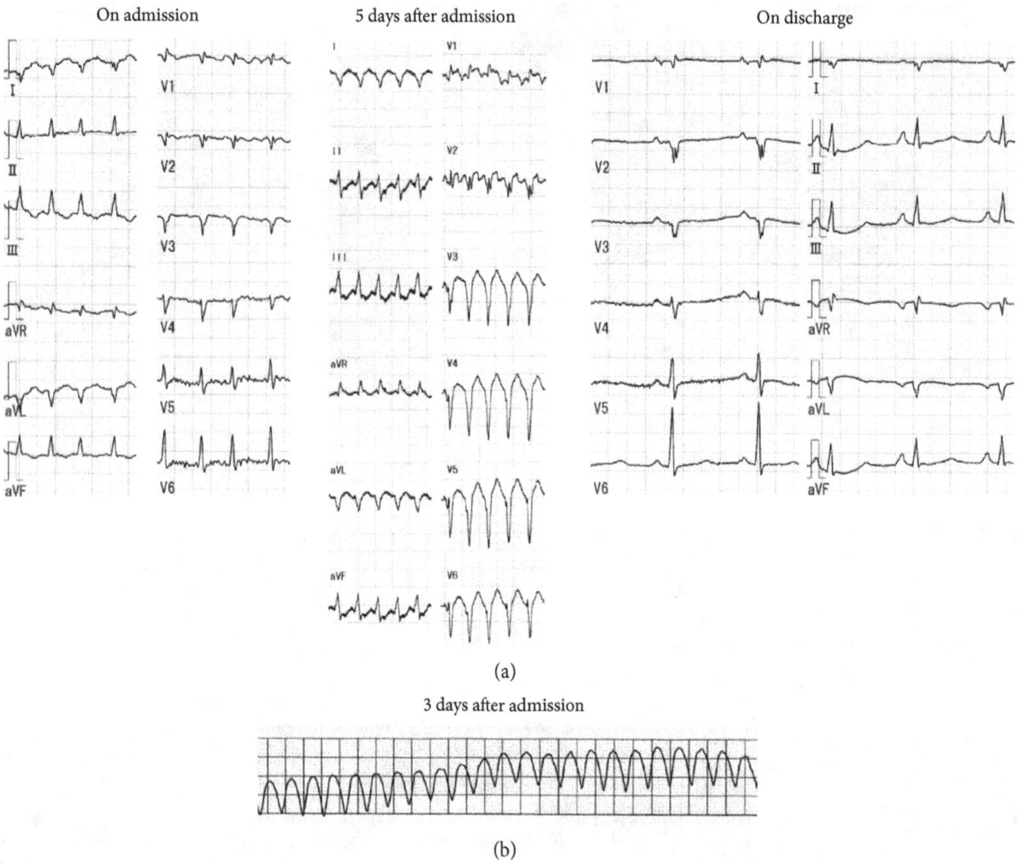

FIGURE 2: Electrocardiogram (ECG) findings at first admission. (a) Rapid atrial fibrillation on admission, atrial tachycardia on day 5, and normal sinus rhythm on discharge. (b) ECG monitor display showing ventricular tachycardia on day 3.

patients with ARVC to prevent arrhythmia, could develop thyrotoxicosis [13]. Previous reports have shown that patients with ARVC treated with amiodarone for long duration developed thyrotoxicosis due to destructive thyroiditis. Although corticosteroid was effective for controlling the thyroid function in some cases [14], thyroidectomy was performed in one case [15] and plasma apheresis and thyroidectomy were required to treat hyperthyroidism in another case [16]. However, precise clinical courses, such as the onset of lethal arrhythmia or whether the case was diagnosed as TS, have not been described in these reports. Moreover, relationships between ARVC and hyperthyroidism were not considered in these reports. Taken together, the precise mechanism by which hyperthyroidism induces arrhythmia in patients with ARVC remains to be elucidated.

We considered that the patient suffered from both-sided heart failure, and the symptoms could have been inconsistent with typical acute left-sided heart failure symptoms observed in TS. Since the function of the right ventricle was originally reduced by ARVC, right ventricular dysfunction may be more predominant. Dilated cardiomyopathy-like features induced by thyrotoxicosis were reported as rare cardiac complications [5]. It may be partly due to tachycardia-induced cardiomyopathy [17]. This patient did not have a dilated left ventricle and had a low cardiac output. We speculate that due to compression by the dilated right ventricle, the dilation of the left ventricle was not apparent. Furthermore, due to the earlier clinical manifestation of right ventricular insufficiency, left ventricular dilatation may not have been apparent at admission. The left ventricular dilatation might have become apparent with time if the treatment for heart failure and TS was not initiated.

In this case, the free T3 level decreased from 26.0 pg/mL on day 2 to 16.4 pg/mL on day 5 (Figure 3). Amiodarone was started on day 3 following admission, and the free T3 level decreased possibly due to amiodarone administration as reported in a previous case [18]. Amiodarone has various effects on thyroid function, and thyroid dysfunction associated with long-term amiodarone administration is hypothyroidism or destructive thyroiditis [13]. However, the short-term effect of amiodarone treatment on thyroid function is yet to be determined. Amiodarone could decrease T3 production or thyroid hormone-related genes and may have a direct toxic effect on thyroid follicular cells as intrinsic effects [19, 20]. Moreover, amiodarone contains large amounts of iodine, and approximately 3% of its mass is actually released into the circulation as free iodine through drug metabolism [21]. Intravenous administration of amiodarone is effective for the emergency treatment of VT, and the total amount of amiodarone is particularly high on the first 2 days of initiation. In our case, 600 mg of amiodarone was administered both on the first and the second

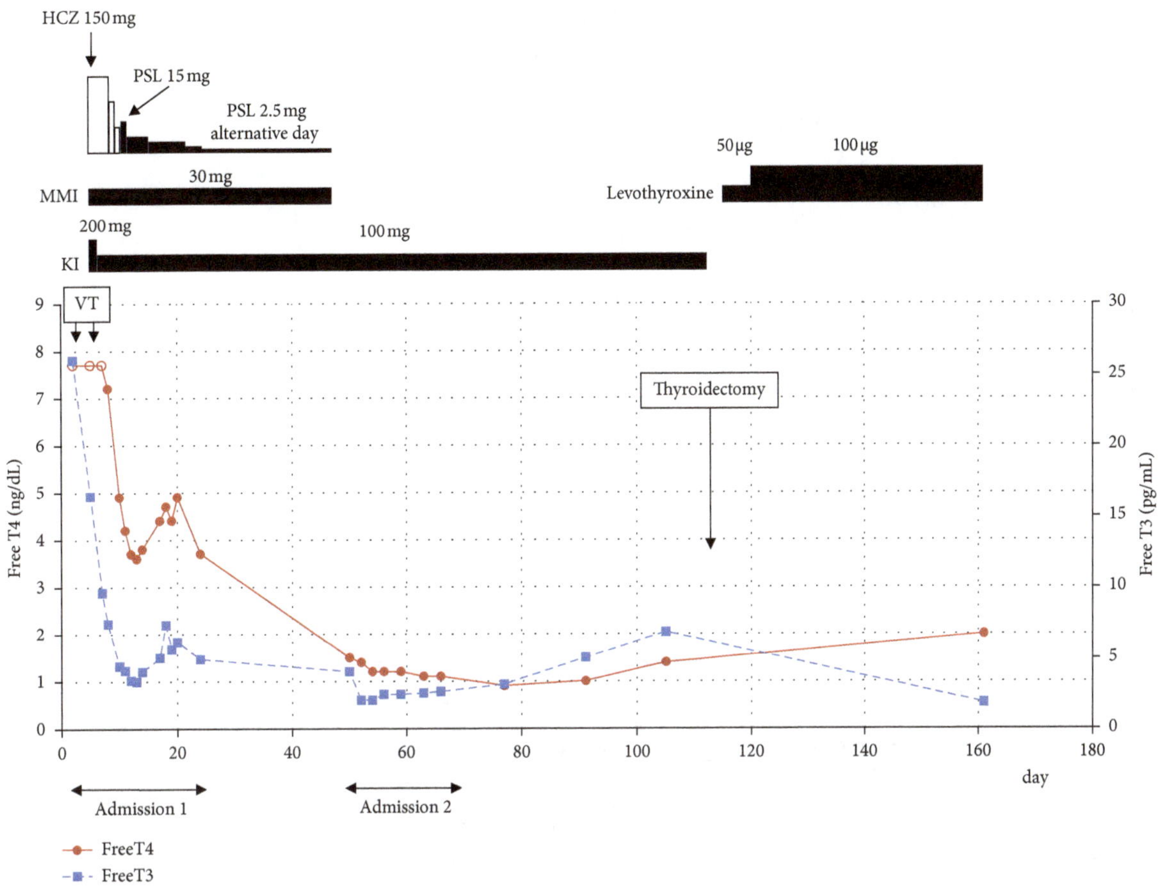

FIGURE 3: Total clinical course of the patient. Open circles indicate the value of free T4 mean more than 7.7 ng/dL. HCZ: hydrocortisone; PSL: prednisolone; MMI: methimazole; KI: potassium iodide; VT: ventricular tachycardia; T3: triiodothyronine; and T4: thyroxine.

days, respectively. Consequently, it was calculated that 18 mg of free iodine was released both on the first and second days of amiodarone administration. KI (50 mg) contains approximately 38 mg of iodine and is frequently used with MMI or propylthiouracil (PTU) to treat Graves' disease. Taken together, we considered that the amount of iodine could be sufficient to decrease thyroid hormone levels as well as intrinsic effects in a short-term treatment of amiodarone. As a previous report, amiodarone might be beneficial for hyperthyroidism-induced VT among patients with Graves' disease for at least a short time [18].

The daily dose of hydrocortisone and MMI for treatment of TS were both less than their recommended doses (300 mg/day intravenous hydrocortisone and 60 mg/day oral MMI) [3]. Since a single and initial administration of 50 mg hydrocortisone and 15 mg oral MMI in addition to 100 mg KI was effective for controlling lethal arrhythmia, we considered that 150 mg/day intravenous hydrocortisone and 30 mg/day oral MMI were enough to treat his TS. Actually, his general condition improved and serum thyroid hormone levels decreased thereafter. The previous guideline stated that corticosteroid overdosing may cause unfavorable hyperglycemia and worsening of general condition; therefore, the dose needs to be carefully determined for individual patients [3]. The recommended dose of oral MMI is 60 mg/day for TS, which is the maximum dose for the treatment of Graves' disease approved by the Ministry of Health, Labor and Welfare of Japan. When large doses of MMI are initiated, the patient should be carefully monitored for potential side effects, which are dose dependent. Agranulocytosis is a rare but life-threatening complication of MMI or PTU treatment in 0.1%–0.5% of patients [22]. Agranulocytosis also shows dose dependency and rarely occurs at low doses of MMI, such as 5–10 mg/day [23]. Genetic predisposition, such as human leukocyte antigentype, has been shown to be associated with the risk of agranulocytosis as well as high dose of antithyroid drugs [24]. Previous reports showing the relationships between ARVC or PKP2 and agranulocytosis have not been identified; thus, we considered that the patient reported in the present study incidentally developed agranulocytosis due to MMI.

Total thyroidectomy was selected for the treatment of Graves' disease instead of radioiodine therapy after the onset of agranulocytosis induced by MMI for the following reasons: (1) KI and amiodarone, which include iodine, should be ceased around radioiodine therapy since there would be decreased uptake of radioactive iodine in the thyroid. The relapse of hyperthyroidism or a decrease in the serum amiodarone concentration could initiate the recurrence of lethal arrhythmia; (2) there is a possibility of elevation of serum levels of thyroid hormone after

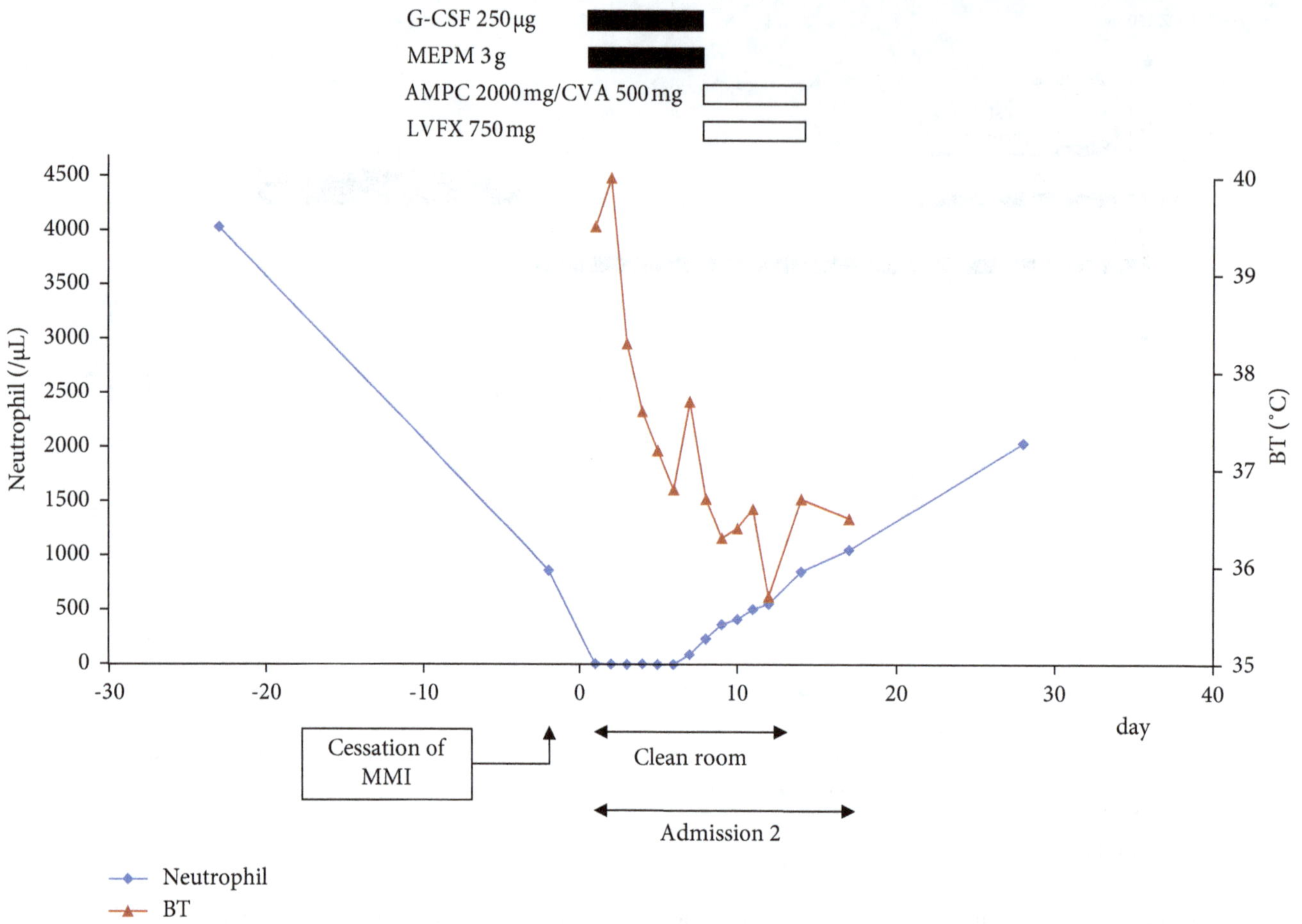

Figure 4: Clinical course of the patient during the second admission due to febrile neutropenia. G-CSF: granulocyte colony-stimulating factor; MEPM: meropenem; AMPC: amoxicillin; CVA: clavulanate; LVFX: levofloxacin; and BT: body temperature.

radioiodine therapy, which could lead to a TS [3]; and (3) repeated radioiodine therapy treatments could be required to control thyroid function for Graves' disease [25]. In particular, uptake of radioactive iodine in the patient's thyroid was expected to decrease due to amiodarone, which could accumulate in the thyroid over a long period regardless of the serum concentration [12]. Hence, single administration of radioactive iodine might be insufficient due to decreased uptake in this case. Therefore, total thyroidectomy was considered to be preferable to radioiodine therapy in this case. Treatment of Graves' disease should be carefully considered in each case when agranulocytosis is induced by antithyroid drugs.

4. Conclusion

Herein, we report the first English report of a patient with ARVC who had a refractory VT induced by TS due to Graves' disease. Furthermore, this patient suffered from biventricular heart failure. The treatment of TS was indeed effective for arrhythmia and heart failure. Clinicians should consider hyperthyroidism as a cause of refractory arrhythmia or biventricular heart failure among patients with ARVC.

Consent

No written consent has been obtained from this patient since no patient identifiable data is included in this case report.

Acknowledgments

The authors would like to thank ENAGO for English proofreading.

References

[1] D. Corrado, M. S. Link, and H. Calkins, "Arrhythmogenic right ventricular cardiomyopathy," *New England Journal of Medicine*, vol. 376, no. 1, pp. 61–72, 2017.

[2] Y. Wada, S. Ohno, T. Aiba, and M. Horie, "Unique genetic background and outcome of non-caucasian Japanese probands with arrhythmogenic right ventricular dysplasia/cardiomyopathy," *Molecular Genetics and Genomic Medicine*, vol. 5, no. 6, pp. 639–651, 2017.

[3] T. Akamizu, T. Satoh, O. Isozaki et al., "Diagnostic criteria, clinical features, and incidence of thyroid storm based on nationwide surveys," *Thyroid*, vol. 22, no. 7, pp. 661–679, 2012.

[4] I. Klein and K. Ojamaa, "Thyroid hormone and the cardiovascular system," *New England Journal of Medicine*, vol. 344, no. 7, pp. 501–509, 2001.
[5] C. Boccalandro, F. Boccalandro, P. Orlander, and C. F. Wei, "Severe reversible dilated cardiomyopathy and hyperthyroidism: case report and review of the literature," *Endocrine Practice*, vol. 9, no. 2, pp. 140–146, 2003.
[6] H. B. Burch and L. Wartofsky, "Life-threatening thyrotoxicosis: thyroid storm," *Endocrinology and Metabolism Clinics of North America*, vol. 22, no. 2, pp. 263–277, 1993.
[7] A. N. Takashi Kurita, H. Abe, K. Ando et al., "JCS/JHRS guideline on non-pharmacotherapy of cardiac arrhythmias," *Circulation Journal*, vol. 85, 2018.
[8] K. Norihiro, "A case in which catheter ablation and sotalol were effective for frequent ventricular tachycardia," *Progress Medical*, vol. 26, pp. 1993–1995, 2006.
[9] I. W. Kenichi Hashimoto, S. Ashino, M. Kobune et al., "Consideration of antiarrhythmic agents for ICD and pacemaker implantable cases for right ventricular dysplasia," *Progress Medical*, vol. 26, pp. 2353–2357, 2006.
[10] L. Fagerberg, B. M. Hallström, P. Oksvold et al., "Analysis of the human tissue-specific expression by genome-wide integration of transcriptomics and antibody-based proteomics," *Molecular and Cellular Proteomics*, vol. 13, no. 2, pp. 397–406, 2014.
[11] A. L. P. Caforio, F. Re, A. Avella et al., "Evidence from family studies for autoimmunity in arrhythmogenic right ventricular cardiomyopathy," *Circulation*, vol. 141, no. 15, pp. 1238–1248, 2020.
[12] B. Biondi and G. J. Kahaly, "Cardiovascular involvement in patients with different causes of hyperthyroidism," *Nature Reviews Endocrinology*, vol. 6, no. 8, pp. 431–443, 2010.
[13] J. Cohen-Lehman, P. Dahl, S. Danzi, and I. Klein, "Effects of amiodarone therapy on thyroid function," *Nature Reviews Endocrinology*, vol. 6, no. 1, pp. 34–41, 2010.
[14] K. Sato, T. Shiga, N. Matsuda et al., "Mild and short recurrence of type II amiodarone-induced thyrotoxicosis in three patients receiving amiodarone continuously for more than 10 years," *Endocrine Journal*, vol. 53, no. 4, pp. 531–538, 2006.
[15] D. Cappellani, P. Papini, A. Pingitore et al., "Comparison between total thyroidectomy and medical therapy for amiodarone-induced thyrotoxicosis," *Journal of Clinical Endocrinology and Metabolism*, vol. 105, 2020.
[16] X. Waintraub and E. Gandjbakhch, "My approach to ventricular tachycardia ablation in patient with arrhythmogenic right ventricular cardiomyopathy/dysplasia," *HeartRhythm Case Reports*, vol. 6, no. 2, pp. 51–59, 2020.
[17] J. S. Shinbane, M. A. Wood, D. N. Jensen, K. A. Ellenbogen, A. P. Fitzpatrick, and M. M. Scheinman, "Tachycardia-induced cardiomyopathy: a review of animal models and clinical studies," *Journal of the American College of Cardiology*, vol. 29, no. 4, pp. 709–715, 1997.
[18] H. Yamamoto, S. Monno, K. Ohta-Ogo, H. Ishibashi-Ueda, and T. Hashimoto, "Delayed diagnosis of dilated thyrotoxic cardiomyopathy with coexistent multifocal atrial tachycardia: a case report," *BMC Cardiovascular Disorders*, vol. 21, no. 1, p. 124, 2021.
[19] R. H. Rao, V. R. McCready, and G. S. Spathis, "Iodine kinetic studies during amiodarone treatment*," *Journal of Clinical Endocrinology and Metabolism*, vol. 62, no. 3, pp. 563–568, 1986.
[20] E. Roti, R. Minelli, E. Gardini, L. Bianconi, and L. E. Braverman, "Thyrotoxicosis followed by hypothyroidism in patients treated with amiodarone," *Archives of Internal Medicine*, vol. 153, no. 7, pp. 886–892, 1993.
[21] S. Basaria and D. S. Cooper, "Amiodarone and the thyroid," *The American Journal of Medicine*, vol. 118, no. 7, pp. 706–714, 2005.
[22] D. S. Cooper, "Antithyroid drugs," *New England Journal of Medicine*, vol. 352, no. 9, pp. 905–917, 2005.
[23] D. S. Ross, H. B. Burch, D. S. Cooper et al., "2013 American thyroid association guidelines for diagnosis and management of hyperthyroidism and other causes of thyrotoxicosis," *Thyroid*, vol. 26, no. 10, pp. 1343–1421, 2016.
[24] S. Nakakura, K. Hosomichi, S. Uchino et al., "HLA-B*39 : 01 : 01 is a novel risk factor for antithyroid drug-induced agranulocytosis in Japanese population," *The Pharmacogenomics Journal*, vol. 21, no. 1, pp. 94–101, 2021.
[25] D. F. Schneider, P. E. Sonderman, M. F. Jones et al., "Failure of radioactive iodine in the treatment of hyperthyroidism," *Annals of Surgical Oncology*, vol. 21, no. 13, pp. 4174–4180, 2014.

23

Giant Parathyroid Tumor: Parathyroid Adenoma versus Parathyroid Carcinoma

Farid Gossili,[1] Allan Carlé,[2] Trine B. Andersen,[1] and Helle D Zacho[1,3]

[1]*Department of Nuclear Medicine, Aalborg University Hospital, Aalborg, Denmark*
[2]*Department of Endocrinology, Aalborg University Hospital, Aalborg, Denmark*
[3]*Department of Clinical Medicine, Aalborg University, Aalborg, Denmark*

Correspondence should be addressed to Farid Gossili; f.gossili@rn.dk

Academic Editor: Osamu Isozaki

Parathyroid adenoma is the most common cause of primary hyperparathyroidism (PHPT). We present the preoperative detection of a giant parathyroid adenoma (GPA) using (^{99m}Tc)-sestamibi parathyroid scintigraphy in a patient presenting with severely elevated parathyroid hormone, hypercalcemia, hypophosphatemia, and vitamin D insufficiency. The patient complained of cerebral symptoms and intermittent abdominal discomfort without constipation. After surgical removal of the hyperactive parathyroid gland and D vitamin supplementation, all blood tests were normalized. The clinical and paraclinical characteristics of GPA may raise the suspicion of parathyroid carcinoma, but not absolutely in this case.

1. Introduction

Primary hyperparathyroidism (PHPT) has an incidence of 0.4 to 82 cases per 100,000 person/year and is characterized mainly by elevated parathyroid hormone (PTH) levels and, consequently, hypercalcemia and hypophosphatemia [1]. The most common cause of PHPT is a solitary parathyroid adenoma (80–85%) [1, 2]. A very enlarged parathyroid adenoma is a rare variation in which the adenoma weighs more than 3500 mg and is known as a giant parathyroid adenoma (GPA) [3, 4]. In addition to clinical complications such as very high levels of calcium and PTH and possible mass effects, GPA can also cause operative challenges during surgical resection [1]. On the other hand, parathyroid carcinoma accounts for approximately 1% of PHPT [1, 2], and suspicion of parathyroid carcinoma increases with increasing adenoma size [5]. Therefore, differentiation with parathyroid carcinoma is very important in cases of giant parathyroid adenoma.

Parathyroidectomy is recommended as the definitive treatment of parathyroid adenoma in cases of young age, high total serum calcium, osteoporosis, renal calcifications, or the presence of symptoms [6]. Minimally invasive parathyroidectomy is considered the best method in terms of reducing surgical complications as well as the cost and length of hospitalization. Consequently, preoperative localization of parathyroid adenoma is very important to allow for minimally invasive surgery [1]. Preoperative diagnosis of parathyroid carcinoma is impossible in the vast majority of patients [7], although very high PTH and calcium levels, as well as palpable tumors and a large amount of tissue, may suggest parathyroid carcinoma. However, due to a lack of preoperative diagnostic modalities, the majority of parathyroid carcinomas are diagnosed postoperatively using pathologic examinations [8].

Parathyroid scintigraphy with (^{99m}Tc)-sestamibi is the gold standard for preoperative localization of the parathyroid tissue, according to some studies [9]. However, several studies have shown that imaging accuracy increases when scintigraphy is combined with ultrasound [1, 10].

The combination of a giant parathyroid mass seen on (^{99m}Tc)-sestamibi scintigraphy and ultrasound, along with severely elevated PTH levels, may raise suspicion for parathyroid carcinoma. This case report is based on a patient presenting all those features.

2. Case Report

A 38-year-old Caucasian woman, previously healthy, was referred to an endocrinology outpatient clinic due to persistent hypercalcemia for one year as well as elevated PTH levels, mild hypophosphatemia, and vitamin D insufficiency. She had psychiatric moans and abdominal discomfort without constipation. She had no familial predisposition to multiple endocrine neoplasias 1 (MEN1). Laboratory tests showed a serum calcium level of 2.93 mmol/l (reference range 2.20–2.55 mmol/l), serum albumin-corrected calcium level of 2.88 mmol/l (reference range 2.20–2.55 mmol/l), serum phosphorus of 0.66 mmol/l (reference range 0.76–1.41 mmol/l), serum 25-hydroxyvitamin D of 17 (reference range 50–160 nmol/l), and a PTH level of 52 pmol/l (reference range 1.3–7.6 pmol/l). The calcium/creatinine clearance ratio was 0.013, which may indicate both familial hypercalcemia hypocalciuric (FHH) and primary hyperparathyroidism [11]. However, gene analysis (CASR, calcium-sensing receptor) was negative for FHH, and primary hyperparathyroidism due to parathyroid adenoma was suspected. CT urography revealed no nephrocalcinosis. Dual-energy X-ray absorptiometry detected osteopenia (T-scores of −2.4/−1.8 in the lower back/femoral neck, respectively).

The patient underwent parathyroid scintigraphy aiming for preoperative localization of the possible parathyroid tumor. Dual-phase (^{99m}Tc)-sestamibi scintigraphy with single-photon emission computed tomography (SPECT) detected a large parathyroid tumor measuring 38 × 18 × 14 mm (craniocaudal x transverse x anteroposterior) located behind the right thyroid lobe compatible with a giant parathyroid adenoma (Figure 1). An ultrasound scan confirmed the scintigraphically detected tissue (Figure 2). The severely elevated PTH levels in this young patient raised the suspicion of a possible parathyroid carcinoma. However, the only slightly increased calcium level indicated otherwise.

The patient underwent minimally invasive parathyroidectomy, and PTH levels (from 34.4 to 3.6 pmol/l), and calcium levels normalized both preoperatively and during follow-up. Vitamin D insufficiency was treated with vitamin D supplementation and serum vitamin D near-normalized during follow-up (from 17 to 47 nmol/l). The postoperative parathyroid adenoma weighed 4 grams. Histopathology revealed a rounded structure with a 1 mm thick connective tissue capsule. The structure consisted of confluent trabecular formations of chief cells with eosinophilic vesicular cytoplasm and relatively small, hyperchromatic nuclei. These changes are representative of a sporadic parathyroid adenoma.

3. Discussion

Giant parathyroid adenoma is a rare cause of PHPT, and consequently, only a few cases of GPA have been reported. A systematic review by Wong et al. identified 62 GPAs from 1952 to 2021 [3]. Reporting a very rare case, namely this case, is important both paraclinically and clinically, as it can contribute to the assessment of this type of patient in possibly challenging situations.

Preoperative differentiation between giant parathyroid adenoma and parathyroid carcinoma is very challenging. The preoperative clinical and paraclinical presentation of giant parathyroid adenoma, especially with severely elevated PTH and calcium levels, may be very similar to that of parathyroid carcinoma [3]. A familial predisposition to MEN1, severely elevated serum corrected calcium level (>3 mmol/l) with several clinical symptoms of hypercalcemia, including nausea, vomiting, abdominal pain, constipation, myopathy and neurocognitive deficit, very high PTH levels (5–10 times more than the upper limit of the reference range), renal and bone involvement, very large tissue and younger age at presentation, can raise the suspicion of parathyroid carcinoma [12–17]. In this case, there was a giant tumor with severely elevated PTH levels in a young woman; however, negative familial disposition to MEN1 only slightly increased corrected calcium levels and no signs of nephrolithiasis or osteoporosis. These characteristics indicate parathyroid adenoma rather than carcinoma. This case demonstrates the importance of a high calcium level with concomitant increasing PTH levels and an enlarged tumor in the preoperative suspicion of parathyroid carcinoma.

According to the international consensus on the management of PHP [18], the preoperative localization of tumor in the parathyroid glands is very important in planning the operation and determining the proper method, especially in minimally invasive surgery. However, the standard of care in the treatment of parathyroid carcinoma is "en bloc" resection of the carcinoma with ipsilateral hemithyroidectomy and reoperation in some patients [8]. Therefore, the differentiation between PTA and parathyroid carcinoma has clinical importance for the choice of the correct surgical method. There is no preoperative modality that can differentiate PTA from parathyroid carcinoma. Therefore, the diagnosis of malignancy before surgery is difficult, and the intraoperative findings including histology are important for all cases of parathyroid tumors. Preoperative fine-needle biopsy is also not recommended due to the increased risk of dissemination and inferiority in differentiation between adenoma and carcinoma [3, 5]. (^{99m}Tc)-sestamibi scintigraphy is recommended as the first-line imaging method, and ultrasound is recommended as a complementary and hopefully confirmatory examination for preoperative localization. With the conformity of both modalities, the positive predictive value for correct localization of the parathyroid tumor is 97% [18]. In addition, ultrasound findings in the form of calcification and high vascularization may indicate parathyroid carcinoma. However, the presence of a thick capsule is most likely suggestive of parathyroid adenoma [12]. In this case, the presence of a thick capsule with minimal internal flow in the Doppler images reduced the likelihood of malignancy. (^{99m}Tc])-sestamibi scintigraphy is based on the accumulation in cells with abundant mitochondria, which display slower wash-out compared to cells with fewer mitochondria, in this way differentiating such cells. Both sporadic parathyroid adenoma and parathyroid carcinoma have such characteristics [12]; therefore, (^{99m}Tc)-sestamibi cannot differentiate between benign and malignant tumors. However, in cases of

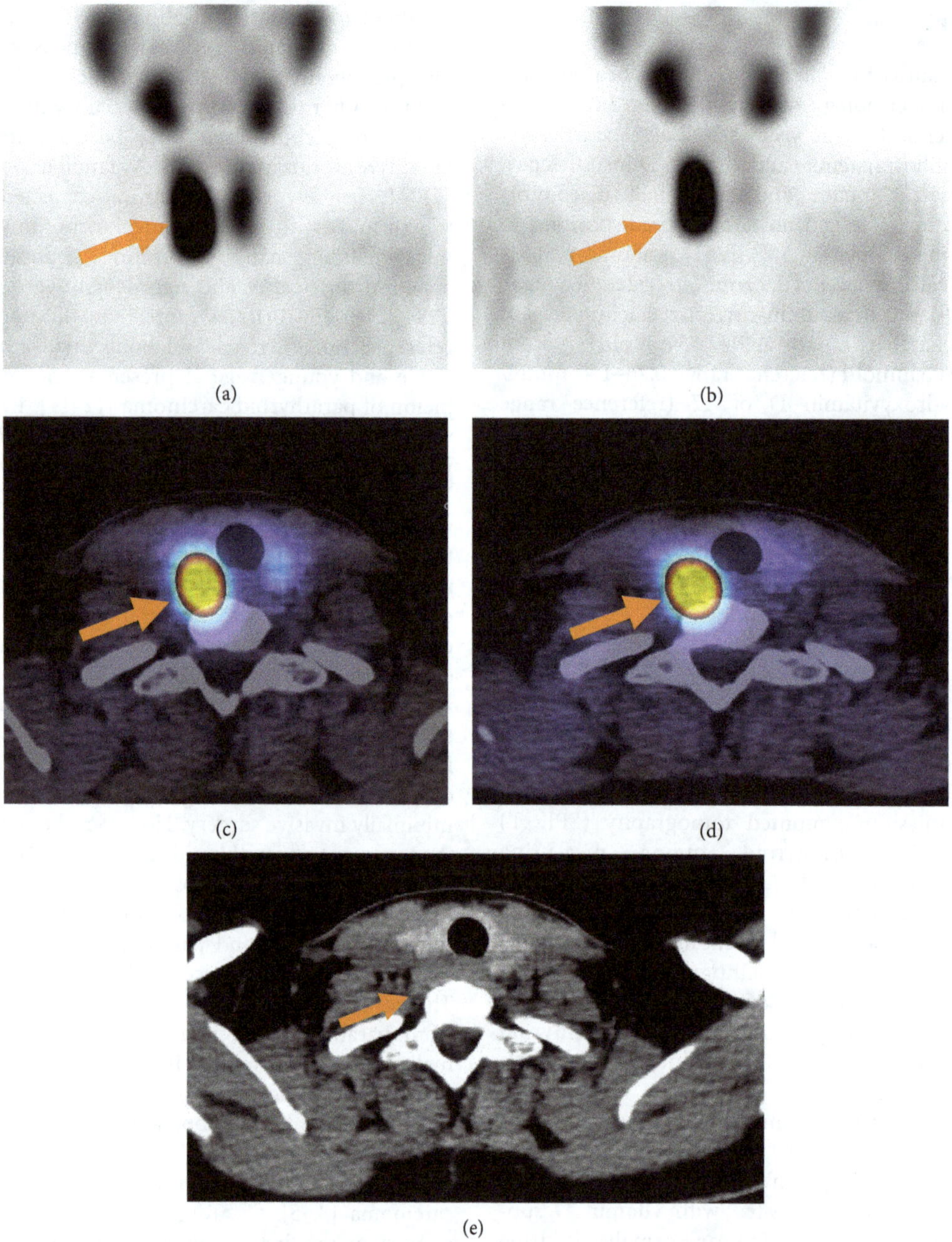

FIGURE 1: A 38-year-old woman with a giant parathyroid adenoma, localized by a sestamibi scan. Immediate (a) and delayed (2-hour) (b) anterior images of (^{99m}Tc)-sestamibi demonstrate a focus of intense sestamibi uptake (arrows). Immediate (c), delayed (2-hour) (d) axial fused SPECT/CT images, and transverse noncontrast CT image (e) localized a circular area with focal uptake posterior to the right thyroid lobe (arrows), which was confirmed histologically to be a giant parathyroid adenoma.

metastatic carcinoma, which accounts for 10–30% of parathyroid carcinoma [14], multiple foci can be detected using scintigraphy [12]. In this case, no other foci on the neck or in the mediastinum were detected.

In the current case, the course of treatment included surgery and follow-up, which were without complications. After approximately 18 months of follow-up, the patient was seen at the endocrinology outpatient clinic with normal calcium and PTH levels, in line with another reported giant parathyroid adenoma [3].

In addition to reporting an extremely rare case, we demonstrated that a very high PTH level might be present in a hyperfunctional giant parathyroid adenoma in a young patient, which can be challenging to differentiate from parathyroid carcinoma. However, in the case of negative familial disposition to MEN1, only mildly increased albumin-corrected calcium levels, lack of nephrolithiasis or osteoporosis, and the presence of a thick capsule on UL, benign adenoma is more likely than carcinoma in the presence of severely elevated PTH.

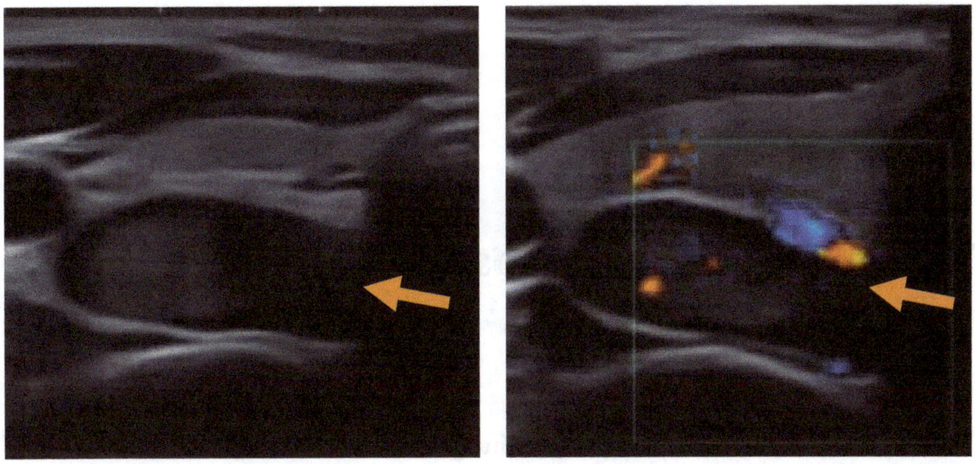

(a) (b)

FIGURE 2: The ultrasound from the patient with a giant parathyroid adenoma. Transverse grayscale images (a) show a giant parathyroid adenoma with a thick capsule and internal echogenic components (arrow). Transverse color doppler images (b) show minimal detectable internal flow (arrow).

Consent

Written informed consent was obtained from the patient to publish this paper.

References

[1] M. D. Walker and S. J. Silverberg, "Primary hyperparathyroidism," *Nature Reviews Endocrinology*, vol. 14, no. 2, pp. 115–125, 2018.

[2] K. Duan, K. Gomez Hernandez, and O. Mete, "Clinicopathological correlates of hyperparathyroidism," *Journal of Clinical Pathology*, vol. 68, no. 10, pp. 771–787, 2015.

[3] H. K. G. Wong, K. Shipman, K. Allan, A. Ghabbour, and F. Borumandi, "Giant parathyroid tumours in primary hyperparathyroidism: a systematic review," *Langenbeck's Archives of Surgery*, vol. 407, no. 2, pp. 501–516, 2022.

[4] P. M. Spanheimer, A. J. Stoltze, J. R. Howe, S. L. Sugg, G. Lal, and R. J. Weigel, "Do giant parathyroid adenomas represent a distinct clinical entity?" *Surgery*, vol. 154, no. 4, pp. 714–719, 2013.

[5] R. Mirza and E. X. Wei, "A giant parathyroid tumor during pregnancy: adenoma versus carcinoma," *Case Reports in Pathology*, vol. 2019, Article ID 4383698, 4 pages, 2019.

[6] J. P. Bilezikian, L. Bandeira, A. Khan, and N. E. Cusano, "Hyperparathyroidism," *The Lancet*, vol. 391, no. 10116, pp. 168–178, 2018.

[7] M. P. Davies, T. W. John Evans, F. Tahir, and S. P. Balasubramanian, "Parathyroid cancer: a systematic review of diagnostic biomarkers," *The Surgeon*, vol. 19, no. 6, pp. e536–e548, 2021.

[8] K. Duan and O. Mete, "Parathyroid carcinoma: diagnosis and clinical implications," *Turkish Journal of Pathology*, vol. 31, pp. 80–97, 2015.

[9] C. C. Juhlin, I. L. Nilsson, H. Falhammar, and J. Zedenius, "Institutional characterisation of water clear cell parathyroid adenoma: a rare entity often unrecognised by TC-99m-sestamibi scintigraphy," *Pathology*, vol. 53, no. 7, pp. 852–859, 2021.

[10] M. Itani and W. D. Middleton, "Parathyroid imaging," *Radiologic Clinics of North America*, vol. 58, no. 6, pp. 1071–1083, 2020.

[11] E. C. Moore, E. Berber, J. Jin, V. Krishnamurthy, J. Shin, and A. Siperstein, "Calcium creatinine clearance ratio is not helpful in differentiating primary hyperparathyroidism from familial herpercalcemic hypocalciuria: a study of 1000 patients," *Endocrine Practice*, 2018.

[12] D. Betea, I. Potorac, and A. Beckers, "Parathyroid carcinoma: challenges in diagnosis and treatment," *Annales d'Endocrinologie*, vol. 76, no. 2, pp. 169–177, 2015.

[13] N. N. Machado and S. M. Wilhelm, "Parathyroid Cancer: A Review," *Cancers*, vol. 11, 2019.

[14] A. L. Fingeret, "Contemporary evaluation and management of parathyroid carcinoma," *JCO Oncology Practice*, vol. 17, no. 1, pp. 17–21, 2021.

[15] A. Mehta, D. Patel, A. Rosenberg et al., "Hyperparathyroidism-jaw tumor syndrome: results of operative management," *Surgery*, vol. 156, no. 6, pp. 1315–1325, 2014.

[16] C. E. Quinn, J. Healy, A. H. Lebastchi et al., "Modern experience with aggressive parathyroid tumors in a high-volume New England referral center," *Journal of the American College of Surgeons*, vol. 220, no. 6, pp. 1054–1062, 2015.

[17] J. M. Sharretts, E. Kebebew, and W. F. Simonds, "Parathyroid cancer," *Seminars in Oncology*, vol. 37, no. 6, pp. 580–590, 2010.

[18] A. A. Khan, D. A. Hanley, R. Rizzoli et al., "Primary hyperparathyroidism: review and recommendations on evaluation, diagnosis, and management. A Canadian and international consensus," *Osteoporosis International*, vol. 28, pp. 1–19, 2017.

24

A Rare Case of Systemic Sarcoidosis in a Middle-Aged Female with a Solitary Thyroid Nodule

Ayrton Bangolo,[1] John Bukasa Kakamba,[2,3] Ali Atoot,[4] Mohammad Jurri,[5] Ashraf Mahmoud,[5] Arthur Oliver Lo,[6] Kunchang Song,[7] Syed Sirajuddin,[4] and Adam Atoot[1]

[1]*Department of Internal Medicine, Hackensack Meridian Health Palisades Medical Center, North Bergen, NJ, USA*
[2]*Endocrine and Metabolic Disorders Department, University Clinics of Kinshasa, Kinshasa, Democratic Republic of the Congo*
[3]*Department of Endocrinology, University of Liege, Liege, Belgium*
[4]*Department of Anesthesia, Hackensack University Medical Center, Hackensack, NJ, USA*
[5]*Department of Family Medicine, Hackensack Meridian Health Palisades Medical Center, North Bergen, NJ, USA*
[6]*University of the East Ramon Magsaysay, Quezon City, Philippines*
[7]*Department of Pathology, Hackensack Meridian Health Palisades Medical Center, North Bergen, NJ, USA*

Correspondence should be addressed to Ayrton Bangolo; ayrtonbangolo@yahoo.com

Academic Editor: Mihail A. Boyanov

Sarcoidosis is a multisystem inflammatory disease characterized by the presence of noncaseating granulomas. Sarcoidosis can affect any organ of the body, the lung being the most affected. Sarcoidosis rarely affects the thyroid gland, and only a few cases of thyroid-related sarcoidosis have been reported in the literature. Herein, we report a case of systemic sarcoidosis with multiple organ involvement in a patient with a solitary left thyroid nodule and benign Fine Needle Aspiration (FNA) findings. The patient was eventually diagnosed with thyroid sarcoidosis using a core needle biopsy of the thyroid nodule. With this case report, we highlight the limitations of the FNA. This case report has the objective to encourage clinicians to include thyroid sarcoidosis in the differential diagnosis of thyroid nodules in patients with systemic sarcoidosis even with unremarkable FNA findings.

1. Introduction

Sarcoidosis is a multisystem granulomatous disorder of unknown etiology that affects individuals worldwide and is characterized pathologically by the presence of noncaseating granulomas in involved organs [1]. Up to 30 percent of patients present with extrapulmonary sarcoidosis [2]. Approximately 8 percent of patients with sarcoidosis present with disease at extrapulmonary sites without lung involvement. In these patients, the skin is the most common site and accounted for nearly half of the patients [3]. Thyroid involvement results in diffuse goiter or solitary thyroid nodule [4]. Most patients with thyroid involvement remain euthyroid and only a few cases have been associated with hypothyroidism [5]. We report the case of a middle-aged female who presented for evaluation of hypercalcemia and was found to have systemic sarcoidosis and a solitary left thyroid nodule. The thyroid nodule was found to be unremarkable on Fine Needle Aspiration (FNA), but sarcoid infiltration of the gland was revealed on Core Needle Biopsy. With this case report, we aim to encourage physicians to include sarcoidosis in the differential diagnosis of thyroid nodules even with normal FNA and recognize the limitations of FNA.

2. Case Presentation

This is a 58-year-old female with a past medical history of Diabetes Mellitus and asthma who presented for evaluation of hypercalcemia. The patient was referred from the Primary Care Physician's office after routine blood work revealed elevated calcium levels. Of note, the patient visited her

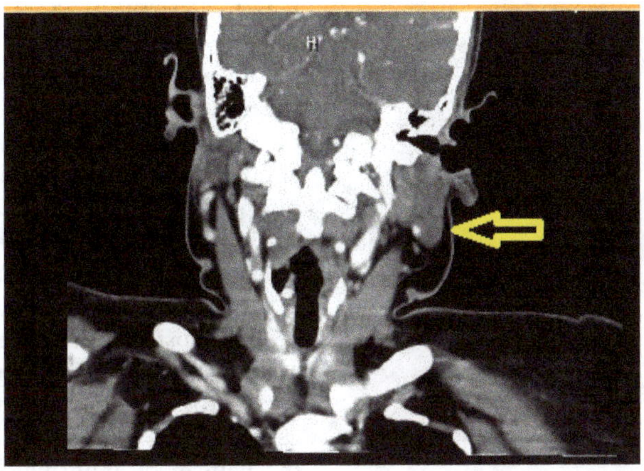

Figure 1: Neck soft tissue computed tomography revealing the left thyroid nodule.

Table 1: Laboratory values on admission.

	Laboratory values
Calcium	**14** milligram/deciliter (mg/dl) (8.6–10.3)
Aspartate aminotransferase	**44** units/liter (U/L) (13–39)
Alanine aminotransferase	47 U/L (7–52)
Parathyroid hormone	**3** picogram/milliliter (pg/ml) (14–64)
Parathyroid hormone-related peptide	20 pg/ml (14–27)
25(OH) vitamin D	22.3 nanogram/milliliter (20–80)
1,25$(OH)_2$ vitamin D	66 pg/ml (18–72)
Phosphorus	3.6 mg/dl (3.0–4.3)
Thyroid-stimulating hormone	2.87 milli-international units per milliliter (0.450–4.50)
Anti-thyroid peroxidase antibody	9 international units per milliliter (IU/mL) (0–34)
Anti-thyroglobulin antibody	<1.00 IU/mL (0.0–0.9)
Alkaline phosphatase (ALP)	**323** U/L (34–104)
Bone specific ALP	**29.6** microgram/milliliter (5.6–29)
Gamma-glutamyl transferase	**282** U/L (9–64)
Angiotensin-1-converting enzyme	**115** U/L (9–67)

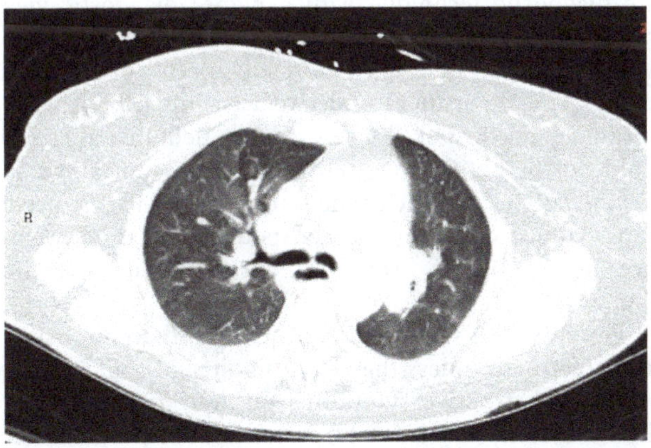

Figure 2: Chest computed tomography revealing mediastinal and hilar lymphadenopathy.

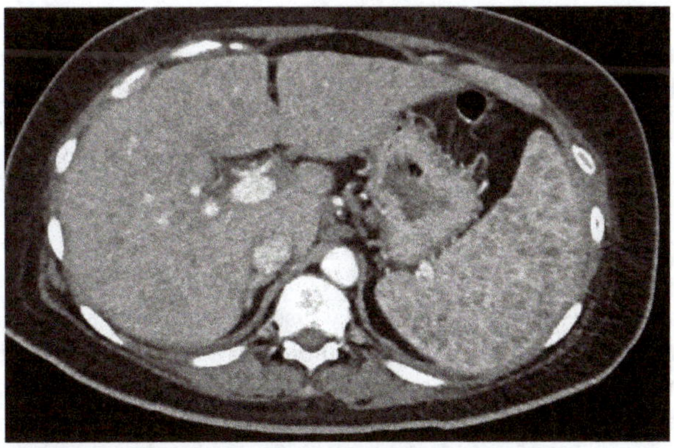

Figure 3: Computed tomography of the abdomen revealing multiple nodules of the liver and spleen.

primary care physician for evaluation of cough and dyspnea one month prior; encounter during which a chest roentgenogram revealed left lobe enlargement with right tracheal deviation. She underwent a subsequent computed tomography (CT) of neck soft tissue which revealed 3.5 centimeters nodule of the left thyroid gland (Figure 1). A fine needle aspiration of the nodule revealed a Bethesda category II, benign. However, the specimen was marginally adequate. She was also diagnosed with hypothyroidism and levothyroxine was initiated. She reported a globus sensation for the past 2 months prior to our encounter. She also reported

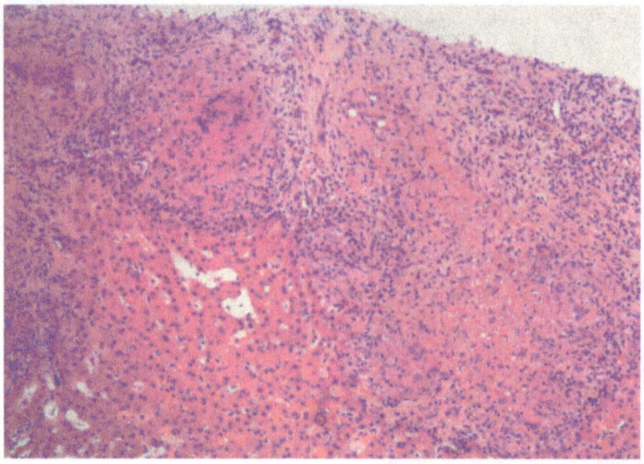

FIGURE 4: Thyroid nodule core biopsy pathology report revealing non-necrotizing granulomatous infiltration consistent with sarcoidosis. Trichrome stain showed no significant fibrosis, and iron stain was negative for iron deposition.

abdominal pain associated with constipation for the past week prior to our encounter. She denied any dysphagia or change in voice.

Upon arrival in the Emergency Department, she was hemodynamically stable. A left thyroid nodule with cervical lymphadenopathy could be felt on physical examination. Her laboratory results revealed an elevated serum calcium, higher normal $1,25(OH)_2$ vitamin D and lower normal 25(OH) vitamin D, and an elevated Angiotensin Converting Enzyme level, as seen in Table 1. A CT of the chest and abdomen revealed mediastinal and hilar lymphadenopathy (Figure 2) and multiple nodules of the liver and spleen (Figure 3). A subsequent biopsy of the liver revealed granulomatous hepatitis consistent with sarcoidosis.

The patient was started on normal saline continuous infusion. Nephrology and oncology were consulted. The patient's calcium level had normalized on day 2 of hospitalization. She eventually underwent a core needle biopsy of the left thyroid nodule which revealed granulomatous infiltration of the gland consistent with sarcoidosis (Figure 4).

She was referred to Ear, Nose, and Throat for a thyroidectomy given the invasive nature of the nodule.

3. Discussion

Sarcoidosis is an inflammatory disease characterized by the presence of noncaseating granulomas. Although sarcoidosis can affect virtually every organ of the body, the lung is most affected. Other organs commonly affected are the liver, skin, and eye [6]. Sarcoidosis rarely affects the thyroid gland. Sarcoidosis can cause diffuse goiter or rarely solitary or multiple thyroid nodules [4] that resemble a malignancy, especially when associated with cervical adenopathy [7]. Although most patients are euthyroid, both hypothyroidism and hyperthyroidism have been reported [8]. Our patient's sarcoidosis has multiple organs involved including the thyroid gland, lymph nodes, liver, spleen, lungs, and mediastinum. She has a solitary thyroid nodule with lymphadenopathy; those findings can mimic a thyroid cancer with metastasis.

Respiratory complaints including cough and dyspnea are the most common presenting symptoms. Fatigue is the most common constitutional symptom [6]. The most common abnormality of liver function is an elevation of the alkaline phosphatase level, consistent with an obstructive pattern. In addition, elevated transaminase levels can occur [6]. Our patient was initially complaining of cough and dyspnea, but a chest roentgenogram failed to show characteristic features of sarcoidosis which delayed the diagnosis. She did not have any constitutional symptoms. The liver profile revealed a cholestatic pattern consistent with sarcoidosis. Hypercalcemia occurs in about 10% of sarcoidosis patients. The mechanism of abnormal calcium metabolism is increased production of 1, 25-dihydroxyvitamin D by the granuloma itself [6]. As seen in our patient, hypercalcemia was associated with higher normal $1, 25(OH)_2$ vitamin D and a lower normal 25(OH) vitamin D. Several conditions can cause mild elevation of Angiotensin Converting Enzyme (ACE) but only a few conditions, including sarcoidosis, will cause an ACE elevation more than 50% of the upper limit of normal [6]. Elevated levels of ACE are reported in 60% of patients with acute disease and only 20% of patients with chronic disease [6]. Our patient had an ACE level elevation of more than 50% of the upper limit of normal, consistent with sarcoidosis.

Thyroid sarcoidosis is diagnosed with fine needle aspiration (FNA) biopsy or thyroidectomy for treatment of goiter demonstrating noncaseating epithelioid granulomas [9]. The false-negative rate of a benign interpretation is 0 to 3 percent [10]. In a retrospective study of nodules with two or more prior nondiagnostic FNAs, core needle biopsy was diagnostic in 86 compared with 29 percent for repeat FNA [11]. Core needle biopsy has low nondiagnostic result rates and high specificity for the diagnosis of malignancy. It is a safe diagnostic technique with a higher diagnostic yield, especially when molecular testing is not available or fine needle aspiration does not yield enough cells for molecular testing [12]. Our patient underwent an initial FNA with a marginally adequate cellularity; thus, a definitive diagnosis could not be obtained. A repeat FNA was warranted but given the higher specificity and sensitivity of the core needle biopsy compared to a repeat FNA; our patient underwent a core needle biopsy. The procedure revealed the final diagnosis.

Patients with sarcoidosis of the thyroid do not usually need treatment unless they have a goiter of sufficient size to cause obstructive symptoms or thyroid dysfunction. Thyroidectomy is generally performed in patients with obstructive symptoms or other absolute indications for surgery, such as thyrotoxicosis or thyroid cancer. Hypothyroidism, if present, should be treated with thyroid hormone therapy [9]. Our patient has dyspnea and tracheal deviation on imaging caused by a large thyroid nodule; thus, she was referred for surgery. The large nodule also caused hypothyroidism for which she is on levothyroxine.

4. Conclusion

Sarcoidosis is a multisystem granulomatous disease that can affect any organ. Some organs are more affected than others. The thyroid gland is one of the least affected organs, and only a few cases of thyroid-related sarcoidosis have been reported in the literature. Fine needle aspiration (FNA) is an important diagnostic tool in the evaluation of thyroid nodules. However, FNA can have limitations in the diagnosis of certain conditions requiring more cells for molecular testing such as sarcoidosis. Core needle biopsy has low non-diagnostic results and should be used in case the FNA sample is marginally adequate. With this case report, we hope to contribute to the growing literature of thyroid-related sarcoidosis and encourage physicians to include such a condition in the differential of thyroid nodules even with unremarkable FNA.

Ethical Approval

This study protocol was reviewed and the need for approval was waived by the ethics committee at Palisades Medical Center Hackensack Meridian Health.

Consent

A written informed consent was obtained from the patient for publication of this case report and any accompanying images.

Authors' Contributions

Ayrton Bangolo searched the literature, wrote, and revised the manuscript. John Bukasa, Ali Atoot, Mohammad Jurri, Ashraf Mahmoud, Arthur Oliver, and Kunchang Song revised and edited the manuscript. Adam Atoot and Syed Sirajuddin revised and approved the final version and are the article's guarantors. All authors certify that they contributed sufficiently to the intellectual content and data analysis. Each author has reviewed the final version of the manuscript and approves it for publication.

References

[1] Y. C. Cozier, J. S. Berman, J. R. Palmer, D. A. Boggs, D. M. Serlin, and L. Rosenberg, "Sarcoidosis in black women in the United States," *Chest*, vol. 139, no. 1, pp. 144–150, 2011.

[2] R. P. Baughman, A. S. Teirstein, M. A. Judson et al., "Clinical characteristics of patients in a case control study of sarcoidosis," *American Journal of Respiratory and Critical Care Medicine*, vol. 164, no. 10, pp. 1885–1889, 2001.

[3] W. E. James, E. Koutroumpakis, B. Saha et al., "Clinical features of extrapulmonary sarcoidosis without lung involvement," *Chest*, vol. 154, no. 2, pp. 349–356, 2018.

[4] A. Vailati, C. Marena, L. Aristia et al., "Sarcoidosis of the thyroid: report of a case and a review of the literature," *Sarcoidosis*, vol. 10, no. 1, pp. 66–68, 1993.

[5] N. Porter, H. L. Beynon, and H. S. Randeva, "Endocrine and reproductive manifestations of sarcoidosis," *QJM: International Journal of Medicine*, vol. 96, no. 8, pp. 553–561, 2003.

[6] R. P. Baughman and E. E. Lower, "Sarcoidosis," in *Harrison's Principles of Internal Medicine, 20e*, J. L. Jameson, A. S. Fauci, D. L. Kasper, S. L. Hauser, D. L. Longo, and J. Loscalzo, Eds., McGraw-Hill Education, New York, NY, USA, 2018.

[7] A. M. Salih, S. M. Fatih, and F. H. Kakamad, "Sarcoidosis mimicking metastatic papillary thyroid cancer," *International Journal of Surgery Case Reports*, vol. 16, pp. 71-72, 2015.

[8] A. Antonelli, P. Fazzi, P. Fallahi, S. M. Ferrari, and E. Ferrannini, "Prevalence of hypothyroidism and Graves disease in sarcoidosis," *Chest*, vol. 130, no. 2, pp. 526–532, 2006.

[9] J. L. Winnacker, K. L. Becker, and S. Katz, "Endocrine aspects of sarcoidosis," *New England Journal of Medicine*, vol. 278, no. 9, pp. 483–492, 1968.

[10] L. Yassa, E. S. Cibas, C. B. Benson et al., "Long-term assessment of a multidisciplinary approach to thyroid nodule diagnostic evaluation," *Cancer*, vol. 111, no. 6, pp. 508–516, 2007.

[11] A. E. Samir, A. Vij, M. K. Seale et al., "Ultrasound-guided percutaneous thyroid nodule core biopsy: clinical utility in patients with prior nondiagnostic fine-needle aspirate," *Thyroid*, vol. 22, no. 5, pp. 461–467, 2012.

[12] C. H. Suh, J. H. Baek, C. Park, Y. J. Choi, and J. H. Lee, "The role of core needle biopsy for thyroid nodules with initially indeterminate results on previous fine-needle aspiration: a systematic review and meta-analysis," *American Journal of Neuroradiology*, vol. 38, no. 7, pp. 1421–1426, 2017.

25

Parathyroid Carcinoma in the Setting of Tertiary Hyperparathyroidism: Case Report and Review of the Literature

Federico Cappellacci,[1] Fabio Medas,[1] Gian Luigi Canu,[1] Maria Letizia Lai,[2] Giovanni Conzo,[3] Enrico Erdas,[1] and Pietro Giorgio Calò[1]

[1]*Department of Surgical Sciences, University of Cagliari, "Policlinico Universitario Duilio Casula", 09042 Monserrato, Italy*
[2]*Department of Cytomorphology, University of Cagliari, Cagliari, Italy*
[3]*Division of Medical Oncology, Department of Internal and Experimental Medicine "F. Magrassi", School of Medicine, University of Campania "Luigi Vanvitelli", Cagliari, Italy*

Correspondence should be addressed to Federico Cappellacci; fedcapp94@gmail.com

Academic Editor: Mihail A. Boyanov

Introduction. Parathyroid carcinoma is one of the rarest cancers in normal population, and it is extremely uncommon in the setting of tertiary hyperparathyroidism. Indeed, only 24 cases have been reported in the literature. *Presentation of the Case.* We report the case of parathyroid carcinoma in a 51-year-old man, with a history of end-stage renal disease due to a horseshoe kidney treated with haemodialysis since 2013. He came to our attention due to an increase in calcium and parathyroid hormone serum levels. Neck ultrasound (US) showed a solid hypodense mass, probably the right inferior parathyroid gland, with an estimated size of $25 \times 15 \times 13$ mm; the 99mTc-sestamibi SPECT/CT scan revealed a large radiotracer activity area in the right cervical region, compatible with a hyperfunctioning right inferior parathyroid gland. So, a tertiary hyperparathyroidism diagnosis was made. In April 2018, resection of three parathyroid glands was performed. Histopathological examination demonstrated the right inferior parathyroid gland specimen to be a parathyroid carcinoma, due to the presence of multiple, full-thickness, capsular infiltration foci, and a venous vascular invasion focus. *Discussion.* Diagnosis of parathyroid carcinoma in tertiary hyperparathyroidism is remarkably complex because of the lack of clinical diagnostic criteria and, in many cases, is made postoperatively at histopathological examination. *Conclusion.* To date, radical surgery represents the mainstay of treatment, with a five- and ten-year survival rates overall acceptable.

1. Introduction

Tertiary hyperparathyroidism (THP) is, most commonly, the outcome of longstanding secondary hyperparathyroidism (SHP) due to chronic kidney disease and is defined as the autonomous and excessive secretion of parathyroid hormone (PTH) by the parathyroid glands, leading to persistent hypercalcemia and elevated PTH serum level, which values do not decrease even when the underlying renal disease is resolved, usually after a renal allograft [1].

SHP is generally caused by diffuse parathyroid hyperplasia, while the onset of THP is usually due to an autonomous PTH-producing adenoma and very rarely to a carcinoma [2].

Indeed, parathyroid carcinoma (PC) is one of the rarest cancers, with a prevalence of 0.005% of all malignancies in the USA [3].

PC is usually associated with primary hyperparathyroidism (PHPT), while it is extremely rare in the setting of secondary or tertiary hyperparathyroidism (THP) [4].

To the best of our knowledge, only 24 cases of THP caused by a PC have been described in the literature [4–10]; herein, we report the case of the 25th patient affected by this disease.

2. Case Report

A 51-year-old man, with a history of 15 years haemodialysis due to a horseshoe kidney, was referred to our surgical unit in April 2018 because of a progressive increase of calcium and parathyroid hormone serum levels.

His past medical history included a right inguinal hernia repair in 1979 and congenital biliary dysplasia.

His medications included sevelamer 800 mg, one pill at breakfast time and two pills at lunch and dinner time; pantoprazole 15 mg daily; bicarbonate 500 mg daily; and polystyrene sulfonate (Kayexalate) one tablespoon every two days. According to our nephrologist, no further therapy with calcimimetic drugs or calcitriol was administered.

The calcium level at the time of our first evaluation was 10.7 mg/dl, while the PTH level was more than 2000 pg/ml. Other biochemical data are summarized in Table 1.

There were no clinical features of hyperparathyroidism, and no parathyroid crisis occurs at the time of diagnosis. Physical examination showed no pathological alteration of the neck.

Preoperative 99mTc-sestamibi SPECT/CT (MIBI scan) revealed a large radiotracer activity area behind the inferior right pole of the thyroid gland, compatible with a hyperfunctioning right inferior parathyroid gland.

Neck ultrasound (US) showed, in the right inferior parathyroid area, a solid hypodense mass with an estimated size of 25 × 15 × 13 mm, compatible with a large parathyroid adenoma, without suspicion of local invasion.

Considering the presence of hypercalcemia and elevated PTH serum level, with US and SPECT/CT evidence of pathological gland, a preoperative diagnosis of tertiary hyperparathyroidism was made.

At surgery, preincision intact PTH, measured with the Future Diagnostics STAT-IntraOperative-Intact-PTH immunoassay kit, was 2582 pg/ml. After the mobilization of the right inferior thyroid lobe, an enlarged right inferior parathyroid was found and surgically removed. Near the right inferior laryngeal nerve, another enlarged mass was discovered and removed. On the left side, a soft mass, presumed to be the left inferior parathyroid gland, was identified and surgically removed.

Twenty minutes after the right inferior parathyroid resection, intact PTH levels, intraoperatively measured, dropped to 334 pg/ml.

At final neck exploration, no other pathological parathyroid glands were found, and there were no signs of local invasion of the surrounding tissues for any of the excised samples.

Histological examination revealed a parathyroid carcinoma on a 2.5 × 2 × 1.3 cm mass confirmed to be the right inferior parathyroid gland specimen. The tumour was circumscribed by a thick fibrous capsule, showing multiple full-thickness infiltration foci (Figure 1) and a venous vascular invasion focus (Figure 2), highlighted by immunohistochemical staining for CD31 (Figure 3). Furthermore, the lesion displayed frequent mitotic figures, with a positive Ki67 index in about 7-8% of the neoplastic element, but no fibrosis or necrosis was found. The pathology report

Table 1: Biochemical data at the time of diagnosis and after surgery.

	BS	1-day AS	2-day AS	3-day AS
Ca (mg/dl)	10.7	6.0	5.9	5.4
P (mg/dl)	6.8	4.3	4.2	4.4
iPTH (pg/ml)	>2000	101.4	226.9	283.9
25OH D (ng/ml)	15.2	—	—	—
Mg (mmol/l)	0.82	—	—	—
K (mEq/l)	5.3	4.6	—	—
Cr (mg/dl)	7.1	6.44	—	—
BUN (mg/dl)	65	52	—	—
ALP (U/l)	604	—	—	—
TSP (g/dl)	7.5	7.4	—	—

BS = before surgery; AS = after surgery. Ca = calcium; P = phosphorus; iPTH = intact parathyroid hormone; Mg = magnesium; K = potassium; Cr = creatinine; BUN = blood urea nitrogen; ALP = alkaline phosphatase; TSP = total serum protein.

confirmed all the other resected tissues to be diffuse parathyroid hyperplasia.

During follow-up, the patient had no postoperative complication.

Calcium and PTH serum levels on the first postoperative day were, respectively, 6.0 mg/dl and 101.4 pg/ml, while three days after the operation, they were 5.4 mg/dl and 283.9 pg/ml, respectively (Table 1).

These values are probably to be attributed to a hungry bone syndrome; therefore, calcium carbonate 2000 mg daily therapy was administered. The patient was finally discharged 3 days after the operation in good condition.

Currently, at 22 months of follow-up, which was performed by our nephrologists and endocrinologists and consisted of regular measurements of calcium and parathyroid hormone values, as well as further instrumental tests, aimed at investigating the possible presence of locoregional recurrence or distant metastases, he is free of disease.

3. Discussion

PC is a rare malignancy and generally presents an indolent but progressive behaviour [11].

According to the USA National Cancer Institute database, in nonrenal patients with PC, the age range at presentation was 15 to 55 years with a mean of 44 years [3]. At the time of diagnosis, the age of the 25 patients with parathyroid carcinoma ranged from 27 to 75 years, with a mean of 50, 4 years [4–10]; our patient received diagnosis when he was 51 years old.

Differently from PC in the setting of primary hyperparathyroidism, women and men are not equally affected: in fact, there is a clear female dominance (16 women and 9 men), but the reason remains unclear [4–12].

It is interesting to note that, as suggested by some authors, considering that almost 3% of PC has been diagnosed in haemodialysis patients, it seems to be more common in end-stage renal disease treated by haemodialysis than expected by chance [6, 13].

PC can be sporadic or in the context of genetic endocrine syndromes, such as hyperparathyroidism-jaw tumour

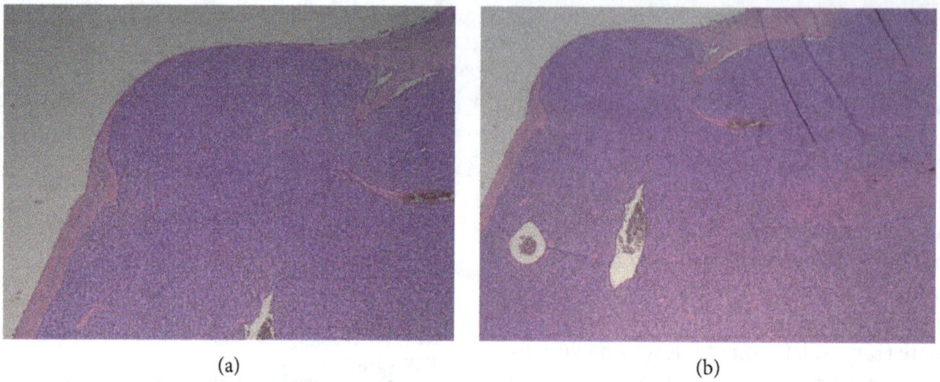

FIGURE 1: Section of the right inferior parathyroid specimen demonstrating a full-thickness capsular invasion (H&E, (a) 4x; (b) 2, 5x).

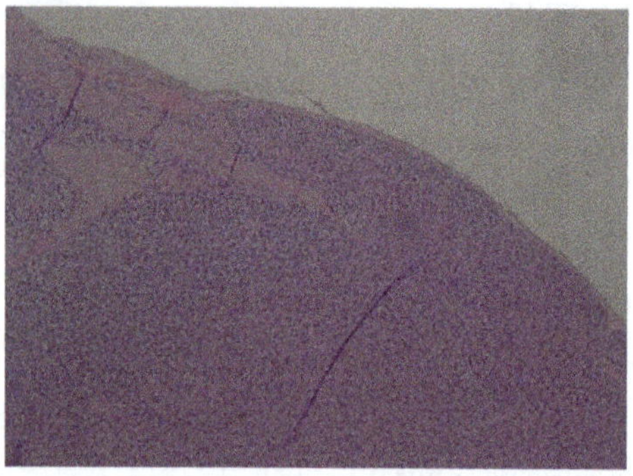

FIGURE 2: Section of the right inferior parathyroid specimen demonstrating a venous vascular invasion focus (H&E, 10x).

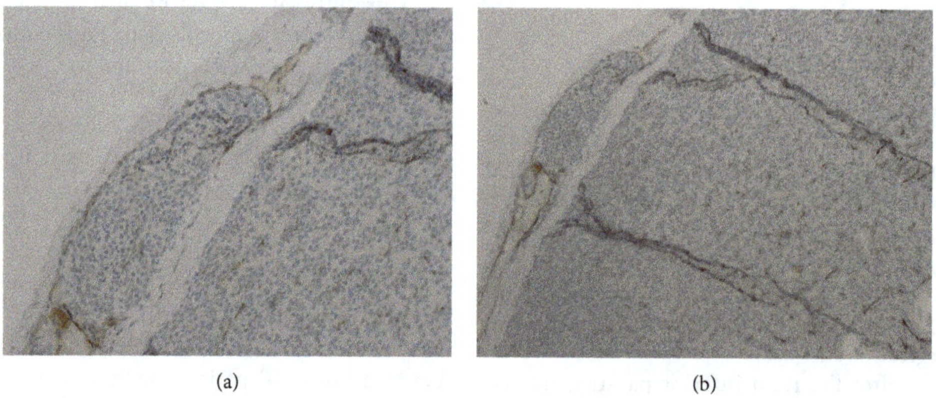

FIGURE 3: Section of the right inferior parathyroid specimen showing a venous vascular invasion focus highlighted by immunohistochemical staining for CD31 ((a) 20x; (b) 10x).

syndrome (HPT-JT), multiple endocrine neoplasia type 1 (MEN 1), multiple endocrine neoplasia type 2A (MEN 2A), and familial isolated hyperparathyroidism (FIHP) [11, 12, 14, 15].

The aetiology of this tumour is unknown, but a genetic background has been established. Genomic alterations identified in PC are mostly represented by CDC73 gene mutations, the same gene involved in HPT-JT, codifying for a protein called parafibromin, which is liable, according to Cetani et al., for up to 70% of sporadic PC [11, 12, 14, 15]. Furthermore, evaluation regarding loss of parafibromin immunohistochemistry could be useful for diagnosis and differentiation of PC from other parathyroid lesions in daily practice, especially in cases with an initial suspicion of malignant potential to avoid excessive numbers of false positives [16–18]. In our patient, given the morphological alterations and other immunohistochemical investigation, our pathologists did not consider to perform parafibromin immunohistochemistry. Furthermore, assuming that the tumour was sporadic, neither the sequencing of CDC73 gene was carry out.

The diagnosis of PC is remarkably complex because of the lack of clinical diagnostic criteria and, in many cases, is made postoperatively at histopathological examination [12].

PC in tertiary hyperparathyroidism patients usually shows up with symptoms and signs of hyperparathyroidism, such as myalgia and arthralgia, weight loss, nephrolithiasis, and with bone disease localized in the spine, long bones, hands, and the skull [4–10].

As some authors suggest, in a patient with PHPT, severe hypercalcemia (>14 mg/dL), very high serum PTH levels (five times above the normal range), concomitant severe renal and skeletal manifestations, and palpable cervical mass should raise suspicion for PC [11, 12]. Nevertheless, calcium and PTH serum levels are not a useful indicator for the presence of PC in patients with THP, due to the end-stage renal disease: in fact, the kidney does not respond to parathyroid hormone in such cases [7].

Imaging techniques, such as neck ultrasound and ^{99m}Tc-sestamibi scintigraphy, are useful for tumour localization but cannot reliably discriminate benign from malignant hyperparathyroidism [11, 12].

In case of preoperative suspicion for malignant disease, some authors recommend that a CT or MR imaging is performed [19]. It has also been suggested that other nuclear medicine techniques, such as 18F-Choline-PET, could be useful in the preoperative management of PC [20].

The finding of metastasis is the only certain criterion of malignancy [12].

Notably, among all cases reported in the literature, only one had preoperative PC suspect: Curto et al. had reported in 2019 a PC with a single pulmonary metastasis in a IV-stage chronic kidney disease patient, which was identified preoperatively with a combination of MIBI scan and PET-CT [10].

To our knowledge, this is the only preoperative diagnosis of PC in tertiary hyperparathyroidism, and in all the other cases, only intraoperative and/or histological findings made it possible to diagnose PC [4–10].

However, it is important to emphasize that also histopathological diagnosis may be difficult. Many pathological characteristics, such as trabecular architecture and mitotic figures, are not exclusive of PC, being also present in benign parathyroid diseases, while other histological features, such as capsular and vascular invasion or necrosis, are not always present in PC. The main challenge at histopathological examination is to distinguish PC from atypical adenoma. The latter tumour shares some histological characteristics with PC, such as fibrous septa, high mitotic activity, and diffuse growth pattern, but lack unequivocal signs of malignancy, as vascular, capsular, and/or perineural invasion [11, 12, 21]. In SHP, histological evaluation could be even challenging, due to the fact that the parathyroid glands tend to become larger, to develop multinodularity, and because of the greater presence of fibrous bands, which can complicate the evaluation of capsular invasion. So, in this setting, it is even more important to investigate the presence of vascular and/or perineural invasion before a PC diagnosis was given, to avoid the risk of false positive results.

As Erickson and Mete suggest, a panel of immunohistochemical markers may help in the histological evaluation of this tumour [22].

In our patient, the pathologist was able to diagnose PC thanks to the presence of multiple full-thickness capsular infiltration foci (Figure 1) and a venous vascular invasion focus (Figure 2), highlighted by immunohistochemical staining for CD31 (Figure 3), but, as we reported earlier, no fibrosis or necrosis was found.

Surgery is the mainstay of treatment, while usefulness of chemotherapy, radiotherapy, and other treatments remains still controversial. The surgical approach mostly suggested consists in an en-bloc resection of the pathological parathyroid gland with the ipsilateral thyroid lobe and any adjacent involved structures. Cervical lymph node dissection is mostly recommended in case of preoperative diagnosis or intraoperative suspicion of metastases [11, 12, 21].

Among the previous 24 patients with parathyroid cancer in the setting of tertiary hyperparathyroidism, 11 underwent parathyroidectomy alone, 5 underwent parathyroidectomy and neck lymphadenectomy, 5 underwent parathyroidectomy with total thyroidectomy, 2 underwent parathyroidectomy, lymphadenectomy, radical neck dissection, and wedge resection of some lung nodules, and 1 underwent parathyroidectomy and thyroid lobectomy [4–10].

In case of parathyroidectomy alone and histopathological diagnosis of PC, the management of the patient becomes more difficult. In this situation, clinical judgment and prompt decision making to choose further neck exploration or surveillance are required. In presence of aggressive histopathological features, such as extensive vascular and capsular invasion, a re-exploration to perform a more radical treatment should be indicated [11, 12, 23].

Restoration of normocalcemia after surgery indicates that all hyperfunctioning tissue has been removed. The use of intraoperative PTH determination could be helpful in surgical management [24–30].

Differently than PHPT, where requirements of success include normalization of PTH in addition to serum calcium levels, in THP the operative endpoint of surgery is not a return of PTH to normal value, but a drop in PTH level higher than 50% is considered sufficient, even if it remains above the normal range. Furthermore, the main objective of surgery for THP is not a normal PTH value, but a normal calcium level at least six months of follow-up [1].

As we reported in our patient, postoperative hypocalcaemia may occur, due to inhibition of remnant parathyroid glands or hungry bone syndrome, and, in this case, hypocalcaemia could be increased because of the chronic renal failure. This condition must be promptly treated with oral or intravenous calcium supplementation [11, 12].

PC recurrence occurs in more than 50% of patients, usually after 2-3 years from surgery, although relapses have been reported up to 23 years after initial treatment. For this reason, in patients with this tumour, follow-up should be careful and life-long [11, 12].

The recurrence site is most frequently locoregional, due to incomplete resection at initial surgery and cervical lymph node metastases; however, also distant metastases are not infrequent. Lymph node metastases occur in about 15–30% of patients at initial presentation. Distant metastases occur in about 25% of patients during follow-up, usually in the lungs, liver, and bone [11, 12]. Seven cases of disease recurrence on the total of 25 PC in the setting of THP are reported: the literature highlights five cases of lung metastasis, one case of liver metastasis, and one case of unknown recurrence origin [4–10].

Primary treatment for disease recurrence is surgical removal, both for local recurrences and, if possible, for distant metastases, even through repeated resection [11, 12, 23].

Five- and ten-year overall survival rates between 77–100 and 49–91%, respectively, have been described. Mortality generally is related to complications of hypercalcemia rather than from tumour burden [11, 12, 21].

In the renal dialysis cases, due to the small number of cases, it is difficult to establish a clear survival rate; however, the longest recorded survival is 9.5 years [31].

Regarding our patient, at 22 months of follow-up, he is alive and free of disease.

In conclusion, parathyroid carcinoma is an extremely rare tumour in the setting of THP, and his clinical diagnosis could be difficult due to the presence of chronic kidney failure, which leads to an increase in PTH blood level. Presence of metastasis is the only certain criterion of malignancies. To date, radical surgery remains the mainstay of treatment.

The recurrence rate of PC is generally high but is notable that 5- and 10-year survival rates are overall acceptable.

Notably in our patient, considering that the definitive diagnosis took place only postoperatively and given the absence of preoperative and intraoperative suspicion for local invasion, radical surgery was not performed.

Consent

Written informed consent was obtained from the patient for publication of this case report and the accompanying images.

References

[1] J. A. Tang, J. Friedman, M. S. Hwang, A. M. Salapatas, L. B. Bonzelaar, and M. Friedman, "Parathyroidectomy for tertiary hyperparathyroidism: a systematic review," *American Journal of Otolaryngology*, vol. 38, no. 5, pp. 630–635, 2017.

[2] K. Duan, K. Gomez Hernandez, and O. Mete, "Clinicopathological correlates of hyperparathyroidism," *Journal of Clinical Pathology*, vol. 68, no. 10, pp. 771–787, 2015.

[3] S. A. Hundahl, I. D. Fleming, A. M. Fremgen, and H. R. Menck, "Two hundred eighty-six cases of parathyroid carcinoma treated in the U.S. between 1985–1995," *Cancer*, vol. 86, no. 3, pp. 538–544, 1999.

[4] M. W. Khan, E. M. Worcester, F. H. Straus, S. Khan, V. Staszak, and E. L. Kaplan, "Parathyroid carcinoma in secondary and tertiary hyperparathyroidism," *Journal of the American College of Surgeons*, vol. 199, no. 2, pp. 312–319, 2004.

[5] I. A. Srouji, A. Resouly, and I. A. Cree, "Case of thymic parathyroid carcinoma in a haemodialysis patient: application of tumour chemosensitivity testing," *The Journal of Laryngology & Otology*, vol. 118, no. 2, pp. 162–164, 2004.

[6] M. Bossola, L. Tazza, A. Ferrante et al., "Parathyroid carcinoma in a chronic hemodialysis patient: case report and review of the literature," *Tumori Journal*, vol. 91, no. 6, pp. 558–562, 2005.

[7] S. K. Byung, S. R. Han, H. K. Kyung, and J. P. Sung, "Parathyroid carcinoma in tertiary hyperparathyroidism," *Asian Journal of Surgery*, vol. 39, no. 4, pp. 255–259, 2016.

[8] M. P. Nasrallah, D. L. Fraker, and V. A. LiVolsi, "Parathyroid carcinoma in the setting of tertiary hyperparathyroidism after renal transplant," *Endocrine Pathology*, vol. 25, no. 4, p. 433, 2014.

[9] A. Pappa and T. Hackman, "Simultaneous incidental parathyroid carcinoma and intrathyroid parathyroid gland in suspected renal failure induced hyperparathyroidism," *Surgery Journal*, vol. 3, no. 1, pp. 23-24, 2017.

[10] L. S. Curto, R. Gervasi, F. Caracciolo, and N. Innaro, "Parathyroid carcinoma presenting with chronic renal failure and single pulmonary metastasis: a case report," *International Journal of Surgery Case Reports*, vol. 65, pp. 322–324, 2019.

[11] A. S. Salcuni, F. Cetani, V. Guarnieri et al., "Parathyroid carcinoma," *Best Practice & Research Clinical Endocrinology & Metabolism*, vol. 32, no. 6, pp. 877–889, 2018.

[12] F. Cetani, E. Pardi, and C. Marcocci, "Parathyroid carcinoma," *Parathyroid Disorders*, vol. 51, pp. 63–76, 2019.

[13] T. B. Drüeke, "Cell biology of parathyroid gland hyperplasia in chronic renal failure," *Journal of the American Society of Nephrology*, vol. 11, no. 6, pp. 1141–1152, 2000.

[14] J. D. Carpten, C. M. Robbins, A. Villablanca et al., "HRPT2, encoding parafibromin, is mutated in hyperparathyroidism-jaw tumor syndrome," *Nature Genetics*, vol. 32, no. 4, pp. 676–680, 2002.

[15] T. M. Shattuck, S. Välimäki, T. Obara et al., "Somatic and germ-line mutations of theHRPT2Gene in sporadic parathyroid carcinoma," *New England Journal of Medicine*, vol. 349, no. 18, pp. 1722–1729, 2003.

[16] F. Cetani, E. Pardi, and C. Marcocci, "Parathyroid carcinoma: a clinical and genetic perspective," *Minerva Endocrinologica*, vol. 43, no. 2, pp. 144–155, 2018.

[17] A. J. Gill, A. Clarkson, O. Gimm et al., "Loss of nuclear expression of parafibromin distinguishes parathyroid carcinomas and hyperparathyroidism-jaw tumor (HPT-JT) syndrome-related adenomas from sporadic parathyroid adenomas and hyperplasias," *The American Journal of Surgical Pathology*, vol. 30, no. 9, pp. 1140–1149, 2006.

[18] C. C. Juhlin, I.-L. Nilsson, K. Lagerstedt-Robinson et al., "Parafibromin immunostainings of parathyroid tumors in clinical routine: a near-decade experience from a tertiary center," *Modern Pathology*, vol. 32, no. 8, pp. 1082–1094, 2019.

[19] S. Fakhran, B. F. Branstetter, and D. A. Pryma, "Parathyroid imaging," *Neuroimaging Clinics of North America*, vol. 18, no. 3, p. 537, 2008.

[20] G. B. Morand, B. M. Helmchen, H. C. Steinert, C. Schmid, and M. A. Broglie, "18F-Choline-PET in parathyroid carcinoma," *Oral Oncology*, vol. 86, pp. 314-315, 2018.

[21] F. Cetani, E. Pardi, and C. Marcocci, "Update on parathyroid carcinoma," *Journal of Endocrinological Investigation*, vol. 39, no. 6, pp. 595–606, 2016.

[22] L. A. Erickson and O. Mete, "Immunohistochemistry in diagnostic parathyroid pathology," *Endocrine Pathology*, vol. 29, no. 2, pp. 113–129, 2018.

[23] V. Ferraro, L. I. Sgaramella, G. Di Meo et al., "Current concepts in parathyroid carcinoma: a single centre experience," *BMC Endocrine Disorders*, vol. 19, no. 1, p. 46, 2019.

[24] P. G. Calò, G. Pisano, G. Loi et al., "Intraoperative parathyroid hormone assay during focused parathyroidectomy: the importance of 20 minutes measurement," *BMC Surgery*, vol. 13, p. 36, 2013.

[25] A. Catania, S. Sorrenti, L. Falvo, M. Santulli, A. Berni, and E. De Antoni, "Validity and limits of intraoperative rapid parathyroid hormone assay in primary hyperparathyroidism treated by traditional and mini-invasive surgery," *International Surgery*, vol. 87, no. 4, pp. 226–232, 2002.

[26] P. G. Calò, G. Pisano, A. Tatti et al., "Intraoperative parathyroid hormone assay during focused parathyroidectomy for primary hyperparathyroidism: is it really mandatory?" *Minerva Chirurgica*, vol. 67, no. 4, pp. 337–342, 2012.

[27] C. P. Lombardi, M. Raffaelli, E. Traini et al., "Intraoperative PTH monitoring during parathyroidectomy: the need for stricter criteria to detect multiglandular disease," *Langenbeck's Archives of Surgery*, vol. 393, no. 5, pp. 639–645, 2008.

[28] M. C. Gioviale, G. Gambino, C. Maione et al., "Use of monitoring intraoperative parathyroid hormone during parathyroidectomy in patients on waiting list for renal transplantation," *Transplantation Proceedings*, vol. 39, no. 6, pp. 1775–1778, 2007.

[29] P. G. Calò, G. Pisano, G. Loi et al., "Surgery for primary hyperparathyroidism in patients with preoperatively negative sestamibi scan and discordant imaging studies: the usefulness of intraoperative parathyroid hormone monitoring," *Clinical Medicine Insights: Endocrinology and Diabetes*, vol. 6, pp. 63–67, 2013.

[30] C. Dobrinja, G. Santandrea, M. Giacca, E. Stenner, M. Ruscio, and N. de Manzini, "Effectiveness of Intraoperative Parathyroid Monitoring (ioPTH) in predicting a multiglandular or malignant parathyroid disease," *International Journal of Surgery*, vol. 41, no. 1, pp. 26–33, 2017.

[31] H. Miki, M. Sumitomo, H. Inoue, S. Kita, and Y. Monden, "Parathyroid carcinoma in patients with chronic renal failure on maintenance hemodialysis," *Surgery*, vol. 120, no. 5, pp. 897–901, 1996.

Delayed Calcium Normalization after Successful Parathyroidectomy in Primary Hyperparathyroidism

Iván Emilio de la Cruz Rodríguez[1], **Elsy Sarahí García Montesinos**[1], **María Fernanda Rodríguez-Delgado**[2], **Guadalupe Vargas Ortega**[1], **Lourdes Balcázar Hernández**[1], **Victoria Mendoza Zubieta**[1], **Victor Hernández Avendaño**[1], and **Baldomero González Virla**[1]

[1]*Endocrinology Department. Hospital de Especialidades, Centro Médico Nacional Siglo XXI, Mexico City 067200, Mexico*
[2]*Faculty of Medicine, Universidad Nacional Autónoma de México, Coordinacion de Servicios a la Comunidad, Programa Comunidad Saludable-Comunidad Solidaria, Mexico City, Mexico*

Correspondence should be addressed to Baldomero González Virla; baldogonzal@hotmail.com

Academic Editor: Michaï¿½l R. Laurent

Introduction. Parathyroidectomy is the curative treatment option in primary hyperparathyroidism (PHPT). The decrease of parathormone (PTH) by 50% or more from levels prior to surgery after excision predicts successful parathyroidectomy. Serum calcium is expected to return to normal within 24–72 hours after the surgery; however, nearly 10% have transient, persistent postoperative hypercalcemia. We present a case report of delayed calcium normalization after successful parathyroidectomy in a 38-year-old patient with PHPT. *Methods.* Parathyroidectomy was performed, with evidence of a decrease in PTH levels of more than 50% in the first 24 hours postoperatively compared to presurgical PTH; however, despite curative parathyroidectomy, a delayed calcium normalization was evidenced, with hypercalcemia persistence up to 120 hours postoperatively. *Results.* After the first month postoperatively, serum calcium remained normal. In conclusion, approximately 10% of patients with curative parathyroidectomy have transient, persistent postoperative hypercalcemia, which is more likely to occur in patients with higher preoperative serum calcium and PTH levels. *Conclusion.* Persistent hypercalcemia after the first month postoperatively is related with persistent PHPT, highlighting the importance of calcium monitoring after parathyroidectomy to predict short-term, medium-term, and long-term outcomes and prognosis.

1. Introduction

Primary hyperparathyroidism (PHPT) is the main cause of hypercalcemia in the outpatient setting. PHPT is a common disorder caused by the autonomous overproduction of the parathyroid hormone (PTH) attributable to hyperfunction of 1 or more glands, related with 4 different pathologic conditions: adenoma (88–90%), hyperplasia (5–7%), multiple adenoma (4–14%), and carcinoma (<1%). Most cases of PHPT are sporadic (90%). PHPT is characterized by the persistent elevation of serum calcium levels with elevated or inappropriately normal PTH levels [1, 2]. PHPT predominates among women, usually in the postmenopause, with a female/male ratio of 3 to 4 : 1. The prevalence varies by country and race [3], with a higher incidence among blacks, followed by whites, Asians, and Hispanics [4].

The clinical presentation is heterogeneous, with a spectrum from an asymptomatic disease to a hypercalcemic crisis. The diagnosis of PHPT is biochemical, and parathyroidectomy is the curative approach [1, 5].

The decrease of PTH by 50% or more from levels prior to surgery after excision predicts a successful parathyroidectomy. Serum calcium is expected to return to normal within 24–72 hours after surgery; however, approximately 10% of patients have transient, persistent postoperative hypercalcemia [6]. We present a case report of delayed calcium normalization after successful parathyroidectomy in a 38-year-old patient with PHPT.

2. Case Presentation

A 38-year-old man with a personal history of hypertension, primary hypothyroidism, and hydronephrosis secondary to urolithiasis was evaluated for hypercalcemia in an endocrinology department of a tertiary health center. There were no familial antecedents of hypercalcemia, lithiasis, or hyperparathyroidism. The patient reported weakness, lack of energy and strength, and mental and physical fatigue. The patient was given levothyroxine 100 mcg and candesartan 16 mg daily.

In the biochemical evaluation, laboratory features included creatinine of 1.4 mg/dL, serum calcium of 13.5 mg/dL, albumin of 4.7 g/dL, albumin-corrected calcium of 12.94 mg/dL, phosphorus of 1.9 mg/dL, vitamin D of 18 ng/mL, and PTH of 383.7 pg/mL, with evidence of hypercalcemia, hypophosphatemia, deficiency of vitamin D, and hyperparathyroidism; PHPT was diagnosed. Tc-99m sestamibi scintigraphy identified an abnormal uptake in the left inferior thyroid pole, corresponding to parathyroid adenoma.

3. Treatment

Neck exploration and parathyroidectomy were performed, with a complete excision of a tumor of 27 × 17 × 8 mm, weight of 2.3 g, and capsule integrity. An intraoperative PTH drop >50% was corroborated after parathyroidectomy, meeting the "Miami criterion." [7] The histopathological reporting evidenced a well-circumscribed lesion with a thin fibrous capsule contained in a vascular capillary network; most of neoplastic cells resembled the normal parathyroid cells; there were uniform polygonal cells with small central nuclei and focal cystic changes, with neither atypia nor increased mitotic figures. The final diagnosis was parathyroid adenoma (Figure 1).

4. Outcome and Follow-Up

During the first 12 hours after parathyroidectomy, a 98% reduction of PTH levels (PTH preoperatory: 383.7 pg/mL vs. PTH postoperatory: 6.5 pg/mL) was evidenced; however, a persistence of elevated serum calcium (12.1 mg/dl) was observed. Magnesium remained normal during evolution. During the first 48 hours after parathyroidectomy, the patient received 1500 ml of 0.9% sodium chloride solution I.V. and 500 ml of water P.O. After this time, he continued with 2000 ml of water P.O. during his follow-up. In the clinical follow-up, the evidence of hypercalcemia and normal PTH levels persisted up to 96 hours, with a delayed calcium normalization up to 120 hours (Figure 2). After the first month postoperatively, serum calcium remained normal; however, the patient currently continues with a strict monitoring of serum calcium and PTH levels.

5. Discussion

We presented a case report of a patient with symptomatic HPTH, who underwent surgery for the presence of renal involvement, age younger than 50 years, and serum calcium level greater than 1 mg/dL above normal, with the histopathological evidence of parathyroid adenoma. We highlighted that, despite a successful parathyroidectomy, serum calcium levels remained elevated for a longer time than reported in the literature, with a delayed calcium normalization up to 120 hours.

Parathyroidectomy is the curative and definitive treatment of PHPT, and it is indicated for all patients with symptomatic PHPT, evidence of renal involvement, osteoporosis, fragility fracture, vertebral fracture, when the serum calcium level is greater than 1 mg/dL, age of 50 years or younger, and when parathyroid cancer is suspected [1]. Parathyroidectomy should be conducted by surgeons with adequate training and experience.

The "Miami criterion" is defined as a PTH decrease >50% from either the highest preincision or pre-excision hormone level in a peripheral blood sample obtained 10 minutes after complete excision of all hyperfunctioning parathyroid tissues. After this, an intraoperative PTH decrease >50% occurs, and the observed hormone dynamic guides the termination of the operation without further exploration. If the 10-minute sample does not meet the criterion, a delayed sample at 20 minutes is measured, and/or further neck exploration is continued until all hypersecreting parathyroid glands are removed, confirmed by another >50% decrease from the highest subsequent pre-excision sample. This protocol was developed and refined at the University of Miami and indicates a successful parathyroidectomy, with a sensitivity of 98%, specificity of 97%, positive predictive value of 99%, negative predictive value of 90%, and overall accuracy of 97% [7].

In the hands of an experienced surgeon, cure rates for parathyroidectomy in sporadic PHPT approach 95% to 99%, with a low complication rate (<1–3%) [1, 5]. Curative parathyroidectomy is defined as the normalization of calcium homeostasis lasting a minimum of 6 months after surgery [1].

Currently, there is no consensus about the time that serum calcium normalizes after parathyroidectomy. After a successful parathyroidectomy, serum calcium levels normalize and reach a nadir at 48–72 hours postoperatively [8, 9]; however, approximately 10% of patients have transient, persistent postoperative hypercalcemia, which is more likely to occur in patients with higher preoperative serum calcium and PTH levels. Most patients with PHPT have normal serum calcium levels within the first two weeks after parathyroidectomy, and 96% will have normal serum calcium levels in the first postoperative month. Hypercalcemia that does not normalize within the first 30 days postoperatively has been associated with persistent PHPT [6], which is defined as a failure to achieve normocalcemia within 6 months after parathyroidectomy [1].

The early biochemical response of PTH and serum calcium levels after parathyroidectomy is the main predictor

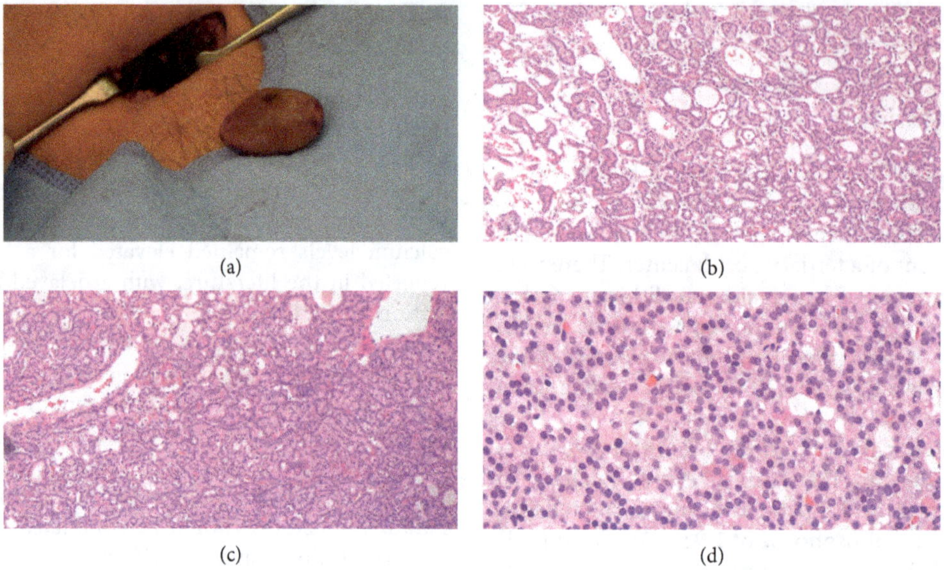

Figure 1: (a) Parathyroid adenoma. Hematoxylin-eosin stain (4x) showed the absence of adipose tissue and follicular (b) and trabecular (c) growth pattern, with a predominance of chief cells and some oxyphilic cells (d).

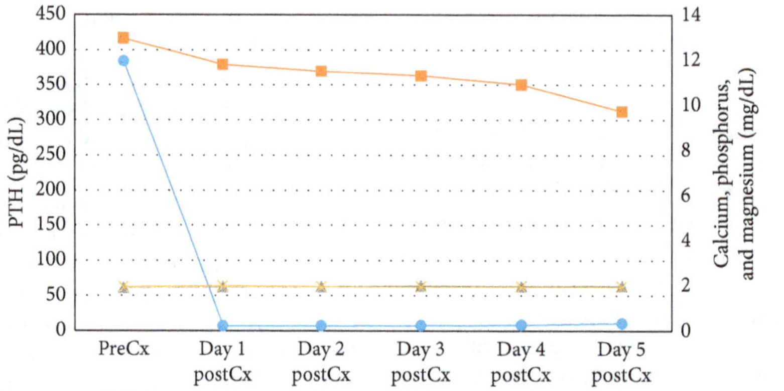

	PreCx	Day 1 postCx	Day 2 postCx	Day 3 postCx	Day 4 postCx	Day 5 postCx
PTH (pg/mL)	383.7	6.5	6.6	7.2	8	10.35
Calcium* (mg/dL)	12.94	11.78	11.48	11.28	10.88	9.7
Phosphorus (mg/dL)	1.9	1.94	1.94	1.98	1.96	1.98
Magnesium (mg/dL)	1.92	1.96	1.94	1.93	1.94	1.93

Figure 2: Evolution of serum PTH, calcium, phosphorus, and magnesium levels before and after parathyroidectomy. PreCx: presurgery. PostCx: postsurgery. *Albumin-corrected calcium.

of persistent or recurrent PTHT after 6 postoperative months. Patients with a partial biochemical response after parathyroidectomy have a greater risk of recurrent hypercalcemia compared to those with complete biochemical response. The postoperative presence of persistently increased PTH but normocalcemia or persistently increased calcium but normal PTH increases 1.6 and 2 times, respectively, the risk of recurrent hypercalcemia [10]. Despite these data, there has been no demonstration of the association between transient hypercalcemia after parathyroidectomy and persistent or recurrent PHPT [6]. The role of transient hypercalcemia and the delayed calcium normalization in the evolution and prognosis of the patient with PHPT represents an important and relevant research topic for long-term studies.

6. Conclusion

Approximately 10% of patients with curative parathyroidectomy have transient, persistent postoperative hypercalcemia, which is more common in patients with higher preoperative serum calcium and PTH levels. Most of these patients achieve calcium normalization within the first postoperative month. Hypercalcemia after the first 30 days postoperatively is related with persistent PHPT, highlighting the importance of calcium monitoring after parathyroidectomy to predict short-term, medium-term, and long-term outcomes and prognosis. There is a lack of information about the association between transient, persistent postoperative hypercalcemia and the development of persistent PHPT; future long-term studies about this research topic are necessary.

Consent

Written informed consent was obtained from the patient for publication of the submitted article and accompanying images.

References

[1] S. M. Wilhelm, T. S. Wang, D. T. Ruan et al., "The American association of endocrine surgeons guidelines for definitive management of primary hyperparathyroidism," *JAMA Surgery*, vol. 151, no. 10, pp. 959–968, 2016.

[2] J. V. Oberger Marques and C. A. Moreira, "Primary hyperparathyroidism," *Best Practice & Research Clinical Rheumatology*, vol. 34, no. 3, Article ID 101514, 2020.

[3] J. P. Bilezikian, "Primary hyperparathyroidism," *The Journal of Clinical Endocrinology & Metabolism*, vol. 103, no. 11, pp. 3993–4004, 2018.

[4] M. W. Yeh, P. H. G. Ituarte, H. C. Zhou et al., "Incidence and prevalence of primary hyperparathyroidism in a racially mixed population," *The Journal of Clinical Endocrinology & Metabolism*, vol. 98, no. 3, pp. 1122–1129, 2013.

[5] A. A. Khan, D. A. Hanley, R. Rizzoli et al., "Primary hyperparathyroidism: review and recommendations on evaluation, diagnosis, and management. A Canadian and international consensus," *Osteoporosis International*, vol. 28, no. 1, pp. 1–19, 2017.

[6] V. Lai, T. W. F. Yen, K. Doffek et al., "Delayed calcium normalization after presumed curative parathyroidectomy is not associated with the development of persistent or recurrent primary hyperparathyroidism," *Annals of Surgical Oncology*, vol. 23, no. 7, pp. 2310–2314, 2016.

[7] Z. F. Khan and J. I. Lew, "Intraoperative parathyroid hormone monitoring in the surgical management of sporadic primary hyperparathyroidism," *Endocrinology and Metabolism*, vol. 34, no. 4, pp. 327–339, 2019.

[8] W. Graf, J. Rastad, G. Åkerström, L. Wide, and S. Ljunghall, "Dynamics of parathyroid hormone release and serum calcium regulation after surgery for primary hyperparathyroidism," *World Journal of Surgery*, vol. 16, no. 4, pp. 625–631, 1992.

[9] Y. Alabdulkarim and E. Nassif, "Delayed serum calcium biochemical response to successful parathyroidectomy in primary hyperparathyroidism," *Journal of Laboratory Physicians*, vol. 2, no. 1, pp. 010–013, 2010.

[10] C. Y. Ryder, A. Jarocki, M. M. McNeely et al., "Early biochemical response to parathyroidectomy for primary hyperparathyroidism and its predictive value for recurrent hypercalcemia and recurrent primary hyperparathyroidism," *Surgery*, vol. 169, no. 1, 2021.

Lingual Thyroid with Subclinical Hypothyroidism in a Young Female

Subash Thapa[1] **and Prakash Khanal**[2]

[1]*Department of Radiology, Nepal Police Hospital, Kathmandu, Nepal*
[2]*Department of ENT-Head and Neck Surgery, Nepal Police Hospital, Kathmandu, Nepal*

Correspondence should be addressed to Subash Thapa; subashthapa.hod@gmail.com

Academic Editor: Osamu Isozaki

Thyroid tissue presenting as a nodule in the base of the tongue due to the embryonic failure to descend to the anterior neck is a rare clinical entity, called lingual thyroid. Clinical presentation varies depending upon the degree of obstruction caused by an enlarged nodule or features related to thyroid function. We report a case of a 27-year-old female who presented with a foreign body sensation in the throat with mild dysphagia for 3 weeks. The patient was diagnosed as lingual thyroid with subclinical hypothyroidism based on clinical findings, imaging, and fine-needle aspiration cytology. Conservative management with hormone suppression can result in size reduction of ectopic thyroid tissue improving symptoms without surgery. Lingual thyroid with mild symptoms and subclinical hypothyroidism can be managed conservatively.

1. Introduction

The thyroid gland is normally located in the pretracheal region of the anterior neck inferior to the thyroid cartilage at the level of the C5-T1 vertebra [1]. The presence of thyroid tissue outside its normal anatomical position due to embryonic failure to descend is called ectopic thyroid tissue (ETT), and when present at the base of the tongue, it is called lingual thyroid (LT). The estimated prevalence of reported ectopic thyroid is 1 per 100,000–300,000 healthy individuals [2–5], which is even more high among the patients with thyroid disease (1 per 4000 to 8000 cases) [3]. The exact prevalence of lingual thyroid is unknown since many asymptomatic patients never come to medical attention; however, a study among 200 consecutive routine necropsies on Caucasian individuals suggested that 10% of adults may harbor asymptomatic thyroid tissue along the path of the thyroglossal duct [3]. Among the patients with thyroid disease, the overall prevalence of lingual thyroid is 1 in 3000 cases [5, 6]. Lingual thyroid is common among females (70–80%) [2, 5, 6]. Most cases of LT are asymptomatic [4–9] unless an increase in gland size occurs resulting in dysphagia, dysphonia, foreign body sensation in the throat, cough, pain, bleeding, and dyspnea [2]. Meticulous diagnostic workup including clinical examination, biochemical profile, imaging tools, radioisotope scanning, and histopathology is necessary to plan the management in lingual thyroid [7, 8, 10]. The approach of size reduction by hormone suppression therapy among mild symptomatic patients with lingual thyroid can resolve symptoms to avoid surgical intervention [4, 7, 10].

2. Case Report

A 27-year-old female presented to the outpatient department with a history of foreign body sensation in the throat with mild dysphagia for 3 weeks. There was no significant medical or surgical history in the past. Throat examination revealed a well-defined nodule in the midline at the base of the tongue with intact smooth mucosa (Figure 1). The thyroid gland could not be appreciated on neck palpation. Chest X-ray was normal. Ultrasonography (USG) neck revealed the absence of a thyroid gland in its orthotopic location. No enlarged cervical lymph nodes were seen. A computed tomography (CT) scan showed a well-defined relatively hyperdense homogeneous enhancing nodule measuring $24 \times 24 \times 22$ mm in the midline at the base of the tongue without calcification. No thyroid gland was seen in the orthotopic location (Figure 2). Thyroid function tests showed normal FT3: 3.3 pg/mL (reference value 1.2–4.1 pg/mL), normal FT4: 13.1 pg/mL (reference value 8.9–17.1 pg/mL), and slightly elevated TSH: 5.7 mIU/mL (reference value 0.3–4.5 mIU/mL). Fine-needle aspiration cytology (FNAC) from the nodule at the base of the tongue showed a cluster of benign-looking thyroid epithelial cells in the background of RBCs (Figure 3). Thyroid scintigraphy with technetium (Tc-99 m) showed uptake of the radiotracer at the region of the base of the tongue. No uptake was seen in the normal thyroid gland location.

Based on the clinical examination, thyroid function test report, USG, and CT findings, a definitive diagnosis of lingual thyroid with subclinical hypothyroidism was made, and the patient was planned for conservative pharmacological management with levothyroxine supplement. Symptoms gradually resolved by 2 months. The patient is now on a regular follow-up.

3. Discussion

The thyroid gland is the first endocrine gland to develop beginning around 20–24 days of gestation [1] from the endoderm of the first and second pharyngeal pouch. It descends anteroinferiorly to reach the pretracheal region inferior to the thyroid cartilage at the level of the C5-T1 vertebra by the 7th week [1, 3, 7]. During its migration, the thyroid gland is attached to the base of the tongue by the thyroglossal duct which solidifies and gradually degenerates by the 10th week of gestation [1]. Failure to descend to the normal anatomical position results in the ectopic location of the thyroid tissue. A few authors state that maternal anti-thyroid immunoglobulins might be responsible for impaired descend during early life [5, 6, 9]. The commonest location of the ectopic thyroid tissue (ETT) in the head and neck region is the lingual [1] and sublingual location followed by the trachea, submandibular gland, lateral cervical region, maxilla, palatine tonsils, carotid bifurcation, iris of the eye, and pituitary gland. ETT may be also found in the cardiac muscle, ascending aorta, thymus, esophagus, duodenum, gall bladder, stomach bed, pancreas, mesentery of the small intestine, porta hepatis, adrenal gland, ovary (strumaovarii), fallopian tube, uterus, and vagina [2, 3]. Lingual thyroid accounts for 90% of ETT [2, 7, 8]. LT was first noticed by Hickmann in 1869 [5, 8–10]. The orthotopic thyroid gland is absent in 70% of cases with lingual thyroid [4, 7, 8, 10]. As in our case, thyroid was absent in a normal location. Hypothyroidism is present in 70% of LT patients [3, 4, 7]. Reported lingual thyroid is more among patients with thyroid disease [3]. LT causes hyperthyroidism rarely and also has malignant potential (1 in 300 cases) [2, 11]. Reported histotypes are papillary, follicular, mixed follicular and papillary, Hurthel cell, and medullary [2, 3]. Increased demand for thyroxine during puberty and pregnancy increases the work of the only functional ectopic tissue and, hence, increases LT size [2, 6, 8, 11]. This explains why the reported lingual thyroid is common among females. The amount of thyroid hormone secretion may not be enough during increasing hormonal demand could have contributed to increased LT size in our patient causing symptoms. Patients with enlarged LT present with dysphagia, dysphonia, foreign body sensation in the throat, cough, pain, bleeding, and dyspnea [4, 8, 11, 12].

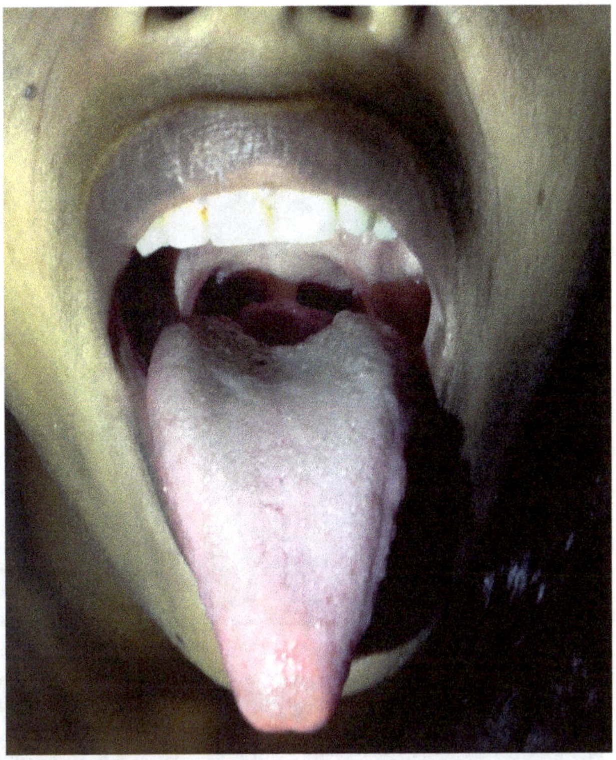

Figure 1: Throat examination showing midline nodule in the base of the tongue.

Examination of the oral cavity to look for the nodule in the base of the tongue and palpation of the neck to assess the thyroid gland in orthotopic location is an essential initial evaluation [7, 11]. High-resolution ultrasonography (USG) is a readily available and noninvasive tool in the evaluation of the thyroid gland in the orthotopic location and detection of the ectopic thyroid nodule [6]. Color Doppler can aid to demonstrate the vascularity of the nodule. Computed tomography (CT) and magnetic resonance imaging (MRI) are valuable tools to define the location of the mass, presence of calcification, relation to the surrounding structure, and degree of luminal obstruction. A contrast-enhanced CT study is helpful to characterize the pattern of enhancement. The presence or absence of the orthotopic thyroid gland can also be defined by CT or MRI [3, 12]. A CT scan can also be helpful to detect possible nodules in mediastinum [2]. 99 m pertechnetate can localize ectopic thyroid tissue with a degree of activity and determine the presence of an orthotopic thyroid gland [3, 7, 11]. Fine-needle aspiration cytology (FNAC) helps to confirm the ectopic thyroid tissue and to rule out malignancy [2–4, 11].

Management of the lingual thyroid depends upon the severity of clinical symptoms and complications. Asymptomatic

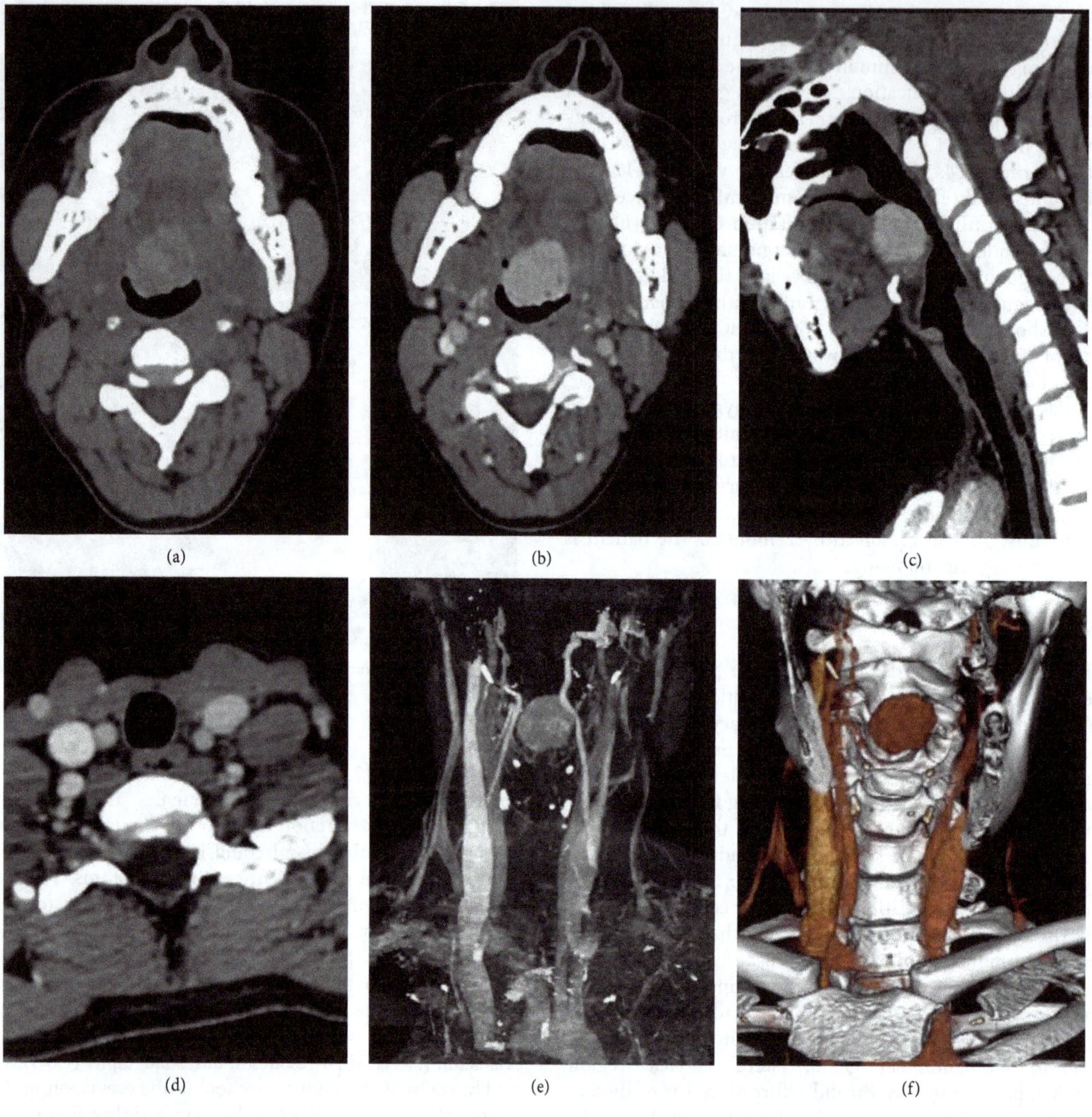

FIGURE 2: Computed tomography (CT) scan of the neck. Axial noncontrast CT image with a well-defined relatively hyperdense nodule in the midline at the base of the tongue (a), axial contrast-enhanced CT showing homogeneous enhancement (b), sagittal contrast-enhanced CT image with an enhancing nodule at the level of C2-C3 vertebra causing narrowing of the oropharyngeal lumen (c), axial contrast-enhanced CT image below the cricoid cartilage without orthotopic thyroid (d), coronal maximum intensity projection (MIP) image with a nodule in the midline (e) with absent orthotopic thyroid, and volume rendered image with a nodule in the midline (f).

euthyroid patients need regular follow-up [3, 10]. Patients with subclinical hypothyroidism with symptoms or overt hypothyroidism are managed conservatively with exogenous thyroid hormone supplement to suppress and reduce the size of the ETT resolving the symptoms [4–11], as in our case. Patients with the only functional lingual thyroid tissue (LT) can be excised and autotransplanted in the muscles of the neck [3–6]. Ablative radioiodine therapy is considered in patients unfit for surgery or refusing intervention [4–9]. Surgical excision is indicated in symptomatic patients not responding to conservative management and patients with severe respiratory tract obstruction, bleeding, ulceration, and malignancy [3–10]. Surgical removal

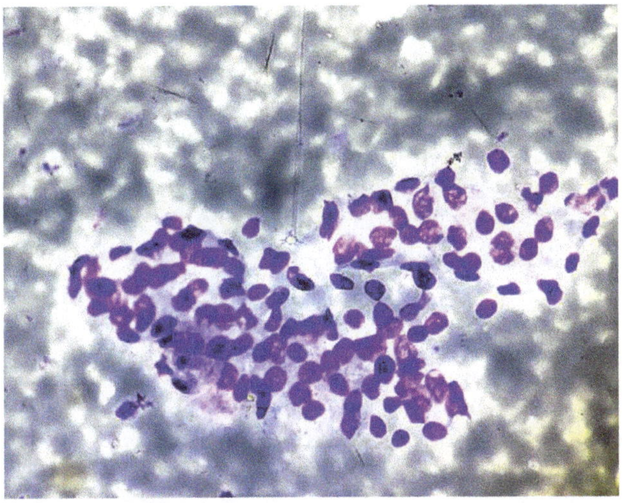

FIGURE 3: Fine-needle aspiration cytology from the nodule showing the cluster of benign-looking thyroid epithelial cells in the background of RBCs (Giemsa stain, 400x).

of the only functioning thyroid tissue needs lifelong hormone replacement therapy [8, 12].

4. Conclusions

Lingual thyroid is a rare clinical entity that presents as a nodule in the base of the tongue. Meticulous diagnostic workup including clinical examination, biochemical profile, imaging tools, radioisotope scanning, and histopathology is necessary to plan the management. Lingual thyroid with mild symptoms and subclinical hypothyroidism can be managed conservatively.

Consent

Written informed consent was obtained from the patient for the publication of this case report.

References

[1] R. D. Rosen and A. Sapra, *Embryology, Thyroid*, StatPearls Publishing, Treasure Island, FL, USA, 2020.

[2] G. Santangelo, G. Pellino, N. De Falco et al., "Prevalence, diagnosis and management of ectopic thyroid glands," *International Journal of Surgery*, vol. 28, pp. S1–S6, 2016.

[3] N. A. Ibrahim and I. O. Fadeyibi, "Ectopic thyroid: etiology, pathology and management," *Hormones (Athens, Greece)*, vol. 10, no. 4, pp. 261–269, 2011.

[4] N. Cruz-Dardíz, N. Rivera-Santana, M. Torres-Torres et al., "Lingual thyroid gland: it's time for awareness," *Endocrinology, Diabetes & Metabolism Case Reports*, vol. 2020, no. 1, 2020.

[5] B. Amr and S. Monib, "Lingual thyroid: a case report," *International Journal of Surgery Case Reports*, vol. 2, no. 8, pp. 313–315, 2011.

[6] G. Koc, I. Taskaldiran, S. Aslan Felek et al., "Ectopic lingual thyroid presenting with massive hematemesis," *Acta Endocrinologica (Bucharest)*, vol. 15, no. 2, pp. 244–246, 2019.

[7] S. S. Kumar, D. M. S. Kumar, and R. Thirunavukuarasu, "Lingual thyroid—conservative management or surgery? A case report," *Indian Journal of Surgery*, vol. 75, no. 1, pp. 118-119, 2013.

[8] G. Thomas, R. Hoilat, J. S. Daniels, and W. Kalagie, "Ectopic lingual thyroid: a case report," *International Journal of Oral and Maxillofacial Surgery*, vol. 32, no. 2, pp. 219–221, 2003.

[9] K. Rao, V. S. Shenoy, P. M. Kamath, and A. Gomati, "A case of lingual thyroid," *Annals of Clinical Investigation*, vol. 1, no. 1, p. 1002, 2020.

[10] D. Kaushal, N. Shakrawal, A. Goyal, N. P. Nair, A. K. Verma, and D. Prakash, "Ectopic lingual thyroid: an entity not to be missed!" *International Journal of Molecular Biology*, vol. 4, no. 4, pp. 132-133, 2019.

[11] R. Ramanathan, J. P. Veerapandian, and S. Sundari, "Lingual thyroid with hypothyroidism in a child," *International Journal of Contemporary Pediatrics*, vol. 6, no. 4, p. 1747, 2019.

[12] P. H. d. Souza Castro, L. E. R. Volpato, J. Tramujas, and A. H. Borges, "Ectopic thyroid at the base of the tongue of a young patient," *Case Reports in Dentistry*, vol. 2016, Article ID 9174970, 4 pages, 2016.

Nephrotic Syndrome as a Cause of Transient Clinical Hypothyroidism

Vânia Benido Silva,[1] Maria Teresa Pereira,[1] Carla Leal Moreira,[2] Sílvia Santos Monteiro,[1] Isabel Inácio,[3] and Maria Helena Cardoso[1]

[1]*Department of Endocrinology, Centro Hospitalar e Universitário do Porto, Porto, Portugal*
[2]*Department of Nephrology, Centro Hospitalar e Universitário do Porto, Porto, Portugal*
[3]*Department of Endocrinology, Centro Hospitalar do Baixo Vouga, Aveiro, Portugal*

Correspondence should be addressed to Vânia Benido Silva; vania.benido@hotmail.com

Academic Editor: Mihail A. Boyanov

Nephrotic syndrome may trigger the onset of hypothyroidism, promoting massive urinary protein losses including thyroxine (T4) and triiodothyronine (T3) along with their binding proteins. At an early stage, a clinical and biochemical euthyroid state is expected. However, in patients with prolonged and severe proteinuria, especially with concomitant low thyroid reserve, urinary losses of free and protein-bound thyroid hormones are sufficiently pronounced to induce a subclinical or overt hypothyroidism. Despite its high prevalence in clinical practice, the literature lacks case reports of newly diagnosed clinical hypothyroidism due to NS in adults, making this condition under-recognized. We report a case of a 23-year-old man with previous normal thyroid function who developed overt hypothyroidism due to a severe nephrotic syndrome, requiring supplementation with levothyroxine (LT). After the patient had undergone bilateral nephrectomy, treatment with LT was discontinued and thyroid function normalized.

1. Introduction

The thyroid and kidney interact with each other in a crucial way to assure the normal functioning of both organs. While the thyroid plays a huge role in renal development and growth, as well as in the tubular and glomerular functions, the kidney is involved in the metabolism and elimination of thyroid hormones [1, 2]. The association between thyroid function abnormalities, particularly hypothyroidism, and chronic kidney disease (CKD) is well established and is highly prevalent in clinical practice [3–7]. In this clinical scenario, thyroid function test results are quite variable depending on the renal disease itself and its severity (including progressive impaired kidney function) [4, 5], but also on the patient's previous history of thyroid disease and thyroid reserve [8], as well as on iatrogenic factors (such as the use of glucocorticoids, furosemide, or others) [9].

Nephrotic syndrome (NS) is one of the most common glomerular diseases and is classically characterized by massive proteinuria (>3.5 g/24 hours), hypoalbuminemia, edema, and hyperlipidemia. Associated excessive urinary protein excretion, justified by marked increase in the glomerular permeability to macromolecules, results in urinary losses of thyroid hormone-binding proteins (thyroxine binding globulin (TBG), transthyretin, and albumin), as well as thyroid hormones (thyroxine (T4) and triiodothyronine (T3)) usually bound to them [8, 10]. Additionally, injury of renal tubules can coexist and compromise the reabsorption of free thyroid hormones [11].

In early stages of the disease, especially when there is no prior history of thyroid disorder, levels of physiologically crucial free T3 (fT3) and T4 (fT4) remain normal and a clinical and biochemical euthyroid state is expected. However, in patients with prolonged and severe proteinuria and with low thyroid reserve, urinary losses of free and protein-bound thyroid hormones are sufficiently pronounced to induce an increase in thyroid-stimulating hormone (TSH) values resulting in subclinical or overt hypothyroidism [2, 4, 5]. Dose increase and frequent adjustments may be needed in patients previously treated with hormone replacement therapy [2, 8, 11].

Other conditions may simultaneously contribute to changes in thyroid function laboratory results in patients with NS. When evaluating and managing challenging NS patients, the use of steroids or other immunosuppressant drugs and the euthyroid sick syndrome, a very common entity in hospitalized ill individuals [9, 12], should be considered.

Several studies linking hypothyroidism to NS patients have been published, mostly in children and in patients with preexisting thyroid dysfunction [11, 13–16]. To date, the literature lacks case reports of newly diagnosed clinical hypothyroidism due to NS in adults, remaining as an underrecognized condition.

We report a case of a 23-year-old man with previous normal thyroid function who developed overt hypothyroidism due to a severe nephrotic syndrome, requiring supplementation with levothyroxine (LT). After the patient had undergone bilateral nephrectomy, he started renal function replacement therapy (hemodialysis) and treatment with LT was discontinued and thyroid function normalized.

2. Case Report

A 23-year-old man was evaluated by his general practitioner for mild asthenia and generalized edema with swelling of the face, abdomen, and lower limbs over the preceding two weeks. He was an active smoker. His past medical history was positive for antiphospholipid syndrome and Raynaud's phenomenon, and he was on treatment with acenocumarol. The physical examination was unremarkable, except for the presence of an exuberant edema of the legs and abdominal wall. His weight was 78 kg, corresponding to a weight gain of 10% in a 3-month period. No evidence of heart failure was noted.

Urinalysis was positive for proteinuria of 53.73 g/L (reference range (RR): 0.00–0.15 g/L), with a protein-to-creatinine ratio of 13.16 g/g (RR: 0.015–0.068 g/g). Blood tests revealed hypoproteinemia of 4.74 g/dL (RR: 6.0–7.3 g/dL), hypoalbuminemia of 2.56 g/dL (RR: 3.5–5.0 g/dL), and hyperlipidemia (triglycerides: 380 mg/dL (RR: 40–160 mg/dL) and total cholesterol: 377 mg/dL (RR: 0–200 mg/dl)). Liver function tests were normal, and renal depuration was preserved (serum creatinine: 0.79 mg/dL (RR: 0.7–1.2 mg/dL); an estimated glomerular filtration rate of 126.6 mL/min/1.73 m^2, according CKD-EPI equation) [17]. At this point, the serum TSH level was 2.77 μUI/mL (RR: 0.30–3.18). Renal ultrasound (US) showed preserved anatomy of the kidneys, except for poor corticomedullary differentiation.

The patient was hospitalized for further investigation of newly diagnosed nephrotic syndrome and underwent a renal biopsy, whose result was consistent with C3 glomerulonephritis. A high dose of glucocorticoids was initiated, and due to poor response, a step-up approach was adopted with cyclosporine and mycophenolate mofetil being added to the therapy strategy. Unfortunately, the patient evolved with anasarca, worsening of renal function, severe hypoalbuminemia, and recurrent episodes of cellulitis.

Two weeks after his admission, abnormalities on thyroid function tests were detected (TSH: 17.40 μUI/mL (RR: 0.3–3.18), total T4: 1.8 μg/dL (RR: 5.56–9.91), fT4: 0.33 μg/dL (RR: 1.01–1.65), total T3: 0.4 ng/mL (RR: 0.83–1.49), fT3: 0.81 pg/mL (RR: 2.66–4.33)) accompanied by worsening of hypoalbuminemia to 1.76 g/dL (RR: 3.5–5.0 g/dL) and occasional proteinuria to 59.59 g/L (RR: 0.00–0.15 g/L), prompting further evaluation from Endocrinology Department. The patient had no personal or family history of thyroid disease. On examination, his thyroid was palpable but not enlarged and no nodules were identified. A complementary thyroid study was conducted: serum anti-thyroid peroxidase and anti-thyroglobulin antibodies titers were both negative and thyroid US revealed a slightly enlarged thyroid gland (upper limit of normal dimensions), homogeneous and regular, without evident nodular lesions.

The diagnosis of clinical hypothyroidism secondary to nephrotic syndrome was assumed, although a possible contribution of euthyroid sick syndrome on thyroid hormone levels was considered. The patient was started on oral LT treatment 50 μg daily, with gradual increase in the dose up to 125 μg (1.5 μg of LT per kg of body weight).

After three months of hospitalization, his clinical condition remained refractory to the immunosuppressive therapy, with a high variability but progressive worsening of urinary protein levels despite prolonged treatment (Figure 1). Due to unresponsiveness to immunosuppression, steroid side effects, and recurrent severe infections, the patient was proposed to bilateral nephrectomy. Full kidney histology was consistent with focal segmental glomerulosclerosis. Thyroid function reassessment performed six days after surgery revealed that TSH was 2.47 μUI/mL (RR: 0.3–3.18), fT4 was 0.93 μg/dL (RR: 1.01–1.65), and fT3 was 1.67 ng/dL (RR: 2.66–4.33), allowing weaning of LT dose to 75 μg daily. Table 1 shows the evolution of thyroid function tests over time under different doses of LT, before and after nephrectomy.

After discharge, the patient remained clinically and analytically euthyroid, with progressively lower dose requirements of LT. Eight months after hypothyroidism diagnosis, the serum TSH level was 1.35 μUI/mL (RR: 0.3–3.18) and fT4 was 1.01 μg/dL (RR: 1.01–1.65) on LT 25 μg replacement and therefore, treatment with LT was discontinued. Four months later, in the absence of LT, thyroid function remained normal (TSH: 0.91 μUI/mL (RR: 0.3–3.18); fT4: 1.39 μg/dL (RR: 1.01–1.65)), with a serum albumin level of 3.92 g/dL (RR: 3.5–5.0 g/dL). Since bilateral nephrectomy, the patient was started on renal function replacement therapy (hemodialysis) and is on a waiting list for renal transplantation.

3. Discussion

Thyroid hormones, T3 and T4, are both poorly soluble in water, and more than 99.5% circulate in the blood bound to proteins: approximately 70% bound to TBG, 20% to

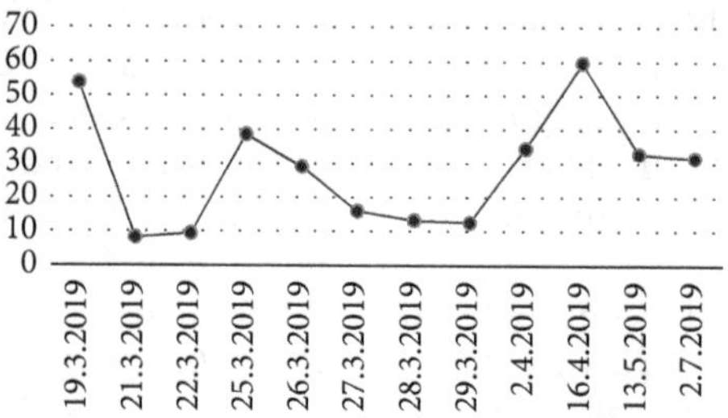

Figure 1: Evolution of proteinuria levels on urinalysis since nephrotic syndrome diagnosis until bilateral nephrectomy.

Table 1: Description of evolution of thyroid function tests over time under different doses of LT, before and after nephrectomy.

Date	15.3.2019	8.4.2019	16.4.2019	29.4.2019	13.5.2019	26.6.2019	*8.7.2019	11.9.2019	20.03.2020
LT dose/day	—	—	50 μg	100 μg	112 μg	125 μg	125 μg	75 μg	—
TSH (μUI/mL) (RR: 0.3–3.18)	2.77	17.40	11.60	7.94	2.66	1.71	2.47	0.15	0.91
fT4 (μg/dL) (RR: 1.01–1.65)		0.33	0.74	0.71	0.77	0.65	0.93	1.29	1.39
fT3 (pg/mL) (RR: 2.66–4.33)		0.81	0.84	0.39	0.53		1.67	2.74	
Total T4 (μg/dL) (RR: 5.56–9.91)		1.8	1.8					5.4	
Total T3 (ng/mL) (RR: 0.83–1.49)		0.4	0.3					0.8	

*Bilateral nephrectomy (2.7.2019).

albumin, and 10% to prealbumin. However, only the low levels of free hormones are metabolically active at the tissues and responsible for all thyroid functions [12, 18].

Under normal conditions, urinary protein losses are insignificant. In NS, on the other hand, there is massive urinary protein losses, including T3 and T4 along with their binding proteins and, to a lesser extent, the free fractions fT3 and fT4 [2, 4, 5, 19]. This is responsible for the frequent abnormalities found in thyroid function in patients with NS representing a renal-endocrine disorder [2]. In early stages of the disease or in milder clinical conditions, serum free hormone levels remain normal and the patient is in euthyroid state, as it was visible in our case, when the patient had already-established NS and the serum TSH value was in the normal range [2, 4]. Nevertheless, in more prolonged situations with worsening of proteinuria and hypoalbuminemia, and especially when associated with a low thyroid reserve, fT3 and fT4 are also significantly reduced and overt hypothyroidism may occur [4, 19]. In this case report, with the massive increase in urinary protein losses and the presence of severe and supplemental-dependent hypoalbuminemia, the patient developed clinical hypothyroidism.

The relationship between thyroid dysfunction and the degree of proteinuria, renal function, and serum albumin levels has been documented in several reports. Jain et al. showed that serum TSH levels in NS patients correlated positively with proteinuria and plasmatic creatinine levels but negatively with serum albumin concentrations as well as glomerular filtration rate [4]. In a study with 317 patients who had been definitively diagnosed with NS, it was proved that high levels of urinary proteins and serum creatinine were independent risk factors for predicting thyroid dysfunction, while a higher level of plasmatic albumin was an independent protective factor [5].

Likewise, some published clinical cases have shown that NS may be the cause behind the increased requirements of LT in patients previously diagnosed with hypothyroidism [8, 11, 15, 16].

In this particular case, the patient had no prior history of thyroid dysfunction, he had negative thyroid autoantibodies, and there were no signs of the typical glandular structural changes suggesting diffuse autoimmune thyroiditis and insufficient functional thyroid reserve. The clinical hypothyroidism was triggered by significant urinary losses of hormones and their binding proteins, requiring LT replacement. Furthermore, we speculate that intestinal edema resulting from severe hypoalbuminemia compromised LT absorption with a progressive need for drug titration. As soon as the huge proteinuria levels were eliminated by performing bilateral nephrectomy, an immediate improvement in thyroid function was documented, and after eight months, it was possible to discontinue LT therapy. The permanent resolution of hypothyroidism following bilateral nephrectomy had already been reported in five children diagnosed with congenital NS [14]. This outcome confirms that there was no intrinsic defect in the thyroid gland contributing to hypothyroidism.

However, in this case scenario, we must consider other potential contributors for the thyroid hormonal profile, particularly the administration of high corticosteroid doses over a four-month period of hospitalization. Corticosteroids could promote thyroid dysfunction by their suppressive effect on serum TSH levels, impairment of peripheral conversion of T4 in T3, and the decrease of TBG production [9].

In addition, euthyroid sick syndrome is a very common entity defined by changes in the thyroid function that occur during a period of critical non-thyroid acute or chronic systemic illness. The typical observed hormonal pattern is low T3 levels, eventually low T4 levels, accompanying with reciprocal high reverse T3 and no significant increase in TSH [20]. The magnitude of the changes is proportional to the severity of illness and length of hospital stay [12, 20].

Considering the extremely low concentrations of thyroid hormones that our patient presented, particularly T3, his severe medical condition, and the prolonged hospitalization, his thyroid dysfunction probably results from an overlapping of this syndrome.

In addition to NS, cases of reversible proteinuria and biopsy-proven glomerulonephritis (GN) including membranous nephropathy, minimal change, membranoproliferative GN, amyloidosis, and IgA nephropathy have been reported in association with hypothyroidism, mainly if autoimmune thyroiditis has been present [2, 21]. Several other mechanisms can justify the higher risk for the development of thyroid dysfunction in CKD patients, such as iodine retention and possible Wolff–Chaikoff effect, the reduced deiodinase activity, or the metabolic acidosis frequently present [2, 21, 22].

In summary, we report a case of a 23-year-old patient without previous thyroid disease, who developed severe steroid-resistant NS and clinical hypothyroidism as a consequence of massive urinary protein losses. Bilateral nephrectomy with consequent anuria allowed LT discontinuation.

Renal disease, with or without kidney failure, is a condition that should be considered in the diagnostic workup of newly diagnosed or worsening of preexisting hypothyroidism, especially in hospitalized ill patients when other causes were excluded. Proteinuria severity, drug interactions, and clinical conditions simultaneously determine thyroid dysfunction severity and therapeutic response.

This case report highlights the importance of a greater awareness of the interactions between thyroid and renal functions, often a challenge for clinicians, and that still remains under-recognized, especially in adult patients. It seems reasonable to test thyroid function when nephrotic syndrome is first diagnosed and then perform serial testing.

Consent

Informed written consent was obtained from the patient, although no patient identifiable data were included in this case report.

References

[1] S. E. Bradley, F. Stéphan, J. B. Coelho, and P. Réville, "The thyroid and the kidney," *Kidney International*, vol. 6, no. 5, pp. 346–365, 1974.

[2] P. Dousdampanis, K. Trigka, G. A. Vagenakis, and C. Fourtounas, "The thyroid and the kidney: a complex interplay in health and disease," *The International Journal of Artificial Organs*, vol. 37, no. 1, pp. 1–12, 2014.

[3] M. Chonchol, G. Lippi, G. Salvagno, G. Zoppini, M. Muggeo, and G. Targher, "Prevalence of subclinical hypothyroidism in patients with chronic kidney disease," *Clinical Journal of the American Society of Nephrology*, vol. 3, no. 5, pp. 1296–1300, 2008.

[4] D. Jain, H. K. Aggarwal, Y. M. Pavan Kumar, and P. Jain, "Evaluation of thyroid dysfunction in patients with nephrotic syndrome," *Medicine and pharmacy reports*, vol. 92, no. 2, pp. 139–144, 2019.

[5] L.-Z. Li, Y. Hu, S.-L. Ai et al., "The relationship between thyroid dysfunction and nephrotic syndrome: a clinicopathological study," *Scientific Reports*, vol. 9, no. 1, p. 6421, 2019.

[6] J. C. Lo, G. M. Chertow, A. S. Go, and C.-Y. Hsu, "Increased prevalence of subclinical and clinical hypothyroidism in persons with chronic kidney disease," *Kidney International*, vol. 67, no. 3, pp. 1047–1052, 2005.

[7] C. M. Rhee, K. Kalantar-Zadeh, E. Streja et al., "The relationship between thyroid function and estimated glomerular filtration rate in patients with chronic kidney disease," *Nephrology Dialysis Transplantation*, vol. 30, no. 2, pp. 282–287, 2015.

[8] V. Chandurkar, J. Shik, and E. Randell, "Exacerbation of underlying hypothyroidism caused by proteinuria and induction of urinary thyroxine loss: case report and subsequent investigation," *Endocrine Practice*, vol. 14, no. 1, pp. 97–103, 2008.

[9] H. B. Burch, "Drug effects on the thyroid," *New England Journal of Medicine*, vol. 381, no. 8, pp. 749–761, 2019.

[10] V. Fonseca, M. Thomas, A. Katrak, P. Sweny, and J. F. Moorhead, "Can urinary thyroid hormone loss cause hypothyroidism?" *The Lancet*, vol. 338, no. 8765, pp. 475-476, 1991.

[11] S. H. Jung, J. E. Lee, and W. Y. Chung, "Changes in the thyroid hormone profiles in children with nephrotic syndrome," *Korean Journal of Pediatrics*, vol. 62, no. 3, pp. 85–89, 2019.

[12] M. J. Maiden and D. J. Torpy, "Thyroid hormones in critical illness," *Critical Care Clinics*, vol. 35, no. 2, pp. 375–388, 2019.

[13] S. Benvenga, R. Vita, F. Di Bari, P. Fallahi, and A. Antonelli, "Do not forget nephrotic syndrome as a cause of increased requirement of levothyroxine replacement therapy," *European Thyroid Journal*, vol. 4, no. 2, pp. 138–142, 2015.

[14] V. Chadha and U. S. Alon, "Bilateral nephrectomy reverses hypothyroidism in congenital nephrotic syndrome," *Pediatric Nephrology*, vol. 13, no. 3, pp. 209–211, 1999.

[15] H. Karethimmaiah and V. Sarathi, "Nephrotic syndrome increases the need for levothyroxine replacement in patients with hypothyroidism," *Journal of Clinical and Diagnostic Research: JCDR*, vol. 10, no. 12, 2016.

[16] S. Soh, O. Aki, O. Manabu, K. Norimasa, K. Hiroshi, and N. Masao, "A case of minimal change nephrotic syndrome with hypothyroidism deterioration," *CEN Case Reports*, vol. 5, no. 1, pp. 95–98, 2016.

[17] A. S. Levey, L. A. Stevens, C. H. Schmid et al., "A new equation to estimate glomerular filtration rate," *Annals of Internal Medicine*, vol. 150, no. 9, pp. 604–612, 2009.

[18] L. Bartalena and J. Robbins, "Thyroid hormone transport proteins," *Clinics in Laboratory Medicine*, vol. 13, no. 3, pp. 583–598, 1993.

[19] A. B. M. Alam, A. N. M. Hasan, A. H. Khan, M. M. U. Quader, S. A. Begum, and S. K. Banik, "Association between primary hypothyroidism and nephrotic syndrome: a case report," *Chattagram Maa-o-Shishu Hospital Medical College Journal*, vol. 12, no. 2, pp. 63–65, 2013.

The Unforeseen Diagnosis: Hyperparathyroidism-Jaw Tumour Syndrome Case Report and Review of the Literature

Maxim Barnett ,[1] Farhan Ahmed,[2] Radu Mihai ,[3] Asha Rattan,[1] and Malik Asif Humayun [2]

[1] *University of Buckingham Medical School, Hunter St, Buckingham MK18 1EG, UK*
[2] *Milton Keynes University Hospital, Standing Way, Eaglestone, Milton Keynes MK6 5LD, UK*
[3] *Oxford Radcliffe Hospitals NHS Foundation Trust, Old Road, Headington, Oxford OX3 7LH, UK*

Correspondence should be addressed to Maxim Barnett; 1500633@buckingham.ac.uk

Academic Editor: Michaël R. Laurent

Hypercalcaemia and its systemic sequelae are a relatively common finding amongst patients in the field of endocrinology. Primary hyperparathyroidism, a frequent cause of hypercalcaemia, is often seen among middle-aged female patients, typically resulting from an underlying single-gland adenoma. Although patients may present with symptoms (nephrolithiasis, musculoskeletal discomfort, dehydration, or mood disturbance, to name a few), hypercalcaemia is rather frequently identified incidentally. In younger patients, a familial form of primary hyperparathyroidism must be considered, with a positive diagnosis mandating familial screening. Hyperparathyroidism-jaw tumour syndrome is one such autosomal dominant familial disorder, characterised by a mutation in the cell division cycle 73 (CDC73; also known as HRPT-2) tumour suppressor gene. This disorder is characterised by multiple pleiotropic phenomena, including recurrent primary hyperparathyroidism (and the effects of hypercalcaemia), neoplasms (such as uterine, renal, mandibular, and maxillary), and infertility. A patient not conforming to the classic candidacy for primary hyperparathyroidism requires consideration for a familial cause. *Case Description.* We present a rare diagnostic entity—hyperparathyroidism-jaw tumour (HPT-JT) syndrome—in a 36-year-old female with recurrent primary hyperparathyroidism, frequent nephrolithiasis, and infertility for 18 years prior to the diagnosis. We aim to promote awareness amongst medical professionals of this rare, but nonetheless essential differential diagnosis through a case report and review of the literature. *Conclusion.* Medical professionals must avoid diagnostic overshadowing and display a low threshold for genetic testing in younger patients with primary hyperparathyroidism. The importance of proper identification extends beyond the patient to their relatives and offspring.

1. Introduction

Hypercalcaemia, defined as a serum calcium level greater than 2.6 mmol/L (10.4 mg/dL) [1], is a frequent finding amongst patients in the field of endocrinology. Whilst most patients are identified incidentally, hypercalcaemia is commonly a manifestation of primary hyperparathyroidism, a condition characterised by excessive parathyroid hormone release. This disorder is common, with an estimated prevalence of 1/1,000, and is typically diagnosed in female adults (average age pooled at 55 years) [2]. In the presence of a young patient with symptoms suggestive of primary hyperparathyroidism, a familial cause must be considered. This paper, which presents a genetically confirmed case of hyperparathyroidism-jaw tumour syndrome, is written to enhance the awareness of this diagnosis and to reaffirm the requirements to screen for a familial cause in adolescent primary hyperparathyroidism.

2. Case Presentation

A 36-year-old female of eastern European origin is reviewed in the urology department in 2018 for a follow-up appointment due to a unique history of eight prior lithotripsy procedures (between the years 2004 and 2011) for prior (recurrent) renal stones. A CT-KUB (computed tomography of the kidneys, ureters, and bladder) had been performed, which identified nephrocalcinosis—not nephrolithiasis. The urology department recommended no further intervention and referred her to the metabolic medicine department for biochemical evaluation.

2.1. Past Medical History. Further history taking in the metabolic medicine clinic identified a prior diagnosis of primary hyperparathyroidism in 2003 (age 21) for symptomatic, uncontrollable hypercalcaemia and severe osteoporosis. A parathyroidectomy had been performed with the removal of a large ectopic parathyroid adenoma located behind the right clavicle, with subsequent calcium and parathyroid hormone normalisation. Despite the uncharacteristically young age of the patient, as there was no family history of primary hyperparathyroidism nor familial neoplastic conditions, a familial cause was considered "unlikely" and was not investigated further. Postparathyroidectomy, the patient was prescribed 2,000 units daily of vitamin D and was placed under annual follow-up. Her annual follow-up remained uneventful; however, over the past three years (2014–2017), her surgical team had identified mild, nonprogressive hypercalcaemia. The hypercalcaemia remained static, and a recurrence of primary hyperparathyroidism was ruled out with an unremarkable sestamibi scan (failing to identify an adenoma) and subsequent dual-energy X-ray absorptiometry scan (demonstrating normal bone densitometry).

Her only other significant past medical history includes the removal of uterine leiomyomas, and she has (unsuccessfully) attempted to conceive on multiple occasions with her husband, for which she is under the care of the obstetrics and gynaecology department for infertility.

2.2. Investigations. Within the metabolic medicine clinic, a comprehensive metabolic panel was requested. Her serum calcium returned elevated (2.65 mmol/L), in addition to an inappropriately increased parathyroid hormone (9.5 pmol/L) and hypophosphataemia (0.7 mmol/L). Although a reduction in renal function was noted (eGFR 57 mL/min), this was a chronic finding and was not considered significant. As her vitamin D levels were replete (99 nmol/L), replacement was not required and further confirmatory tests were ordered, including a urine calcium-to-creatinine ratio, 24-hour urinary calcium, and fractional excretion of calcium, all of which returned elevated, consistent with a recurrence of primary hyperparathyroidism (Table 1).

Despite an absent positive family history of primary hyperparathyroidism, a genetic panel was requested due to her young age and recurrence of the disease. She was referred to Churchill Hospital (Oxford), whereby MLPA (multiplex ligation-dependent probe amplification) analysis was performed, assessing for eight known genetic mutations responsible for familial forms of primary hyperparathyroidism (Table 2).

To our surprise, the analysis returned with a demonstration of a heterozygous deletion of exons 8-9 (CDC73 (HRPT-2) gene), confirming hyperparathyroidism-jaw tumour (HPT-JT) syndrome. The patient was confused as to why there are no other family members afflicted if this is a familial disorder; it was explained the disease may have occurred from a "de novo" mutation or is present in a family member with incomplete penetrance. The patient's family members have been notified and have undergone screening for the mutation.

Table 1: Laboratory results.

Investigations	Level	Reference range
Corrected calcium (mmol/L)	**2.65**	2.2–2.6 mmol/L
PTH (pmol/L)	**9.5**	1.3–9.3 pmol/L
PO_4 (mmol/L)	**0.7**	0.8–1.5
Vit D (nmol/L)	99	Optimal: >70 nmol/L
eGFR (mL/min/1.73 m^2)	**57**	85–125 mL/min
Urine Ca-Cr	**0.71**, **0.86**, and **0.73**	Indicative of increased calcium excretion based on body weight of 50 kg
FE-Ca (%)	**2.58**	
Urine calcium (mmol/24 hour)	**7.16**	

PTH: parathyroid hormone; PO_4: phosphate; Vit D: 25-hydroxyvitamin D; eGFR: estimated glomerular filtration rate; urine Ca-CR: urinary calcium-to-creatinine ratio; FHH: familial hypocalciuric hypercalcaemia; FE-Ca: fractional excretion of calcium. Bold signifies blood levels outside of the normal reference range.

Table 2: Genetic mutations assessed.

Genetic mutation
MEN1
CDC73
CDKN1A
CDKN1B
RET
AP2S1
CASR
GCM2

MEN1: multiple endocrine neoplasia 1; CDC73: cell division cycle 73; CDKN1A: cyclin-dependent kinase inhibitor 1A; CDKN1B: cyclin-dependent kinase inhibitor 1B; RET: rearranged during transfection; AP2S1: adaptor-related protein complex 2 subunit sigma 1; CASR: calcium sensing receptor; GCM2: glial cells missing transcription factor 2.

2.3. Treatment and Outcome. A repeat sestamibi-SPECT (single-photon emission computed tomography) scan was performed, demonstrating a 5 mm enhancing nodule deep to the right thyroid lobe. During the second parathyroidectomy procedure (October 2020) however, the surgical team identified a mass on the right side of the thymus (and not deep to the thyroid lobe as the scan had suggested), which was fully excised and sent for histopathological analysis; the mass was confirmed to be an ectopic parathyroid adenoma. Successful removal was confirmed by the precipitous drop in serum parathyroid hormone levels postoperatively (Figure 1).

Following successful recovery from the operation, our patient was placed under six-monthly follow-up in the endocrine and clinical genetic clinic, with serial MRI

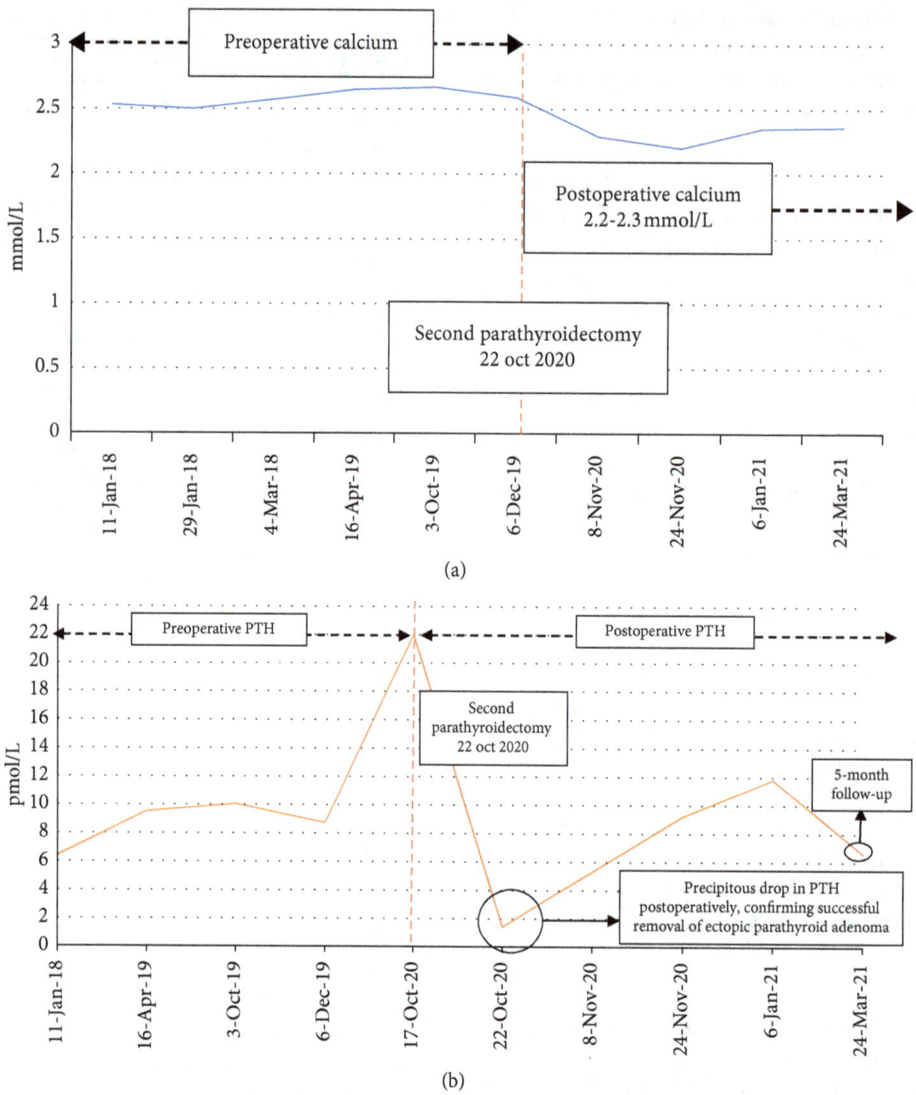

FIGURE 1: Calcium and parathyroid hormone (PTH) before and after second parathyroidectomy.

(magnetic resonance imaging) of her abdomen and pelvis. The obstetrics and gynaecology department has been notified of the diagnosis and its strong association with uterine lesions (and infertility), for which she is receiving interval follow-up. An updated pelvic ultrasound has identified three additional intramural fibroids. As HPT-JT syndrome is associated with an increased risk for renal disorders, an MRI (magnetic resonance imaging) of the abdomen was performed, from which multiple renal cysts were identified. Finally, an OPG (orthopantomogram) was performed, which ruled out any jaw lesions.

3. Discussion

Inherited primary hyperparathyroidism must be considered (and assessed for) in young patients (below 40 years of age) or in those with a positive family history presenting with primary hyperparathyroidism [3–5]. The estimation of primary hyperparathyroidism is present at one per thousand in the population, and 10% of these cases are considered to be familial; therefore, one per ten thousand cases are due to inherited hyperparathyroidism [2, 4]. Genetic causes of familial hyperparathyroidism include multiple endocrine neoplasia (MEN1, MEN2A, and MEN4), familial isolated hyperparathyroidism, and hyperparathyroidism-jaw tumour (HPT-JT) syndrome [4, 6].

HPT-JT syndrome is inherited in an autosomal dominant fashion [6]. Demonstration of the CDC73 (also known as HRPT-2) gene mutation is diagnostic of the condition [7]; CDC73 is a tumour suppressor gene, involved in regulating the cell cycle (cell division cycle 73) [3]. The CDC73 gene is located on chromosome one and encodes parafibromin, a 531-long amino acid exerting antiproliferative capabilities [3, 8]. Parafibromin promotes cell cycle arrest as well as functioning to regulate the expression of various genes and chromatin structure (via RNA polymerase-II associated factor 1 complex) [9–12].

Due to the scarcity of this condition, a true prevalence cannot be determined; however, estimates include 200 cases reported within the medical literature since its debut in 1958 [13, 14]. Although the disorder is inherited in an autosomal dominant pattern, the penetrance is incomplete (70%); however, it is noted to increase with age [3–5, 15–17]. Furthermore, penetrance is reduced in females for reasons which are unclear [6, 18–20].

The most common manifestation of HPT-JT syndrome is primary hyperparathyroidism, in which single-gland adenoma (typically cystic) involvement is predominant (15% of cases arise from a carcinoma) [3, 6, 12, 15, 19, 21, 22]. A distinction is noted in relation to other familial hyperparathyroidism disorders, which demonstrate multiglandular involvement [3, 23–26]. The mean age at diagnosis of primary hyperparathyroidism in HPT-JT syndrome is 27 (12–58 years) [15, 27], with the earliest recorded case in a seven-year-old patient [15, 28]. The primary hyperparathyroidism may be mild and can often go unnoticed; however, if severe (or the presence of a hypercalcaemic crisis), a carcinoma must be considered [3, 29]. Recurrence of primary hyperparathyroidism is common in HPT-JT syndrome, as demonstrated in our case report [3]. With the prolonged, mild hypercalcaemia, our patient demonstrated, as well as the minimal increase in parathyroid hormone levels and initial normalisation of serum calcium (and parathyroid hormone) postoperatively, these findings are suggestive of benign (and not malignant) primary hyperparathyroidism.

Suggestions for differentiating an adenoma from a carcinoma include parathyroid hormone levels threefold above the upper limit of normal; severe hypercalcaemia; and lesions greater than three centimetres in size [3, 15, 30, 31].

Rather infrequently, children with a CDC73 gene mutation may demonstrate malignant primary hyperparathyroidism [3]. Moreover, a palpable mass will be evident with a carcinoma, in addition to systemic symptoms such as cachexia. As the carcinoma progresses, dysphonia and dysphagia may occur, as well as hypercalcaemic symptomatology (nausea, vomiting, confusion, bone pain, and fractures) [3, 7, 15, 17, 32–34].

Succeeding primary hyperparathyroidism, the next most frequent manifestation involves neoplasms of uterine origin (50%), which can be either benign (leiomyoma, hyperplasia, adenomyosis, adenofibroma, or multiple adenomyomatous polyps) or malignant (adenosarcomas) [3, 4, 16]. Moreover, Mullerian duct tumours have been described [3]. Common to patients with HPT-JT syndrome (and seen in our patient), there is an increased frequency of miscarriages and infertility [3, 35].

Contradictory to the nomenclature, jaw tumours are not prominent in this disorder and are prevalent in no more than 30% of individuals [3]. Better known as "ossifying fibromas," these lesions (from either the maxilla or mandible) arise from periodontal ligaments within the premolar or molar areas and are typically observed prior to the third decade [3, 15, 19]. Although benign (with a risk of malignant degeneration below one percent) [15, 36, 37], the local destruction of tissue incorporates functional limitations (such as breathing difficulties, dentition abnormalities, periorbital swelling, and cosmetic concerns) necessitating its removal [3, 36, 38]. These lesions can be bilateral and multifocal and may also recur; therefore, monitoring for recurrence is essential [3, 39]. These fibromas can be distinguished from sporadic causes on an X-ray, with HPT-JT syndrome demonstrating radiolucency, as opposed to mixed radiolucency/radiopaque [3, 15, 40].

Less frequent demonstrations include renal anomalies (15–20%) with cysts being the commonest lesions [3, 15]. Other renal anomalies include hamartomatous lesions, Wilms' tumour, mixed epithelium-stromal tumour (MEST), and papillary renal carcinoma [3, 5, 21]. Cysts can vary from minimal lesions to polycystic-like disease presentation (leading to renal failure) [12, 15, 41].

Other uncommon neoplasms have been observed in HPT-JT syndrome; however, debate ensues regarding the increased frequency of some of the neoplasms due to limited available data: pancreatic, testicular, thyroid (Hürthle cell), colon, cholangiocarcinoma, pituitary cysts, and chronic lymphocytic leukaemia [3, 5, 15, 21, 42].

3.1. Management. With this infrequent diagnosis, there are no formal guidelines in the diagnosis and management of HPT-JT syndrome; however, genetic analysis is confirmatory [3, 15, 36]. Surgery remains the ultimate management of the primary hyperparathyroidism (total, subtotal, or limited parathyroidectomy); however, there is as of yet no gold standard [3]. Total parathyroidectomy risks hypoparathyroidism (of permanent duration) and is best avoided; limited parathyroid excision is preferred due to an unlikely risk of hypoparathyroidism and decreased morbidity. Total parathyroidectomy has been attempted in the setting of autotransplantation (typically the forearm); however, this can potentially disseminate tumorous cells should a carcinoma be present [3, 31]. If patients are poor surgical candidates, cinacalcet has demonstrated efficacy in treating primary hyperparathyroidism [3, 15]. Should a carcinoma be confirmed, "en bloc" resection is the gold standard, with the removal of the ipsilateral thyroid, parathyroid, fatty tissue, and lymph nodes; a biopsy is contraindicated due to the risk of seeding the tumour [3, 5, 15, 29, 31, 43]. Postoperative complications are best avoided with preoperative treatment of vitamin D (to limit hypocalcaemia) and antiemetics (dehydration promotes devascularisation of the remaining parathyroid gland) [15]; it is imperative to inform the patient, however, that despite the surgical approach used, baseline risk of recurrence (25%) remains for primary hyperparathyroidism [3].

Obstetric and gynaecological manifestations are managed on an individual basis, as are renal anomalies. Female patients are encouraged to attain normocalcaemia prior to pregnancy to prevent foetal and maternal complications (otherwise, likely to require surgery within the second trimester); furthermore, a hysterectomy may be required in the presence of certain uterine lesions; however, this should be a last resort to preserve the potential for conception [3, 15].

Surveillance is recommended from genetic confirmation of diagnosis, including the following [3, 15]:

(i) Annual calcium, parathyroid hormone, and vitamin D

(ii) Periodic ultrasound examination of the parathyroid gland

(iii) Panoramic X-ray dental imaging (with neck shielding) at least 5-yearly

(iv) Renal imaging (ultrasound/MRI/CT) at least 5-yearly

(v) Regular gynaecological evaluation (at least pelvic ultrasound)

Family members must be screened for this diagnosis [3, 15, 36]; in the case report presented, our patient was advised to inform her family, who have undergone screening and are awaiting the results. Lifelong biochemical monitoring is mandatory as the risk of recurrence for hyperparathyroidism is around one-quarter, with a second lesion either occurring synchronously or metachronously any time after identification of the first adenoma [3, 5, 15]. Reoperations are considered on an individual basis [44].

This case report further reinforces the limitations of nuclear imaging for the identification of a hyperfunctioning parathyroid adenoma. As with our patient, her parathyroid adenoma was not identified upon the sestamibi-SPECT scan, and a false-positive was noted deep to her thyroid gland (no histopathological abnormality identified). Small adenomas and diminished oxyphil expression are well-documented factors associated with poor localisation with sestamibi scanning [45].

4. Conclusion

Although a rare diagnostic entity, hyperparathyroidism-jaw tumour syndrome must be considered in early-onset, familial, atypical, or recurrent primary hyperparathyroidism. Genetic analysis is the gold standard for confirming the diagnosis, and patients must be continually monitored and reassessed to detect recurrence and other systemic manifestations of the disorder. Surgical treatment is the favoured approach to managing primary hyperparathyroidism, and all family members must be screened for the genetic mutation.

With the myriad of phenotypes displayed by hyperparathyroidism-jaw tumour syndrome, patients may initially present to departments other than endocrinology or metabolic medicine, including obstetrics and gynaecology (for infertility), urology (for renal stones), or maxillofacial (for jaw tumours). This case report aims to enhance the awareness of hyperparathyroidism-jaw tumour syndrome and its various associations across all medical domains. Moreover, as with our patient, this report serves as a reminder of the limitations with nuclear imaging (sestamibi) for the detection of adenomas.

Consent

The consent form was signed by the patient.

Acknowledgments

The authors thank the Milton Keynes University Hospital Obstetrics & Gynaecology, Urology, Endocrinology, and Metabolic Medicine Departments and the Churchill Hospital (Oxford) for their support in the care of this patient.

References

[1] R. Carroll and G. Matfin, "Review: endocrine and metabolic emergencies: hypercalcaemia," *Therapeutic Advances in Endocrinology and Metabolism*, vol. 1, no. 5, pp. 225–234, 2010.

[2] A. E. Kearns and G. B. Thompson, "Medical and surgical management of hyperparathyroidism," *Mayo Clinic Proceedings*, vol. 77, no. 1, pp. 87–91, 2002.

[3] F. Torresan and M. Iacobone, "Clinical features, treatment, and surveillance of hyperparathyroidism-jaw tumor syndrome: an up-to-date and review of the literature," *International Journal of Endocrinology*, vol. 2019, Article ID 1761030, 8 pages, 2019.

[4] M. Iacobone, B. Carnaille, F. F. Palazzo, and M. Vriens, "Hereditary hyperparathyroidism-a consensus report of the European society of endocrine surgeons (ESES)," *Langenbeck's Archives of Surgery*, vol. 400, no. 8, pp. 867–886, 2015.

[5] M. Iacobone, G. Masi, L. Barzon et al., "Hyperparathyroidism-jaw tumor syndrome: a report of three large kindred," *Langenbeck's Archives of Surgery*, vol. 394, no. 5, pp. 817–825, 2009.

[6] F. Tonelli, T. Marcucci, F. Giudici, A. Falchetti, and M. L. Brandi, "Surgical approach in hereditary hyperparathyroidism," *Endocrine Journal*, vol. 56, no. 7, pp. 827–841, 2009.

[7] J. D. Carpten, C. M. Robbins, A. Villablanca et al., "HRPT2, encoding parafibromin, is mutated in hyperparathyroidism-jaw tumor syndrome," *Nature Genetics*, vol. 32, no. 4, pp. 676–680, 2002.

[8] A. Cascón, C. V. Huarte-Mendicoa, L. Javier Leandro-García et al., "Detection of the first gross CDC73 germline deletion in an HPT-JT syndrome family," *Genes, Chromosomes and Cancer*, vol. 50, no. 11, pp. 922–929, 2011.

[9] O. Rozenblatt-Rosen, C. M. Hughes, S. J. Nannepaga et al., "The parafibromin tumor suppressor protein is part of a human Paf1 complex," *Molecular and Cellular Biology*, vol. 25, no. 2, pp. 612–620, 2005.

[10] A. Yart, M. Gstaiger, C. Wirbelauer et al., "The HRPT2 tumor suppressor gene product parafibromin associates with human PAF1 and RNA polymerase II," *Molecular and Cellular Biology*, vol. 25, no. 12, pp. 5052–5060, 2005.

[11] P. J. Newey, M. R. Bowl, and R. V. Thakker, "Parafibromin—functional insights," *Journal of Internal Medicine*, vol. 266, no. 1, pp. 84–98, 2009.

[12] F. Bringhurst, M. Demay, and H. Kronenberg, "Hormones and disorders of mineral metabolism," in *William's Textbook of Endocrinology*, pp. 1232–1304, Elsevier, Philadelphia, PA, USA, 12th edition, 2011.

[13] MedlinePlus.Gov, "Hyperparathyroidism-jaw tumor syndrome: medlineplus genetics," 2020, https://medlineplus.gov/genetics/condition/hyperparathyroidism-jaw-tumor-syndrome/#frequency.

[14] C. E. Jackson, "Hereditary hyperparathyroidism associated with recurrent pancreatitis," *Annals of Internal Medicine*, vol. 49, no. 4, pp. 829–36, 1958.

[15] S. M. Hyde, T. A. Rich, S. G. Waguespack et al., "CDC73-related disorders," in *GeneReviews®*, pp. 1993–2020, University of Washington, Seattle, Seattle, WA, USA, 2008.

[16] K. J. Bradley, M. R. Hobbs, I. D. Buley et al., "Uterine tumours are a phenotypic manifestation of the hyperparathyroidism-jaw tumour syndrome," *Journal of Internal Medicine*, vol. 257, no. 1, pp. 18–26, 2005.

[17] K. van der Tuin, C. M. J. Tops, M. A. Adank et al., "CDC73-related disorders: clinical manifestations and case detection in primary hyperparathyroidism," *The Journal of Clinical Endocrinology & Metabolism*, vol. 102, no. 12, pp. 4534–4540, 2017.

[18] T. Clerici, M. Brandie, J. Lange, G. M. Doherty, and P. G. Gauger, "Impact of intraoperative parathyroid hormone monitoring on the prediction of multiglandular parathyroid disease," *World Journal of Surgery*, vol. 28, no. 2, pp. 187–192, 2004.

[19] J. D. Chen, C. Morrison, C. Zhang, K. Kahnoski, J. D. Carpten, and B. T. Teh, "Hyperparathyroidism-jaw tumour syndrome," *Journal of Internal Medicine*, vol. 253, no. 6, pp. 634–642, 2003.

[20] B. T. Teh, F. Farnebo, U. Kristoffersson et al., "Autosomal dominant primary hyperparathyroidism and jaw tumor syndrome associated with renal hamartomas and cystic kidney disease: linkage to 1q21–q32 and loss of the wild type allele in renal hamartomas," *The Journal of Clinical Endocrinology & Metabolism*, vol. 81, no. 12, pp. 4204–4211, 1996.

[21] C. J. Haven, F. K. Wong, E. W. C. M. van Dam et al., "A genotypic and histopathological study of a large Dutch kindred with hyperparathyroidism-jaw tumor syndrome," *The Journal of Clinical Endocrinology & Metabolism*, vol. 85, no. 4, pp. 1449–1454, 2000.

[22] M. H. Kivlen, D. L. Bartlett, S. K. Libutti et al., "Reoperation for hyperparathyroidism in multiple endocrine neoplasia type 1," *Surgery*, vol. 130, no. 6, pp. 991–998, 2001.

[23] B. M. Cavaco, L. Barros, A. Pannett et al., "The hyperparathyroidism-jaw tumour syndrome in a Portuguese kindred," *QJM*, vol. 94, no. 4, pp. 213–222, 2001.

[24] C. Jackson, R. Norum, S. Boyd et al., "Hereditary hyperparathyroidism and multiple ossifying jaw fibromas: a clinically and genetically distinct syndrome," *Surgery*, vol. 108, no. 6, pp. 1006–1012, 1990.

[25] J. Szabó, B. Heath, V. Hill et al., "Hereditary hyperparathyroidism-jaw tumor syndrome: the endocrine tumor gene HRPT2 maps to chromosome 1q21–q31," *American Journal of Human Genetics*, vol. 56, no. 4, pp. 944–950, 1995.

[26] J. S. Dinnen, R. H. Greenwoood, J. H. Jones, D. A. Walker, and E. D. Williams, "Parathyroid carcinoma in familial hyperparathyroidism," *Journal of Clinical Pathology*, vol. 30, no. 10, pp. 966–975, 1977.

[27] L. Bricaire, M.-F. Odou, C. Cardot-Bauters et al., "Frequent large GermlineHRPT2 deletions in a French national cohort of patients with primary hyperparathyroidism," *The Journal of Clinical Endocrinology & Metabolism*, vol. 98, no. 2, pp. E403–E408, 2013.

[28] A. R. Pichardo-Lowden, A. Manni, B. D. Saunders, and M. J. Baker, "Familial hyperparathyroidism due to a germline mutation of the Cdc73 gene: implications for management and age-appropriate testing of relatives at risk," *Endocrine Practice*, vol. 17, no. 4, pp. 602–609, 2011.

[29] M. Iacobone, F. Lumachi, and G. Favia, "Up-to-date on parathyroid carcinoma: analysis of an experience of 19 cases," *Journal of Surgical Oncology*, vol. 88, no. 4, pp. 223–228, 2004.

[30] V. Guarnieri, A. Scillitani, L. A. Muscarella et al., "Diagnosis of parathyroid tumors in familial isolated hyperparathyroidism with HRPT2 mutation: implications for cancer surveillance," *The Journal of Clinical Endocrinology & Metabolism*, vol. 91, no. 8, pp. 2827–2832, 2006.

[31] M. Iacobone, V. Camozzi, C. Mian et al., "Long-term outcomes of parathyroidectomy in hyperparathyroidism-jaw tumor syndrome: analysis of five families with CDC73 mutations," *World Journal of Surgery*, vol. 44, no. 2, pp. 508–516, 2019.

[32] F. Cetani, E. Pardi, S. Borsari et al., "Genetic analyses of theHRPT2Gene in primary hyperparathyroidism: germline and somatic mutations in familial and sporadic parathyroid tumors," *The Journal of Clinical Endocrinology & Metabolism*, vol. 89, no. 11, pp. 5583–5591, 2004.

[33] T. M. Shattuck, S. Välimäki, T. Obara et al., "Somatic and germ-line mutations of the HRPT2 gene in sporadic parathyroid carcinoma," *New England Journal of Medicine*, vol. 349, no. 18, pp. 1722–1729, 2003.

[34] F. Cetani, E. Ambrogini, P. Viacava et al., "Should parafibromin staining replace HRTP2 gene analysis as an additional tool for histologic diagnosis of parathyroid carcinoma?" *European Journal of Endocrinology*, vol. 156, no. 5, pp. 547–554, 2007.

[35] K. J. Bradley, B. M. Cavaco, M. R. Bowl et al., "Parafibromin mutations in hereditary hyperparathyroidism syndromes and parathyroid tumours," *Clinical Endocrinology*, vol. 64, no. 3, pp. 299–306, 2006.

[36] H. du Preez, A. Adams, P. Richards, and S. Whitley, "Hyperparathyroidism jaw tumour syndrome: a pictoral review," *Insights into Imaging*, vol. 7, no. 6, pp. 793–800, 2016.

[37] Y. Liu, H. Wang, M. You et al., "Ossifying fibromas of the jaw bone: 20 cases," *Dentomaxillofacial Radiology*, vol. 39, no. 1, pp. 57–63, 2010.

[38] N. Zegalie, P. M. Speight, and L. Martin, "Ossifying fibromas of the jaws and craniofacial bones," *Diagnostic Histopathology*, vol. 21, no. 9, pp. 351–358, 2015.

[39] Y. Chen, D. Hu, T. Wang et al., "CDC73 gene mutations in sporadic ossifying fibroma of the jaws," *Diagnostic Pathology*, vol. 11, no. 1, 2016.

[40] M. J. Aldred, A. A. Talacko, R. Savarirayan et al., "Dental findings in a family with hyperparathyroidism-jaw tumor syndrome and a novel HRPT2 gene mutation," *Oral Surgery, Oral Medicine, Oral Pathology, Oral Radiology, and Endodontology*, vol. 101, no. 2, pp. 212–218, 2006.

[41] M. Tan and B. Teh, "Renal neoplasia in the hyperparathyroidism-jaw tumor syndrome," *Current Molecular Medicine*, vol. 4, no. 8, pp. 895–897, 2004.

[42] V. Guarnieri, M. Bisceglia, N. Bonfitto et al., "Re: familial hyperparathyroidism: surgical outcome after 30 years of follow-up in three families with germline HRPT2 mutations," *Surgery*, vol. 144, no. 5, pp. 839-840, 2008.

[43] M. Iacobone, C. Ruffolo, F. Lumachi, and G. Favia, "Results of iterative surgery for persistent and recurrent parathyroid carcinoma," *Langenbeck's Archives of Surgery*, vol. 390, no. 5, pp. 385–390, 2005.

Graves' Disease Presenting with Complete Atrioventricular Block

Young Sil Eom and Pyung Chun Oh

Department of Internal Medicine, Gil Medical Center, Gachon University College of Medicine, Incheon, Republic of Korea

Correspondence should be addressed to Pyung Chun Oh; likemed@gilhospital.com

Academic Editor: Mihail A. Boyanov

Hyperthyroidism commonly causes tachyarrhythmias such as sinus tachycardia and atrial fibrillation. Impaired atrioventricular conduction is a very rare complication of hyperthyroidism. We report a case of a patient with hyperthyroidism due to Graves' disease presenting with syncope and complete atrioventricular block. Because lack of awareness of atypical presentation in patients with hyperthyroidism may delay diagnosis and treatment, the recognition that hyperthyroidism can be one of the reversible causes of complete atrioventricular block is important.

1. Introduction

Although thyrotoxicosis commonly causes tachyarrhythmias including sinus tachycardia and atrial fibrillation, atrioventricular (AV) block is very rarely described in patients with hyperthyroidism. Here, we report a case of a patient who presented with syncope due to complete AV block, was diagnosed with Graves' disease, and completely recovered on antithyroid treatment.

2. Case Presentation

A 28-year-old female patient had presented with dizziness a week ago. While she was waiting for medical consultation at a primary care clinic, she suddenly lost consciousness and had involuntary convulsive-like movements for 10 seconds. She had a history of acute otitis media 7 days ago and had taken medications including antibiotics for 3 days. The electrocardiogram performed at the primary care clinic showed complete AV block with supraventricular rhythm, followed by long ventricular asystole over 4.4 seconds (Figure 1(a)). Initial blood pressure and pulse rate were 128/70 mmHg and 30 per minute, respectively. Follow-up electrocardiography at the emergency room revealed complete AV block with the ventricular escape rhythm (Figure 1(b)). A temporary transvenous ventricular pacing was applied through the internal jugular vein. Serum electrolyte levels were within the normal clinical range, and renal function was normal. She did not take other or herbal medications except for drugs for acute otitis media including cefditoren, erdosteine, and levocetirizine. The thyroid gland was diffusely enlarged, and bilateral exophthalmos was identified. The level of the thyroid-stimulating hormone was very low, less than 0.008 μIU/mL (reference range, 0.55–4.78 μIU/mL), and the levels of free T4 and T3 were 6.4 ng/dL and 511.0 ng/dL, respectively (reference range, 0.89–1.78 ng/dL and 60–180 ng/dL, respectively). Propylthiouracil 300 mg daily was started. Thyroid ultrasound noted diffuse thyroid enlargement with heterogenous parenchymal echogenicity. Radioiodine scan showed intense increased thyroid uptake, consistent with hyperthyroidism (Figure 2). Echocardiography reported normal cardiac function without structural abnormalities. Coronary computed tomography angiography or cardiac catheterization was not performed because she did not have any risk factors for coronary artery disease, and myocardial ischemia was less likely to be the cause of complete AV block in this patient. At the eighth hospital day, the levels of free T4 and T3 decreased to 2.9 ng/dL and 222.3 ng/dL, respectively. Complete AV block was recovered to sinus rhythm with rates of 75 per

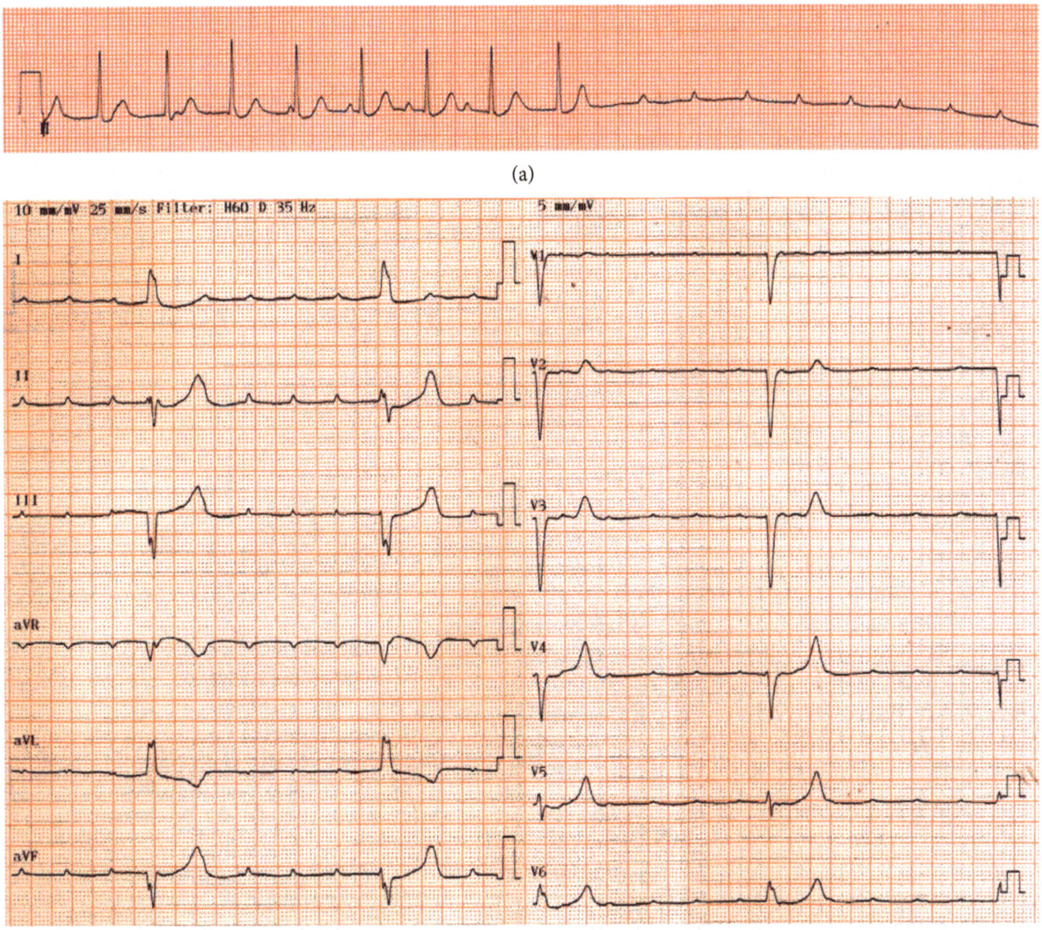

FIGURE 1: (a) Electrocardiography performed at the primary care clinic showing complete atrioventricular block with supraventricular rhythm, followed by long ventricular asystole over 4.4 seconds. (b) Follow-up electrocardiography at the emergency room revealing complete AV block with ventricular escape rhythm.

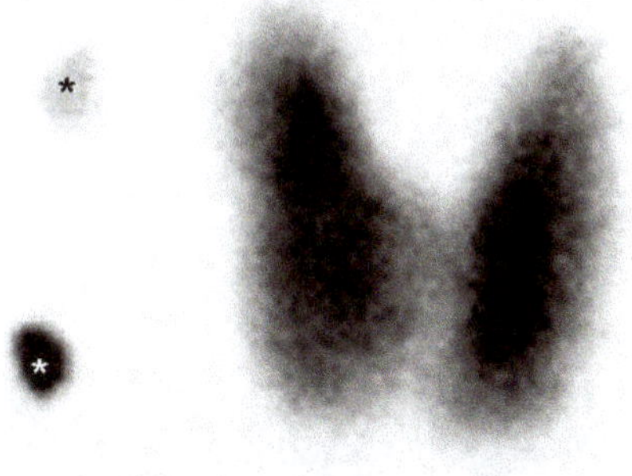

FIGURE 2: Radioiodine scan showing intense increased thyroid uptake, consistent with hyperthyroidism.

minute (Figure 3), and transvenous pacing lead was removed. She was discharged with medications for hyperthyroidism without the recurrence of the AV block.

3. Discussion

Complete AV block results from various pathologic states causing an anatomical or functional impairment in the conduction system. The common causes of complete AV block include degenerative diseases characterized with progressive fibrosis of the conduction system, cardiac diseases such as ischemic heart disease or cardiomyopathies, and medications impairing AV conduction. In addition, electrolyte disturbance (especially, hyperkalemia) or thyroid disease can lead to AV block.

Thyroid hormones are known to have direct inotropic, chronotropic, and dromotropic effects such as tachycardia and increased cardiac output. Therefore, hyperthyroidism commonly causes tachyarrhythmias such as sinus tachycardia and atrial fibrillation, and bradyarrhythmias occur more commonly in association with hypothyroidism. Complete atrioventricular block can be present in patients with hypothyroidism, which resolves after levothyroxine therapy [1]. In addition, thyrotoxic periodic paralysis rarely causes AV block, which is related with hypokalemia [2].

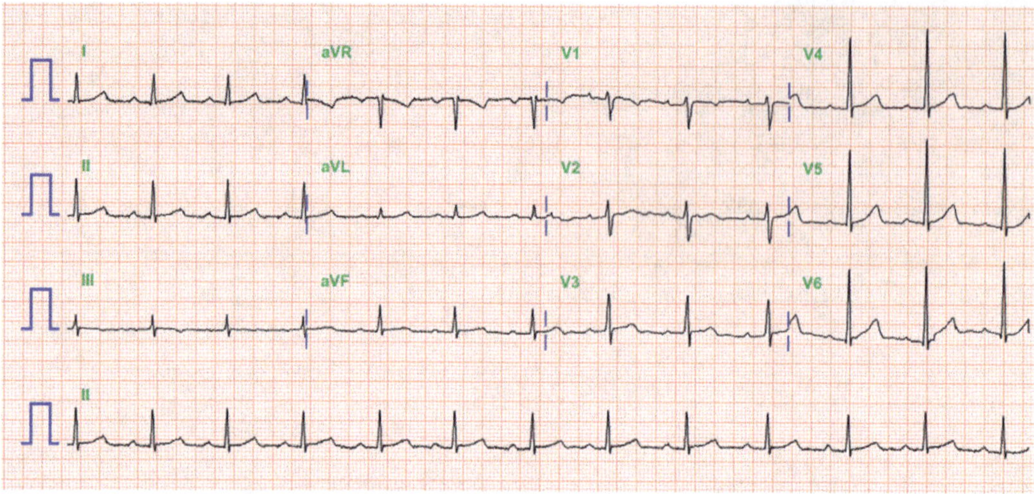

FIGURE 3: 8-day follow-up electrocardiography after decreasing the level of free T4 and T3 with propylthiouracil showing sinus rhythm.

Impaired AV conduction is a very rare complication of thyrotoxicosis [3, 4]. Bradyarrhythmias complicating hyperthyroidism have been commonly associated with acute infectious disease, hypercalcemia, thyroid storm, or underlying structural heart disease [5–7]. In our patient, acute otitis media had been preceded before the development of complete AV block. The exact mechanism of complete AV block in thyrotoxicosis has not been elucidated. Interstitial inflammation of the AV node or focal myocarditis around the AV node has been reported in a patient with hyperthyroidism [8, 9]. Autopsies in patients with fatal hyperthyroidism showed myocyte hypertrophy, myocyte necrosis, interstitial and perivascular fibrosis, and myocardial edema, which has been postulated to result in AV block [10].

In conclusion, we report a case of a patient with hyperthyroidism due to Graves' disease presenting with syncope and complete AV block. Complete AV block rarely occurs in thyrotoxicosis. Because lack of awareness of atypical presentations in patients with hyperthyroidism may delay diagnosis and treatment, the recognition that hyperthyroidism can be a reversible cause of complete AV block is important.

References

[1] N. Schoenmakers, W. E. de Graaff, and R. H. J. Peters, "Hypothyroidism as the cause of atrioventricular block in an elderly patient," *Netherlands Heart Journal*, vol. 16, no. 2, pp. 57–59, 2008.

[2] H.-F. Wang, S.-C. Tsai, M.-S. Pan, and C.-C. Shiao, "Complete heart block during potassium therapy in thyrotoxic periodic paralysis," *The Journal of Emergency Medicine*, vol. 44, no. 1, pp. 61–64, 2013.

[3] M. R. Kramer, S. Shilo, and C. Hershko, "Atrioventricular and sinoatrial block in thyrotoxic crisis," *Heart*, vol. 54, no. 6, pp. 600–602, 1985.

[4] S. A. Eraker, R. Wickamasekaran, and S. Goldman, "Complete heart block with hyperthyroidism," *JAMA: The Journal of the American Medical Association*, vol. 239, no. 16, pp. 1644–1646, 1978.

[5] M. P. Stern, R. L. Jacobs, and G. W. Duncan, "Complete heart block complicating hyperthyroidism," *JAMA: The Journal of the American Medical Association*, vol. 212, no. 12, pp. 2117–2119, 1970.

[6] A. L. Muggia, M. Stjernholm, and T. Houle, "Complete heart block with thyrotoxic myocarditis," *New England Journal of Medicine*, vol. 283, no. 20, pp. 1099-1100, 1970.

[7] L. Sataline and G. Donaghue, "Hypercalcemia, heart-block, and hyperthyroidism," *JAMA: The Journal of the American Medical Association*, vol. 213, no. 8, p. 1342, 1970.

[8] K. Yusoff and B. A. Khalid, "Conduction abnormalities in thyrotoxicosis--a report of three cases," *Annals of the Academy of Medicine, Singapore*, vol. 22, no. 4, pp. 609–612, 1993.

[9] C. Ortmann, H. Pfeiffer, A. Du Chesne, and B. Brinkmann, "Inflammation of the cardiac conduction system in a case of hyperthyroidism," *International Journal of Legal Medicine*, vol. 112, no. 4, pp. 271–274, 1999.

[10] J. Shirani, M. M. Barron, M.-L. Y. Pierre-Louis, and W. C. Roberts, "Congestive heart failure, dilated cardiac ventricles, and sudden death in hyperthyroidism," *The American Journal of Cardiology*, vol. 72, no. 3, pp. 365–368, 1993.

31

Severe Hypothyroidism Complicated by Myopathy and Neuropathy with Atypical Demyelinating Features

Malgorzata Monika Brzozowska,[1,2] **Shraddha Banthia,**[1] **Simon Thompson,**[3] **Manisha Narasimhan,**[4,5] **and James Lee**[4,6]

[1]*Department of Endocrinology, Sutherland Hospital, Sydney, NSW, Australia*
[2]*The University of New South Wales Sydney, Faculty of Medicine, Sydney, NSW, Australia*
[3]*Department of Chemical Pathology, NSW Health Pathology, Prince of Wales Hospital, Sydney, NSW, Australia*
[4]*Department of Neurology, Sutherland Hospital, Sydney, NSW, Australia*
[5]*The University of Sydney, Brain and Mind Centre, Sydney, NSW, Australia*
[6]*Department of Neurology, Royal North Shore Hospital, Sydney, NSW, Australia*

Correspondence should be addressed to Malgorzata Monika Brzozowska; m.brzozowska@unsw.edu.au

Academic Editor: Toshihiro Kita

Autoimmune hypothyroidism may result in a wide range of neuromuscular disorders. The frequently observed neurological manifestations of acquired hypothyroidism include mild to moderate myopathy and sensorimotor neuropathy, which usually resolve by clinical and electrophysiological criteria, in adults treated with thyroid hormone replacement. We report a case of a 30-year-old male with severe hypothyroidism secondary to chronic autoimmune thyroiditis who presented with a 2-year history of progressive fatigue, upper and lower limb weakness, myalgia, and intermittent paraesthesia. His neurological exam demonstrated proximal and distal muscle weakness, lower limb areflexia, and relatively intact sensory modalities. The patient's biochemistry revealed unusually and profoundly raised the thyroid stimulating hormone (TSH) level of 405.5 mIU/L (reference range (RR): 0.27–4.2 mIU/L) and creatine kinase (CK) level of 20,804 U/L (RR: 45–250 U/L), while his nerve conduction studies (NCS) demonstrated severe sensorimotor polyneuropathy with both axonal and demyelinating features. Thyroid hormone replacement therapy over the first 3 months resulted in biochemical normalization of his extremely deranged thyroid function tests (TFTs) and CK levels. At 12 months, despite maintaining euthyroidism and noticeable improvement in strength, his nerve conduction studies (NCS) demonstrated the continued absence of distal motor and sensory responses in his lower limbs with only partial improvement in sensory amplitudes and conduction velocities in his upper limbs. This report highlights the potential for severe neuromuscular consequences from advanced and chronic autoimmune hypothyroidism. The patient's myopathy has resolved over a period of three months with prompt normalization of CK levels. Concerningly, the patient achieved significant but incomplete recovery from his mixed axonal and demyelinating neuropathy with residual mild distal weakness and areflexia in his lower limbs and persistent motor and sensory impairments on his NCS. The severity and incomplete resolution of our patient's neurological manifestations emphasize the importance of early diagnosis and the need for prompt therapeutic intervention for hypothyroidism.

1. Introduction

Chronic autoimmune thyroiditis (also known as Hashimoto's disease) is the most common cause of hypothyroidism in iodine-sufficient areas [1]. Neurological features of hypothyroidism include myopathy, mono- and polyneuropathy, cognitive impairment, rarely cerebellar ataxia, and in more extreme presentations, myxoedema coma. The prevalence of neuromuscular manifestations associated with thyroid disorders has varied significantly between studies [2]. Myopathy is a frequent manifestation of hypothyroidism (between 20% and 80% of reported cases), manifesting clinically as weakness, cramps, and myalgias often associated with mild to moderate elevations in creatine kinase [2, 3]. The estimates of neuropathy in hypothyroidism range between 10% and 70% [2] with nerve conduction studies in hypothyroid neuropathy most commonly demonstrating a mild sensory axonal neuropathy [2, 4]. We present a patient with severe hypothyroidism due to Hashimoto's disease, with associated rhabdomyolysis complicated by severe mixed axonal and demyelinating polyneuropathy, with significant but incomplete response to levothyroxine treatment at 12 months after initial presentation.

2. Case Presentation

A 30-year-old male presented with a 2-year history of insidious and progressive fatigue, generalised weakness, myalgias, muscle cramps, and intermittent paraesthesiae in his upper and lower limbs. The patient reported impaired concentration and low mood due to mild depression, and he denied any alcohol intake or recreational drug use. The patient's father and his brother were subsequently diagnosed with Hashimoto's thyroiditis.

2.1. Examination and Investigations. The patient had loss of hair at the outer third of the eyebrows as well as over his shins, minimal periorbital oedema, and yellow palmar discolouration consistent with hypercarotenemia and macroglossia, with an absence of a palpable goitre or thyroid nodules. The patient's voice was hoarse in quality with slow speech and a delayed response latency when asked questions. There was no evidence of hepatosplenomegaly, lymphadenopathy, or skin hyperpigmentation. Neurological exam demonstrated proximal muscle weakness of grade 4/5 with an inability to rise from a seated position, as well as distal weakness of grade 3/5 in his lower limbs with significant weakness of ankle dorsiflexion bilaterally and absent ankle and knee jerk reflexes. In contrast, surprisingly, all sensory modalities (pinprick, vibration, light touch, and proprioception) appeared relatively spared by clinical examination. He did, however, have a wide-based high stepping gait with bilateral foot drop.

Initial laboratory results (September 2019) showed significantly deranged thyroid function tests (TFT) with an elevated thyroid stimulating hormone (TSH) level of 405.5 mIU/L (reference range (RR): 0.27–4.2 mIU/L), low free thyroxine (fT4) level of 1.6 pmol/L (RR: 12.0–22.0 pmol/L), and undetectable free triiodothyronine (FT3) level < 1.5 pmol/L (RR: 3.1–6.8 pmol/L) with raised thyroid peroxidase (TPO) antibody level of >600 IU/mL, consistent with Hashimoto's thyroiditis. The TSH level was measured by immunoassay with electrochemiluminescent detection (Roche Diagnostics, North Ryde, NSW, Australia). The assay is a sandwich immunoassay with a linear range between 0.005 mIU/L and 100 mIU/L. As TSH level of 405.5 mIU/L was significantly beyond the assay's analytical range, the examined sample required additional dilution in a validated matrix to obtain a numerical result. The initial creatine kinase (CK) level was elevated at 20,804 U/L (RR: 45–250 U/L); however, he had normal renal function. The patient's serial measurements of folate levels have remained within midnormal range with values up to 45.5 nmol/L (05/06/20). Further investigations (September 2019) revealed negative autoimmune screening including ANA, dsDNA, ENA, antinuclear antibodies, myositis-specific antibodies, myositis-associated antibodies, antimyelin-associated glycoprotein, and acetylcholine receptor antibodies. He had normal levels. There was a possible mild vitamin B12 deficiency with a holotranscobalamin level of 42.8 pmol/L (RR: 50.1–165 pmol/L). There was no evidence of monoclonal paraprotein on serum protein electrophoresis (EPG) (03/10/19). The patient's initial biochemistry is given in Table 1 with boldface highlighting abnormal results.

The patient's thyroid ultrasound (September 2019) revealed a normal-sized thyroid gland with a 9 mm nodule in the right lobe confirmed on fine needle aspiration biopsy to be lymphocytic thyroiditis. His nerve conduction studies (NCS) and electromyography (EMG) (18 September 2019) demonstrated an absence of distal lower limb motor and sensory responses and markedly prolonged upper limb distal motor latencies and conduction velocities, sensory nerve conduction velocities, and F-wave latencies. EMG confirmed acute denervation changes in distal muscles alongside widespread chronic partial denervation and reinnervation. The overall pattern was of severe generalised length-dependent sensorimotor neuropathy with both axonal and demyelinating features. An MRI of the brain (November 2019) was normal with no evidence of demyelinating, atrophic, or ischaemic features.

2.2. Treatment and Outcomes. The patient's clinical findings were suggestive of hypothyroidism-associated myopathy and polyneuropathy. He was commenced on levothyroxine at an initial dose of 100 μg daily, with partial and gradual improvement in his neurological presentation. He was also administered vitamin B12 replacement. Following 2.5 weeks of thyroxine replacement, the patient's TSH level had decreased to 183 mIU/L with a decline in CK level to 3203 U/L (Figure 1), and improvement in his proximal strength was observed to grade 5/5 power. There was persistent distal lower limb weakness with bilateral footdrop. His ankle and knee reflexes remained absent.

At two months post levothyroxine initiation (November 2019), his TFT had significantly improved with the TSH level of 15.1 mIU/L, fT4 of 18.7 pmol/L, and fT3 of 5.1 pmol/L with normalization of his liver function tests, likely due to resolved rhabdomyolysis and improved total vitamin B12 levels to 266 pmol/L (RR: 150–700). Repeat NCS at this time continued to demonstrate severe sensorimotor neuropathy with mixed axonal and demyelinating features. After three months of thyroxine replacement, the patient reported improvement in his lower limb muscle strength and gait, mood and concentration, energy levels, and in his speech quality. There was persistent distal lower limb weakness and lower limb areflexia.

Table 1: Results of initial laboratory tests (September 2019).

Parameters	Parameter value	Reference interval
Sodium (mmol/L)	140	135–145
Potassium (mmol/L)	4.0	3.5–5.2
eGFR (mL/min/1.73 m^2)	>90	>90
Fasting glucose (mmol/L)	3.9	3.0–5.5
Albumin (g/L)	46	33–48
Alanine aminotransferase (U/L)	**197**	<51
Aspartate aminotransferase (U/L)	**345**	<36
Alkaline phosphatase (U/L)	45	30–110
γ-Glutamyl transferase (U/L)	12	5–50
Bilirubin (μmol/L)	6	0–20
Corrected calcium (mmol/L)	2.3	2.1–2.6
Magnesium (mmol/L)	0.95	0.7–1.1
Phosphate (mmol/L)	1.25	0.75–1.5
Holotranscobalamin (pmol/L)	**42.8**	50.1–165
Folate (nmol/L)	19.3	8.83–60.8
Creatine kinase (U/L)	**20,804**	45–250
Total cholesterol (mmol/L)	**7.9**	3–5.5
Free T4 (pmol/L)	**1.6**	12–22
Free T3 (pmol/L)	<1.5	3.1–6.8
TSH (mIU/L)	**405.5**	0.27–4.2
Haemoglobin (g/L)	142	130–180
Platelets ($\times 10^9$/L)	270	150–450
White cell count ($\times 10^9$/L)	7.67	3.5–11
Thyroid peroxidase (TPO) antibodies (IU/mL)	**>600**	≤35
Thyroglobulin antibodies (IU/mL)	**152**	0–115
Intrinsic factor antibodies	Negative	
Gastric parietal cell antibodies	Negative	
Antinuclear antibodies	Negative	
Double stranded DNA antibodies	Negative	
ENA screen	Not detected	
Myositis antibodies screen	Not detected	
Antimyelin-associated glycoprotein	Not detected	
Acetylcholine receptor antibodies	Not detected	

Values in bold represent abnormal results

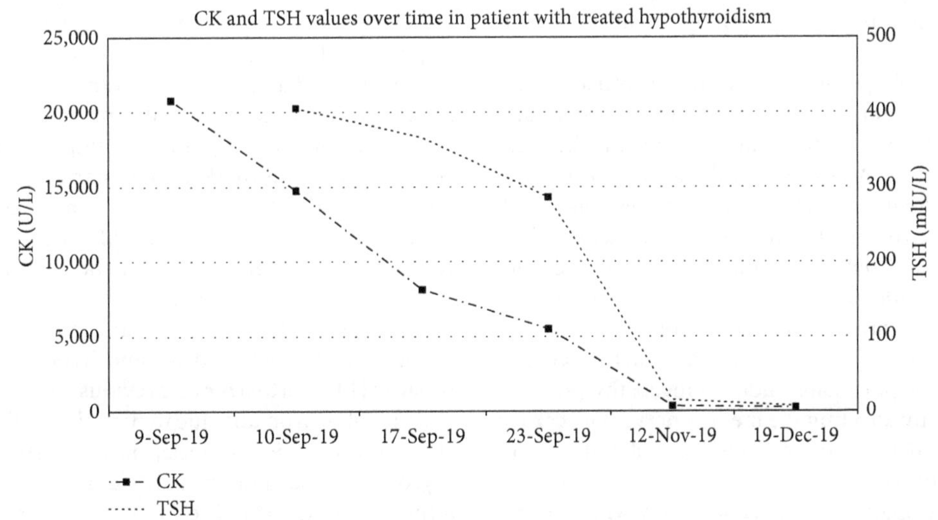

Figure 1: CK and TSH values over time in patient with treated hypothyroidism.

Follow-up clinical assessment at 12 months after his diagnosis (September 2020) revealed significant improvement in lower limb strength with persistent areflexia. Congruently, with physical findings, his repeat NCS revealed some improvement in sensory amplitudes and conduction velocities in patient's arms; however,

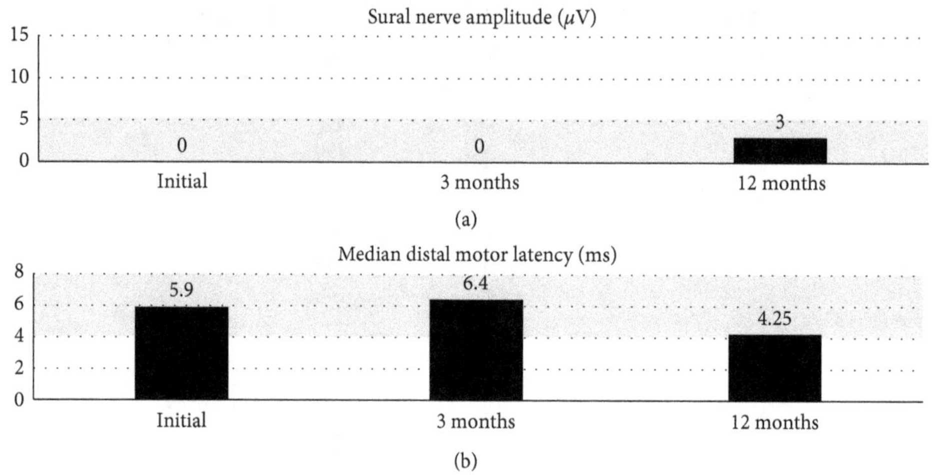

FIGURE 2: Serial nerve conduction values over time. (a) Sural nerve amplitude (μV). (b) Median distal motor latency (ms).

motor and sensory responses in his legs remained largely absent (Figure 2). Figure 2(a) demonstrates the trend of sural sensory nerve amplitudes, whilst Figure 2(b) depicts median distal motor nerve latency over three studies performed at baseline, 3 months, and 12 months after diagnosis. The abnormal ranges for these values are shaded in grey, with values trending towards normal at the 12-month study.

3. Discussion

The neuromuscular manifestations of hypothyroidism frequently occur in conjunction with common systemic features such as fatigue, weight gain, cold intolerance, and dry skin [1]. Rarely, as in the presented case, muscle and nerve dysfunction may flag the presence of hypothyroidism, highlighting the importance of considering thyroid dysfunction in any patient presenting with new neuromuscular symptomatology [2].

The pathophysiology of hypothyroid myopathy, although incompletely understood, is thought to be secondary to an altered metabolic state, which results in aberrant glycogen and oxidative metabolism in the actin-myosin unit [3, 5]. Severe or prolonged oxidative damage causes muscle cell injury and rhabdomyolysis. The muscle involvement in hypothyroidism ranges from asymptomatic CK elevation to proximal myopathy mimicking inflammatory myositis and rarely, frank rhabdomyolysis [6, 7] and necrotising myopathy [8]. Furthermore, patients with primary hypothyroidism are more at risk of developing statin-induced myopathy [9].

Mononeuropathy affecting the median nerve (i.e., carpal tunnel syndrome) is the most common peripheral neurological complication of hypothyroidism [4]. Hypothyroid-associated polyneuropathy presents commonly with length-dependent symmetric sensory neuropathy and predominantly axonal neuropathy [2, 4] without unique distinguishing features [10]. Interestingly, although polyneuropathy occurs commonly in hypothyroidism, at times, it may not be detected on clinical exam unless diagnosed via electrophysiological criteria [11].

The physiological mechanisms involved in polyneuropathy due to hypothyroidism are not well understood but are possibly related to axonal degeneration, deposition of mucopolysaccharides in the endoneurial interstitium and perineurial sheath with segmental demyelination and remyelination changes [11], and metabolic alterations affecting Schwann cells. Electrophysiological studies have reported resistance to the conduction of impulses with increased response latencies and decreased conduction velocity.

Our patient presented with severe neuropathy with mixed axonal and demyelinating features including electrodiagnostic findings suggestive of demyelination on his NCS. While metabolic neuropathies are usually thought to be axonal, demyelinating neuropathies are less frequently documented in the literature in association with hypothyroidism [12, 13].

Our patient's repeat NCS results, which were expected to improve following thyroid hormone replacement [10], remained unchanged at 2 months after the diagnosis of hypothyroidism. Despite achieving and maintaining clinical euthyroidism and significant improvement in muscle strength, his NCS markers only partially corrected after 12 months of thyroid hormone replacement. Furthermore, vitamin B12 levels at the time of repeat NCS testing were replete, making vitamin B12 deficiency an unlikely contributor to his presentation.

The literature highlights an association between the duration of hypothyroidism and hypothyroid-related neuropathy [14]. Furthermore, previous studies have shown that peripheral neuropathy due to hypothyroidism, diagnosed by electrophysiological criteria, occurs early in the course of thyroid disease and initially remains latent and asymptomatic [11, 15, 16]. The presented patient had significant neuropathy with persistent distal weakness and bilateral footdrop gait. His profound elevations of TSH levels, to values which are rarely seen in clinical practice, are suggestive of a prolonged period of overt hypothyroidism, possibly accounting for the severity of our patient's electrodiagnostic findings and his persistent neurological deficit.

Importantly, in previous studies, over one-third of patients affected by hypothyroidism had residual polyneuropathy after 12 months of adequate thyroid replacement therapy [2], with a reported case of severe hypothyroid neuropathy which had only resolved after 6 years of thyroid hormone replacement [17].

Previous reports have pointed to an association between Hashimoto's thyroiditis and autoimmune demyelinating neuropathies such as Guillain–Barré syndrome, chronic inflammatory demyelinating polyneuropathy, and multifocal motor neuropathy, likely due to an underlying shared genetic susceptibility to autoimmune conditions [18–22]. The significant clinical improvement in our patient's distal weakness together with partial improvement in his NCS findings after 12 months of thyroxine therapy and the absence of other systemic involvements make the presence of an autoimmune demyelinating neuropathy a less likely diagnosis. Furthermore, an absence of hepatosplenomegaly, lymphadenopathy, skin hyperpigmentation, clonal plasma cell disorder, or lymphoproliferative disease excluded the presence of POEMS syndrome [23].

The majority (57–90%) of individuals with hypothyroidism present with mild to moderate elevations of serum creatine kinase (CK) to values less than 5000 U/L [24]. The reported patient presented with CK values more than one hundred times the reference range (RR: 45–250 U/L), likely consistent with rhabdomyolysis [25] and more commonly described in immune-mediated myopathies. The detailed laboratory evaluation of inflammatory myopathies was negative, excluding other myopathic disorders. Previous case studies of patients with hypothyroid-induced myopathy have shown that successful treatment with thyroxine therapy results in clinical and biochemical recovery [24, 26]. In the present case, following the resolution of hypothyroidism, the patient's CK level had normalised with a complete restoration of power in his proximal muscles.

An interesting aspect of this case is the biochemical severity of patient's hypothyroidism. Importantly, we have obtained a numerical result of patient's TSH concentration which allowed for accurate biochemical assessment of the patient's response to therapy.

When faced with extreme and unusual laboratory results, it is important to consider the possibility of analytical interferences. Interferences with immunoassays are common and are easily missed unless clinical and laboratory personnels are vigilant when reviewing biochemistry results. Common causes of TSH immunoassay interferences include the presence of cross-reacting (heterophile) antibodies, exogenous biotin in the sample, and macroanalyte complexes (analyte molecules bound together by immunoglobulin) which have delayed clearance from the plasma and therefore are present in higher concentrations [27]. In the present case, the pattern of exceedingly high TSH values with low concentrations of both thyroid hormones, positive anti-TPO antibody status, and clinical features consistent with a severe hypothyroid state improved the confidence in the analytical accuracy of the results.

In conclusion, the presented case highlights the severe neuromuscular consequences of profound and likely long-standing chronic autoimmune hypothyroidism. The patient presented with severe myopathy, which resolved over a period of two months with the introduction of thyroxine therapy. Despite early diagnosis and successful treatment of the biochemical hypothyroidism, the patient achieved only partial recovery from his sensorimotor peripheral neuropathy with residual distal weakness and areflexia in his lower limbs and ongoing motor and sensory impairments on his NCS at 12 months. The severity and incomplete resolution of the patient's neurological manifestations emphasises the importance of early diagnosis and prompt therapeutic intervention for hypothyroidism.

The routine screening of patients presenting with neuromuscular symptoms for thyroid dysfunction would lead to timely administration of thyroid replacement therapy with a subsequent reduction in their serious neuromuscular comorbidities. Importantly, physicians need to be aware about long-term neuromuscular sequelae which may complicate untreated hypothyroidism. Therefore, we hope to increase diagnostic awareness for an early recognition and treatment of neurological complications arising from thyroid hormone deficiency.

References

[1] L. Chaker, A. C. Bianco, J. Jonklaas, and R. P. Peeters, "Hypothyroidism," *The Lancet*, vol. 390, no. 1, pp. 1550–1562, 2017.

[2] R. F. Duyff, J. Van den Bosch, D. M. Laman, B. J. van Loon, and W. H. Linssen, "Neuromuscular findings in thyroid dysfunction: a prospective clinical and electrodiagnostic study," *Journal of Neurology, Neurosurgery & Psychiatry*, vol. 68, no. 6, pp. 750–755, 2000.

[3] H. A. Horak and R. Pourmand, "Endocrine myopathies," *Neurologic Clinics*, vol. 18, no. 1, pp. 203–213, 2000.

[4] F. Eslamian, A. Bahrami, N. Aghamohammadzadeh, M. Niafar, Y. Salekzamani, and K. Behkamrad, "Electrophysiologic changes in patients with untreated primary hypothyroidism," *Journal of Clinical Neurophysiology*, vol. 28, no. 3, pp. 323–328, 2011.

[5] A. Sindoni, C. Rodolico, M. A. Pappalardo, S. Portaro, and S. Benvenga, "Hypothyroid myopathy: a peculiar clinical presentation of thyroid failure," *Review of the literature and Reviews in Endocrine and Metabolic Disorders*, vol. 17, no. 4, pp. 499–519, 2016.

[6] C. G. Seo, K. J. Kim, E. Park et al., "Untreated primary hypothyroidism with simultaneous rhabdomyolysis, pericardial effusion, and sudden sensorineural hearing loss: a case report," *BMC Endocr Disord*, vol. 19, no. 1, p. 52, 2019.

[7] N. Salehi, E. Agoston, I. Munir, and G. J. Thompson, "Rhabdomyolysis in a patient with severe hypothyroidism," *American Journal of Case Reports*, vol. 18, pp. 912–918, 2017.

[8] E. Tiniakou and A. L. Mammen, "Necrotizing myopathy caused by central hypothyroidism," *Muscle & Nerve*, vol. 52, no. 1, pp. 152-153, 2015.

[9] J. Peringat, R. G. Manappallil, and U. Karadan, "Rhabdomyolysis: a rare complication of Hashimoto's thyroiditis precipitated by statin therapy," *BMJ Case Reports*, vol. 2018, 2018.
[10] M. Laycock and R. Pascuzzi, "The neuromuscular effects of hypothyroidism," *Seminars in Neurology*, vol. 11, no. 03, pp. 288–294, 1991.
[11] E. Beghi, M. L. Delodovici, G. Bogliun et al., "Hypothyroidism and polyneuropathy," *Journal of Neurology, Neurosurgery & Psychiatry*, vol. 52, no. 12, pp. 1420–1423, 1989.
[12] J. D. Pollard, J. G. McLeod, T. G. A. Honnibal, and M. A. Verheijden, "Hypothyroid polyneuropathy," *Journal of the Neurological Sciences*, vol. 53, no. 3, pp. 461–471, 1982.
[13] C. Meier and A. Bischoff, "Polyneuropathy in hypothyroidism," *Journal of Neurology*, vol. 215, no. 2, pp. 103–114, 1977.
[14] R. Nemni, E. Bottacchi, R. Fazio et al., "Polyneuropathy in hypothyroidism: clinical, electrophysiological and morphological findings in four cases," *Journal of Neurology, Neurosurgery & Psychiatry*, vol. 50, no. 11, pp. 1454–1460, 1987.
[15] S. Sharma, V. Tobin, P. R. J. Vas, and G. Rayman, "The ldiflare and ccm methods demonstrate early nerve fiber abnormalities in untreated hypothyroidism: a prospective study," *The Journal of Clinical Endocrinology & Metabolism*, vol. 103, no. 8, pp. 3094–3102, 2018.
[16] E. M. Khedr, L. F. El Toony, M. N. Tarkhan, and G. Abdella, "Peripheral and central nervous system alterations in hypothyroidism: electrophysiological findings," *Neuropsychobiology*, vol. 41, no. 2, pp. 88–94, 2000.
[17] C. F. Torres and R. T. Moxley, "Hypothyroid neuropathy and myopathy: clinical and electrodiagnostic longitudinal findings," *Journal of Neurology*, vol. 237, no. 4, pp. 271–274, 1990.
[18] A. Toscano, C. Rodolico, S. Benvenga et al., "Multifocal motor neuropathy and asymptomatic Hashimoto's thyroiditis: first report of an association," *Neuromuscular Disorders*, vol. 12, no. 6, pp. 566–568, 2002.
[19] A. Polizzi, M. Ruggieri, I. Vecchio, S. Genovese, L. Rampello, and R. Raffaele, "Autoimmune thyroiditis and acquired demyelinating polyradiculoneuropathy," *Clinical Neurology and Neurosurgery*, vol. 103, no. 3, pp. 151–154, 2001.
[20] R. S. Kohli, W. Bleibel, and H. Bleibel, "Concurrent immune thrombocytopenic purpura and Guillain-Barre syndrome in a patient with Hashimoto's thyroiditis," *American Journal of Hematology*, vol. 82, no. 4, pp. 307-308, 2007.
[21] S. Raghavendra, S. Sanjay, R. Somashekar, R. Ashalatha, and S. K. Shankar, "CIDP, Hashimoto's thyroiditis and nephropathy: autoimmune syndrome complex?" *Canadian Journal of Neurological Sciences/Journal Canadien des Sciences Neurologiques*, vol. 36, no. 3, pp. 382–384, 2009.
[22] C. Bairactaris, G. Stouraitis, E. Papalias, N. Fakas, G. Papatheodorou, and P. Gourtzelidis, "Early neurophysiological evolution of chronic inflammatory demyelinating polyneuropathy in a patient with Hashimoto's thyroiditis," *Muscle & Nerve*, vol. 38, no. 5, pp. 1518–1522, 2008.
[23] A. Dispenzieri, "POEMS Syndrome: 2019 Update on diagnosis, risk-stratification, and management," *American Journal of Hematology*, vol. 94, no. 7, pp. 812–827, 2019.
[24] J. Finsterer, C. Stöllberger, C. Grossegger, and A. Kroiss, "Hypothyroid myopathy with unusually high serum creatine kinase values," *Hormone Research in Paediatrics*, vol. 52, no. 4, pp. 205–208, 1999.
[25] K. Stahl, E. Rastelli, and B. Schoser, "A systematic review on the definition of rhabdomyolysis," *Journal of Neurology*, vol. 267, no. 4, pp. 877–882, 2020.
[26] K. R. Scott, Z. Simmons, and P. J. Boyer, "Hypothyroid myopathy with a strikingly elevated serum creatine kinase level," *Muscle & Nerve*, vol. 26, no. 1, pp. 141–144, 2002.
[27] J. Tate and G. Ward, "Interferences in immunoassay," *The Clinical Biochemist Reviews*, vol. 25, no. 2, pp. 105–120, 2004.

32

Headache in a Child with Pseudohypoparathyroidism: An Alarming Symptom Not to Miss

Sarah Wing-yiu Poon, Brian Hon-yin Chung, Anita Man-ching Tsang, and Grace Wing-kit Poon

Department of Paediatrics and Adolescent Medicine, Queen Mary Hospital, LKS Faculty of Medicine, The University of Hong Kong, Pok Fu Lam, Hong Kong

Correspondence should be addressed to Sarah Wing-yiu Poon; sarahpoonwy@gmail.com

Academic Editor: Toshihiro Kita

Background. While the endocrine manifestations of pseudohypoparathyroidism are well known, less is known about the associated brain and spine abnormalities. These abnormalities may present with nonspecific symptoms in the paediatric population, and lack of awareness to these uncommon manifestations of the disease may result in a delay in necessary intervention. *Case Presentation.* We herein present a case of known pseudohypoparathyroidism type 1a who presented initially with minor head injury. She later developed progressive worsening headache, increased irritability, and vomiting. Repeated imaging showed hydrocephalus and Chiari malformation type 1 necessitating emergency craniectomy. *Conclusion.* Growth hormone deficiency, a common manifestation of pseudohypoparathyroidism type 1a, results in underdevelopment of the posterior cranial fossa and may account for the higher incidence of Chiari malformation in this group of patients. Other associated neurological features reported in pseudohypoparathyroidism type 1a include spinal stenosis, syringomyelia, and craniosynostosis. While less commonly seen, awareness to these associations is important in order to optimize the multidisciplinary care to this group of patients.

1. Background

Pseudohypoparathyroidism (PHP) and related disorders comprise a spectrum of disorders characterized by parathyroid hormone (PTH) resistance. Based on different molecular abnormalities and clinical features, PHP can be divided into several subtypes. Pseudohypoparathyroidism type 1a (PHP1A) is caused by heterozygous inactivating mutations on the maternal allele of the guanine nucleotide-binding protein, alpha subunit (*GNAS*) gene. These mutations result in impaired G-protein coupled receptor signalling and end-organ resistance to PTH, thyrotropin-stimulating hormone (TSH), gonadotropins, and growth hormone-releasing hormone (GHRH) [1]. While it is known that PHP1A is associated with Albright hereditary osteodystrophy (AHO), less is known about the association with brain and spine abnormalities.

In this report, we present a case of known PHP1A who required emergency craniectomy as a result of hydrocephalus and Chiari malformation type 1 (CM-1). It is important to highlight this rare association such that prompt imaging can be performed in any child with PHP1A who presents with symptoms of raised intracranial pressure.

2. Case Presentation

This girl was the first child born full term to a Chinese nonconsanguineous couple with body weight 1.73 kg (<3rd centile), body length 38 cm (<3rd centile), and head circumference 31 cm (<3rd centile). Apart from short stature (140 cm), her mother also has brachydactyly, spinal stenosis, and mild mental retardation (Figure 1). Antenatal checkup for this pregnancy showed short long bones, and the finding was confirmed on newborn assessment. Newborn screening also showed congenital hypothyroidism with elevated TSH, presence of normal thyroid gland but absent uptake on thyroid technetium scintiscan. She was thus started on

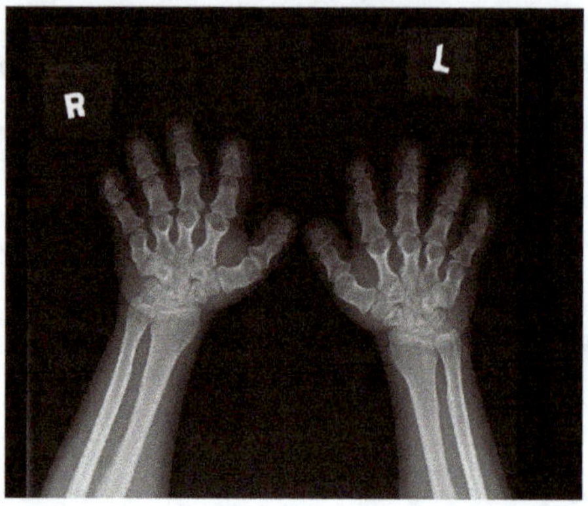

Figure 1: Patient's mother's X-ray hand demonstrating brachydactyly.

thyroxine replacement since 2 months of age. She had rapid weight gain during infancy, and her weight-for-height rose to 97th centile at 5 months.

During the first year of life, her PTH was elevated (9.1–16 pmol/L, ref: 1.3–6.8 pmol/L), while her calcium and phosphate were normal. She started to develop hyperphosphataemia (2.81 mmol/L, ref: 1.20–1.80 mmol/L) and hypocalcaemia (1.75 mmol/L, ref: 2.17–2.51 mmol/L) since 14 months and was started on oral calcium gluconate and alfacalcidol. Physical examination showed round facies, acral shortening of the long bones, and brachydactyly (Figure 2). In view of clinical features of AHO and PTH resistance, PHP1A was suspected. Genetic analysis at 1.5 years of age confirmed the diagnosis of PHP1A with heterozygous mutation of the *GNAS* gene (*NM_001077488.c.C394G.p.(L132V)*). Her mother was also found to have the same mutation.

Magnetic resonance imaging (MRI) of the brain was performed at 2 years of age for suspected central sleep apnoea, which revealed no abnormalities. At the age 4 years, she presented to the emergency department for minor head injury. Skull *X*-ray showed no skull fracture, and she was discharged. Six months later, she presented with increasing headache, irritability, and occasional vomiting. Upon admission, her vital signs were stable and neurological assessment was normal. Urgent MRI of the brain showed hydrocephalus with obstruction at the craniocervical junction. The posterior cranial fossa was small with severe crowding of the foramen magnum and inferior herniation of the cerebellar vermis causing cervicomedullary kinking (Figure 3). Emergency posterior fossa craniectomy for decompression was performed. On reviewing the skull X-ray taken 6 months prior to this hospital admission, generalized prominent gyri with copper beaten skull appearance was noted (Figure 4).

She had an uneventful postoperative course, and there was no recurrence of headache. Repeated MRI brain 5 months after operation showed interval improvement of her hydrocephalus and much reduced crowding at the foramen magnum. Upon follow-up, she was gaining height even though she was still below the 3rd centile and her body weight remained along the 75th centile. Clonidine and

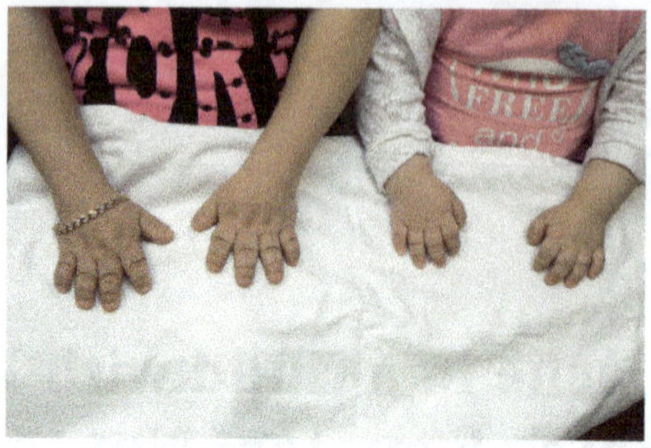

Figure 2: Patient's (left) and her mother's (right) hands demonstrating brachydactyly.

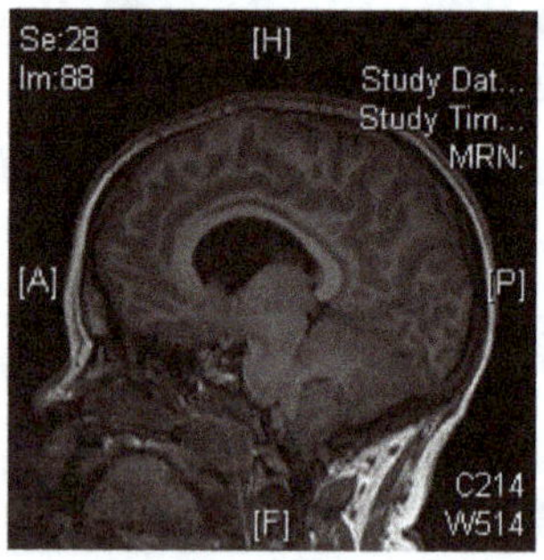

Figure 3: MRI brain showing hydrocephalus with obstruction at the craniocervical junction.

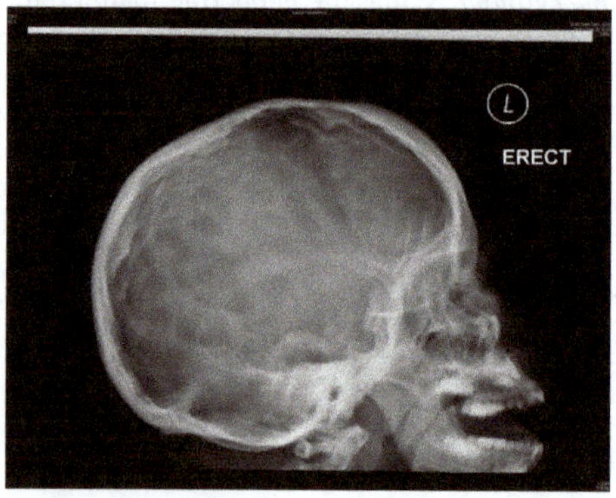

Figure 4: Skull X-ray showing copper beaten skull appearance.

glucagon stimulation tests confirmed growth hormone deficiency (GHD), and she was started on growth hormone (GH) replacement therapy at 5 years of age.

Regular monitoring of her PTH, calcium, phosphate, and thyroid function showed satisfactory parameters. The girl has global developmental delay and is currently receiving extra training at a special school with satisfactory developmental progress.

3. Discussion and Conclusions

We hereby report a case of PHP1A who developed hydrocephalus with CM-1.

CM-1 is defined as caudal displacement of the cerebellar tonsils below the foramen magnum and can result in life-threatening complications as a result of cerebellar compression, spinal cord dysfunction, or central sleep apnoea.

In our case, lack of awareness to the association of PHP1A and CM-1 resulted in a delay in diagnosis on the initial skull X-ray and subsequent neurosurgical emergency. While endocrine defects in PHP1A are well known, nonendocrine features of PHP1A are less commonly described. Shoemaker et al. described the nonclassic features of PHP1A including various orthopedic complications and ear-nose-throat findings [2]. Specific dental and craniofacial features in patients with PHP1A and maternal *GNAS* mutation have also been described in a systematic analysis, with high rate of patients showing dental anomalies and alteration in craniofacial bone development [3]. Association of neurologic dysfunction with PHP1A is not well appreciated. Two cases on the association of PHP1A and CM-1 have been reported in the literature [4, 5]. Martínez-Lage et al. reported a girl with PHP1A who also complained of mild headache, with imaging showing cerebellar tonsillar descent. In contrast to our case, tonsillar descent regressed with time [4]. In another report by Kashani et al., a younger patient with PHP1A had MRI brain performed for evaluation of developmental delay at 34 months, which revealed CM-1 with hydrocephalus requiring neurosurgical intervention. Similar to our patient, he had a normal MRI brain earlier in life [5]. These cases demonstrated that CM-1 may develop with time presenting with nonspecific symptoms, and hence, a low threshold in performing brain imaging should be adopted.

Multiple theories have been proposed for Chiari malformation (CM), one of which is the small posterior fossa theory. In our patient, MRI brain also showed a small posterior fossa volume with reduced craniocaudal height and crowding of the foramen magnum. The small posterior fossa theory was initially described by Marin-Padilla in 1981, where it was hypothesized that a mismatch between the size of the posterior fossa and its content leads to neural element compression and caudal herniation [6]. As such, GHD may also contribute to the underdevelopment of the posterior fossa. GH has an important role on cartilage growth, and a study showed that GH excess or deficiency may affect cartilaginous growth loci at cranial base [7]. In fact, Hamilton et al. performed MRI on 35 patients with GHD, and up to 20% of them have Chiari malformations [8]. With impaired responsiveness of somatotrophs to GHRH, PHP1A patients are thus at higher risk of CM due to GHD. Our patient, who was confirmed to have GHD at 5 years of age, had a normal MRI brain at 2 years of age. This demonstrated that underdevelopment of the posterior fossa might evolve with time and normal brain imaging earlier in life might not rule out the possibility of neurological abnormalities as the child grows.

Other associated neurological features reported in PHP1A include spinal stenosis, syringomyelia, and craniosynostosis. Our patient's mother suffers from chronic low back pain and lower limb numbness as a result of diffuse spinal stenosis. This highlights the importance to attend to the nonendocrine manifestation of the disease, as well as the need to offer multidisciplinary evaluation and therapy in PHP1A patients at all stages of life.

Abbreviations

PHP: Pseudohypoparathyroidism
PHP1A: Pseudohypoparathyroidism type 1a
PTH: Parathyroid hormone
GNAS: Guanine nucleotide-binding protein, alpha subunit
TSH: Thyrotropin-stimulating hormone
GHRH: Growth hormone-releasing hormone
AHO: Albright hereditary osteodystrophy
CM-1: Chiari malformation type 1
CM: Chiari malformation
MRI: Magnetic resonance imaging
GHD: Growth hormone deficiency
GH: Growth hormone.

Consent

Informed consent for publication has been obtained from the patient's mother.

Authors' Contributions

SWYP drafted and revised the manuscript. BHYC provided support in genetic analysis of the case. BHYC, AMCT, and GWKP supervised the preparation of the manuscript, and all authors approved the final manuscript.

References

[1] S. Turan and M. Bastepe, "The G N AS c o mplex l o cus and human diseases associated with loss-of-function mutations or epimutations within this imprinted gene," *Hormone Research in Paediatrics*, vol. 80, no. 4, pp. 229–241, 2013.

[2] A. H. Shoemaker and H. Jüppner, "Nonclassic features of pseudohypoparathyroidism type 1A," *Current Opinion in Endocrinology, Diabetes, and Obesity*, vol. 24, no. 1, pp. 33–38, 2017.

[3] E. Le Norcy, C. Reggio-Paquet, M. de Kerdanet, B. Mignot, A. Rothenbuhler, and C. Chaussain, "Dental and craniofacial features associated with GNAS loss of function mutations," *European Journal of Orthodontics*, vol. 42, no. 5, 2019.

[4] J. F. Martínez-Lage, E. Guillén-Navarro, A. L. López-Guerrero, M. J. Almagro, B. Cuartero-Pérez, and P. de la Rosa, "Chiari type 1 anomaly in pseudohypoparathyroidism type Ia: pathogenetic hypothesis," *Child's Nervous System*, vol. 27, no. 12, pp. 2035–2039, 2011.

[5] P. Kashani, M. Roy, L. Gillis, O. Ajani, and M. C. Samaan, "The association of pseudohypoparathyroidism type ia with chiari malformation type i: a coincidence or a common link?" *Case Reports in Medicine*, vol. 2016, Article ID 7645938, 2016.

[6] M. Marin-Padilla and T. M. Marin-Padilla, "Morphogenesis of experimentally induced arnold-chiari malformation," *Journal of the Neurological Sciences*, vol. 50, no. 1, pp. 29–55, 1981.
[7] S. Pirinen, A. Majurin, H. L. Lenko, and K. Koski, "Craniofacial features in patients with deficient and excessive growth hormone," *Journal of Craniofacial Genetics and Developmental Biology*, vol. 14, no. 3, pp. 144–152, 1994.
[8] J. Hamilton, S. Blaser, and D. Daneman, "MR imaging in idiopathic growth hormone deficiency," *American Journal of Neuroradiology*, vol. 19, no. 9, pp. 1609–1615, 1998.

Pulmonary Hypertension and Hypocholesterolemia Secondary to Thyrotoxicosis

Narangoda Liyanage Ajantha Shyamali[1] **and Chandrike Ponnamperuma**[2]

[1]*University of Sri Jayewardenepura, Gangodawila, Nugegoda, Sri Lanka*
[2]*National Hospital of Sri Lanka, Colombo 10, Sri Lanka*

Correspondence should be addressed to Narangoda Liyanage Ajantha Shyamali; ajaliyanage@yahoo.com

Academic Editor: Lucy Mastrandrea

Background. Thyroid disorders commonly affect the cardiovascular system. Thyrotoxicosis leading to pulmonary hypertension has been increasingly reported during recent years. Thyroid dysfunction affects the lipid metabolism, and thyrotoxicosis can be associated with low lipid levels. Thyrotoxicosis presenting with right ventricular dysfunction is rare, and only few cases had been reported. *Case Presentation.* A 53-year-old woman presented with progressive shortness of breath and swelling of body for four months. Examination showed generalized oedema and a systolic murmur over the left sternal border. Transthoracic echocardiography confirmed pulmonary hypertension with tricuspid regurgitation. Investigations revealed thyrotoxicosis and very low cholesterol levels. Diagnosis of Graves' disease was confirmed with detection of thyrotropin receptor antibodies. Pulmonary pressure was normalized six months after antithyroid therapy. *Conclusion.* Thyrotoxicosis is a recognized cause of reversible pulmonary hypertension and acquired hypocholesterolemia. However, most clinicians are not aware of these associations. This case illustrates the importance of assessing thyroid function in patients presenting with pulmonary hypertension.

1. Introduction

Thyrotoxicosis is well known to associate with left ventricular dysfunction due to long-standing effects of thyroid hormones. However, the association of hyperthyroidism with right ventricular dysfunction secondary to pulmonary hypertension has been reported in the literature since 1980 [1]. The exact mechanism of pulmonary hypertension in thyrotoxicosis is ill-defined [2, 3]. Several studies have reported the resolution of pulmonary hypertension secondary to thyrotoxicosis with antithyroid therapy [4]. The association of hypothyroidism with hyperlipidemia has been well known for a long period. However, low cholesterol level secondary to thyrotoxicosis is not widely appreciated. Only few cases of Graves' thyrotoxicosis with pulmonary hypertension and hyperlipidemia have been reported in the literature.

2. Case Presentation

A 53-year-old previously healthy woman presented with fever for 3 days associated with a four-month history of progressive shortness of breath and generalized body swelling. She has also noted increased sweating which she considered as a perimenopausal symptom. On examination, she was febrile with a heart rate of 101/min and oxygen saturation of 98% on room air. She had bilateral ankle oedema and extensive abdominal wall oedema. Jugular venous pressure was elevated, and there was a pansystolic murmur over the left sternal border. Respiratory system examination was clinically normal.

Her basic blood investigations of full blood count, erythrocyte sedimentation rate, C-reactive protein levels, renal function tests, and liver function tests were normal. She was found to have low cholesterol levels with total

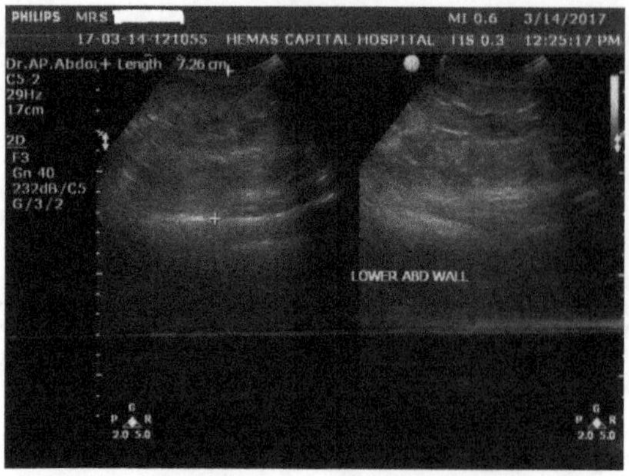

Figure 1: Ultrasound scan of the abdomen showing extensive abdominal wall oedema.

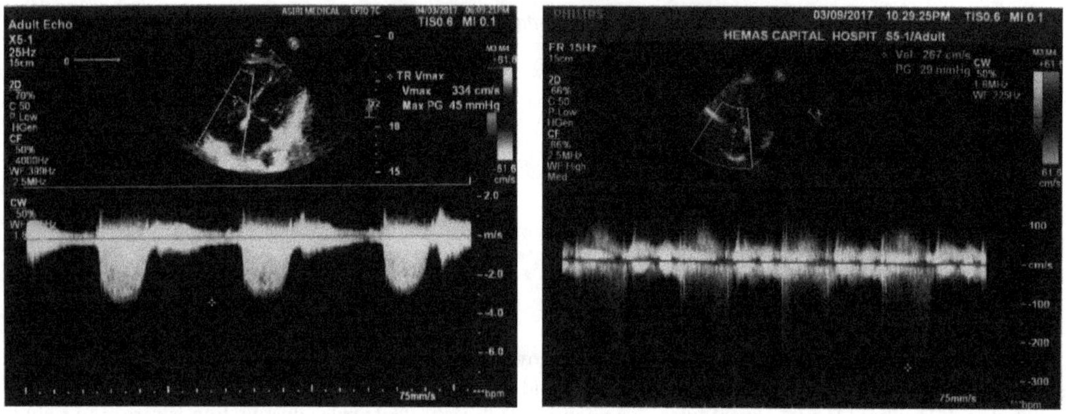

(a) (b)

Figure 2: Transthoracic echocardiography demonstrating pulmonary artery pressures before (a) and after (b) the treatment of thyrotoxicosis.

cholesterol of 61 mg/dl (normal range: 140–239), low-density lipoprotein cholesterol (LDLC) of 26 mg/dl (normal range: 75–159), and high-density lipoprotein cholesterol (HDLC) of 20 mg/dl (normal range: 35–85). Thyroid-stimulating hormone (TSH) level was 0.004 μIU/ml (normal range: 0.4–4.0) with free thyroxin (FT4) 5.48 ng/dl (normal range: 0.89–1.76) and free triiodothyronine (FT3) 11.48 pg/dl (normal range: 1.5–4.1). TSH receptor antibodies were positive with 4.39 IU/L (normal < 2 IU/L). Ultrasound of the thyroid showed diffusely enlarged glands with increased vascularity, and ultrasound scan of the abdomen revealed marked lower abdominal wall oedema without organomegaly (Figure 1). Transthoracic echocardiography showed right ventricular enlargement with tricuspid regurgitation. The systolic pulmonary artery pressure gradient was 45 mmHg (normal < 25 mmHg) (Figure 2(a)).

Graves' thyrotoxicosis was diagnosed, and she was started on antithyroid medication. She underwent computed tomographic pulmonary angiography (CT-PA) ten days after starting thyrostatic drugs which did not show evidence of chronic thromboembolic pulmonary hypertension or abnormalities of lung parenchyma. After six months of treatment, her symptoms improved. The systolic pulmonary artery pressure gradient was reduced to 29 mmHg in repeated transthoracic echocardiography (Figure 2(b)). TSH level increased to 0.48 μIU/ml with normalization of thyroid hormone levels. Her serum lipid levels returned to normal with total cholesterol of 185 mg/dl, LDLC of 109 mg/dl, and HDLC of 61 mg/dl.

3. Discussion

The association of thyrotoxicosis with right ventricular dysfunction was first reported in the literature in 1973 [5]. Thyrotoxicosis as a cause for pulmonary hypertension and reduction of pulmonary artery pressure with treatment of antithyroid medication have been clearly established recently [6, 7]. Therefore, most clinicians are not aware of this important association.

In a study of 23 patients with Graves' thyrotoxicosis, 65% of patients had pulmonary hypertension which normalized with definitive treatment, and a recent single-center cross-sectional study carried out in Ethiopia showed that 30% of patients with hyperthyroidism have echocardiographic evidence of pulmonary hypertension [4, 8]. Although the underlying pathophysiology for this complication is unclear, several mechanisms have been hypothesized: endothelial injury secondary to high cardiac output, immune-mediated endothelial damage, and enhanced metabolism of intrinsic pulmonary vasodilators [3, 9].

Increased expression of low-density lipoprotein (LDL) receptors and activity of lipoprotein lipase by thyroid hormones decrease the circulating levels of lipoproteins. Consequently, decreased levels of HDLC and LDLC are seen in patients with hyperthyroidism [10, 11]. The action of thyroid hormones in the liver is responsible for the reduction of LDLC levels, which is caused by enhanced transcription of LDL receptors in the liver. Therefore, the extent of LDLC level reduction is proportional to free thyroid hormone levels [11]. Hyperthyroidism is recognized as a significant cause of acquired hypocholesterolemia and unanticipated improvement of lipid levels in hyperlipidemic patients [12].

Thyrotoxicosis is an overlooked, reversible cause of pulmonary hypertension, and there is a high prevalence of pulmonary hypertension among hyperthyroid patients [13]. Thus, patients presenting with thyrotoxicosis and dyspnea should be screened for pulmonary hypertension [14]. All clinicians should be aware of this association, and this case highlights the importance of assessing thyroid function tests in patients with pulmonary hypertension.

Abbreviations

LDLC: Low-density lipoprotein cholesterol
HDLC: High-density lipoprotein cholesterol
TSH: Thyroid-stimulating hormone
FT4: Free thyroxin
FT3: Free triiodothyronine.

Consent

The authors obtained written informed consent from the patient to report and publish about her illness anonymously.

Authors' Contributions

NLA Shyamali was involved in the history taking, examination, diagnosis, and management of the patient's condition and prepared the manuscript for publication. C Ponnamperuma performed and reported echocardiography and was involved in diagnosis and management of the patient's condition. All authors read and approved the final manuscript.

Acknowledgments

The authors acknowledge the support from the staff of Asiri Medical Hospital, Sri Lanka, in the management of this patient's condition.

References

[1] M. Shimazaki, T. Mitsuhashi, and K. Hasegawa, "Idiopathic pulmonary hypertension associated with hyperthyroidism—an autopsy case," *Nihon Rinsho. Japanese Journal of Clinical Medicine*, vol. 38, no. 3, pp. 1783–1786, 1980.

[2] M. Conradie, C. Koegelenberg, M. Conradie, B. Ascott-Evans, and F. Hough, "Pulmonary hypertension and thyrotoxicosis," *Journal of Endocrinology, Metabolism and Diabetes of South Africa*, vol. 17, no. 2, pp. 101–104, 2014.

[3] F. Rashidi, H. Sate, E. Faraji, and S. Tahsini Tekantapeh, "Thyrotoxicosis presenting as exertional dyspnea and pulmonary hypertension: case report and review of literature," *SAGE Open Medical Case Reports*, vol. 5, 2017.

[4] M. Marvisi, P. Zambrelli, M. Brianti, G. Civardi, R. Lampugnani, and R. Delsignore, "Pulmonary hypertension is frequent in hyperthyroidism and normalizes after therapy," *European Journal of Internal Medicine*, vol. 17, no. 4, pp. 267–271, 2006.

[5] M. J. Dougherty and E. Craige, "Apathetic hyperthyroidism presenting as tricuspid regurgitation," *Chest*, vol. 63, no. 5, pp. 767–772, 1973.

[6] S. L. Teasdale, W. J. Inder, M. Stowasser, and T. Stanton, "Hyperdynamic right heart function in Graves' hyperthyroidism measured by echocardiography normalises on restoration of euthyroidism," *Heart, Lung and Circulation*, vol. 26, no. 6, pp. 580–585, 2017.

[7] C. S. Singarayar, F. S. Hui, N. Cheong, and G. S. En, "Right ventricular dysfunction and pulmonary hypertension: a neglected presentation of thyrotoxicosis," *Endocrinology, Diabetes & Metabolism Case Reports*, vol. 2018, 2018.

[8] H. A. Mulatu, "Pattern and presentation of thyro-cardiac disease among patients with hyperthyroidism attending a tertiary hospital in Ethiopia: a cross sectional study," *Ethiopian Journal of Health Sciences*, vol. 29, no. 1, pp. 887–894, 2019.

[9] M. O. Hegazi, A. El Sayed, and H. El Ghoussein, "Pulmonary hypertension responding to hyperthyroidism treatment," *Respirology*, vol. 13, no. 6, pp. 923–925, 2008.

[10] Y. Chen, X. Wu, R. Wu et al., "Changes in profile of lipids and adipokines in patients with newly diagnosed hypothyroidism and hyperthyroidism," *Scientific Reports*, vol. 6, Article ID 26174, 2016.

[11] Y. Bonde, O. Breuer, D. Lütjohann, S. Sjöberg, B. Angelin, and M. Rudling, "Thyroid hormone reduces PCSK9 and stimulates bile acid synthesis in humans," *Journal of Lipid Research*, vol. 55, no. 11, pp. 2408–2415, 2014.

[12] C. V. Rizos, M. Elisaf, and E. Liberopoulos, "Effects of thyroid dysfunction on lipid profile," *The Open Cardiovascular Medicine Journal*, vol. 5, no. 1, pp. 76–84, 2011.

[13] E. Berta, I. Lengyel, S. Halmi et al., "Hypertension in thyroid disorders," *Frontiers in Endocrinology*, vol. 10, p. 482, 2019.

[14] S. Vallabhajosula, S. Radhi, R. Alalawi, R. Raj, K. Nugent, and C. Cevik, "Hyperthyroidism and pulmonary hypertension: an important association," *The American Journal of the Medical Sciences*, vol. 342, no. 6, pp. 507–512, 2011.

Methimazole-Induced Pleural Effusion in the Setting of Graves' Disease

Le Yu Khine,[1] Dong Won Kim,[2] Omolola Olajide,[1] Chelsey White,[3] Yousef Shweihat,[3] and Henry Driscoll[1]

[1]*Division of Endocrinology, Marshall University, Joan C. Edwards School of Medicine, USA*
[2]*Division of Internal Medicine, University of Maryland School of Medicine, USA*
[3]*Division of Pulmonary and Critical Care and Sleep Medicine, Marshall University, Joan C. Edwards School of Medicine, USA*

Correspondence should be addressed to Le Yu Khine; khinel@marshall.edu

Academic Editor: John Broom

Methimazole is a thionamide drug that inhibits the synthesis of thyroid hormones by blocking the oxidation of iodine in the thyroid gland. We report a case of methimazole-induced recurrent pleural effusion. A 67-year-old female with recently diagnosed Graves' disease on methimazole 20mg daily was admitted with dyspnea and new onset atrial fibrillation with rapid ventricular rate. Chest X-ray revealed a unilateral right pleural effusion, which was consistent with a transudate on thoracocentesis. She was managed as a case of congestive heart failure and methimazole dose was increased to 30 mg daily. She was readmitted twice with recurrent right pleural effusion. The fluid revealed an exudative process on repeat thoracocentesis. CT scan of the chest with contrast showed mediastinal lymphadenopathy and a diffuse ground glass process involving the right lower lobe suggestive of pneumonitis. Bronchoalveolar lavage showed neutrophil predominant fluid, and cytology and adenosine deaminase were negative. Patient also had an endobronchial ultrasound guided biopsy of the lymph nodes (EBUS). She was treated empirically with steroids 40 mg for 10 days and the methimazole was also discontinued. The antinuclear antibodies (ANA) came back positive with a speckled pattern; antineutrophil cytoplasmic antibody (c-ANCA) and antimyeloperoxidase were also positive. The effusion resolved but recurred on rechallenge with methimazole. She was referred for urgent thyroidectomy. The patient's repeat chest X-ray showed complete resolution of the pleural effusion after stopping the methimazole. Few weeks later, repeat ANCA and antimyeloperoxidase antibody were both negative. Our case report highlights the importance of the recognition of a rare side effect of methimazole. Timely diagnosis would ensure that appropriate treatment is given.

1. Introduction

Methimazole is a thionamide drug that inhibits the synthesis of thyroid hormones by blocking the oxidation of iodine in the thyroid gland. It has been associated with a significant number of side effects. ANCA-associated vasculitis is a well-known complication of propylthiouracil, another thionamide drug. Methimazole has been recently implicated in inducing ANCA vasculitis [1].

There are reported cases of methimazole-induced pulmonary hemorrhage; however, other complications such as pleural effusion are very rare with methimazole [2–4]. There have been two reported cases of methimazole associated pleural effusions [2, 3]. We report a case of methimazole-induced recurrent pleural effusion in a woman with Graves' Disease.

2. Case Presentation

We present a 67-year-old female admitted with dyspnea and new onset atrial fibrillation with rapid ventricular rate. She was diagnosed with Graves' disease 3 weeks earlier and had been started on 20 mg of methimazole daily. Thyroid function tests showed suppressed TSH with elevated Free T3 and Free T4. Details of lab results are given in Table 1. Pro-BNP was elevated at 1762. Chest X-ray revealed unilateral

Table 1: Detailed laboratory and procedures.

Thyroid Function Tests	Initial Presentation: TSH <0.005 (0.358-3.740) Free T4 2.78 (0.76-1.46) Free T3 7.35 (2.18-3.98) 9 days after medical optimization: TSH <0.005 Free T4 1.54 Free T3 2.80 Hospital Course: TSH <0.005, Free T4 1.87, free T3 2.56
ANA	>1:80, positive and speckled pattern
Anti-Double stranded antibody	Negative
Antimyeloperoxidase antibody	Positive
c-ANCA	Positive⟶normal one and a half weeks after methimazole was discontinued.
p-ANCA	Negative
CT chest	Pleuritic, pneumonitis and mediastinal lymphadenopathy
CT abdomen	Ruled out intraabdominal etiologies such as malignancies
Bronchoscopy with EBUS	Negative for granulomatous disease, infection or malignancy
Bronchoalveolar Lavage (BAL)	Neutrophil predominant fluid with bacterial, fungal and AFB cultures negative. Cytology negative
Mediastinal Lymph Node Biopsy	Negative

right pleural effusion which was subsequently drained by thoracentesis and was consistent with transudative effusion. She was managed as a case of congestive heart failure. Her heart rate control was optimized and the dose of methimazole was increased to 30 mg once daily. She was discharged home but readmitted 2 days later with recurrent dyspnea. A repeat chest X-ray showed recurrence of the right pleural effusion. Transthoracic echocardiogram was done showing normal ejection fraction and diastolic function. Her heart rate was controlled. Repeat thyroid function tests showed a normal free T3 and almost normal free T4. Patient was diuresed, and the unilateral right pleural effusion was drained again. The fluid characteristics showed a transformation from transudative to exudative likely in the setting of recent diuretic use.

She was then discharged home after she had improved clinically only to be readmitted again with worsening dyspnea attributed to reaccumulation of the right pleural fluid a few days later. A repeat drainage with pleural catheter was performed, and the fluids revealed an exudative process with elevated LDH. This was further evaluated with a CT scan of the chest with contrast (Figures 1 and 2) which showed mediastinal lymphadenopathy and a diffuse ground glass process involving the right lower lobe suggestive of pneumonitis. A bronchoscopy was also performed. The bronchoalveolar lavage showed neutrophil predominant fluid, and cytology and adenosine deaminase were negative. Patient also had an endobronchial ultrasound-guided biopsy of the lymph nodes (EBUS). A work-up at this time was begun for drug induced vasculitis. She was treated empirically with steroids 40 mg for 10 days, and the methimazole was also discontinued. The antinuclear antibodies (ANA) came back positive with a speckled pattern; antineutrophil cytoplasmic antibody (c-ANCA) and antimyeloperoxidase MPO were also positive, but anti-double stranded DNA (DS-DNA) was negative. The

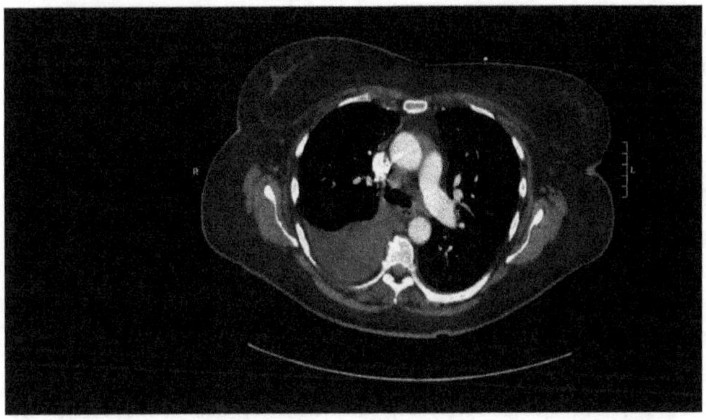

Figure 1: CT of chest showing mediastinal lymphadenopathy with presence of pleural effusion.

clinical picture was in keeping with a drug-induced vasculitic picture which is unusual with the use of methimazole. The patient improved remarkably without recurrence of the pleural effusion. She was restarted on methimazole as it was not definite it was the cause of the pleural effusion. On a subsequent outpatient visit a couple of weeks after restarting the methimazole, the effusion recurred but did not require drainage. Methimazole was discontinued. She was referred for urgent thyroidectomy. Repeat chest X-ray showed complete resolution of the pleural effusion after stopping the methimazole. Repeat ANCA and antimyeloperoxidase antibody were both negative one and a half weeks after methimazole was discontinued.

2.1. Laboratory and Procedures. See Table 1.

2.2. Imaging. See Figures 1 and 2.

TABLE 2: Summary of all the case reports of thioamide-induced pleural effusion.

Cases	Characteristics of pleural effusion	Thionamide	Treatment
Pedro Gaspar-da-Costa [3]	Eosinophils	Methimazole	Discontinued Methimazole
Gautam Das [5]	Exudative	Carbimazole	Switched to propylthiouracil (PTU)
Carol D Cardona Attard [6]	Exudative	Carbimazole	Switched to PTU and later total thyroidectomy
Ihteshamul Haq I [7]	Exudative	Carbimazole	Discontinued carbimazole and started prednisone
P. Sen [2]	Neutrophil predominant	Methimazole	Discontinued methimazole
Emmy YF Lau [4]	Pulmonary hemorrhage	Methimazole	Discontinued Methimazole and started prednisone

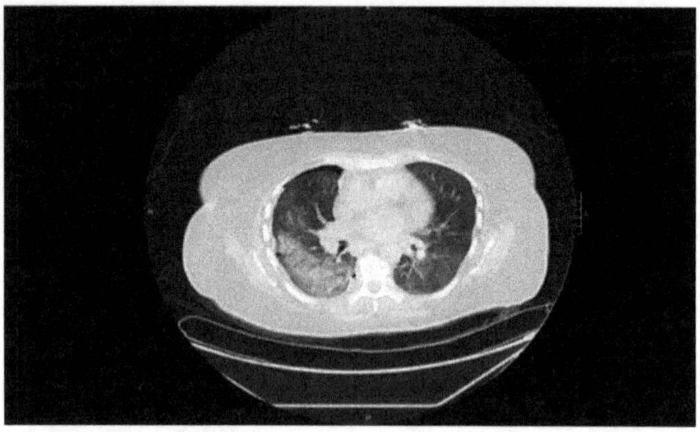

FIGURE 2: Presence of ground glass opacity suggesting pneumonitis after removal of pleural fluid.

3. Discussion

This is the third published case of methimazole related pleural effusion [2, 3]. In our case, the unilateral pleural effusion was initially managed in the setting of atrial fibrillation with rapid ventricular rhythm. The consensus was that the dyspnea was from uncontrolled hyperthyroidism likely causing CHF exacerbation. However, even with optimization including rate control, thoracentesis, and antithyroid treatment, the patient was readmitted twice for a recurring unilateral pleural effusion. At the time of the second and third admission, the pleural effusion was exudative with neutrophilic predominance. The initial extensive work-up was largely negative, but, by the third admission, there was a suspicion that the effusion was related to the methimazole. She also tested positive for c-ANCA and MPO. Discontinuation of the methimazole with concomitant systemic steroids led to resolution of pleural effusion. Restarting the drug caused reaccumulation of the effusion, and withdrawing it caused its resolution without recurrence.

There are several notable differences among the three reported cases. For our case, the fluid was neutrophilic predominant. This may be explained in the context that the methimazole led to ANCA associated vasculitis leading to pleural effusion. This differs from the Gaspar-da-Costa et al.'s (BMC) case, which had eosinophilic exudative effusion with likely hypersensitivity immune drug reaction, and ANCA negative work-up [3]. The Sen et al.'s case showed a neutrophilic predominant effusion, but there is no mention of ANCA being tested. They had a histopathologic diagnosis of leukocytoclastic vasculitis; ANA was positive with a homogenous pattern but had negative anti-DS and anti-histone antibody [2]. Our patient had a positive ANA but with a speckled pattern without any other features concerning for lupus. Anti-DS DNA was negative also. These three cases show different profiles and possible mechanisms leading to the proposed methimazole-induced pleural effusion.

Thionamide side effects are uncommon and include fever, rash, arthralgias, agranulocytosis, and hepatitis as well as SLE like symptoms. Pleural manifestations associated with thionamides are relatively rare with only two cases associated with methimazole, two with PTU, and three with carbimazole. Propylthiouracil-induced vasculitis has been well described in several case reports, and most of them presented with pulmonary hemorrhage.

Doses of methimazole were not clearly mentioned in two case reports. Our patient was initially taking methimazole 20 mg daily prior to her first admission, but the dose was then increased to 30 mg daily during her first hospital stay. On review of other literature (Table 2), pleural effusion was reported starting from a dose of 10 mg of carbimazole.

Onset of pleural effusion may vary. It can be as short as 6 days, but it could also be long after thionamide therapy was started. The longest duration reported in the literature was 5 years after methimazole was initiated.

For control of our patient's hyperthyroid state, she received an urgent thyroidectomy due to concerns for worsening symptoms. Other thionamides were considered, but there was concern for recurrence of the pleural effusion as both PTU and Carbimazole have more reports of related pleural effusion. Radioactive iodine was considered, but the patient had a recent CT scan with contrast. In the ATS case, the patient also went for thyroidectomy. In the BMC case, the patient had type II amiodarone induced thyrotoxicosis, and no further treatment was needed after discontinuation of amiodarone. Detailed summary is provided in Table 2.

4. Conclusion

Our case report highlights the importance of the recognition of a rare side effect of methimazole. Timely diagnosis would ensure that appropriate treatment is given including corticosteroid administration, surgery, or radioiodine.

Table 2 is the summary of all the case reports of thioamide-induced pleural effusion.

References

[1] D. R. Thickett, A. G. Richter, N. Nathani, G. D. Perkins, and L. Harper, "Pulmonary manifestations of anti-neutrophil cytoplasmic antibody (ANCA)-positive vasculitis," *Rheumatology*, vol. 45, no. 3, pp. 261–268, 2006.

[2] P. Sen and M. J. Dunn, "Its never lupus: a rare case of methimazole induced pleural effusion," *American Journal of Respiratory and Critical Care Medicine*, vol. 197, Article ID A6619, 2018.

[3] P. Gaspar-da-Costa, F. Duarte Silva, J. Henriques et al., "Methimazole associated eosinophilic pleural effusion: a case report," *BMC Pharmacology & Toxicology*, vol. 18, no. 1, article 16, 2017.

[4] E. Y. F. Lau, S. Y. So, E. Chan, J. Kwok, J. Ma, and A. W. C. Kung, "Methimazole-induced antineutrophil cytoplasmic antibody-associated diffuse alveolar haemorrhage in a Chinese woman with Graves' disease," *Hong Kong Medical Journal*, vol. 15, no. 3, pp. 209–212, 2009.

[5] G. Das, S. E. R. S. Stanaway, and L. Brohan, "Carbimazole induced pleural effusion: a case report," *Case Reports in Endocrinology*, vol. 2012, Article ID 941241, 3 pages, 2012.

[6] C. D. C. Attard, M. Gruppetta, J. Vassallo, and S. Vella, "Carbimazole-induced exudative pleural effusions," *BMJ Case Reports*, 2016.

[7] I. Haq, M. D. Sosin, S. Wharton, and A. Gupta, "Carbimazole-induced lupus," *BMJ Case Reports*, 2013.

35

Thyroiditis after mRNA Vaccination for COVID-19

Arunava Saha,[1] **Sanjita Chittimoju**,[2] **and Nitin Trivedi**[2]

[1]*PGY2 Internal Medicine, Saint Vincent Hospital, Worcester, MA, USA*
[2]*Endocrinology and Metabolic Medicine, Saint Vincent Hospital, Worcester, MA, USA*

Correspondence should be addressed to Arunava Saha; saha.arunava100@gmail.com

Academic Editor: Wayne V. Moore

Background. SARS-CoV-2 has been known to cause multisystemic involvement, gaining entry through ACE-2 and TMPRSS2 receptors. COVID-19 vaccine-associated thyroiditis cases are now being reported. *Case Report. Case 1.* A 36-year-old woman with a history of right hemithyroidectomy for a benign thyroid nodule, on a stable dose of levothyroxine with euthyroid labs, presented with progressively worsening left neck pain, episodic palpitations, and heat intolerance after the second dose of mRNA1273 (Moderna) vaccine. Examination revealed an enlarged and tender left lobe of the thyroid with suppressed TSH but normal free T4 and ESR, signifying subacute thyroiditis. She was managed conservatively without corticosteroids or beta-blockers, and her symptoms resolved. A follow-up revealed increasing TSH, and levothyroxine was restarted. *Case 2.* A 33-year-old man with a history of anxiety disorder on Sertraline, presented with a two-week history of palpitations, heat intolerance, and 10-pound weight loss after the second dose of BNT162b2 (Pfizer-BioNTech) vaccine. Examination revealed a normal thyroid gland with no tenderness with elevated thyroid peroxidase and thyroglobulin antibodies. Ultrasound showed a diffusely heterogeneous thyroid with increased vascularity, suggesting silent thyroiditis. Follow-up revealed a hypothyroid phase with high TSH for which levothyroxine supplementation was started. *Discussion.* COVID-19 vaccine-associated subacute and silent thyroiditis have occurred following all three kinds of available vaccines, characterized by an initial thyrotoxic phase, followed by a hypothyroid phase and a recovery phase. Hypotheses include an immune response triggering thyroid inflammation or cross-reactivity with viral proteins. *Conclusions.* COVID-19 vaccine-associated thyroiditis is rare, but long-term monitoring of these patients is essential to ensure appropriate diagnosis and management of the potential hypothyroid phase.

1. Introduction

The novel coronavirus disease 2019 (COVID-19) caused by severe acute respiratory syndrome coronavirus-2 (SARS-CoV-2) has affected more than 250 million people worldwide [1]. It uses the angiotensin-converting enzyme 2 (ACE-2) and transmembrane protease serine-2 (TMPRSS2) receptors for entry that are expressed widely throughout the body including the endocrine glands. Hence, COVID-19 can have multisystemic involvement with a range of severity [2, 3].

Several effective vaccines have been introduced, and currently, mass vaccination drives are underway. The inactivated vaccines use adjuvants such as aluminum salts and toll-like receptor (TLR) agonists to increase the immunogenic response to vaccination [4]. However, in genetically susceptible individuals, adjuvants may lead to autoimmune/inflammatory syndrome induced by adjuvants (ASIA syndrome). Possible mechanisms include disrupting the immunological balance and molecular mimicry-triggering polyclonal activation of B lymphocytes [5]. Subacute thyroiditis following COVID-19 vaccination has been described with ASIA syndrome and also following mRNA and adenovirus vaccines that do not have an adjuvant.

We report two cases of thyroiditis that developed soon after receiving the second dose of the mRNA COVID-19 vaccine. The article's objective is to create awareness about

Table 1: Laboratory test results.

	Case 1	Case 2
At diagnosis		
TSH (0.35–4.94 mIU/L)	<0.01	<0.01
FT4 (0.9–1.8 ng/dl)	1.8	1.71
T3 (100–200 ng/dl)	188	139
Anti-TPO (<10 IU/ml)	7	147
Anti-TG (<14 IU/ml)	Negative	1296.1
TRAB (<1.75 IU/L)	<1.10	<1.10
ESR (<20 mm/hr)	2	—
TSI antibodies	—	<0.10
CRP (<5.0 mg/L)	—	25
WBC (4.0–11.0) $\times 10^3$/ml	—	5.3
Follow-up 4th week		
TSH	14.23	25
FT4	0.90	0.40
T3	—	—

a possible association between thyroiditis and the COVID-19 mRNA vaccines.

2. Case 1

A 36-year-old woman with a history of right hemithyroidectomy for a benign thyroid nodule six years ago, presented with a 6-week history of progressively worsening left-sided neck pain accompanied by palpitations and heat intolerance. She developed transient myalgia and neck pain after her first dose of mRNA1273 (Moderna COVID-19 vaccine). Her current symptoms started 2 weeks after receiving the second dose of the vaccine. She had been euthyroid on a stable dose of levothyroxine for the last 6 years. She denied any history of viral or respiratory illness prior to the onset of symptoms. She had no family history of thyroid disorders or autoimmune conditions. Laboratory evaluation revealed suppressed TSH at urgent care triggering a consultation with an endocrinologist, which took place in a few weeks, by when her symptoms were spontaneously resolving.

On physical examination, her heart rate was 88/min, the temperature was 37.7°C, her blood pressure was 110/65, and her respiratory rate was 20/min. A neck examination revealed an enlarged and tender left thyroid lobe. There was no palpable lymphadenopathy, exophthalmos, pharyngeal erythema, irregular heart rhythm, hepatosplenomegaly, edema, tremors, or skin lesions. Laboratory investigations revealed a TSH of less than 0.01 mIU/L with a free T4 of 1.8 ng/dl on the upper limit of normal (Table 1). Antithyroglobulin, anti-thyroid peroxidase, and antibodies to thyrotropin receptor were negative, and the erythrocyte sedimentation rate (ESR) was normal. She was diagnosed with subacute thyroiditis. Levothyroxine was held in view of suppressed TSH and elevated free T4. Corticosteroid treatment was not recommended given the mild nature of the symptoms. Her symptoms gradually subsided over the subsequent few weeks, and TSH levels started rising. Levothyroxine therapy was restarted when the TSH level increased above the normal range.

3. Case 2

A 33-year-old man with a past history of anxiety disorder treated with sertraline presented with a two-week history of persistent palpitations, heat intolerance, and 10 pounds of weight loss. He reported no past or family history of thyroid disorders. He did not have any history of COVID-19 infection and was vaccinated with both doses of BNT162b2 (Pfizer-BioNTech COVID-19 vaccine) 4 weeks apart. Soon after receiving the second vaccine dose, he developed a high-grade fever at 102.5 F, myalgia, and sore throat, which persisted for 2 weeks. Subsequently, he experienced palpitations, diaphoresis, and heat intolerance along with generalized weakness. An endocrinology referral was triggered as he was found to have suppressed TSH along with elevated CRP at his primary care provider's office (Table 1). On physical examination, his heart rate was 86/min, blood pressure was 143/71, and respiratory rate was 18. A thyroid examination revealed a normal thyroid gland with no significant tenderness. He had no extrathyroidal features of Graves' disease. Repeat laboratory investigations revealed an undetectable TSH with normal T3 and T4 levels. Additional lab investigations revealed elevated thyroid peroxidase and thyroglobulin antibodies but undetectable levels of thyroid receptor antibodies and thyroid-stimulating immunoglobulin antibodies. An ultrasound of the thyroid showed a diffusely heterogeneous gland with increased vascularity and no nodules. The clinical features were consistent with silent thyroiditis. There were a few large benign-appears lymph nodes, which were resolved on follow-up ultrasound. His symptoms improved with NSAIDs without corticosteroid treatment. Repeat laboratory evaluation 4 weeks later revealed elevated TSH and low free T4 suggestive of a hypothyroid phase. He was transiently treated with levothyroxine because of severe fatigue and relative bradycardia with a heart rate of 50 s. Levothyroxine was subsequently discontinued as his TSH normalized. He currently remains euthyroid and asymptomatic without levothyroxine supplementation.

4. Discussion

We describe two cases of thyroiditis associated with the COVID-19 vaccine, subacute thyroiditis for the first case and silent thyroiditis for the second case. Both patients had an initial thyrotoxic phase followed by a hypothyroid phase which required levothyroxine supplementation.

Subacute and silent thyroiditis is a self-limiting thyroid disorder. They are more prevalent in women. Viral infections and immune-modulatory drugs have been implicated as etiological factors. Characteristically, they have an initial destructive thyrotoxic phase, followed by a hypothyroid phase and a recovery phase, leading to the normalization of thyroid functions [6].

The endocrine system has been found to be involved in COVID-19, causing hypopituitarism, adrenal necrosis, pancreatic beta-cell damage, gonadal dysfunction, and thyroiditis [7]. The exact pathogenesis is unknown, but the hypothesis involves an immune-mediated hormonal dysfunction, direct virus entry into cells causing cell destruction or cellular dysfunction caused by inflammation [7, 8].

Along with the common viruses such as CMV and HSV, cases of thyroiditis have emerged in association with COVID-19. The ACE-2 and TMPRSS2 that allow SARS-CoV-2 to infiltrate human cells are highly expressed in the thyroid follicular cells [9].

A recent study by Muller et al. suggested silent thyroiditis induced by COVID-19 occurs in an underlying setting of nonthyroidal illness in critically ill male patients. This was usually followed by a permanent hypothyroid phase [10]. However recent systematic reviews have demonstrated several cases of subacute thyroiditis secondary to COVID-19 infection, amongst which 92% presented with neck pain and the majority were female patients [11, 12]. This suggests that thyroiditis caused by COVID-19 infection can have varied clinical presentations.

Additionally, an increasing number of cases of COVID-19 vaccine-associated thyroiditis are now being reported. These cases have occurred following all three kinds of available vaccines, inactivated SARS-CoV-2 vaccine, mRNA-based vaccine, and vector-based vaccine. Most cases that developed after the inactivated vaccine have been attributed to adjuvants, triggering adverse reactions in genetically predisposed individuals, and causing ASIA syndrome [13–15]. In a case report of two cases of subacute thyroiditis postvaccination from Germany, symptoms were attributed to the adenovirus vector vaccine and the mRNA vaccine. Both the patients had classic symptoms and fine-needle aspiration cytology showed lymphocytic infiltrate and multinucleated giant cells consistent with subacute thyroiditis [16].

A few other cases have been described, including a 42-year-old female who developed painful hyperthyroid symptoms five days after the first dose of the BNT162b2 vaccine and required a short course of steroids and beta-blockers with which her symptoms improved [15]. Similarly, a 46-year-old female developed neck pain after the second dose of the Moderna vaccine and was diagnosed to have subacute thyroiditis. She was managed with analgesics, oral steroids, and beta-blockers and was found to have normal thyroid function at follow-up [17].

Adenovirus-vector vaccines stimulate innate immunity sensors whereas mRNA vaccines encode the viral spike S glycoprotein, causing a potent immunological response. The vaccine is formulated in lipid particles which enable the delivery of RNA into the host cells to allow expression of the SARS-CoV-2 S antigen. This process elicits an immune response to the S antigen, which protects against COVID-19 infection [18].

The mechanism of postvaccination-associated thyroiditis remains unknown. It has been hypothesized that vaccinations may be responsible for producing an immune response that triggers thyroid inflammation in predisposed patients. Another hypothesis includes the SARS-CoV-2 spike protein, nucleoprotein, and membrane protein which cross-reacts with thyroid peroxidase [19].

There has been some recent understanding regarding the potential immune upheaval due to mRNA COVID-19 vaccination and its role in causing myocarditis, particularly in young men. The mechanism may include molecular mimicry between the spike protein of SARS-CoV-2 and self-antigens, increased cytokine expression secondary to dysregulated immune pathways, or an exaggerated immune response to viral mRNA [20].

In these two cases of thyroiditis after the mRNA COVID-19 vaccination, although a direct causal relationship could not be established, however, no other causes could be identified and temporality with the administration of the mRNA COVID-19 vaccine is very strongly suggestive. Up to 10% of patients with subacute thyroiditis develop permanent hypothyroidism. Hence, it is important that these patients are followed long-term [21]. Overall, further data are needed to determine the association between subacute thyroiditis and COVID-19 vaccinations.

5. Conclusion

COVID-19 vaccine-induced thyroiditis can range from subacute to silent presentation and is a rare phenomenon. The purpose of this report is to raise awareness among providers about the same. It is important for clinicians to be aware of this presentation to recognize COVID-19 vaccine-related immune effects in the thyroid to accurately manage the relevant stages of thyroiditis. Long-term monitoring of these patients is essential to ensure an appropriate diagnosis of the potential hypothyroid phase in them. Further investigation is needed to determine possible predisposing factors and mechanisms leading to thyroiditis after the COVID-19 vaccine.

References

[1] World Health Organization, WHO Coronavirus (COVID-19) Dashboard, https://www.COVID19.who.int.

[2] M. Hoffmann, H. Kleine-Weber, S. Schroeder et al., "SARS-CoV-2 cell entry depends on ACE2 and TMPRSS2 and is blocked by a clinically proven protease inhibitor," *Cell*, vol. 181, no. 2, pp. 271–280.e8, 2020.

[3] M. Y. Li, L. Li, Y. Zhang, and X. S. Wang, "Expression of the SARS-CoV-2 cell receptor gene ACE2 in a wide variety of human tissues," *Infectious Diseases of Poverty*, vol. 9, no. 1, p. 45, 2020.

[4] K. Xing, X. Y. Tu, M. Liu et al., "Efficacy and safety of COVID-19 vaccines: a systematic review," *Zhong Guo Dang Dai Er Ke Za Zhi*, vol. 23, no. 3, pp. 221–228, 2021.

[5] B. G. İremli, "Three cases of subacute thyroiditis following SARS-CoV-2 vaccine: post-vaccination ASIA syndrome," *Journal of Clinical Endocrinology and Metabolism*, 2021.

[6] A. Brancatella, D. Ricci, N. Viola, D. Sgrò, F. Santini, and F. Latrofa, "Subacute thyroiditis after sars-COV-2 infection," *Journal of Clinical Endocrinology and Metabolism*, vol. 105, no. 7, pp. 2367–2370, 2020.

[7] M. K. Garg, M. Gopalakrishnan, P. Yadav, and S. Misra, "Endocrine involvement in COVID-19: mechanisms, clinical features, and implications for care," *Indian Journal of Endocrinology and Metabolism*, vol. 24, no. 5, pp. 381–386, 2020.
[8] E. Lazartigues, M. M. F. Qadir, and F. Mauvais-Jarvis, "Endocrine significance of SARS-CoV-2's reliance on ACE2," *Endocrinology*, vol. 161, no. 9, 2020.
[9] M. Rotondi, F. Coperchini, G. Ricci et al., "Detection of SARS-COV-2 receptor ACE-2 mRNA in thyroid cells: a clue for COVID-19-related subacute thyroiditis," *Journal of Endocrinological Investigation*, vol. 44, no. 5, pp. 1085–1090, 2021.
[10] I. Muller, D. Cannavaro, D. Dazzi et al., "Early follow-up of atypical thyroiditis induced by SARS-CoV-2," *Journal of the Endocrine Society*, vol. 5, no. Supplement_1, p. A61, April-May 2021.
[11] A. Khatri, E. Charlap, and A. Kim, "Subacute thyroiditis from COVID-19 infection: a case report and review of literature," *European Thyroid Journal*, vol. 9, no. 6, pp. 324–328, 2020.
[12] P. Trimboli, C. Cappelli, L. Croce, L. Scappaticcio, L. Chiovato, and M. Rotondi, "COVID-19-associated subacute thyroiditis: evidence-based data from a systematic review," *Frontiers in Endocrinology*, vol. 12, Article ID 707726, 2021.
[13] J. Schimmel, E. L. Alba, A. Chen, M. Russell, and R. Srinath, "Letter to the editor: thyroiditis and thyrotoxicosis after the SARS-CoV-2 mRNA vaccine," *Thyroid*, vol. 31, no. 9, p. 1440, 2021 Sep.
[14] O. Vera-Lastra, A. O. Navarro, M. P. C. Domiguez, G. Medina, T. I. S. Valadez, and L. J. Jara, "Two cases of graves' disease following SARS-CoV-2 vaccination: an autoimmune/inflammatory syndrome induced by adjuvants," *Thyroid*, vol. 31, no. 9, pp. 1436–1439, 2021.
[15] S. O. Oyibo, "Subacute thyroiditis after receiving the adenovirus-vectored vaccine for coronavirus disease (COVID-19)," *Cureus*, vol. 13, no. 6, Article ID e16045, 2021.
[16] C. Bornemann, K. Woyk, and C. Bouter, "Case report: two cases of subacute thyroiditis following SARS-CoV-2 vaccination," *Frontiers of Medicine*, vol. 8, Article ID 737142, 24 August 2021.
[17] S. Franquemont and J. Galvez, "Subacute thyroiditis after mRNA vaccine for COVID-19," *Journal of the Endocrine Society*, vol. 5, p. A956, 2021.
[18] S. P. Kaur and V. Gupta, "COVID-19 vaccine: a comprehensive status report," *Virus Research*, vol. 288, Article ID 198114, 2020.
[19] M. Patel, M. Shahid, A. Khawaja, C. Ejike, and K. Vemuri, "Subacute thyroiditis secondary to moderna COVID-19 vaccine: a case report of a rare manifestation," *Advances in Clinical Medical Research and Healthcare Delivery*, vol. 1, no. 2, 2021.
[20] A. Simone, J. Herald, A. Chen et al., "Acute myocarditis following COVID-19 mRNA vaccination in adults aged 18 years or older," *JAMA Internal Medicine*, vol. 181, no. 12, p. 1668, 2021.
[21] M. Aemaz Ur Rehman, H. Farooq, M. M. Ali, M. Ebaad Ur Rehman, Q. A. Dar, and A. Hussain, "The association of subacute thyroiditis with COVID-19: a systematic review," *SN Comprehensive Clinical Medicine*, vol. 3, no. 7, pp. 1515–1527, 2021.

Severe Hypothyroidism and Large Goiter due to Iodine Deficiency in an Adolescent Male in the United States: A Case Report and Review of the Literature

Claire E. Moore,[1] Sabitha Sasidharan Pillai,[1,2] Juliana Austin,[3,4] Meghan E. Fredette,[1,2] and Monica Serrano-Gonzalez[1,2]

[1]*Department of Pediatrics, The Warren Alpert Medical School of Brown, Providence, RI, USA*
[2]*Division of Pediatric Endocrinology, Hasbro Children's Hospital, Providence, RI, USA*
[3]*Center for Endocrinology, Diabetes and Metabolism, Children's Hospital Los Angeles, Los Angeles, CA, USA*
[4]*Department of Pediatrics, Keck School of Medicine, University of Southern California, Los Angeles, CA, USA*

Correspondence should be addressed to Monica Serrano-Gonzalez; monica_serrano@brown.edu

Academic Editor: Toshihiro Kita

Acquired hypothyroidism due to iodine deficiency is extremely rare in the United States due to the introduction of table salt iodization in the 1920s (Leung et al., 2012). We present the case of an adolescent male with a history of mild autism spectrum disorder and an extremely restrictive diet who was found to have iodine deficiency as the etiology for his rapidly enlarging goiter and antibody-negative hypothyroidism. Thyroid-stimulating hormone (TSH) was 416 μIU/mL (0.350–5.500 μIU/mL), free thyroxine (T4) was <0.1 ng/dL (0.80–1.80 ng/dL), and triiodothyronine (T3) was 41 ng/dL (82–213 mg/dL) at diagnosis. The patient's 24-hour urinary iodine was undetectable. He was started on iodine supplementation with rapid visible improvement of goiter within two weeks and normalization of thyroid function tests within four weeks. Thorough dietary history and nutritional screening are important in cases of acquired hypothyroidism and/or goiter. Alternatively, diets that are low in iodized salt, dairy, bread, and seafood should raise concern for iodine deficiency, and patients with suspected or proven iodine deficiency should be screened for hypothyroidism.

1. Introduction

Iodine deficiency is uncommon in the United States and hence an uncommon cause of hypothyroidism. Trends in median urinary excretion of iodine as tracked by the National Health and Nutrition Examination Survey (NHANES) demonstrated that while the average individual in the United States is iodine sufficient, the median urinary iodine content has been decreasing over time. Fortunately, children's median urinary iodine excretion has been relatively stable (mean value of 190 μg/L from 2011-2014 data) [2].

Because there is no public-health mandate for salt iodization in the United States, personal dietary choices determine iodine sufficiency. A transition to less iodized forms of salt and health trends encouraging decreased salt intake may be two factors contributing to a reduction in iodide intake [3]. While primary sources of dietary iodine include fish, seafood, grains, and iodized salt, children and adolescents receive 53–70% of their daily iodide intake from dairy [4]. Iodine deficiency is diagnosed by urine iodine concentrations less than 100 mcg/L [5]. Iodine is necessary for the production of thyroid hormones (T3 and T4) and its deficiency leads to hypothyroidism [6].

We report the case of a 13-year-old male presenting with a rapidly enlarging goiter who was found to have markedly elevated TSH, undetectable free T4 and low total T3 levels, and negative autoimmune thyroiditis antibodies. Iodine deficiency was identified as the ultimate etiology of his

TABLE 1: Reported cases of dietary restriction causing iodine deficiency hypothyroidism.

	Kanaka et al. 1992 [7]	Leniszewski et al. 2009 [8]	BrooksMJ et al. 2014 [9]	Cheetham et al. 2015 [10]	Booms et al. 2016 [11]		Yeliosof et al. 2018 [12]	Our patient
					Case 1	Case 2		
Age at diagnosis	7.5 months	12 years	9 years	4 years	5 years	2 years	23 months	13 y
Cause of dietary restriction	Developmental delay, hypotonia, and vegan diet	Autism, multiple food allergies	Eosinophilic esophagitis and food allergies	Multiple food allergies	Autism, gluten, and casein free diet	Picky eater and dairy-free diet due to eczema	Strict vegan diet	Autism
Physical examination	Goiter	Goiter	Goiter	Goiter	Goiter	Normal thyroid gland	Goiter	Goiter
TSH (μIU/mL)	378 (0.3–4)	16.5 (0.5–4.5)	150.4 (0.6–4.84)	9.1 (0.3–4.7)	355 (0.47–4.53)	222.43 (0.30–5.50)	382 (0.7–5.9)	416 (0.35–5.50)
Free T4 (ng/dl)	0.2253 (0.77–2)	0.2 (0.8–2)	0.18 (0.9–1.68)	0.4894 (0.74–1.63)	0.18 (0.84–2.26)	0.24 (0.76–1.70)	<0.2 (0.85–1.75)	<0.1 (0.8–1.8)
Total T4 (ug/dl)		1.6 (4.5–10)					<0.5 (4.5–12)	
Free T3 (ng/dl)	0.4883 (0.20–0.55)	0.48 (0.34–0.48)			0.253 (0.2–0.5)			
Total T3 (ng/dl)							59(83–230)	41 (81–213)
TPO antibodies	Negative	Negative	Negative		Negative	Negative	Negative	Negative
Tg antibodies	Negative	Negative	Negative		Negative	Negative	Negative	Negative
Urine iodine (μg/L)	3.03 (6.58–42.66)	<10 (100–460)	—	10.1 (50–240)	11 (100–199)	20 (100–199)	—	<5 (26–705)
Thyroid ultrasound	—	Right lobe 7.4 × 4.0 × 2.6 cm, total volume 41 cc. Left lobe 7.8 × 3.2 × 2.9 cm, total volume 38 cc	Simple goiter	Thyroid gland enlargement with hypervascularity on doppler	Enlarged hyperemic gland, suggesting Hashimoto's thyroiditis	—	Right lobe −1.5 × 1.7 × 3.3 cm, left lobe 1.2 × 1.1 × 2.4 cm	Right lobe 8.3 × 3.7 × 4.6 cm. Left lobe 8.6 × 3.2 × 4.5 cm. Heterogeneous in echotexture with a lobular contour and diffuse hyperemia

hypothyroidism. We performed a literature review and identified 6 case reports from developed nations, describing 7 children aged 7.5 months to 12 years with hypothyroidism due to iodine deficiency (Table 1) [7–12].

2. Case Presentation

A 13-year-old male with a history of mild autism spectrum disorder, anxiety, and attention-deficit hyperactivity disorder presented to his pediatrician with neck swelling in the setting of two months of fatigue. He had been sleeping over twelve hours per day and did not have sufficient energy to complete his schoolwork. Based on the review of family photographs, thyroid enlargement may have started about two months prior to the initial clinic visit. The pediatrician noted significant goiter. Laboratory workup revealed elevated TSH of 416 μIU/mL (0.350–5.500 μIU/mL), low free T4 < 0.1 ng/dL (0.80–1.80 ng/dL), and low T3 41 ng/d (82–213 ng/dL). The complete blood count was normal. Ultrasound of the thyroid was interpreted by radiology as consistent with autoimmune thyroiditis (see Table 1 for detailed description and thyroid gland dimensions); however, thyroid peroxidase (TPO) and thyroglobulin (Tg) antibodies were negative. He was referred to pediatric endocrinology for further evaluation and management.

A review of the growth charts revealed growth deceleration starting at 10 years old, with height percentiles decreasing from the 60th to the 35th percentile and weight percentiles declining from the 75th to the 25th percentile. The mother reported a very restrictive diet. He ate specific brands of bread and peanut butter, neither of which contained iodine. His diet included some chicken but no seafood, fish, dairy, or processed or canned foods. He did not consume iodized table salt. Restriction of diet was largely related to the patient's preference for certain foods in the context of his autism spectrum disorder. In addition, a year prior to the presentation, the family had eliminated dairy from the patient's diet due to presumed lactose intolerance.

On examination, vital signs were within normal limits. Height was at the 36th percentile and weight was at the 54th percentile. Physical examination revealed symmetric, firm thyromegaly without distinct nodules. The right lobe measured 8 cm, and the left lobe measured 8.5 cm (Figure 1(a)).

Given his severe dietary restrictions, the possibility of iodine deficiency was considered. The patient was initially started on a low dose of levothyroxine (25 mcg daily [0.5 mcg/kg/day]) with a plan for slow, stepwise increases while his 24-hour urinary iodine was pending. Urinary iodine concentration from 24-hour collection resulted as <5.0 μg/L (26–705.0 μg/L), confirming severe iodine deficiency. He has been prescribed iodine supplementation of 150 mcg daily. Given his very restrictive diet, iron studies and vitamin levels were assessed. He was found to have mild iron deficiency (elevated total-iron binding capacity −505 μg/dL-with normal iron, ferritin, and hemoglobin) and vitamin C deficiency (serum vitamin C undetectable at <5 μmol/liter) and was started on a multivitamin with iron. Vitamins D and B12 were not deficient because he had already been receiving supplementation prior to the presentation.

Two weeks after iodine replacement, the family reported significant improvement in the size of his goiter, as well as his energy level (Figure 1(b)). Eggs were reintroduced successfully into his diet. Repeated laboratory evaluation one month after iodine initiation showed normalization of values with TSH of 0.707 μIU/mL (0.350–5.500 uIU/mL) and free T4 of 1.45 ng/dL (0.80–1.80 ng/dL). The small dose of levothyroxine was discontinued following these test results, and thyroid function remained normal on subsequent follow-ups after 2 months. On follow-up examination 5 months after iodine supplementation was started, the patient had a much decreased albeit persistent goiter, with the left lobe measuring 6.5 centimeters and the right lobe measuring 6.0 centimeters.

3. Discussion

Iodine is a necessary component for the synthesis of T3 and T4. Initially, with mild iodine deficiency, there is upregulation of sodium-iodide symporters to increase iodine uptake into the thyroid gland, and renal iodine excretion is reduced. As the severity of deficiency worsens, there is a preferential synthesis of T3 over T4. Severe and prolonged deficiency of dietary iodine leads to a decreased production of both T3 and T4 with a subsequent appropriate elevation of TSH [5]. TSH has the secondary effect of inducing hypertrophy and hyperplasia of the thyroid follicular cells that leads to goiter [15]. Initially, goiters are smooth; however, with long-standing deficiency, patients can develop thyroid nodules which are associated with an increased risk of thyroid cancer [16].

The necessary iodine intake to maintain sufficiency varies by age. The World Health Organization recommends 90 μg per day for children under 5 years, 120 μg per day for children aged 6–12,150 μg per day for adolescents over the age of 12 and adults, and 250 μg per day for pregnant and lactating women. For our adolescent patient, a target supplementation of 100–299 μg would avoid both insufficiency and excess [5].

When unacknowledged, iodine deficiency not only leads to hypothyroidism but can impair growth and cognitive development [17]. There are few modern case reports of iodine deficiency in developed nations secondary to diets restricted for autism spectrum disorder, food aversion, and food allergies (Table 1) [7–12]. All except two patients were treated with iodine supplementation. One patient was treated with kelp capsules containing 400 ug of iodine/capsule per parental request [9] and another with oral aversion was given nasogastric feeds rich in iodine content resulting in the normalization of thyroid function tests [11]. Ikomi et al. reported iodine deficiency in 85% (17/20) and acquired hypothyroidism in 33% (8/27) of patients younger than 17 years on parenteral nutrition for more than 6 months. No significant association was observed between the duration of parenteral nutrition and iodine deficiency or hypothyroidism [18].

Because the body relies exclusively on iodide ingestion through diet or supplementation to achieve iodine sufficiency, changes in personal or family dietary patterns would

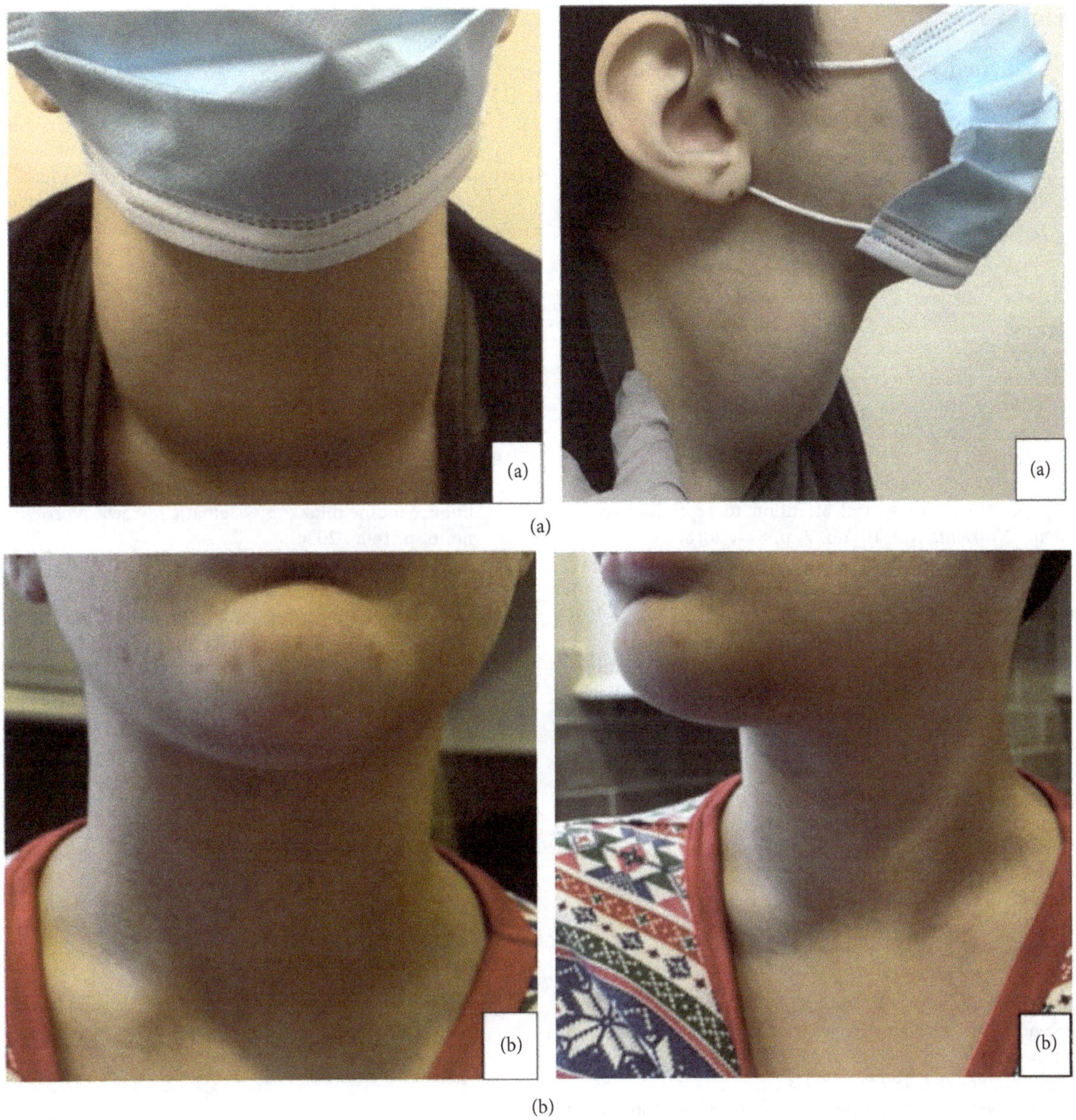

Figure 1: (a) Visible goiter at the initial endocrinology visit and (b) virtual follow-up two weeks after treatment initiation.

explain why some children are iodine deficient. In addition to health concerns about excessive salt consumption, there have been trends toward more specialized diets recently. Patients with vegan diets rely primarily on iodized table salt or foods such as seaweed for their iodine content [19] and are thus at high risk for iodine deficiency. A study on women in Boston found that a majority of vegetarians and vegans studied had not consumed iodized table salt in the last 24 hours and were not on an iodine-containing multivitamin [20].

Management of iodine deficiency involves reintroducing iodine into the diet. Thyroid function tests rapidly normalize after repletion, and levothyroxine, if started, can be discontinued. The patients' large goiters also improve quickly with near resolution noted at three-monthfollow-up visits [8, 21]. Ongoing monitoring of thyroid function tests should be performed as thyrotoxicosis can develop secondary to iodine supplementation [21].

The present case highlights the importance of thorough dietary history and nutritional screenings in cases of hypothyroidism and/or goiter. Diets that are low in iodized salt, dairy, bread, and seafood should raise concern for iodine deficiency and prompt urinary testing by 24-hour urine collection, which produces more reliable values than testing from spot urine collections [22]. Patients with suspected or proven iodine deficiency due to restrictive diets or parenteral nutrition should be screened for hypothyroidism. Repletion and maintenance of dietary iodine are expected to lead to prompt resolution of symptoms of hypothyroidism.

Abbreviations

TSH: Thyroid-stimulating hormone
T4: Thyroxine
T3: Triiodothyronine
NHANES: National health and nutrition examination survey
TPO: Thyroid peroxidase
Tg: Thyroglobulin.

References

[1] A. M. Leung, L. E. Braverman, and E. N. Pearce, "History of U.S. iodine fortification and supplementation," *Nutrients*, vol. 4, no. 11, pp. 1740–1746, 2012.

[2] K. A. Herrick, C. G. Perrine, Y. Aoki, and K. L. Caldwell, "Iodine status and consumption of key iodine sources in the U.S. population with special attention to reproductive age women," *Nutrients*, vol. 10, no. 7, p. 874, 2018.

[3] A. G. Ershow, J. Gahche, N. Potischman, J. Spungen, and P. Pehrsson, "Abstract P359: assessment of household salt types, iodine intake, and iodine status in 2019-2020 NHANES," *Circulation*, vol. 141, no. 1, 2020.

[4] C. W. Murray, S. K. Egan, H. Kim, N. Beru, and P. M. Bolger, "US food and drug administration's total diet study: dietary intake of perchlorate and iodine," *Journal of Exposure Science and Environmental Epidemiology*, vol. 18, no. 6, pp. 571–580, 2008.

[5] World Health Organization, United Nations Children's Fund, and International Council for the Control of Iodine Deficiency Disorders, *Assessment of Iodine Deficiency Disorders and Monitoring their Elimination*, WHO, Geneva, Switzerland, 3rd edition, 2007.

[6] M. B. Zimmermann and K. Boelaert, "Iodine deficiency and thyroid disorders," *Lancet Diabetes & Endocrinology*, vol. 3, no. 4, pp. 286–295, 2015.

[7] C. Kanaka, B. Schütz, and K. A. Zuppinger, "Risks of alternative nutrition in infancy: a case report of severe iodine and carnitine deficiency," *European Journal of Pediatrics*, vol. 151, no. 10, pp. 786–788, 1992.

[8] S. Leniszewski and R. Mauseth, "Goiter and multiple food allergies," *International Journal of Pediatric Endocrinology*, vol. 2009, Article ID 628034, 3 pages, 2009.

[9] M. J. Brooks and E. M. Post, "Acquired hypothyroidism due to iodine deficiency in an American child," *Journal of Pediatric Endocrinology and Metabolism*, vol. 27, no. 11-12, pp. 1233–1235, 2014.

[10] T. Cheetham, E. Plumb, J. Callaghan, M. Jackson, and L. Michaelis, "Dietary restriction causing iodine-deficient goitre," *Archives of Disease in Childhood*, vol. 100, no. 8, pp. 784–786, 2015.

[11] S. Booms, E. Hill, L. Kulhanek, J. Vredeveld, and B. Gregg, "Iodine deficiency and hypothyroidism from voluntary diet restrictions in the US: case reports," *Pediatrics*, vol. 137, no. 6, Article ID e20154003, 2016.

[12] O. Yeliosof and L. A. Silverman, "Veganism as a cause of iodine deficient hypothyroidism," *Journal of Pediatric Endocrinology and Metabolism*, vol. 31, no. 1, pp. 91–94, 2018.

[13] E. N. Pearce, A. P. Farwell, and L. E. Braverman, "Thyroiditis," *New England Journal of Medicine*, vol. 348, no. 26, pp. 2646–2655, 2003.

[14] M. Rotondi, L. de Martinis, F. Coperchini et al., "Serum negative autoimmune thyroiditis displays a milder clinical picture compared with classic Hashimoto's thyroiditis," *European Journal of Endocrinology*, vol. 171, no. 1, pp. 31–36, 2014.

[15] M. B. Zimmermann, P. L. Jooste, and C. S. Pandav, "Iodine-deficiency disorders," *The Lancet*, vol. 372, no. 9645, pp. 1251–1262, 2008.

[16] M. B. Zimmermann and V. Galetti, "Iodine intake as a risk factor for thyroid cancer: a comprehensive review of animal and human studies," *Thyroid Research*, vol. 8, no. 1, p. 8, 2015.

[17] K. L. Caldwell, A. Makhmudov, E. Ely, R. L. Jones, and R. Y. Wang, "Iodine status of the U.S. population, national health and nutrition examination survey, 2005–2006 and 2007–2008," *Thyroid*, vol. 21, no. 4, pp. 419–427, 2011.

[18] C. Ikomi, C. R. Cole, E. Vale, M. Golekoh, J. C. Khoury, and N. H. Y. Jones, "Hypothyroidism and iodine deficiency in children on chronic parenteral nutrition," *Pediatrics*, vol. 141, no. 4, Article ID e20173046, 2018.

[19] E. R. Eveleigh, L. J. Coneyworth, A. Avery, S. J. M. Welham, Vegetarians, and Omnivores, "How does dietary choice influence iodine intake? a systematic review," *Nutrients*, vol. 12, no. 6, p. 1606, 2020.

[20] A. M. Leung, A. Lamar, X. He, L. E. Braverman, and E. N. Pearce, "Iodine status and thyroid function of Boston-area vegetarians and vegans," *The Journal of Clinical Endocrinology & Metabolism*, vol. 96, no. 8, pp. E1303–E1307, 2011.

[21] I. Goyal, M. R. Pandey, and R. Sharma, "Hypothyroidism and goiter in a young male with suspected dietary iodine deficiency followed by thyrotoxicosis after iodine supplementation," *AACE Clinical Case Reports*, vol. 6, no. 1, pp. e19–e22, 2020.

[22] W. Chen, Y. Wu, L. Lin et al., "24-hour urine samples are more reproducible than spot urine samples for evaluation of iodine status in school-age children," *The Journal of Nutrition*, vol. 146, no. 1, pp. 142–146, 2016.

A Case Report of Subacute Thyroiditis following mRNA COVID-19 Vaccine

Leidy Plaza-Enriquez,[1] **P. Khatiwada**,[1] **M. Sanchez-Valenzuela**,[2] **and A. Sikha**[1]

[1]*Department of Internal Medicine, Memorial Healthcare System, Hollywood, FL, USA*
[2]*Internal Medicine Residency, St. Barnabas Hospital, Bronx, NY, USA*

Correspondence should be addressed to Leidy Plaza-Enriquez; leidyplaza94@hotmail.com

Academic Editor: Wei Wu

Background. Subacute thyroiditis has been reported after administration of influenza vaccine. We describe a case of a patient who developed subacute thyroiditis after administration of. Moderna mRNA COVID-19 vaccine. *Case Presentation.* A 42-year-old female, with a past medical history of stage IIIB pT3N1aM0 right adenocarcinoma of colon status, after right hemicolectomy on 01/2020, followed by adjuvant chemotherapy, paroxysmal supraventricular tachycardia, iron deficiency anemia, chemotherapy-induced neuropathy, and lumbar radiculopathy, presented to our clinic with anterior neck pain that started 6 days after the second dose of Moderna mRNA COVID-19 vaccine. She was diagnosed with subacute thyroiditis and treated conservatively with pain medications. *Conclusion.* Subacute thyroiditis could represent one of the side effects of Moderna mRNA COVID-19 vaccine. Further reports are lacking.

1. Introduction

Subacute thyroiditis is a well-known clinical diagnosis, usually presenting one to two weeks after an acute viral infection, including COVID-19 [1,2]. Symptoms fluctuate in intensity and last for 3 to 6 weeks. Laboratory investigations show high erythrocyte sedimentation rate (ESR), elevated C-reactive protein (CRP), and suppressed TSH with elevated free T4 and T3 [2]. Treatment with analgesics is recommended, and prednisone if poor improvement [2,3].

Subacute thyroiditis has been reported after administration of influenza and COVID-19 vaccines [1,4–6]. We present a case of subacute thyroiditis after administration of an mRNA COVID-19 vaccine. To our knowledge, this is the first case report of subacute thyroiditis after Moderna mRNA COVID-19 vaccine.

2. Case Report

A 42-year-old African American female with a past medical history of stage IIIB pT3N1aM0 right adenocarcinoma of colon status after right hemicolectomy on 01/2020, followed by adjuvant chemotherapy, paroxysmal supraventricular tachycardia, iron deficiency anemia, chemotherapy-induced neuropathy, and lumbar radiculopathy, presented to our primary-care clinic on the first week of March 2021 complaining of bilateral ear pain for 2 weeks. The patient was treated with 9 cycles of FOLFOX regimen (fluorouracil, oxaliplatin, and leucovorin) for her colon carcinoma and completed her chemotherapy on 09/2020. She received her 1st dose of Moderna mRNA COVID-19 vaccine on 02/05/2021 and the second dose on 03/05/2021. Symptoms started about 5–6 days after the vaccination. She began experiencing right-sided and then left-sided earache radiating down to the lateral and anterior neck and bilateral lower jaw. The pain was exacerbated by turning her head, swallowing, and coughing. She denied fever, fatigue, malaise, anorexia, myalgia, dysphagia, dysphonia, dyspnea cough, rhinorrhea, lacrimation, and ear discharge. She has no history of thyroid disease and/or head and neck radiation exposure. The patient denied any family history of head and neck cancer. She denied smoking cigarettes, but drinks alcohol socially. Her home medications included Metoprolol 25 mg two times a day, vitamin B12 1000 mcg once daily, ferrous sulfate 325 mg two times a day, and multivitamin capsule 1 capsule daily.

Her vitals at the time of presentation were a temperature of 35.9°C, pulse 88 beats/min, blood pressure 111/75 mm of Hg, respiratory rate 17 breaths/min, and oxygen saturation 97% on room air. Physical examination was notable for anterior neck swelling about 3 cm in size which was tender on palpation.

Routine laboratory investigations showed WBC 6.4 (3.5–10.0 1000/uL), hemoglobin 13.2 g/dL (1.4–15.4 g/dL), platelets 207 (150–450 1000/uL), BUN 10 mg/dL (7–18 mg/dL) creatinine 0.43 (0.51–0.95 mg/dL), and normal electrolyte level and liver function test. Laboratory investigations were significant for low serum TSH < 0.0005 IU/ml (0.350–4.000 IU/ml), low serum T3 1.90 ng/dL (0.60–1.81 ng/mL), and normal free T4-1.51 ng/dL (0.80–2.00 ng/dL). TSH the week prior to COVID-19 vaccination, obtained as a part of fatigue workup, was 2.030 IU/ml (0.350–4.000 IU/ml). ESR was elevated 81 mm/hour. Thyroid peroxidase antibodies were negative <10 (<35 IU/ml). Ultrasound of the thyroid revealed a 1.6 × 1.4 × 3.4 cm heterogeneous mass in the right lobe and a 1.6 × 1.8 × 3.4 cm hypoechoic and moderately heterogeneous mass in the left lobe (Figures 1 and 2) without calcifications, associated with mildly enlarged inferior left paratracheal lymph nodes.

The patient was treated with analgesics as needed for pain, until she underwent ultrasound-guided fine-needle aspiration biopsy of the bilateral 3.4 cm thyroid masses in April 2021. Biopsy results showed scattered multinucleated giant cells (some with ingested colloid), scattered epithelioid granulomas, groups of follicular cells, scattered lymphocytes, and karyorrhexis. These features were consistent with a benign hyperplastic nodule suggestive of subacute (de Quervain) thyroiditis. Cytopathology was benign (Bethesda Category II). During this time period, she had minimal symptoms and was treated with NSAIDs as needed for pain. On a subsequent follow-up visit, 2 months after the biopsy, previously described anterior neck discomfort and earache radiating to the neck resolved. Her follow-up labs obtained on 06/2021 showed TSH 8.80 (0.350–4.000 IU/ml), free T4 0.65 ng/dL (0.80–2.00 ng/dL), total T3 1.20 ng/ml (0.60–1.81 ng/ml), and ESR 14 mm/hour.

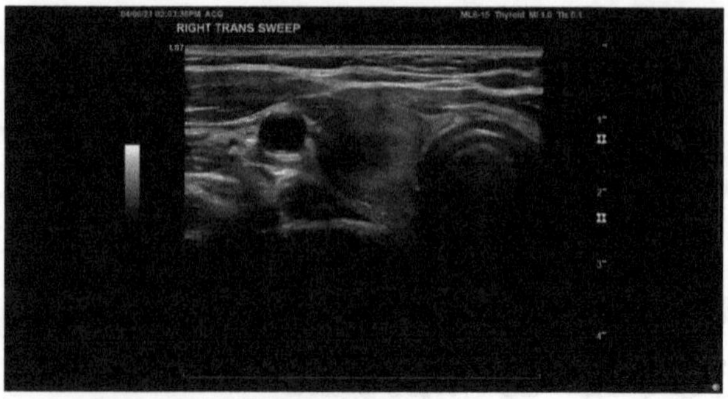

Figure 1: Ultrasound of the right thyroid lobe showing a heterogeneous mass.

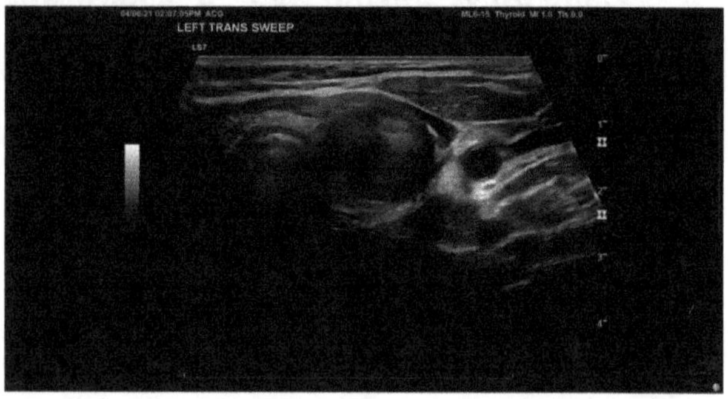

Figure 2: Ultrasound of the left thyroid lobe showing a heterogeneous mass.

3. Discussion

Subacute thyroiditis is a relatively uncommon cause of hyperthyroidism that has been associated with upper respiratory viruses, such as influenza, mumps, and other respiratory viruses, but few cases have been reported after inactivated viral vaccines or live-attenuated vaccines such as those for influenza [1,4,5]. This condition is characterized by neck pain, a tender goiter, and a thyroid dysfunction. We present a case of a female with classic symptoms of subacute thyroiditis after Moderna mRNA COVID-19 vaccine administration. Thyroiditis has been reported as a possible side effect of COVID-19 vaccine in 4 cases thus far [3,5], one case after CoronaVac® administration [5] and the other with Pfizer mRNA COVID-19 vaccine [3]. Cross recognition between the coronavirus spike protein targeted with mRNA vaccine and thyroid cell antigens is likely the mechanism. Differential diagnosis includes Graves' disease, toxic multinodular goiter, and pharyngitis, but after the administration of a vaccine, subacute thyroiditis should be suspected. Further reports are lacking; however, clinicians should consider subacute thyroiditis after administration of mRNA COVID-19 vaccines as a possible side effect.

Abbreviations

ESR: Erythrocyte sedimentation rate
CRP: C-reactive protein
TSH: Thyroid-stimulating hormone
T3: Triiodothyronine
T4: Thyroxine.

Consent

Informed consent for publication was obtained from the patient.

Acknowledgments

This work was supported by the Graduated Medical Education Department of Memorial Healthcare System, Florida.

References

[1] P. Trimboli, C. Camponovo, S. Franscella, E. Bernasconi, and N. Buetti, "Subacute thyroiditis during the COVID-19 pandemic: searching for a clinical association with SARS-CoV-2," *International Journal of Endocrinology*, vol. 2021, Article ID 5588592, 4 pages, 2021.

[2] H. Jv, *Subacute Thyroiditis*, K. R. Feingold, B. Anawalt, and A. Boyce, Eds., MDText.Com, Inc., South Dartmouth, MA, USA, 2000.

[3] S. Franquemont and J. Galvez, "Subacute thyroiditis after mRNA vaccine for covid-19," *Journal of the Endocrine Society*, vol. 5, no. 1, p. A956, 2021.

[4] C. M. Girgis, R. R. Russo, and K. Benson, "Subacute thyroiditis following the H1N1 vaccine," *Journal of Endocrinological Investigation*, vol. 33, no. 7, p. 506, 2010.

[5] B. G. İremli, S. N. Şendur, and U. Ünlütürk, "Three cases of subacute thyroiditis following SARS-CoV-2 vaccine: postvaccination ASIA syndrome," *Journal of Clinical Endocrinology & Metabolism*, vol. 106, no. 9, 2021.

[6] M. Şahin Tekin, S. Şaylısoy, and G. Yorulmaz, "Subacute thyroiditis following COVID-19 vaccination in a 67-year-old male patient: a case report," *Human Vaccines & Immunotherapeutics*, pp. 1–3, 2021.

38

Thyrotoxic Periodic Paralysis Causing Back Pain and Leg Weakness: An Unusual Presentation of Hyperthyroidism

Henrik Elenius, Marie Cesa, Corina C. Nava Suarez, Abhishek Nimkar, Prasanta Basak, and Nandita Sinha

Montefiore New Rochelle Hospital, 16 Guion Pl, New Rochelle, NY 10801, USA

Correspondence should be addressed to Henrik Elenius; melenius@montefiore.org

Academic Editor: Osamu Isozaki

Thyrotoxic periodic paralysis (TPP) is a rare muscular disorder, characterized by muscle weakness and hypokalemia triggered by thyrotoxicosis. In Asian populations, 2% of patients with thyrotoxicosis are affected, compared to only 0.1–0.2% of non-Asians. The vast majority of patients are male. Muscle weakness ranges in severity from very mild to life-threatening, due to respiratory compromise. We present a case of a previously healthy 39-year-old Hispanic male who presented with sudden quadriparesis and quickly recovered after being treated for hypokalemia and thyrotoxicosis. TPP, although unusual, is important to recognize as it is a potentially fatal condition that requires close monitoring and is readily reversible with appropriate therapy. Any cause of thyroid hormone excess can cause TPP, with Graves' disease being the most common etiology. Acute treatment includes potassium repletion, while long-term management focuses on determining and treating the cause of thyrotoxicosis, since maintaining a euthyroid state will prevent further episodes of TPP.

1. Introduction

Periodic paralysis is a rare group of muscular disorders characterized by episodes of muscle weakness in combination with hypo- or hyperkalemia. Most cases are familial, but a small subset of cases, designated thyrotoxic periodic paralysis (TPP), are acquired with thyrotoxicosis triggering episodes of paralysis and hypokalemia. While hyperthyroidism is more common in females, >95% of patients with TPP are male. TPP is also significantly more common in Asian populations, affecting 2% of Asians with thyrotoxicosis, compared to 0.1–0.2% of non-Asians [1]. Although unusual, it is important to recognize TPP, as it is a potentially fatal condition which is readily reversible with appropriate therapy.

We present a case of a 39-year-old Hispanic male with no past medical history who presented with sudden quadriparesis and quickly recovered after being treated for hypokalemia and thyrotoxicosis.

2. Case Presentation

A 39-year-old Venezuelan man with no past medical history presented to the emergency room with recurring, cramping pain in his lower back and legs, along with mild bilateral leg weakness for 1 month. These symptoms would return every afternoon, when the patient came home from his job in demolition, and then resolve by the following morning. Over the same period of time, he had also experienced intermittent palpitations at rest, hand tremors and excessive sweating. The day before presentation, his pain and weakness got significantly worse, causing a fall while walking. On the morning of presentation, he was unable to ambulate without support due to severe leg weakness. His lower back pain was described as sharp, 8/10 intensity, exacerbated by movement and radiating down his legs to both feet. Prior to his symptoms starting in the preceding month, he had never experienced similar episodes in the past. The patient also noted a 5 kg unintentional weight loss over 4 months. He denied any recent injuries, constipation, diarrhea, problems with urination, vomiting, recent travel, recent illness, new medications or supplements. He had no heredity for muscle or thyroid problems. He had never had any thyroid issues, and blood work as part of a routine check up had reportedly been normal 5 months prior, although these results were not available for review.

Vital signs were only notable for a heart rate of 98 beats per minute. Physical exam was notable for proximal weakness in all extremities, with the patient only being able to move his limbs against minimal resistance. Additionally, decreased range of motion was seen on bilateral hip flexion and right shoulder abduction owing to sharp pain on movement. Deep tendon reflexes were reduced in all extremities. Sensation was intact. Symmetrical hand tremors were noted with arms outstretched. Bilateral exophthalmos was noted. Cranial nerves were intact, and no diplopia was seen. Thyroid exam was unremarkable, without any enlargement, nodules or tenderness noted. No further abnormalities were noted on systemic examination.

A CT of the lumbar spine was unremarkable, with no significant central canal stenosis or neural foraminal narrowing. Laboratory findings, reviewed in Table 1, revealed low levels of potassium, 1.7 mmol/L; magnesium, 1.3 mEq/L; and phosphorus, 1.5 mg/dL. A complete blood count and the remainder of the comprehensive metabolic panel were both normal. Thyroid function tests showed a low thyroid-stimulating hormone (TSH), 0.010 mIU/mL as well as elevated free T4, 2.98 ng/mL and total T3, 399 ng/dL. Further thyroid testing revealed elevated thyroid-stimulating immunoglobulin (TSI); 278% of baseline; thyroglobulin antibodies, 20.0 IU/mL; and thyroid peroxidase antibodies, 180.0 IU/mL. An ECG was notable for inverted T-waves followed by U-waves in leads II, III, AvF, and V3–V6 (Figure 1).

The patient was given a total of 90 mEq of oral potassium chloride on the day of admission. Magnesium and phosphorus were repleted as well. In addition, he was started on oral methimazole (40 mg, twice daily) and propranolol (40 mg, three times daily) on admission. By the next morning, his potassium level had normalized, and his weakness and back pain had resolved completely. He was discharged on beta-blockers and methimazole. After discharge, the patient struggled with medication compliance due to financial constraints. As of the last follow-up, three months after discharge, he had resumed his medications with reported resolution of all symptoms. He was planned to receive radioactive iodine therapy, but was eventually lost to follow-up.

Table 1: Initial laboratory investigations.

Lab	Value	Reference	Units
Potassium	1.7	3.5–5.0	mmol/L
Magnesium	1.3	1.5–2.2	mEq/L
Phosphorus	1.5	2.6–4.9	mg/dL
TSH	0.010	0.450–5.330	mIU/ml
Free T4	2.98	0.58–1.64	ng/mL
Total T3	399	76–181	ng/dL
TSI	278	<140	% of baseline
Thyroglobulin antibodies	20.0	≤1	IU/mL
Thyroid peroxidase antibodies	180.0	<9	IU/mL

3. Discussion

This case highlights TPP, a rare condition, especially in a patient without Asian heritage. TPP is characterized by episodes of sudden generalized weakness, with the age of onset being 20–39 in 80% of patients, unlike familial cases of periodic paralysis, which usually debut in childhood or adolescence. Symptoms of hyperthyroidism develop around the onset of TPP in around 25% of patients, but can also appear years earlier or later [2]. Our patient had symptoms for a few months prior to developing TPP, with weight loss, palpitations, heat intolerance and tremors noted. The muscle weakness in TPP is predominant in proximal muscles, with legs being more affected than arms. Decreased muscle tone with decreased reflexes is typical [3]. Myalgia is seen in around 40% of patients and can occur before or concurrently with the paralytic attack [4]. Episodes typically last from several hours to days. Apart from hypokalemia, both hypomagnesemia and hypophosphatemia are common, as seen in our patient. ECG findings include those consistent with hypokalemia (decreased T-wave amplitudes, U-waves, and widened QRS-complexes), but also sinus tachycardia, 1st degree AV block and arrhythmias, including atrial and ventricular fibrillation [3].

While not completely understood, TPP is thought to be caused by skeletal muscle ion channel dysfunction. Varying degrees of hypokalemia are seen, with the severity often correlating with the degree of muscle weakness [2]. The inwardly rectifying potassium channel Kir2.6, which contributes to the resting potential of mainly skeletal muscle, has been linked to TPP, with up to 33% of patients in certain populations having mutations in its gene, KCNJ18. Notably, the gene has a thyroid response element in its promoter, suggesting that thyrotoxicosis would alter its transcription [5]. Skeletal muscle Na/K ATPase overactivity has also been suggested, leading to an excessive intracellular shift of potassium and inexcitability of muscle fibers. Thyroid hormone increases Na/K ATPase activity both by itself and also indirectly by increasing sensitivity to beta-adrenergic stimulation [1]. It has been hypothesized that patients with TPP have mild ion channel defects which only become significant enough to cause symptoms in the setting of thyrotoxicosis, through the mechanisms described above [6]. In addition, insulin and testosterone are both thought to act synergistically to increase Na/K ATPase activity, with the latter providing a potential explanation for why TPP is seen almost exclusively in males [4]. One study [7] found that patients with TPP had higher levels of testosterone and an increased release of insulin in response to glucose as compared to hyperthyroid patients without TPP, further pointing to the contributory roles of these hormones. Episodes of TPP are sometimes triggered by intense exercise and high-carbohydrate meals, which could be explained by increased levels of beta-adrenergic agonists and insulin, respectively [1, 4]. With this in mind, it is interesting to note that our patient had a physically strenuous job and would regularly experience leg weakness after coming home from work in the weeks leading up to his admission.

Our patient presented with a history of back pain and leg weakness suggestive of nerve root or spinal compression, but no signs of either were seen on a CT of the lumbar spine. While myalgia is not a hallmark of TPP, it does occur and can be misleading. Our patient was noted to be weak in his upper extremities as well. While other causes for acute quadriparesis

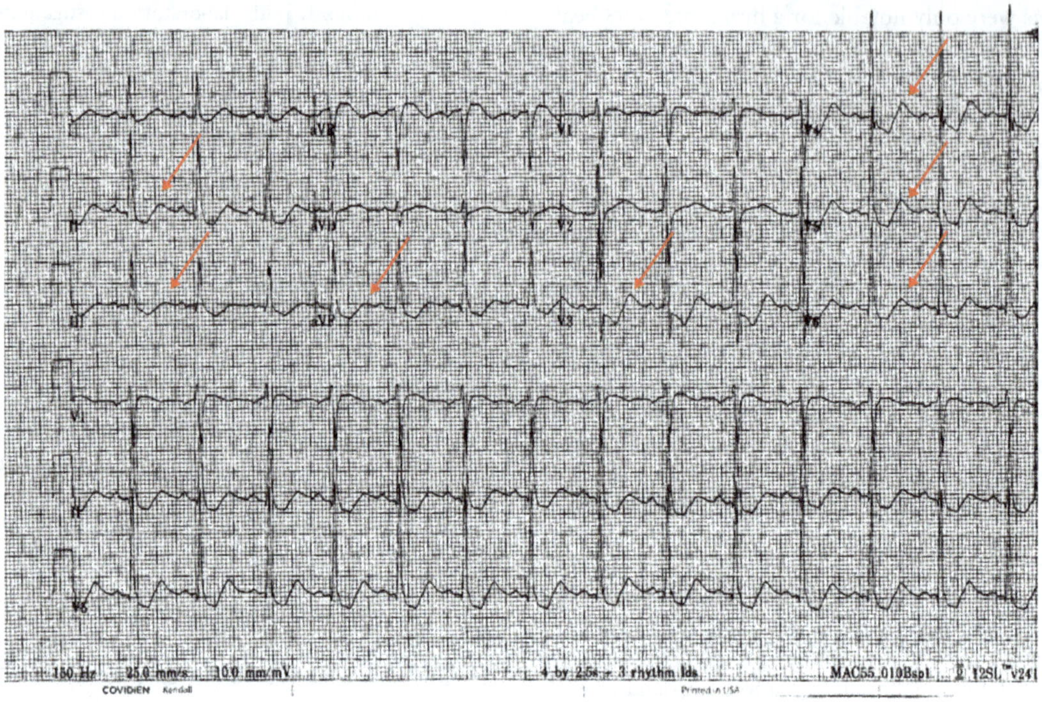

Figure 1: Admission ECG showing inverted T-waves followed by U-waves (red arrows) in leads II, III, AvF, and V3–V6, a sign of hypokalemia.

(e.g., myasthenia gravis or Guillain–Barré syndrome) must be considered, concurrent hypokalemia should alert the clinician to consider TPP and hypokalemic periodic paralysis, a hereditary, more common diagnosis which presents virtually identically. Thyroid function tests should be obtained to distinguish between these two conditions. Muscle weakness in TPP can range from mild to severe and, rarely, life-threatening due to respiratory compromise. Potassium repletion shortens the time to recovery, with muscle strength usually returning to normal once normokalemia is achieved. A maximum of 90 mEq oral potassium is recommended per 24-hour period to prevent rebound hyperkalemia, which is seen in around half of patients. Refractory hypokalemia can be treated with nonselective beta-blockers (e.g., propranolol), which may also be beneficial for potential concurrent symptoms of thyrotoxicosis [3]. Cardiac monitoring is recommended during treatment since fatal arrhythmias (e.g., sinus arrest and ventricular fibrillation) secondary to hypokalemia have been described, although rare. Any cause of thyrotoxicosis, including exogenous hyperthyroidism, can cause TPP. Graves' disease, as seen in our patient, is the most common underlying disorder. Once stabilized, the goal is to investigate the etiology of thyrotoxicosis and provide appropriate treatment since maintaining a euthyroid state will prevent further episodes of TPP [1].

4. Conclusion

Thyrotoxic periodic paralysis is a muscular disorder which can complicate thyrotoxicosis of any etiology. Due to its rare nature, a high index of suspicion is required for diagnosis in patients who present with muscle weakness, hypokalemia and symptoms of thyrotoxicosis. Patients need to be closely monitored due to the risks of respiratory failure and cardiac arrhythmias. Acute episodes will resolve with restoration of normokalemia, while treatment of the underlying cause of thyrotoxicosis will prevent recurrence.

Acknowledgments

This research was conducted as part of the employment of the authors at Montefiore New Rochelle Hospital, New Rochelle, NY.

References

[1] S.-H. Lin, "Thyrotoxic p eriodic p aralysis," *M ay oC linic Proceedings*, vol. 80, no. 1, pp. 99–105, 2005.

[2] K. P. Ober, "Thyrotoxic periodic paralysis in the united states. report of 7 cases and review of the literature," *Medicine*, vol. 71, no. 3, pp. 109–120, 1992.

[3] L. Lam, R. J. Nair, and L. Tingle, "Thyrotoxic p eriodic paralysis," *Bay lor University Medical Center Proceedings*, vol. 19, no. 2, pp. 126–129, 2006.

[4] M.-J. Hsieh, R.-K. Lyu, W.-N. Chang et al., "Hypokalemic thyrotoxic periodic paralysis: clinical characteristics and predictors of recurrent paralytic attacks," *European Journal of Neurology*, vol. 15, no. 6, pp. 559–564, 2008.

[5] D. P. Ryan, M. R. Dias da Silva, T. W. Soong et al., "Mutations in potassium channel Kir2.6 cause susceptibility to thyrotoxic hypokalemic periodic paralysis," *Cell*, vol. 140, no. 1, pp. 88–98, 2010.
[6] E. J. Gallagher, "Is thyrotoxic periodic paralysis a "channelopathy"?" *Journal of Emergency Medicine*, vol. 17, no. 1, pp. 123–128, 1999.
[7] W. Li, C. Changsheng, F. Jiangfang et al., "Effects of sex steroid hormones, thyroid hormone levels, and insulin regulation on thyrotoxic periodic paralysis in Chinese men," *Endocrine*, vol. 38, no. 3, pp. 386–390, 2010.

39

Acute Bacterial Suppurative Thyroiditis following Fine Needle Aspiration: A Case Report and Review of the Literature

Zaw Win Htet,[1] **E. Shyong Tai**,[2] **and Samantha Peiling Yang**[2]

[1]*Division of Endocrinology, Department of Medicine, National University Hospital, Level 10, NUHS Tower Block, 1E Kent Ridge Road, Singapore 119228*
[2]*Division of Endocrinology, Department of Medicine, Yong Loo Lin School of Medicine, National University of Singapore, Level 10, NUHS Tower Block, 1E Kent Ridge Road, Singapore 119228*

Correspondence should be addressed to Zaw Win Htet; win_htet_zaw@nuhs.edu.sg

Academic Editor: Osamu Isozaki

Background. Fine needle aspiration (FNA) of thyroid nodules is a simple, reliable, and inexpensive procedure performed on suspicious thyroid nodules found in thyroid ultrasound (US). Acute bacterial suppurative thyroiditis is an uncommon complication of FNA which, however, can be life threatening. *Case Presentation.* A 49-year-old lady presented with fever and neck pain 1 month after FNA with biochemical evidence of thyrotoxicosis. Repeat US of the thyroid showed interval enlargement of the thyroid nodule, and the culture of the cystic fluid of repeat FNA grew *Propionibacterium acnes*. She responded well to bedside aspiration and 2 weeks of antibiotic therapy without requiring surgical intervention. *Discussion.* Acute bacterial suppurative thyroiditis following FNA has been increasingly reported in immunocompetent hosts. There are 2 peculiar features in our case: a smoldering course caused by an indolent organism and a significant time lag between initial FNA and clinical presentation. On literature review, it was found that the onset of acute bacterial suppurative thyroiditis after FNA can range from a few days to up to 3 months. Clinicians should be aware of this complication even if FNA has been performed a few months ago. Thyroid US and US-guided FNA are useful initial investigations. Conventional management of acute bacterial suppurative thyroiditis has been surgery combined with antimicrobial therapy. However, recently, a more conservative approach has been reported to be effective in the treatment of acute bacterial suppurative thyroiditis as well. *Conclusion.* Proper infection control practices are necessary in performing the FNA. Initial management (conservative versus surgical) of acute bacterial thyroiditis should be based on the patient's clinical status and the extent of infective focus.

1. Introduction

Fine needle aspiration (FNA) of thyroid nodules is a simple, reliable, and inexpensive procedure performed on suspicious thyroid nodules found in thyroid ultrasound (US) [1]. We present an unusual complication of FNA causing acute bacterial thyroiditis. Our case is the second case of anaerobic acute bacterial thyroiditis following FNA reported in the available literature. This patient's clinical presentation is peculiar as she presented with thyrotoxicosis and had no known congenital piriform sinus fistula and immunodeficiency risk factors. We also reviewed the available literature on acute bacterial thyroiditis following FNA and outlined its pathophysiology and management.

2. Case Presentation

A 49-year-old female with the background history of hypertension, hyperlipidaemia, and presumed transient ischemic attack (TIA) presented to our endocrine clinic in November 2017 with an anterior neck lump of 1-year duration. The baseline thyroid function test was normal, and fine needle aspiration cytology (FNAC) of the thyroid nodule previously performed in another hospital revealed scanty yield of follicular cells consistent with nodular goitre. The initial US thyroid report and prior thyroid nodule dimension were unavailable. On examination, a right thyroid nodule was noted, measuring 3 cm by 4 cm. There was no palpably enlarged cervical lymph node, or tracheal deviation, and Pemberton's sign was negative. US thyroid performed in November 2017 showed a 4.7 cm × 3.1 cm × 1.7 cm mixed solid-cystic thyroid nodule in the right mid to lower pole, with comet-tail artefact and peripheral vascularity (Figure 1). In view of the size of the thyroid nodule and the lack of objective measure of growth (baseline nodule size not known), a repeat US-guided FNAC of this thyroid nodule was performed on 7 Feb 2018, and this showed a benign colloid nodule with cystic degeneration. As such, a follow-up plan at 1 year was made. The patient represented to our clinic on 6 March 2018, complaining of pain over the thyroid nodule and fever of 39 degree Celsius for 1-day duration. Upper respiratory tract infective symptoms were also present. Oral antibiotics (cloxacillin and clarithromycin) were started for the presumptive diagnosis of infected thyroid cyst. In view of the presence of pain from a patient with pre-existing thyroid cyst, the differential diagnosis was that of haemorrhage into the thyroid cyst. She was planned for close outpatient follow-up. However, the patient presented to the Emergency Department on 13 March 2018 for persistent fever and neck pain and was admitted for further treatment.

On admission, the patient had hand tremors and tenderness over her right thyroid nodule without any overlying skin changes or palpable cervical lymph nodes. She did not have any signs of airway compression. She was not in respiratory distress, had no tracheal deviation, and Pemberton's sign was negative. There were no features of thyroid eye disease. Vital signs were stable with a temperature of 36.6 degree Celsius, blood pressure of 140/77 mmHg, heart rate of 65/min, which was regular in rhythm, and oxygen saturation of 99% on room air. Investigations on admission showed a raised white cell count of 13.85×10^9/L (reference range, 3.84–10.01 × 10^9/L) with neutrophilia, raised ESR of 105 mm/hr (reference range, 3–9 mm/hr), raised fT4 of 25.7 pmol/L (reference range, 8–16 pmol/L), and suppressed TSH of 0.04 mIU/L (reference range, 0.45–4.5 mIU/L). TSH receptor antibody (TRAb), thyroid peroxidase antibody (anti-TPO Ab), and thyroglobulin antibody (anti-Tg) were negative. A thyroid uptake scan showed generalized reduced thyroid uptake suggestive of destructive thyroiditis and a large cold nodule in the right mid to lower pole of the thyroid gland. Repeat US thyroid revealed interval enlargement of the thyroid nodule which measured 5.0 cm × 4.1 cm × 3.0 cm with interval development of isoechoic debris in the cystic fluid (Figure 2). We were only able to aspirate 30 ml of fluid from the thyroid cyst under strict aseptic condition. Nonpurulent reddish-brown cystic thyroid fluid was sent for Gram stain and culture.

The patient was treated with intravenous Augmentin, nonsteroidal anti-inflammatory drugs (NSAIDs), and low-dose propranolol 20 mg two times a day with the presumptive diagnosis of infected thyroid cyst with thyrotoxicosis from destructive thyroiditis. Gram stain smear of the cystic fluid revealed numerous white blood cells and moderate Gram-positive rods. The cystic fluid culture grew *Propionibacterium acnes*. The patient remained afebrile and clinically stable. She completed 7 days of intravenous Augmentin after which she was discharged, and 7 day of

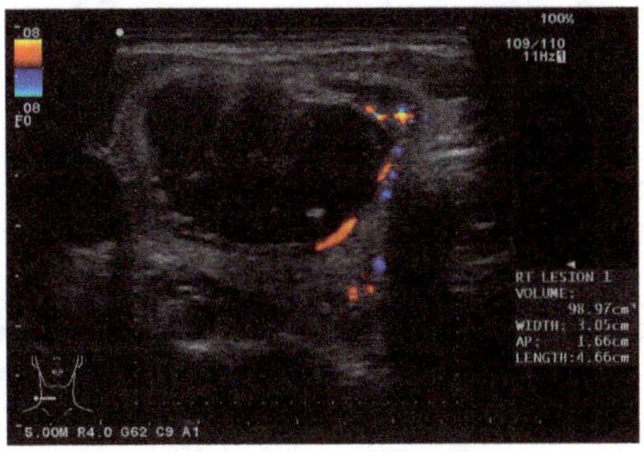

FIGURE 1: Ultrasound image before presentation showing the right mid to lower pole mixed cystic-solid thyroid nodule measuring 4.66 × 3.05 × 1.66 cm, with a well-defined margin and comet-tail artefact (consistent with the colloid nodule).

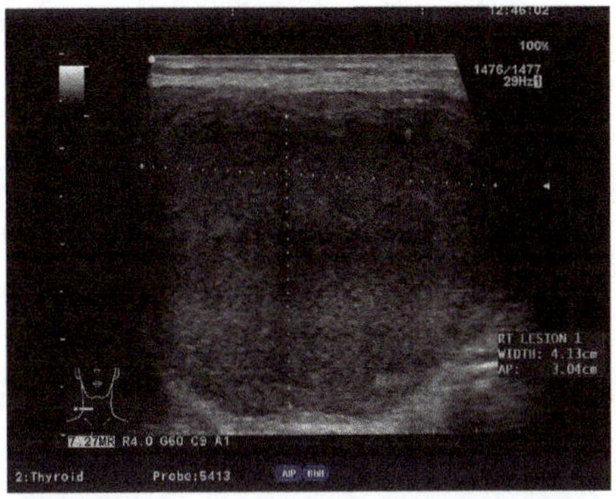

FIGURE 2: Ultrasound image at the time of presentation with neck pain and fever, showing the same thyroid nodule with increase in size measuring 4.95 × 4.13 × 3.04 cm and with interval development of isoechoic debris in the cystic fluid.

oral amoxicillin was continued as outpatient treatment. At follow-up visit 1 week later, the patient was afebrile, clinically euthyroid, and her neck swelling was stable in size and no longer tender. The thyroid function test and inflammatory markers had normalized at follow-up review 3 weeks after discharge. She remained euthyroid and well without any recurrence of neck tenderness. Repeat US thyroid at 1 year showed markedly smaller right solid-cystic thyroid nodule, measuring 1.3 cm in the greatest dimension, and on US thyroid performed at 2 years, it remained stable in size.

3. Discussion and Literature Review

Our case represents a case of acute bacterial thyroiditis caused by *Propionibacterium acnes,* which featured two atypical clinical presentations: a smoldering course caused by an indolent organism and a significant time lag between initial FNA and clinical presentation.

We did a literature search on the PubMed database, as well as the Google search engine using the search terms, "FNA", "thyroiditis," and "abscess". References were selected based on the identification of the relevance of the topic by the authors. The previous case reports of acute bacterial thyroiditis following FNA are presented in Table 1.

Table 1: Case reports of acute bacterial thyroiditis following FNA in the literature.

Author	Published year	Causal organism	Risk factor	Thyroid function status at presentation	Time of FNA to presentation	Management
Isenberg [22]	1994	*Staphylococci*	Diabetes mellitus	Not stated	Not available	Not available
Wang et al. [14]	1997	*Escherichia coli*	On adjuvant chemotherapy for colon cancer and leukopenic	Euthyroid	3 months	Semiemergent thyroidectomy
Sun et al. [9]	2001	*Propionibacterium acnes*	No known risk factors	Not stated	Not stated	Pus aspiration 3 times and antibiotics for 28 days
Nishihara et al. [21]	2005	*Staphylococcus aureus*	Severe atopic dermatitis	Thyrotoxic	4 days	Antibiotics for 1 month followed by resection of the affected thyroid lobe due to persistent fever, raised inflammatory markers, and leukocytosis
Chen et al. [18]	2005	Sterile	Papillary thyroid cancer (PTC)	Euthyroid	Within a week	Parenteral antibiotics for 2 weeks followed by total thyroidectomy for PTC
Halenka et al. [17]	2008	*Escherichia coli*	No known risk factors	Euthyroid	3 days	Drainage of abscess with parenteral antibiotics followed by total thyroidectomy
Yildar et al. [20]	2014	Methicillin-sensitive *Staphylococcus aureus*	Diabetes mellitus	Thyrotoxic on the 7th day of treatment(Increased uptake in the thyroid gland surrounding the abscess in thyroid scintigraphy) etiology of hyperthyroidism was not discussed in the article	15 days	Needle aspiration of abscess 3 times and parenteral antibiotics for 14 days followed by oral antibiotics. Drainage with a 6F pigtail catheter on the 12th day after the end of parenteral antibiotics, due to further enlargement of the nodule. In view of sterile culture, no antibiotics were given at the time of catheter drainage
Unluturk U et al. [15]	2014	Sterile	No known risk factors	Not stated	3 days	Empirical antibiotics for 10 days
Tartaglia et al. [16]	2017	Not done	Psoriasis on methotrexate	Euthyroid	10 days	Parenteral empiric antibiotics (ceftazidime and teicoplanin) for 11 days followed by oral amoxicillin/clavlanic acid and levofloxacin for 10 days
Ar et al. [19]	2018	Staphylococci	No known risk factors	Thyrotoxic	3 weeks	Parenteral antibiotics, open drainage of the abscess, and excision of the cyst wall and right lobe of the thyroid on the 2nd day of admission due to failed aspiration and persistent fever in spite of antibiotic therapy

Acute bacterial suppurative thyroiditis is a rare disorder of the thyroid gland, representing only 0.1–0.7% of all thyroid disease [2]. Although infrequent, it can sometimes lead to serious life-threatening endocrine emergency, endangering the airway, causing cardiac arrhythmias and systemic sepsis, with or without thyrotoxicosis. Thyroid gland is relatively resistant to infections due to its rich vascularity, lymphatic supply, presence of complete fibrous capsule separating it from other nearby structures, high iodine, and hydrogen peroxide content. Infections of the thyroid gland usually occur in patients with underlying thyroid abnormalities such as multinodular goiter, thyroid neoplasms, autoimmune thyroiditis, or persistence of piriform sinus fistula (a tract extending from the apex of the piriform sinus in the hypopharynx to the thyroid gland, usually left-sided, and patients present at a younger age) or in immunocompromised patients such as those who are on immunosuppressant and those with HIV infection, diabetes, or inherited immunodeficiency [2, 3]. Most common organisms causing acute suppurative thyroiditis are Gram-positive aerobes (*Staphylococcus aureus* and *Streptococcus* sp.), followed by Gram-negative aerobes. These two groups constitute nearly 70% of all cases of acute suppurative thyroiditis. Anaerobes constitute only about 12% of all cases. Acute suppurative thyroiditis can rarely be caused by mycobacterial and fungal infections [3].

In earlier reviews, underlying thyroid abnormalities and immunocompromised status were two important risk factors for the development of acute suppurative thyroiditis [3, 4]. However, in a recent case series, spontaneous acute bacterial suppurative thyroiditis has been increasingly reported in immunocompetent patients without underlying structural abnormality such as pyriform sinus fistula [5]. Also, these patients had a more favorable prognosis than the earlier case series. This can be related to improved diagnostic ability in the recent years or under-reporting of acute bacterial thyroiditis in immunocompetent hosts in the previous years. In our patient, although recent FNA and the underlying thyroid nodule could be considered as risk factors for the development of acute bacterial thyroiditis, she did not have any immunodeficiency conditions. Therefore, acute bacterial suppurative thyroiditis following thyroid FNA should be considered as a rare but possible complication even in an immunocompetent host.

We reviewed our infection control practice after this incident. In our institution, thyroid FNA is performed only by experienced practitioners who run FNA clinic every week. The skin is cleaned with 70% alcohol, and we use a sterile disposable transducer probe cover. Although sterile gloves are not used, we ensure no-touch technique to the cleaned skin surface. Our technique is the same as that used in the United States and Europe [6, 7]. Our thyroid FNA service, which started in 2011, had performed an average of 236 thyroid nodule FNAs per year in the past 5 years, and this case is the first case of acute bacterial thyroiditis encountered. For the year of 2018, there were 247 thyroid nodule FNAs performed. As such, the rate of acute bacterial thyroiditis in our clinic in 2018 was 0.4%. No similar cases occurred after the index case.

In our patient, the acute bacterial thyroiditis is caused by *Propionibacterium acnes,* a slow-growing aero-tolerant anaerobic Gram-positive bacillus. It is a commensal of the human skin, gastrointestinal tract, conjunctiva, and external ear. Apart from its well-known link to pathogenesis of acnes vulgaris, it is now recognized as an opportunistic pathogen causing infection of prostheses, ventricular shunts, cardiovascular devices, the heart valves, and the eye [8]. Our case is the second case of acute bacterial thyroiditis due to *Propionibacterium acnes,* according to the available literature [9]. In both of the cases caused by *Propionibacterium acnes*, the presentation is more subtle compared to the typical presentation of acute bacterial thyroiditis. There was no spiking fever, overlying skin change, airway compressive symptoms, or sudden drastic increase in size of the thyroid nodules. All of these features can be contributed to the slow-growing nature and low pathogenic potential of *Propionibacterium acnes. Propionibacterium* species are susceptible to betalactam antibiotics, macrolides, lincosamides, tetracyclines, and fluoroquinolones. Penicillin G is the drug of choice. Resistant strains have developed to macrolides, lincosamides, and tetracyclines. [10].

Possible differential diagnoses in our patient include, but are not limited to, De Quervain's thyroiditis, hemorrhage into the thyroid cyst, acute suppurative thyroiditis, and aggressive thyroid cancer or thyroid lymphoma [11]. Release of thyroid hormones from damaged thyroid follicles can lead to thyrotoxicosis and reduced radioiodine uptake in destructive thyroiditis or acute suppurative thyroiditis. Neck tenderness or neck swelling progression and elevated circulating inflammatory markers can be present in all these conditions and cannot be used as discriminatory factors. Thyroid US and US-guided FNA are the most useful investigations in this clinical setting. Thyroid US features in acute bacterial thyroiditis may include heterogeneous echotexture of the thyroid gland and interval development of hypo-to hyperechoic debris in the thyroid cystic fluid. US-guided FNA will show blood in the case of hemorrhage, polymorphonuclear cell infiltration in the case of acute suppurative thyroiditis, multinucleated giant cells and mononuclear cell infiltration in the case of De Quervain's thyroiditis, and atypical or malignant cells in the case of malignancy. Gram stain smear and culture of FNA material will give additional information as in our patient. However, initial stabilization of the patient must always take precedence, and the role of other imaging such as neck CT scan to delineate the extent and complexity of abscesses or neck anatomy should be considered, especially when the size of the infective focus is large [2]. In the case of pediatric presentation, endoscopic hypopharyngoscopy, neck CT scan with trumpet maneuver, and barium swallow can identify piriform sinus fistula that predisposes to thyroid abscess development [2, 12, 13].

Another peculiar feature in our patient is the time lag of 1 month between the time of FNA and the time of presentation with fever and neck pain. In the available literature, the onset of acute bacterial suppurative thyroiditis after FNA can range from a few days to 3 months [14]. Prolonged subclinical course or subtle presentation was seen in cases of immunocompromised hosts or infection with a low virulent organism as in our case. The suspicion of acute suppurative thyroiditis in a patient with neck pain, swelling, and fever should always be borne in mind, especially if the patient has undergone FNA even a few months ago.

Conventional management of acute bacterial suppurative thyroiditis has been surgery combined with antimicrobial therapy [14]. Recently, a more conservative approach has been reported to be effective [9, 15, 16]. When we reviewed the case reports of acute bacterial suppurative thyroiditis following thyroid FNA, most used parenteral broad spectrum empirical antibiotic therapy with or without needle aspiration drainage as the initial management, similar to our case. Definitive surgery (open drainage or thyroidectomy) were required in a few cases, with main indications being impending airway obstruction in 2 cases [14, 17], underlying papillary thyroid cancer (PTC) in 1 case [18], and failed aspiration due to thick content of cyst in 1 case [19]. These scenarios underlined the importance of personalized management of acute bacterial suppurative thyroiditis based on clinical status of patients. Two case reports required surgery a few weeks after the initial presentation (catheter drainage in one case [20] due to recollection of pus and lobectomy in another case [21] due to persistent fever, leukocytosis, and elevated inflammatory markers). These cases demonstrate the importance of close follow-up in patients who are initially managed conservatively.

4. Conclusions

Acute bacterial suppurative thyroiditis following thyroid FNA is a rare but possible complication even in immunocompetent patients with no known risk factors. Hence, a proper infection control practice is necessary when performing the procedure. The presentation can be subtle and prolonged, sometimes mimicking subacute thyroiditis; it can also present as an emergency endangering the airway, with sepsis and/or thyrotoxicosis. Thyroid US and US-guided FNA are useful initial investigation modalities. Initial management (conservative versus surgical) should be based on the patient's clinical status and the extent of infective focus. Even in patients who are initially managed conservatively, the need for surgery should always be evaluated closely.

References

[1] B. R. Haugen, E. K. Alexander, K. C. Bible et al., "American thyroid association management guidelines for adult patients with thyroid nodules and differentiated thyroid cancer: the American thyroid association guidelines task force on thyroid nodules and differentiated thyroid cancer," *Thyroid*, vol. 26, no. 1, pp. 1–133, 2016.

[2] J. E. Paes, K. D. Burman, J. Cohen et al., "Acute bacterial suppurative thyroiditis: a clinical review and expert opinion," *Thyroid*, vol. 20, no. 3, pp. 247–255, 2010.

[3] S. A. Berger, J. Zonszein, P. Villamena, and N. Mittman, "Infectious diseases of the thyroid gland," *Clinical Infectious Diseases*, vol. 5, no. 1, pp. 108–122, 1983.

[4] E. H. Yu, W. Ko, Y. Chuang, and T. Wu, "Suppurative acinetobacter baumanii thyroiditis with bacteremic pneumonia: case report and review," *Clinical Infectious Diseases*, vol. 27, no. 5, pp. 1286–1290, 1998.

[5] H. Falhammar, G. Wallin, and J. Calissendorff, "Acute suppurative thyroiditis with thyroid abscess in adults: clinical presentation, treatment and outcomes," *BMC Endocrine Disorders*, vol. 19, no. 1, 2019.

[6] H. Gharib, "Fine-needle aspiration biopsy of thyroid nodules: advantages, limitations, and effect," *Mayo Clinic Proceedings*, vol. 69, no. 1, pp. 44–49, 1994.

[7] J. Feldkamp, D. Führer, M. Luster, T. J. Musholt, C. Spitzweg, and M. Schott, "Fine needle aspiration in the investigation of thyroid nodules," *Dtsch Aerzteblatt Online*, vol. 113, no. 20, pp. 353–359, 2016.

[8] A. Perry and P. Lambert, "Propionibacterium acnes: infection beyond the skin," *Expert Review of Anti-Infective Therapy*, vol. 9, no. 12, pp. 1149–1156, 2011.

[9] J. H. Sun, H. Y. Chang, K. W. Chen, K. D. Lin, J. D. Lin, and C. Hsueh, "Anaerobic thyroid abscess from a thyroid cyst after fine-needle aspiration," *Head Neck*, vol. 24, no. 1, pp. 84–86, 2002.

[10] Brook I. Propionibacterium Acnes - Infectious Disease and Antimicrobial Agents. http://www.antimicrobe.org/new/b225.asp.

[11] D. A. Meier and C. E. Nagle, "Differential diagnosis of a tender goiter," *The Journal of Nuclear Medicine*, vol. 37, no. 10, pp. 1745–1747, 1996.

[12] K. H. Kim, M. W. Sung, S. H. Oh, T. Y. Koh, and I. S. Kim, "Pyriform sinus fistula: management with chemocauterization of the internal opening," *Annals of Otology, Rhinology & Laryngology*, vol. 109, no. 5, pp. 452–456, 2000.

[13] S. L. Smith and K. D. Pereira, "Suppurative thyroiditis in children: a management algorithm," *Pediatric Emergency Care*, vol. 24, no. 11, 2008.

[14] Y.-C. Wang, T.-S. Yeh, and J. -Der Lin, "Gram-negative thyroid abscess resulting from fine-needle aspiration in an immunosuppressed patient," *Clinical Infectious Diseases*, vol. 25, no. 22, pp. 953–41661, 1997.

[15] U. Ünlütürk, K. Ceyhan, and D. Çorapçıoğlu, "Acute suppurative thyroiditis following fine-needle aspiration biopsy in an immunocompetent patient," *Journal of Clinical Ultrasound*, vol. 42, no. 4, pp. 215–218, 2014.

[16] N. Tartaglia, P. Cianci, R. Iadarola et al., "Acute suppurative thyroiditis after fine needle aspiration. case report and literature review," *Chirurgia (Bucur)*, vol. 30, no. 3, pp. 89–94, 2017.

[17] M. Halenka, I. Skodova, D. Horak, L. Kucerova, D. Karasek, and Z. Frysak, "Thyroid abscess as a complication of fine-needle aspiration biopsy," *Endocrinologist*, vol. 18, no. 6, pp. 263–265, 2008.

[18] H.-W. Chen, F.-Y. Tseng, D.-H. Su, Y.-L. Chang, and T.-C. Chang, "Secondary infection and ischemic necrosis after fine needle aspiration for a painful papillary thyroid carcinoma: a case report," *Acta Cytologica*, vol. 50, no. 2, pp. 217–220, 2006.

[19] A. Ar, A. Turki, A. Quarshi, A. Mohamed, A. Mutairi, and A. Saud, "Thyroid abscess rare complication of thyroid FNA: case report and literature review," *Scholars Journal Medical Case Reports*, vol. 6, no. 2, pp. 101–107, 2018.

[20] M. Yildar, G. Demirpolat, and M. Aydın, "Acute suppurative thyroiditis accompanied by thyrotoxicosis after fine-needle aspiration: treatment with catheter drainage," *Journal of Clinical and Diagnostic Research*, vol. 8, no. 11, pp. ND12–ND14, 2014.

[21] E. Nishihara, A. Miyauchi, F. Matsuzuka et al., "Acute suppurative thyroiditis after fine-needle aspiration causing thyrotoxicosis," *Thyroid*, vol. 15, no. 10, pp. 1183–1187, 2005.

[22] S. F. Isenberg, "Thyroid abscess resulting from fine-needle aspiration," *Otolaryngol-Head Neck Surg*, vol. 111, no. 6, pp. 832-833, 1994.

Apathetic Thyroid Storm with Cardiorespiratory Failure, Pulmonary Embolism and Coagulopathy in a Young Male with Graves' Disease and Myopathy

Abuobeida Ali,[1] **Wail Mostafa**,[2] **Cornelius Fernandez**,[3] **Habib Ahmad**,[1] **and Nyi Htwe**[3]

[1]*Department of Acute Medicine, Pilgrim Hospital, Boston PE21 9QS, UK*
[2]*Department of Gastroenterology, Pilgrim Hospital, Boston PE21 9QS, UK*
[3]*Department of Endocrinology, Pilgrim Hospital, Boston PE21 9QS, UK*

Correspondence should be addressed to Abuobeida Ali; abuobeida.ali@ulh.nhs.uk

Academic Editor: Wayne V. Moore

A 38-year-old gentleman presented with thyroid storm with multiorgan involvement in the form of heart failure (thyrotoxic cardiomyopathy), respiratory failure (respiratory muscle fatigue), hepatic dysfunction, fast atrial fibrillation, pulmonary embolism, and disseminated intravascular coagulation (DIC). His Graves' disease (GD) remained undiagnosed for nearly 8 months because apart from weight loss, he has not had any other symptoms of thyrotoxicosis. The presentation of thyroid storm was atypical (apathetic thyroid storm) with features of depression and extreme lethargy without any fever, anxiety, agitation, or seizure. There were no identifiable triggers for the thyroid storm. Apart from mechanical ventilation and continuous veno-venous renal replacement therapy in the intensive care unit, he received propylthiouracil (PTU), esmolol, and corticosteroids, which were later switched to carbimazole and propranolol with steroids being tapered down. He was diagnosed with thyrotoxic myopathy which, like GD, remained undiagnosed for long (fatigability). A high index of suspicion and a multidisciplinary care are essential for good outcome in these patients.

1. Case Presentation

A 38-year-old gentleman presented to the emergency department (ED) with worsening shortness of breath, chest tightness, and dry cough of 3-day duration. Apart from these symptoms, he has been experiencing frequent watery diarrhoea for 2 weeks associated with intermittent vomiting, fatigue, extreme lethargy, and a depressed mood. He has had a weight loss of nearly 6-7 kg over 8 months, which the patient considered as intentional. There was no history of fever, palpitation, abdominal pain, haematemesis, malaena, jaundice, loss of appetite, agitation, confusion, or seizure. He had a past medical history of bronchial asthma, well controlled on a salbutamol inhaler. Social history revealed a high-risk sexual behaviour that has resulted in a penile sore which was investigated in the genitourinary outpatient clinic. While in ED, he has had an episode of frank haemoptysis.

On examination, he was alert, but ill looking, cachectic, dyspnoeic, and tachypneic. Observations were as follows: pulse rate of 151 beats/minute, blood pressure (BP) of 109/82 mmHg, respiratory rate of 28/minute, oxygen saturation (SPO_2) of 98% on 2 litres of oxygen, and temperature of 36.2 C. Cardiorespiratory examination showed grossly congested neck veins, with bibasal crackles. His Glasgow Coma Scale (GCS) was 15/15, and there was no focal neurological deficit. His abdomen was soft, mildly distended, with normal bowel sounds. He had no lower limb oedema or deep vein thrombosis. Genital examination showed penile cellulitis which has been an ongoing problem for last few weeks.

2. Investigations

ECG showed evidence of atrial fibrillation (AF) with a ventricular rate of 155 beats/minute. The arterial blood gas done on 2 litres of oxygen showed a pH of 7.392 (7.35–7.45),

PO_2 of 10.43 kPa (10.67–13.33), PCO_2 of 2.88 kPa (4.67–6), lactate of 3.9 mmol/L (1–2.5), bicarbonate of 12.9 mmol/L (22–28), and base excess −10.01 mmol/L (−2 to +2). Bedsides, echo done by FAST (focused assessment with sonography for trauma) by a trained emergency physician revealed right ventricular dilation. Hence, a provisional diagnosis of possible pulmonary embolism (PE), with PE triggered AF, was considered. However, in view of cachexia, underlying malignancy or immunodeficiency was to be excluded. The serial blood results are given in Figures 1–3.

CT pulmonary angiogram along with CT abdomen-pelvis was done which revealed evidence of acute peripheral pulmonary embolism involving the segmental and sub-segmental branches of the right lower lobe pulmonary artery associated with significant cardiomegaly, bilateral moderate basal pleural effusion, congestive hepatomegaly, mild-to-moderate ascites, and significant subcutaneous oedema in the abdominopelvic region. In view of the AF and CT evidence of heart failure, additional tests like the thyroid function test and NT-proBNP (*N*-terminal probrain natriuretic peptide) were sent. He received intravenous digoxin and furosemide with therapeutic dose of enoxaparin.

3. Diagnosis and Treatment

His general condition rapidly deteriorated with respiratory muscle fatigue and an impending respiratory arrest. Hence, he was transferred to the intensive care unit (ICU). He rapidly became haemodynamically unstable with profound metabolic acidosis necessitating electrical cardioversion (for fast AF with haemodynamic compromise), rapid sequence intubation, and mechanical ventilation. The cardioversion successfully reverted AF to sinus tachycardia. His profound metabolic acidosis and fluid overload (heart failure) were treated with continuous veno-venous renal replacement therapy (CRRT).

His additional blood tests showed TSH <0.01 mU/L (0.27–4.5), free T4 >100 pmol/L (11–23), free T3 10.16 pmol/L (3.1–6.8), and NT-proBNP 19,398 ng/L (0–300). Accordingly, the ITU team has started the patient on carbimazole and hydrocortisone with a diagnosis of thyrotoxic crisis with AF. Patient's liver function got worse even before starting carbimazole. Hence, it was attributed to congestive hepatomegaly. A diagnosis of thyroid storm with the Burch–Wartofsky Point Scale (BWPS) of 80, heart failure secondary to cardiomyopathy, and deranged liver function tests secondary to congestive hepatomegaly were agreed by the endocrine team. They suggested to switch carbimazole to propylthiouracil (PTU) and hydrocortisone to dexamethasone. Additionally, they advised to seek the cardiology opinion to choose the most appropriate β-blocker in view of heart failure and to do the thyroid peroxidase antibody (TPO), TSH receptor antibody (TRAb), thyroid ultrasound, and formal echocardiogram (ECHO).

The formal ECHO showed that the left ventricle was moderately dilated with severe global hypokinesia with an ejection fraction (EF) of 27%. Right ventricle was of normal size, but with severely impaired systolic function. The gastroenterologist and cardiologist agreed with the diagnosis of congestive heart failure secondary to thyrotoxic cardiomyopathy and deranged liver function tests caused by congestive hepatomegaly. Tests for HIV, *Treponema pallidum*, covid-19, and tuberculosis were negative. The cardiologist suggested to use esmolol until stable thyroid and cardiac functions are achieved and then to switch to propranolol 20 mg three times daily. A follow-up ECHO repeated 2 weeks later showed an improvement in EF to 36%.

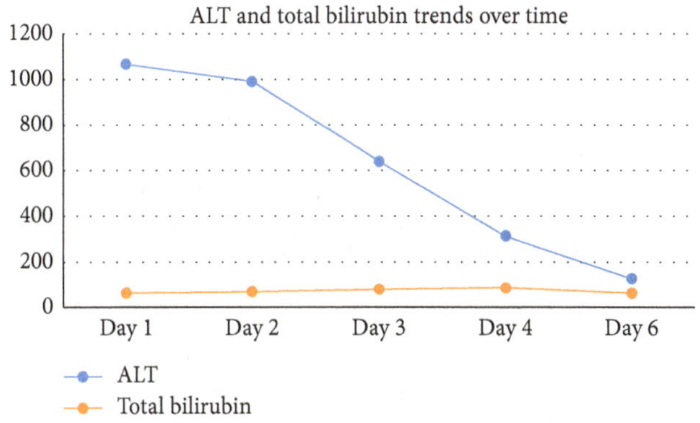

FIGURE 1: Trends of ALT and total bilirubin in the first 6 days of hospitalisation.

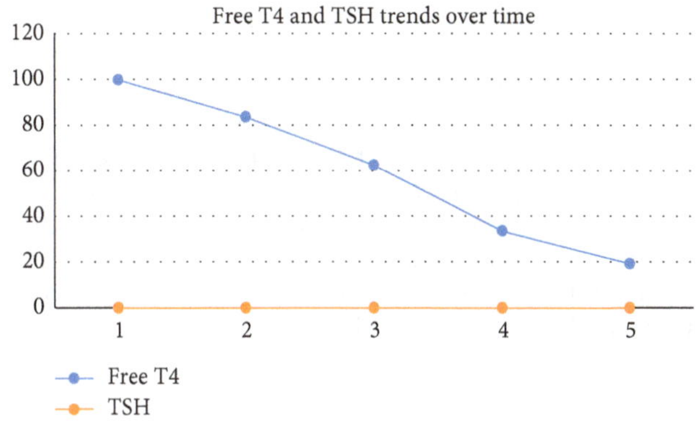

FIGURE 2: Trends of free T4 and TSH in the first 6 days of hospitalisation.

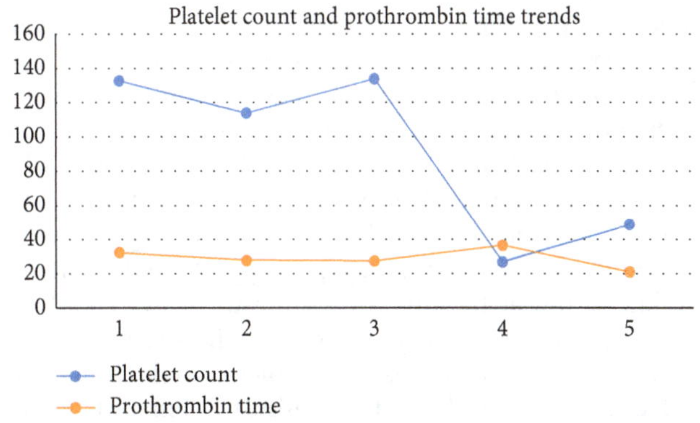

FIGURE 3: Trends of platelet count and prothrombin time in the first 6 days of hospitalisation.

Infective hepatitis screen and autoimmune liver screen were negative.

Thyroid ultrasound demonstrated a bulky thyroid with retrosternal extension and heterogeneous echotexture, with moderately increased vascularity suggestive of thyroiditis. A review of the CT pulmonary angiogram by the radiologist revealed a disproportionately enlarged left thyroid lobe, with mild tracheal deviation towards the right. The TRAb came as 8.16 U/L (0–1.74) and TPO came as 593 IU/ml (0–34). On the 5th day of admission, his free T4 was 19.3 pmol/L (11–23), free T3 was 2.94 pmol/L (3.1–6.8), and TSH was <0.01 mU/L (0.27–4.5). The endocrinology team advised to continue PTU for a total of 6 weeks and then switch to carbimazole.

During the ICU stay, he had persistent thrombocytopenia (lowest 27 × 109/L), persistently prolonged prothrombin time (highest 36.9 seconds), occasionally prolonged activated partial thromboplastin time (highest 40.2 seconds), with persistently high D-dimer levels (highest 6,713 ng/mL), and a reduced Clauss fibrinogen level of 1.4 g/L. On the International Society on Thrombosis and Haemostasis (ISTH) criteria for DIC, he scored 7 which was compatible with a diagnosis of DIC, and he was treated with frozen plasma and vitamin K under haematology supervision. He developed a hospital-acquired pneumonia with *Pseudomonas* grown on the sputum culture and received piperacillin-tazobactam and nebulised colomycin with microbiology input.

4. Outcome of Treatment

In two weeks, he was extubated and stepped down to the medical ward, where he was found to have evidence of significant proximal myopathy associated with a significant difficulty in swallowing. Assessment by the Speech and Language Therapy (SALT) team observed an evidence of severe oesophageal dysphagia. He was on nasogastric feeding due to high risk of aspiration pneumonia. For the neuromuscular issues, he was seen by the neurologist who has made a provisional diagnosis of thyrotoxic myopathy which was later confirmed by electromyography. He is currently receiving physiotherapy support for his muscle weakness, and at the time of writing this case report, his muscle power was slowly improving. His swallowing has already improved, and he is able to tolerate oral feeding. The endocrine team has planned to continue carbimazole (CBZ) for a period of 12–18 months, and if the hyperthyroidism relapses, he will be considered for radioactive iodine (RAI) or thyroidectomy.

5. Discussion

5.1. Introduction. Thyroid storm (TS), also known as thyrotoxic crisis or thyroid crisis, is a life-threatening hypermetabolic thyrotoxicosis, presenting as multiorgan dysfunction with or without a known precipitating cause [1]. This is a rare condition with an annual incidence of 0.57–0.76/100,000 persons in community residents, whereas among hospitalized patients, the annual incidence is 4.8–5.6/100,000 patients [1]. Thyroid storm is associated with 12-fold higher hospital mortality compared to thyrotoxicosis without storm (1.2–3.6% vs. 0.1–0.4%), longer hospital stays (4.8–5.6 vs. 2.7–3.4 mean days), and increased treatment costs [1].

Various physical or mental stressors can act as triggers to induce thyroid storm in patients with diagnosed or undiagnosed thyrotoxicosis [2]. Common triggers include infection, acute illness (myocardial infarction, stroke, hypoglycaemia, and diabetic ketoacidosis), emotional stress, noncompliance with antithyroid drugs, thyroidectomy, neck trauma (strangulation), nonthyroidal surgery, pregnancy, delivery, iodinated contrast, high-dose iodine, and radioiodine treatment [2]. Rare triggers include thyroid palpation, thyroid fine needle aspiration, subacute thyroiditis, thyroid hormone over dosage, metastatic thyroid cancer, gestational trophoblastic disease, struma ovarii, intense exercise, and finally drugs including anaesthetics, salicylates, pseudoephedrine, amiodarone, α-interferon, interleukin-2, methamphetamine, sorafenib, and ipilimumab. In nearly 25–45% of patients, no definite trigger is identified [2].

5.2. Pathophysiology. Thyroid storm occurs in 1-2% of subjects with untreated/poorly controlled hyperthyroidism. Thyroid storm is commonly associated with Graves' disease. Nevertheless, it can happen with toxic adenoma or toxic multinodular goitre [2]. Even though uncertain, the pathophysiology of thyroid storm is thought to be due to an acutely increased release, decreased metabolism (increasing intracellular levels), decreased plasma protein binding (increasing free hormone levels), or augmented peripheral response of thyroid hormones, activation of the β-adrenergic system, and relative adrenal insufficiency caused by the hypermetabolic state [3]. The thyroid function tests in thyrotoxic subjects with storm are not different from those without storm, and there are no absolute thyroid hormone level cutoffs to diagnose thyroid storm [3].

5.3. Clinical Features and Diagnosis. The diagnosis of thyroid storm is purely clinical, and an accurate diagnosis is crucial to improve the morbidity and mortality. The clinical features of thyroid storm are that of an exaggerated hyperthyroidism associated with multiorgan dysfunction [2]. The Burch–Wartofsky Point Scale (BWPS) proposed in 1993 for diagnosis of thyroid storm provides a quantitative diagnostic aid where increasing points are given for greater severity of dysfunction [4]. According to the BWPS (Table 1), a score ≥45 provides a diagnosis of thyroid storm, a score of 25–44 suggests impending thyroid storm, and a score <25 makes the thyroid storm unlikely [4].

Another nonquantitative criteria proposed by the Japan Thyroid Association known as Akamizu criteria (Table 2) categorize patients into definite or suspected thyroid storm based on presence of defined clinical features [6]. It is advised to use both criteria for the accurate diagnosis [5]. Nevertheless, inappropriate use of either can lead to misdiagnosis [5]. The BWPS has superior sensitivity for diagnosing thyroid storm compared to the Akamizu criteria [7],

Table 1: The Burch–Wartofsky Point Scale for diagnosis of thyroid storm [5].

Thermoregulatory dysfunction	Temperature (°C)	37.2–37.7	5 points
		37.8–38.3	10
		38.4–38.8	15
		38.9–39.3	20
		39.4–39.9	25
		≥40	30
Cardiovascular dysfunction	Tachycardia (beats/minute)	90–109	5
		110–119	10
		120–129	15
		130–139	20
		≥140	25
	Atrial fibrillation (AF)	Absent	0
		Present	10
Congestive heart failure (CHF)	Status	Absent	0
		Mild	5
		Moderate	10
		Severe	15
Gastrointestinal (GI) and hepatic dysfunction	No gastrointestinal manifestations	Absent	0
	Vomiting, diarrhoea, abdominal pain	Moderate	10
	Jaundice	Severe	20
Central nervous system (CNS) disturbance	No nervous system manifestations	Absent	0
	Agitation	Mild	10
	Delirium, psychosis, extreme lethargy	Moderate	20
	Seizure, coma	Severe	30
Precipitating event	Status	Absent	0
		Present	10 points
Total score	≥45	Thyroid storm	
	25–44	Impending storm	
	<25	Storm unlikely	

Table 2: The Akamizu criteria for the diagnosis of thyroid storm [5].

Prerequisite for diagnosis

(i) Presence of thyrotoxicosis with high free triiodothyronine (FT3) or free thyroxine (FT4)

Symptoms

(1) CNS manifestations: restlessness, delirium, psychosis, somnolence/lethargy, coma (≥1 on the Japan Coma Scale or ≤14 on the Glasgow Coma Scale)

(2) Fever: ≥38°C

(3) Tachycardia: ≥130 beats/minute or heart rate ≥130 in AF

(4) CHF: pulmonary oedema, crackles over > half of the lung field, cardiogenic shock, or class IV by the New York Heart Association or ≥ class III in the Killip classification

(5) GI/hepatic manifestations: nausea, vomiting, diarrhoea, or a total bilirubin ≥3 mg/dL

Diagnosis

TS grade	Combinations	Requirements for diagnosis
TS1	First combination	Thyrotoxicosis and at least 1 CNS manifestation and fever, tachycardia, CHF, or GI/hepatic manifestations
TS1	Alternate combination	Thyrotoxicosis and at least 3 combinations of fever, tachycardia, CHF, or GI/hepatic manifestations
TS2	First combination	Thyrotoxicosis and a combination of 2 of the following: fever, tachycardia, CHF, or GI/hepatic manifestations
TS2	Alternate combination	Patients who met the diagnosis of TS1 except that serum FT3 or FT4 level is not available

but it is less specific for the diagnosis [8]. The thyroid storm patients with CNS dysfunction derive the greatest benefit from aggressive treatment [8]. The diagnosis of apathetic thyroid storm (thyroid storm without fever and agitation) is challenging. Though apathetic thyroid storm is a disease of elderly [9], there are occasional case reports in young adults [10] and children [11].

According to the Akamizu criteria, thyroid storm should not be considered if there are other underlying diseases that can clearly explain the symptoms. However, if a physician cannot accurately differentiate the exact origin of symptoms, whether from trigger or thyroid storm, consider that symptoms are due to thyroid storm caused by the trigger and the treatment should be given for both. For example, in a patient with antithyroid drug- (ATD-) associated agranulocytosis, the symptoms could either be due to sepsis [12] or be due to the thyroid storm triggered by sepsis [13]. Here, treatment should be given for both sepsis and thyroid storm [12].

5.4. Cardiac Failure and Cardiomyopathy. Thyrotoxicosis could have both central and peripheral effects on the cardiovascular system [14]. The central effects include direct effect on the sinoatrial node causing atrial tachyarrhythmias and direct effect on the heart muscle causing increased myocardial contractility. In the peripheral circulation, it causes vasodilatation leading to a fall in peripheral vascular resistance, after load and diastolic blood pressure. Reduction in renal perfusion secondary to vasodilatation causes an activation of the renin-angiotensin-aldosterone system (RAAS) with resultant sodium retention, increase in circulating volume, preload, and stroke volume. The increase in myocardial contractility associated with decrease in peripheral vascular resistance leads to an increase in cardiac output (2-3-fold) and systolic hypertension with a wide pulse pressure [14].

When the circulating volume significantly increases, it decreases the myocardial contractile reserve leading on to high-output heart failure [15] (HF). Nearly, 6% of thyrotoxic patients would develop high-output HF and 1% would develop thyrotoxic cardiomyopathy (TCMP), a form of dilated cardiomyopathy having low cardiac output with impaired left ventricular systolic and diastolic functions [14]. Mechanisms for TCMP apart from the direct effect of tachycardia include autoimmune or lymphocytic myocarditis [16]. Rarely, stress-induced reversible cardiomyopathy (Takotsubo) characterized by apical hypokinesia has been reported with thyrotoxicosis [17]. Isolated right ventricular dysfunction with pulmonary hypertension has been reported with thyrotoxicosis. An explanation is the increased cardiac output increasing the right ventricular preload, which in turn causing pulmonary vascular endothelial sheer stress, stimulating pulmonary vasoconstriction, pulmonary hypertension, and right ventricular dysfunction [18].

5.4.1. Respiratory Fatigue/Failure. Inspiratory muscle fatigue and failure causing respiratory acidosis, necessitating mechanical ventilation, is not uncommon with thyroid storm, as thyrotoxicosis is known to decrease the muscle mass by 20% and muscle strength by 40% [19]. Various mechanisms for acute respiratory failure include pulmonary oedema [19], pulmonary embolism [20], thyrotoxic myopathy, thyrotoxic periodic paralysis, rhabdomyolysis, polymyositis, or coexisting myasthenia gravis [21].

5.4.2. Renal Failure and Rhabdomyolysis. Renal failure could be due to hypoperfusion, infection, or rhabdomyolysis, with the latter due to fever, agitation, hypermetabolism, hypoperfusion, hypokalaemia, infection, or steroids [21

5.4.3. Venous and Arterial Thromboembolism. Thyrotoxicosis is a hypercoagulable state characterized by increased fibrinogen, FVIII, and vWF activity (due to a direct effect on gene transcription of coagulation proteins) associated with decreased fibrinolysis [22]. Other mechanisms include contact system activation, neutrophil extracellular trap formation, or immune-mediated inflammatory response [22]. Thyroid storm could be associated with deep vein thrombosis with pulmonary embolism [23], cerebral venous sinus thrombosis [24], or extensive systemic venous thromboembolism [25]. It could also cause ischaemic stroke by arterial thrombosis or by embolism from atrial fibrillation [26].

5.4.4. Atrial Fibrillation. AF has a prevalence of 10–20% in thyrotoxicosis and 30–40% in thyroid storm [23]. Even though thyroid storm is a hypercoagulable state, there is no consensus regarding therapeutic anticoagulation even when thyroid storm is associated with AF, as thyrotoxicosis is not included in the CHA_2DS_2-VASc score. However, few authors have recommended that anticoagulation should be considered in patients with thyroid storm or impending storm irrespective of the CHA_2DS_2-VASc score [23]. Moreover, few others have recommended that anticoagulation should be considered in all cases of thyroid storm even in the absence of AF [25].

5.4.5. Hepatic Manifestations. Deranged liver function tests in thyroid storm could be due to multiple mechanisms including heart failure-induced congestive hepatomegaly [27], peripheral vasodilatation-induced hepatic ischaemia [27], thyrotoxicosis-induced direct hepatocyte toxicity [27], concomitant autoimmune hepatic diseases (autoimmune hepatitis and primary biliary cirrhosis) [27], or effect of antithyroid drugs [28]. Hyperthyroidism as the cause of deranged liver function can only be considered after all those aetiologies are ruled out [29

Congestive hepatomegaly is associated with moderate (2- or 3-fold) transaminase levels with bilirubin levels that are rarely >50 μmol/L, whereas ischaemic hepatitis is associated with extremely high bilirubin (~250 μmol/L) and transaminase (>10-fold) levels [30]. Fulminant hepatitis is a rare, life-threatening complication of thyroid storm associated with multiorgan failure and poor prognosis [27]. Orthotopic liver transplantation is the treatment of choice for thyroid storm-associated fulminant hepatitis [27].

5.4.6. Haematological Manifestations. In the euthyroid state, thyroid hormones stimulate haematopoietic stem cells increasing blood cell formation. Thyrotoxicosis causes anaemia (34%), leukopenia (5.8%), and thrombocytopenia (3.3%). But, pancytopenia is rare [30]. Mechanisms include thyrotoxicosis-induced direct bone marrow toxicity, ineffective haematopoiesis [31], or reduced lifespan of blood components by stimulation of the reticuloendothelial system [32], autoimmune mechanisms [32] (pernicious anaemia and immune thrombocytopenic purpura), or by a β-adrenergic mechanism [32]. Moreover, thionamides are associated with leucopenia or agranulocytosis. Direct bone marrow toxicity of the thyroid storm is suggested when thionamide improves leucopenia. Though many triggers for thyroid storm including infection, surgery, and trauma can provoke DIC (disseminated intravascular coagulation), thyroid storm could directly cause it through systemic inflammatory response syndrome. The resultant DIC could worsen the thrombocytopenia caused by thyroid storm [33].

5.4.7. Neurological Manifestations. Though commonly associated with acute confusion [34] or agitation [34] which resolves within 2 weeks after normalization of thyroid function [35], thyroid storm might present with protracted loss of consciousness [35], psychosis [36], status epilepticus [37], extreme lethargy [10], or coma [38].

5.5. Treatment of Thyroid Storm. A multidisciplinary care, with specialist inputs from endocrinology, cardiology, neurology, hepatology, and haematology, is needed in the management of thyroid storm [3]. The treatment targets involve biochemical control of thyrotoxicosis, control of symptoms and signs, control of multiorgan involvement, treatment of triggers, and definitive treatment of thyrotoxicosis [3]. The various treatment modalities involve drugs like antithyroid drugs, corticosteroids, beta-blockers, and inorganic iodine (Table 3), along with volume resuscitation, aggressive cooling with antipyretics or cooling blankets, nutritional support, respiratory care, and ICU monitoring [39].

5.5.1. Antithyroid Drugs (ATDs). The ATDs are carbimazole (CBZ), methimazole (MMI), and propylthiouracil (PTU). MMI is the active metabolite of CBZ [40]. CBZ/MMI is at least 10 times potent than PTU [40]. Moreover, MMI has longer half-life (6–8 hours vs. 90 minutes) and duration of action (>24 hours vs. 8–12 hours), compared to PTU [41]. This enables once daily administration of CBZ/MMI, whereas PTU needs multiple daily dosing [41]. PTU is the preferred ATD in thyroid storm due to additional inhibition of peripheral deiodinase-mediated T4 to T3 conversion [42]. When used in standard doses, ATDs could cause agranulocytosis (0.2–0.5%), hepatic dysfunction (0.03% for CBZ/MMI and 0.05% for PTU), rash (6% for CBZ/MMI and 3% for PTU), antineutrophilic cytoplasmic antibody positive vasculitis (PTU), and antithyroid arthritis syndrome (CBZ/MMI) [40].

Both agranulocytosis and hepatic dysfunction are dose related for CBZ/MMI but not for PTU [40]. The high doses that are required in thyroid storm are unlikely to cause harm with PTU than with CBZ/MMI. As there is 15.2% cross-reaction between CBZ and PTU for agranulocytosis, patients with PTU-induced agranulocytosis should not be given CBZ/MMI, and vice versa. In such scenarios, radioactive iodine (RAI) or thyroidectomy should be considered. Transaminase elevations are seen in one-third of thyrotoxicosis patients [40]. A hepatitic pattern is seen with PTU, whereas a cholestatic pattern occurs with CBZ/MMI [40]. Worsening of transaminase levels or new transaminase elevation that is >3 times the upper limit of normal is an indication to stop the ATD. Though severe cases of PTU-induced hepatic dysfunction should be considered for RAI or thyroidectomy, mild cases can be managed by a switch to CBZ/MMI [43]. Though PTU is known to worsen the hepatic dysfunction of thyroid storm, it is still the preferred drug due to added effect [42]. But, careful liver function monitoring is indicated.

5.5.2. Beta-Blockers. Thyroid hormones increase the β-adrenergic receptor density by increased formation and decreased degradation [44]. Hyperthyroidism has increased sensitivity to catecholamine and increased sympathetic tone. Noncardio selective beta-blockers (NCBB) like propranolol were traditionally used in thyroid crisis as they could not only overcome the hyperadrenergic state and control the peripheral symptoms, but also could block the T4 to T3 conversion [44]. Thyroid storm patients with clinical or subclinical TCMP might develop an exaggerated response to propranolol resulting in cardiogenic shock [44]. Hence, it is advisable to use intravenous cardio selective β-blockers like esmolol (short-acting) or landiolol (ultrashort-acting) that would allow easy titration and rapid cessation of β-blocking effect without the risk of prolonged cardiac depression [44]. The half-life and $\beta1/\beta2$ selectivity for esmolol versus landiolol were 9.19 minutes versus 3.96 minutes and 33 versus 255, respectively [45]. Bisoprolol is preferred over propranolol for tachycardia in thyroid storm [5]. It is preferable to use either PTU or inorganic iodides for inhibiting T4 $\longrightarrow$ T3 conversion rather than using NCBB for this purpose.

5.5.3. Inorganic Iodide. Acting through the Wolff–Chaikoff effect, inorganic iodide (saturated solution of potassium iodide or SSKI as well as Lugol's solution) reduces the thyroid hormone much faster than ATDs and corticosteroids [5]. However, their effect might disappear after 1-2 weeks in some patients [5]. Inorganic iodide can either be given 1 hour after [40] or simultaneously with [5] ATD administration. Once stable, the inorganic iodide should be reduced before tapering dose of ATD [5].

5.5.4. Cholestyramine. Thyrotoxicosis is associated with an abnormal increase in enterohepatic circulation of thyroid hormones [46]. Cholestyramine could bind these thyroid hormones and remove them from the enterohepatic circulation [46]. The drug could be used in refractory hyperthyroidism, iodine-induced hyperthyroidism, and in whom the ATDs are contraindicated [46].

TABLE 3: Drugs used in the management of thyroid storm [3, 6, 39].

Drug name	Treatment dose	Mechanism of action and comments
Propylthiouracil	500–1000 mg stat, then 200–250 mg every 4 hours	Blocks thyroid hormone synthesis Blocks T4 $\longrightarrow$ T3 conversion (>400 mg/day)
Carbimazole	25–30 mg every 4 hours	Blocks thyroid hormone synthesis
Methimazole	15–20 mg every 4 hours	Blocks thyroid hormone synthesis
Propranolol	60–80 mg every 4 hours	Ameliorates the β-adrenergic symptoms
Bisoprolol	2.5–5 mg/day	Blocks T4 $\longrightarrow$ T3 conversion (at high doses: propranolol >160 mg/day) Aims heart rate (HR) <130/minute Needs invasive monitoring in HF patients Asthma: use diltiazem/verapamil
Esmolol	1 mg/kg IV over 30 seconds, 150 μg/kg/minute infusion	
Landiolol	1 μg/kg/min as IV infusion Dose range 1–10 μg/kg/min	
Digoxin	0.125–0.25 mg intravenous	Use only with normal renal function
Lugol's solution	5 drops or 0.25 mL or 250 mg every 6 hours	Blocks thyroid hormone synthesis and release. Administer 1 hour after ATD use
Lithium carbonate	300 mg every 8 hours	Blocks iodination and release
Cholestyramine	4 gm 3-4 times daily	Binds iodothyronines and removes them from the enterohepatic circulation
Hydrocortisone	300 mg IV stat, then 100 mg every 8 hours	Inhibits release and T4 $\longrightarrow$ T3 conversion Prevents relative adrenal insufficiency Promotes vascular stability
Dexamethasone	2 mg IV every 6 hours	

5.5.5. Corticosteroids. Corticosteroids, in large doses, inhibit thyroid hormone release, block conversion to T4 to T3, promote vascular stability, and prevent relative adrenal insufficiency which is associated with the hypermetabolic state of thyroid storm. Hydrocortisone and dexamethasone, the commonly used corticosteroids in thyroid storm, are associated with improved survival [47]. Corticosteroids should be continued until resolution of thyroid storm. The corticosteroid dose should be appropriately tapered depending on the duration of the corticosteroid therapy. In those who were on corticosteroids for long duration, the drug should be stopped only after confirming that adrenals have recovered [47]. Dexamethasone is preferred by some authors due to its less frequent dosing and availability of intravenous, oral, and nasogastric formulations [48]. Hydrocortisone is preferred by few as it has both mineralocorticoid and glucocorticoid effects (1 : 1), whereas dexamethasone has only a negligible mineralocorticoid effect [49]. Inconsistency in recommendations exists even in standard pharmacology text books [50]. Hence, as per latest papers, either dexamethasone or hydrocortisone can be used in patients with thyroid storm [5].

5.5.6. Therapeutic Plasma Exchange (TPE). TPE improves the thyroid storm by rapidly removing the large molecular weight substances like thyroid hormones, TSH receptor antibodies, catecholamines, and cytokines [51]. Similarly, TPE would help to replace the thyroid-binding proteins. Fresh frozen plasma (FFP) is preferred as the replacement fluids compared to albumin, as it contains higher levels of TBG to bind to thyroid hormones [51]. Absolute indication for TPE is acute liver failure associated with thyroid storm, whereas relative indication is lack of clinical improvement after 24–48 hours of ATDs, β-blockers, corticosteroids, and inorganic iodide, treatment of triggers, and complications [51]. Moreover, when ATDs are not effective or contraindicated, TPE is used as a bridge to control the thyroid hormones until the curative treatment is introduced [5].

5.5.7. Radioactive Iodine (RAI) and Thyroidectomy. After successful management of thyroid storm, definitive treatments like thyroidectomy or RAI should be considered to prevent recurrence of thyroid storm [5]. These are considered when the thyroid storm is refractory to medical management or when ATDs are contraindicated [5]. Patients undergoing thyroidectomy should be made euthyroid by giving CBZ/MMI along with β-blockade [39] (and iodide for Graves' disease). The ATDs should be stopped at the time of surgery and β-blockers weaned following surgery [39]. High-risk patients (elderly/cardiovascular disease) undergoing RAI should be made euthyroid by giving CBZ/MMI along with β-blockade [3, 39]. The ATDs should be discontinued 2-3 days before RAI and restarted after 5–7 days [3], with an intention to taper down in 6 weeks to 6 months [39].

5.6. Prognosis. Commonest causes of death from thyroid storm were multiorgan failure, heart failure, respiratory failure, arrhythmia, DIC, gastrointestinal perforation, hypoxic brain syndrome, and sepsis [52]. Though the mortality has come down, as per the latest studies, to 3.6% from 10%, an early accurate diagnosis and multidisciplinary care are the key to the improved outcomes [1].

5.7. Learning Points

(i) Thyroid storm can be the first presentation of thyrotoxicosis

(ii) Apathetic thyroid storm, though common in elderly, can rarely occur in young adults
(iii) Diagnosis of thyroid storm is purely clinical, and early diagnosis improves the outcomes
(iv) Atrial fibrillation and arterial and venous thrombosis are common in thyroid storm
(v) Cardiorespiratory failure is the commonest cause of mortality in thyroid storm
(vi) PTU is the preferred ATD in thyroid storm, though it might worsen the hepatic function
(vii) Cardio selective β-blockers are preferred over NCBB in thyroid storm with TCMP
(viii) Corticosteroids (hydrocortisone or dexamethasone) should be used in thyroid storm

Authors' Contributions

A.A., W.M., and C.F. collected the data and prepared the initial draft under the supervision of H.A; C.F. modified the draft under the supervision of N.H.

References

[1] R. J. Galindo, C. R. Hurtado, F. J. Pasquel, R. García Tome, L. Peng, and G. E. Umpierrez, "National trends in incidence, mortality, and clinical outcomes of patients hospitalized for thyrotoxicosis with and without thyroid storm in the United States, 2004-2013," *Thyroid*, vol. 29, no. 1, p. 36, 2019.

[2] M. Chiha, S. Samarasinghe, and A. S. Kabaker, "Thyroid storm," *Journal of Intensive Care Medicine*, vol. 30, no. 3, p. 131, 2015.

[3] T. Akamizu, "Thyroid storm: a Japanese perspective," *Thyroid*, vol. 28, no. 1, p. 32, 2018.

[4] H. B. Burch and L. Wartofsky, "Life-threatening thyrotoxicosis: thyroid storm," *Endocrinology and Metabolism Clinics of North America*, vol. 22, no. 2, p. 263, 1993.

[5] T. Suzuki, O. Isozaki, A. Suzuki et al., "2016 guidelines for the management of thyroid storm from the Japan thyroid association and Japan endocrine society (first edition)," *Endocrine Journal*, vol. 63, no. 12, p. 1025, 2016.

[6] T. Akamizu, T. Satoh, O. Isozaki et al., "Diagnostic criteria, clinical features, and incidence of thyroid storm based on nationwide surveys," *Thyroid*, vol. 22, no. 7, p. 661, 2012.

[7] M. L. Wakino, G. Szuman, M. F. Scoscia et al., "The challenge of diagnosing thyroid storm: a comparison of the Japanese thyroid association criteria to de Burch Wartofsky point scale," in *Proceedings of the 19th European Congress of Endocrinology: Endocrine Abstracts*, Lisbon, Portugal, May 2017.

[8] T. E. Angell, M. G. Lechner, C. T. Nguyen, V. L. Salvato, J. T. Nicoloff, and J. S. LoPresti, "Clinical features and hospital outcomes in thyroid storm: a retrospective cohort study," *The Journal of Clinical Endocrinology & Metabolism*, vol. 100, no. 2, p. 451, 2015.

[9] P. L. Samantha, P. H. Wu, B. H. Tey, and C. K. Tan, "A patient with thyroid storm presenting with apathetic thyrotoxicosis and features of meningoencephalitis," *Thyroid*, vol. 21, no. 6, p. 675, 2011.

[10] D. Y. Tan, J. Kepchar, R. Sartori, and M. Sarkar, "Painless thyroiditis presenting as apathetic hyperthyroidism in a young male," *Military Medicine*, vol. 173, no. 6, pp. 609–611, 2008.

[11] A. Grossman and S. S. Waldstein, "Apathetic thyroid storm in a 10-year-old child," *Pediatrics*, vol. 28, pp. 447-451, 1961.

[12] S. G. Rayner, F. Hosseini, and A. A. Adedipe, "Sepsis mimicking thyroid storm in a patient with methimazole-induced agranulocytosis," *BMJ Case Reports*, vol. 2013, 2013.

[13] M. Stumpf, G. C. A. Schrut, M. Ramthun et al., "Methimazole-induced agranulocytosis and sepsis: was thyroid storm present or just being mimicked?" *Acta Endocrinologica (Bucharest)*, vol. 15, no. 4, p. 522, 2019.

[14] S. Ertek and A. F. Cicero, "Hyperthyroidism and cardiovascular complications: a narrative review on the basis of pathophysiology," *Archives of Medical Science*, vol. 9, no. 5, pp. 944–295, 2013.

[15] G. M. Taylor, A. M. C. Pop, and E. L. McDowell, "High-output congestive heart failure: a potentially deadly complication of thyroid storm," *Oxford Medical Case Reports*, vol. 2019, no. 6, 2019.

[16] K. Sourial, S. M. Borgan, J. E. Mosquera et al., "Thyroid storm-induced severe dilated cardiomyopathy and ventricular tachycardia," *Cureus*, vol. 11, no. 7, p. e5079, 2019.

[17] M. Eliades, D. El-Maouche, C. Choudhary, B. Zinsmeister, and K. D. Burman, "Takotsubo cardiomyopathy associated with thyrotoxicosis: a case report and review of the literature," *Thyroid*, vol. 24, no. 2, p. 383, 2014.

[18] C. S. Zinsmeister, F. Siew Hui, N. Cheong et al., "Right ventricular dysfunction and pulmonary hypertension: a neglected presentation of thyrotoxicosis," *Endocrinology, Diabetes & Metabolism Case Reports*, vol. 2018, pp. 18–0012, 2018.

[19] Q. Nai, M. Ansari, S. Pak et al., "Cardiorespiratory failure in thyroid storm: case report and literature review," *Journal of Clinical Medicine Research*, vol. 10, no. 4, p. 351, 2018.

[20] C. Tian, S. Aoki, T. Takahashi, and F. Hirahara, "Acute respiratory failure due to thyroid storm developing immediately after delivery," *Clinical Case Reports*, vol. 3, no. 12, p. 997, 2015.

[21] P.-H. Hirahara, X.-S. Dong, C. Li et al., "Acute severe asthma with thyroid crisis and myasthenia: a case report and literature review," *The Clinical Respiratory Journal*, vol. 11, no. 6, p. 671, 2017.

[22] L. P. B. Bao, E. Fliers, and S. C. Cannegieter, "The influence of thyroid function on the coagulation system and its clinical consequences," *Journal of Thrombosis and Haemostasis*, vol. 16, no. 4, p. 634, 2018.

[23] T. Min, S. Benjamin, and L. Cozma, "Thromboembolic complications of thyroid storm," *Endocrinology, Diabetes & Metabolism Case Reports*, vol. 2014, 2014.

[24] N. Tanabe, E. Hiraoka, M. Hoshino et al., "Progressive ischemic stroke due to thyroid storm-associated cerebral venous thrombosis," *American Journal of Case Reports*, vol. 18, p. 194, 2017.

[25] A. C. Deshpande and D. G. S. L. Tan, "A case of thyroid storm with systemic thromboembolism," in *Proceedings of the*

Annual Meeting of the Endocrine Society, San Francisco, CA, USA, March 2020.

[26] S. Snyder and M. Joseph, "The perfect storm: a case of ischemic stroke in the setting of thyroid storm," *Cureus*, vol. 12, no. 5, p. e7992, 2020.

[27] Y. Tanaka, T. Uchida, H. Yamaguchi, Y. Kudo, T. Yonekawa, and M. Nakazato, "Fulminant hepatitis, and elevated levels of sIL-2R in thyroid storm," *Endocrinology, Diabetes & Metabolism Case Reports*, vol. 2019, 2019.

[28] N. Tufton, N. Hashim, C. Sze, and M. Waterhouse, "A case of thyroid storm complicated by acute hepatitis due to propylthiouracil treatment," *Endocrinology, Diabetes & Metabolism Case Reports*, vol. 2015, 2015.

[29] M. Amir, M. N. Rahhal, and J. Calles-Escandon, "Rapid resolution of hyperthyroidism induced hepatic dysfunction with methimazole," in *Proceedings of the Annual Meeting of the Endocrine Society*, San Francisco, CA, USA, March 2020.

[30] R. D. Wickramasinghe, W. A. Luke, B. S. Sebastiampillai, M. P. M. L. Gunathilake, and R. Premaratna, "Thyrotoxic crisis presenting with jaundice," *BMC Research Notes*, vol. 9, no. 1, p. 320, 2016.

[31] P. Jha, Y. P. Singh, B. Ghimire, and B. K. Jha, "Pancytopenia in a surgical patient, a rare presentation of hyperthyroidism," *BMC Surgery*, vol. 14, p. 108, 2014.

[32] Y. Tokushima, Y. Sakanishi, K. Nagae et al., "Thyroid storm complicated by bicytopenia and disseminated intravascular coagulation," *American Journal of Case Reports*, vol. 15, pp. 312–316, 2014.

[33] Y. Shimoda, T. Satoh, H. Takahashi et al., "A case of thyroid storm with a markedly elevated level of circulating soluble interleukin-2 receptor complicated by multiple organ failure and disseminated intravascular coagulation syndrome," *Endocrine Journal*, vol. 61, no. 7, p. 691, 2014.

[34] S. Katano-Toki, L. Marino, J. Ayari et al., "Thyroid storm: a rare and life-threatening cause of acute neurological manifestations during urgent percutaneous coronary intervention for acute coronary syndrome," *Cardiology Journal*, vol. 24, no. 3, p. 342, 2017.

[35] C. Namatame, T. Sonoo, K. Fukushima, H. Naraba, H. Hashimoto, and K. Nakamura, "A thyroid storm patient with protracted disturbance of consciousness and reversible lesion in the splenium of corpus callosum: a case report," *Medicine*, vol. 97, no. 7, p. e9949, 2018.

[36] Y. Naraba, T. Sugawa, H. Kaneko et al., "The delayed diagnosis of thyroid storm in patients with psychosis," *Internal Medicine*, vol. 58, no. 15, p. 2195, 2019.

[37] T. G. Hiroshima-Hamanaka, C. K. Ha, and B. H. Lim, "Thyroid storm presenting as status epilepticus and stroke," *Postgraduate Medical Journal*, vol. 73, no. 855, p. 61, 1997.

[38] L. A. Burmeister, "Coma in thyroid storm: review of aggregated English-language case reports," *Journal of the Endocrine Society*, vol. 3, no. 7, p. 1261, 2019.

[39] R. Bahn, H. Burch, D. Cooper et al., "Hyperthyroidism and other causes of thyrotoxicosis: management guidelines of the American thyroid association and American association of clinical endocrinoloigists," *Endocrine Practice*, vol. 17, no. 3, p. 456, 2011.

[40] H. B. Garber and D. S. Cooper, "Antithyroid drug therapy: 70 years later," *European Journal of Endocrinology*, vol. 179, no. 5, p. R261, 2018.

[41] G. J. Kahaly, L. Bartalena, L. Hegedüs, L. Leenhardt, K. Poppe, and S. H. Pearce, "2018 European thyroid association guideline for the management of Graves' hyperthyroidism," *European Thyroid Journal*, vol. 7, no. 4, p. 167, 2018.

[42] R. Leenhardt and G. Matfin, "Review: endocrine and metabolic emergencies: thyroid storm," *Therapeutic Advances in Endocrinology and Metabolism*, vol. 1, no. 3, pp. 139–145, 2010.

[43] LiverTox, *Clinical and Research Information on Drug-Induced Liver Injury*, National Institute of Diabetes and Digestive and Kidney Diseases, Bethesda, MD, USA, 2012.

[44] H. Abubakar, V. Singh, A. Arora, and S. Alsunaid, "Propranolol-induced circulatory collapse in a patient with thyroid crisis and underlying thyrocardiac disease: a word of caution," *Journal of Investigative Medicine High Impact Case Reports*, vol. 5, no. 4, 2017.

[45] H. Tsuchiya and M. Mizogami, "Characteristic interactivity of landiolol, an ultra-short-acting highly selective β_1-blocker, with biomimetic membranes: comparisons with β_1-selective esmolol and non-selective propranolol and alprenolol," *Frontiers in Pharmacology*, vol. 4, p. 150, 2013.

[46] W.-C. Tsai, D. Pei, T.-F. Wang et al., "The effect of combination therapy with propylthiouracil and cholestyramine in the treatment of Graves' hyperthyroidism," *Clinical Endocrinology*, vol. 62, no. 5, p. 521, 2005.

[47] N. Wu, L. Preechasuk, and T. Kunavisarut, "Nonthionamide drugs for the treatment of hyperthyroidism: from present to future," *International Journal of Endocrinology*, vol. 2018, Article ID 5794054, 10 pages, 2018.

[48] Empalife.com. Thyroid-storm: a life-threatening disease that requires rapid stabilization, 2020 http://www.empalife.com/thyroid-storm.

[49] M. Misra, A. Singhal, and D. Campbell, "Thyroid storm," 2020, https://emedicine.medscape.com/article/925147-medication#5.

[50] G. Bhutani, S. Kalra, and P. Dhamija, "Academic heterogeneity: a tale of management of thyrotoxicosis across textbooks—a bibliometric review," *Thyroid Research and Practice*, vol. 13, no. 1, pp. 5–8, 2016.

[51] A. Miller and K. D. Silver, "Thyroid storm with multiorgan failure treated with plasmapheresis," *Case Reports in Endocrinology*, vol. 2019, Article ID 2475843, 5 pages, 2019.

[52] O. Isozaki, T. Satoh, S. Wakino et al., "Treatment and management of thyroid storm: analysis of the nationwide surveys: the taskforce committee of the Japan thyroid association and Japan endocrine society for the establishment of diagnostic criteria and nationwide surveys for thyroid storm," *Clinical Endocrinology*, vol. 84, no. 6, pp. 912–918, 2016.

41

Henoch–Schönlein Purpura (IgA Vasculitis) in Association with Thyrotoxicosis

Mojgan Sanjari,[1] **Mohammadreza Shakibi**,[2] **and Moeinadin Safavi**[3,4]

[1]*Department of Endocrinology, Afzalipour Medical Faculty and Endocrinology and Metabolism Research Center, Institute of Basic and Clinical Physiology Sciences, Kerman University of Medical Sciences, Kerman, Iran*
[2]*Rheumatology Department, Afzalipour Medical Faculty and Physiology Research Center, Institute of Neuropharmacology, Kerman University of Medical Sciences, Kerman, Iran*
[3]*Pathology Department, School of Medicine, Kerman University of Medical Sciences, Kerman, Iran*
[4]*Pathology Department, School of Medicine, Tehran University of Medical Sciences, Tehran, Iran*

Correspondence should be addressed to Moeinadin Safavi; msafavi@sina.tmu.ac.ir

Academic Editor: Toshihiro Kita

Graves' disease is the most common cause of hyperthyroidism, which is characterized by thyroid antibodies and the following clinical manifestations: goiter, ophthalmopathy, and pretibial myxedema. On the other hand, Henoch–Schönlein purpura is an IgA-mediated small-vessel vasculitis. Review of the literature showed a relationship between propylthiouracil overdose and the following Henoch–Schönlein purpura (IgA vasculitis) as a side effect. The patient was a 31-year-old woman with a chief complaint of tremor and significant weight loss who contracted pruritic palpable purpura during her disease course. Then, she underwent the treatment of hyperthyroidism by methimazole which intensified her cutaneous lesions. The diagnosis of Henoch–Schönlein purpura (IgA vasculitis) was confirmed after skin biopsy. Finally, she was treated with colchicine, prednisolone, and radioiodine ablation, which caused her lesions to disappear. The temporal priority of pruritic palpable skin lesions to hyperthyroidism treatment with methimazole suggested that Henoch–Schönlein purpura (IgA vasculitis) was related to hyperthyroidism and was intensified by antithyroid agents in this patient.

1. Introduction

Graves' disease is the most common cause of hyperthyroidism, which is characterized by thyroid antibodies (TSI, antimicrosomal, antithyroglobulin, and ANA) and the following clinical manifestations: goiter, ophthalmopathy, and pretibial myxedema. [1] On the other hand, Henoch–Schönlein purpura is an IgA-mediated small-vessel vasculitis, which is characterized by the following criteria (2 of 4 is 87% sensitive and 89% specific) [2]: (1) palpable purpura, (2) age ≤20 at disease onset, (3) bowel angina, and (4) biopsy showing granulocytes in the walls of arterioles and venules.

Review of the literature showed a relationship between propylthiouracil overdose and the following Henoch–Schönlein purpura (IgA vasculitis) as a side effect. [3] It has been well documented that propylthiouracil could induce antineutrophil cytoplasmic antibody (ANCA)-positive vasculitis, which predominantly affects small vessels. [4, 5] However, the causal relationship between Henoch–Schönlein purpura (IgA vasculitis) and Grave's disease or antithyroid drugs has been remained unclear yet [6].

2. Case Report

The patient was a 31-year-old woman with a chief complaint of hand tremor and significant weight loss (20 kg during 5 months). She also developed pruritis 5 months later, which led to palpable purpuric rash of both the legs and arms extended to the palms and soles during 2 weeks (Figure 1).

More evaluation of the patient by lab tests revealed mild anemia (Hb = 11.3 g/dL) and hyperthyroidism (T4 > 24.86 μg/dL, T3 = 483 ng/dL, and TSH = 0.01 mIU/mL). Thus, the

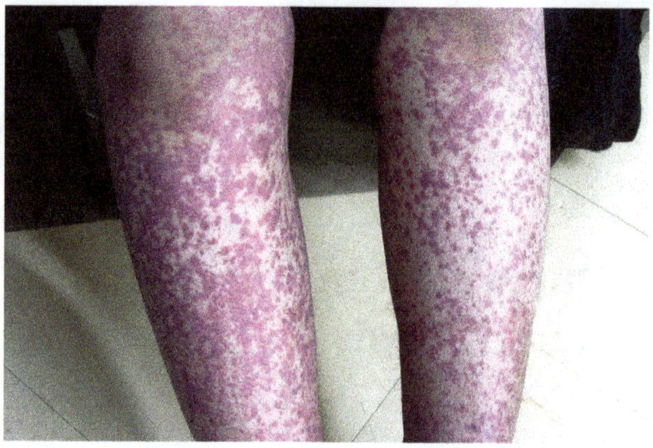

FIGURE 1: Palpable purpura with more intensity on the lower extremities.

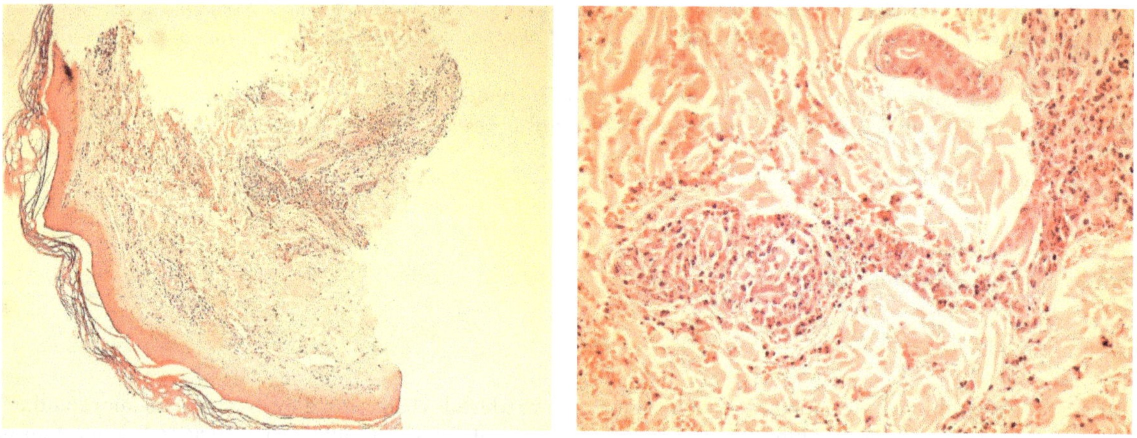

(a) (b)

FIGURE 2: Perivascular neutrophilic infiltration, impinging vessel walls, RBC extravasation, and nuclear dust with endothelial cell plumping in the dermis (hematoxylin and eosin, 40x and 100x magnification, respectively).

patient underwent the treatment with methimazole thereafter. During the disease course, the purpuric lesions extended to the abdominal skin. Therefore, she was referred to a dermatologist for a more comprehensive workup. According to his opinion, a skin biopsy was performed with the impression of vasculitis. The pathology report showed hyperkeratosis of the *epidermis* and perivascular neutrophilic infiltration, impinging vessel walls, RBC extravasation, and nuclear dust with endothelial cell plumping in the dermis. All these findings were strongly suggestive of Henoch–Schönlein purpura (IgA vasculitis) (Figures 2(a) and 2(b)).

Based on the findings, a complete autoimmune antibody study was performed which yielded the following results: anti-ds-DNA = 40.7 (<100 negative), ANA = 1/20(up to1/10), ANA (pattern) = homogenous, IgA = 3.3 g/l (0.86–3.2), c-ANCA = 0.7 RU/ml (<20 negative), p-ANCA = 1.9 RU/ml (<20 negative), and cryoglobulin = negative.

The result of urine analysis was negative for hematuria and proteinuria. Further lab data including lipid profile and renal and liver function tests were all in the normal range. After consultation with a rheumatologist, treatment with colchicine (10 mg) and prednisolone (100 mg) was started which caused the skin lesions to disappear. Gradual tapering of prednisolone to 25 mg could control the cutaneous lesions. Nevertheless, a lower dose of prednisolone could not resolve the lesion. Therefore, the patient received 10 mCi radioiodine due to the possibility of an allergic reaction to methimazole. Cutaneous lesions disappeared after radioiodine therapy. Three months later, laboratory tests revealed hypothyroidism (TSH = 98 μg/dL) after radioiodine therapy. Therefore, levothyroxine was prescribed for her. Seven months later, skin lesions recurred and laboratory findings showed concomitant hyperthyroidism (TSH = 0.005 μg/dL). Thus, levothyroxine dose was tapered to half and led to skin lesion resolution. Thereafter, the patient was euthyroid, and cutaneous lesions did not recur.

3. Discussion

Traditionally, vasculitis is a well-known side effect of Graves' disease treatment with antithyroid drugs such as propylthiouracil and methimazole. It manifests as a systemic sickness with several cutaneous presentations from erythema to necrosis. Leukocytoclastic vasculitis along with fibrinoid necrosis of vessel walls is the most common histopathologic findings in this phenomenon [7]. The pathogenesis of antithyroid drug-associated vasculitis is unclear yet. However, induction of antineutrophilic cytoplasmic antibodies (ANCA) such as antimyeloperoxidase by antithyroid drugs has been proposed as a possible underlying cause. [8].

During the recent decade, few cases of Henoch–Schönlein purpura (IgA vasculitis) have been reported in patients with Graves' disease with or without usual doses of antithyroid drugs suggesting Graves' disease as a triggering factor for Henoch–Schönlein purpura (IgA vasculitis). [9] On the other hand, few cases of Henoch–Schönlein purpura (IgA vasculitis) have been reported with subsequent development of autoimmune thyroiditis or transient hyperthyroidism and a possible immunologic relationship between these two conditions has been postulated [6, 10].

In the described case, the temporal precedence of Henoch–Schönlein purpura (IgA vasculitis) to treatment beginning with methimazole in the background of Graves' disease suggested that these two conditions are associated. However, treatment with methimazole augmented the vasculitis lesions in this case. It is very interesting that vasculitis relapsed under thyrotoxicosis caused by L-thyroxin overdose. Therefore, there are two episodes of hyperthyroidism of different causes, both leading to a vasculitis flare. These findings may show that hyperthyroidism per se irrespective of pathogenesis may cause vasculitis in susceptible individuals. Indeed, the vasculitis resolved after radioiodine therapy and after dose reduction of L-thyroxin, which strongly supports that view.

In conclusion, Henoch–Schönlein purpura (IgA vasculitis) might be occasionally related to thyrotoxicosis and can be intensified by antithyroid agents.

References

[1] D. S. Cooper, "Hy perthy roidism,"*The L ancet*, v ol. 362, no. 9382, pp. 459–468, 2003.

[2] J. A. Mills, B. A. Michel, D. A. Bloch et al., "The American college of rheumatology 1990 criteria for the classification of Henoch-Schönlein purpura," *Arthritis & Rheumatism*.vol. 33, no. 8, pp. 1114–1121, 1990.

[3] J. E. Lee, C. H. Jeon, D. K. Chang, M.-S. Lee, and H. Y. Oh, "Henoch-Schönlein purpura associated with propylthiouracil overdose," *Nephrology Dialysis Transplantation*, vol. 21, no. 8, 2006.

[4] K. M. Dolman, A. E. G. K. Von Dem Borne, R. Goldschmeding et al., "Vasculitis and antineutrophil cytoplasmic autoantibodies associated with propylthiouracil therapy," *The Lancet*, vol. 342, no. 8872, pp. 651-652, 1993.

[5] L. Harper, P. Cockwell, and C. O. Savage, "Case of propy lthiouracil-induced ANCA associated small vessel vasculitis," *Nephrology Dialysis Transplantation*, vol. 13, no. 2, pp. 455–458, 1998.

[6] J. I. Shin, J. M. Park, J. S. Lee, D. H. Kim, and H. J. Jeong, "Development of graves' disease during cyclosporin treatment for severe Henoch-Schönlein nephritis," *Nephrology Dialysis Transplantation*, vol. 20, no. 9, pp. 2014-2015, 2005.

[7] N. C. Pietszkowski, G. A. D. Carvalho, H. N. D. Souza et al., "Auto-imunidade ANCA (anticorpo anti-citoplasma de neutrófilos) positiva induzida por propiltiouracil: relato de caso e revisão da literatura," *Arquivos Brasileiros de Endocrinologia & Metabologia*, vol. 51, no. 1, pp. 136–141, 2007.

[8] K. Ahmed, S. Rao, and V. Simha, "Antineutrophil cytoplasmic antibody-positive vasculitis in a patient with graves disease: cross-reaction between propylthiouracil and methimazole," *Endocrine Practice*, vol. 16, no. 3, pp. 449–451, 2010.

[9] J. I. Shin, J. M. Park, J. H. Kim et al., "Association of Henoch-Schönlein purpura and graves' disease," *Nephrology Dialysis Transplantation*, vol. 21, no. 10, p. 2997, 2006.

[10] C. Garcia-Porrua, M. Gonzalez-Gay, M. Botana, and A. Sanchez-Andrade, "Henoch-Schönlein purpura in adults and autoimmune thyroiditis," *The Journal of Rheumatology*, vol. 27, no. 5, p. 1326, 2000.

Delayed Diagnosis of Congenital Hypothyroidism in a Child with Trisomy 21 and Biotinidase Deficiency and Successful use of Levothyroxine Sodium Oral Solution

Matthew M. Feldt

Pediatric Endocrinologist, Children's Mercy Hospital, Kansas City, MO, USA

Correspondence should be addressed to Matthew M. Feldt; mmfeldt@cmh.edu

Academic Editor: Wei Wu

Endocrine disorders are more common and appear earlier in people with trisomy 21 (T21) than in the general population, with thyroid dysfunction being the most common, including both congenital and acquired hypothyroidism. The treatment for biotinidase deficiency, a condition that occurs in approximately 1 : 110,000 people, is with biotin (vitamin B7) supplementation. However, biotin can interfere with endocrine laboratory assays and cause falsely low thyroid-stimulating hormone (TSH) and elevated free thyroxine (FT4) levels. This can interfere with the timely diagnosis and subsequent treatment of congenital hypothyroidism (CH). This case report describes an infant with partial biotinidase deficiency that was confirmed on day 10 of life. Routine screening erroneously reported "normal" TSH that caused delayed diagnosis of CH due to interference with the TSH assay from concurrent biotin use. Once the biotin treatment was withheld for 4 days and the thyroid function tests repeated, an elevated TSH became apparent. Treatment with tablet levothyroxine (L-T4) was started and subsequently changed to L-T4 oral solution (Tirosint®-SOL) to overcome treatment administration difficulties encountered with the tablet form. This resulted in improved TSH control due to more accurate and consistent dosing compared with the tablet formulation. This is the first report of the use of L-T4 oral solution in an infant with T21 and biotinidase deficiency.

1. Introduction

Trisomy 21 (T21), or Down syndrome, affects both the physical and intellectual development of the individual [1, 2]. Endocrine disorders are more common and appear earlier in people with T21 than in the general population [3]. Of the many endocrine disorders associated with T21, thyroid dysfunction is the most common and includes both congenital and acquired hypothyroidism [3–6]. Biotinidase deficiency is a relatively rare condition occurring in approximately 1 : 110,000 [7]. Biotin (vitamin B7) supplementation is the treatment in biotinidase deficiency but can interfere with many laboratory assays [8], causing falsely low levels of thyroid-stimulating hormone (TSH) and elevated free thyroxine (FT4) levels [9]. This can interfere with the timely diagnosis of congenital hypothyroidism (CH) [10]. Levothyroxine (L-T4), in tablet form, is considered the standard of care for treatment of hypothyroidism [11].

The therapeutic administration of tablet L-T4 in patients with T21 may prove challenging due to the often-associated occurrence of global developmental delay [2] and gastrointestinal problems, including functional and anatomical anomalies [1]. There is a paucity of literature about concomitant CH and biotinidase deficiency, and no prior literature describing the use of levothyroxine sodium oral solution (L-T4 oral solution), Tirosint®-SOL, which has recently become available in the United States for the treatment of hypothyroidism [12]. Prior European studies on the use of L-T4 oral solution in CH have shown initial improvements in TSH and/or maintenance of euthyroidism over time versus tablets [13–15]. These observations may be linked to higher absorption and bioequivalence for liquid L-T4 solution compared with tablets [13–15].

This case report describes a patient with "normal" TSH on routine screening that caused delayed diagnosis of CH due to interference with the TSH assay from concurrent biotin use. Once biotin treatment was withheld for 4 days and thyroid function tests repeated, an elevated TSH became apparent and CH was diagnosed. Treatment with tablet L-T4 was started and subsequently changed to L-T4 oral solution to overcome administration difficulties. This resulted in easier administration, accurate dosing, improved compliance, and biochemical euthyroidism.

2. Case Presentation

The patient is a white, non-Hispanic, full-term, infant female with T21. Pertinent family history includes both parents being confirmed carriers for biotinidase deficiency. TSH-based newborn screening was performed and not flagged as abnormal for hypothyroidism. The patient was confirmed with partial biotinidase deficiency (2.0 U/L; reference range: 3.5–13.8 U/L) on day of life 10 and started on biotin 1000 μg daily. At 2 weeks of life (WOL), thyroid function was tested while receiving biotin: TSH was 3.39 mIU/mL and FT4 was elevated at 5 ng/dL. Autoimmune evaluations for hyperthyroidism in the mother and child were negative. At 3 WOL, biotin was withheld for 3 days and repeat thyroid function tests showed a TSH of 5.1 mIU/mL and that FT4 had normalized to 2.4 mIU/mL. At 8 WOL, after biotin was withheld for 4 days, TSH was now elevated and FT4 remained in the reference range. Congenital hypothyroidism was diagnosed at that time and the child was started on the tablet form of L-T4 25 μg. The patient's parents reported difficulty in administering the dose via a crushed tablet in a bottle of formula. At 16 WOL, biotin was withheld for 4 days and repeat thyroid function tests showed that TSH was suppressed and FT4 was slightly elevated. The dose of L-T4 was reduced to 12.5 μg (half tablet) and at 20 WOL, after biotin was withheld for 4 days, repeat thyroid testing again showed suppressed TSH and elevated FT4. The parents still reported difficulty with cutting and crushing the L-T4 tablet, resulting in inconsistent dosing. A referral to pediatric endocrine care was then initiated and the L-T4 tablet formulation was changed to oral solution 13 μg daily. The parents reported that administration was much easier with the oral formulation. At 24 WOL, biotin was again withheld for 4 days and repeat thyroid function tests showed normalization in both TSH (1.75 mIU/mL) and FT4 (1.96 ng/dL). At 28 WOL, after biotin was withheld for 4 days, both TSH and FT4 were still normal and the family reported being very happy with the L-T4 oral solution. A timeline of treatments administered along with outcomes is shown in Table 1 and Figure 1.

3. Discussion

The prognosis for children with CH has improved significantly due to the implementation of neonatal screening methods and a more focused therapeutic approach [16]. Studies on cognitive function in patients with CH treated soon after birth have shown that normal development can be achieved in most patients, although cognitive development depends on the severity of the disorder and the age at which the hormone replacement therapy with L-T4 is started [16, 17]. Most neonatal screening methods in the United States use a combination of TSH, FT4, or both [18].

Biotinidase deficiency, the major cause of late-onset biotin-responsive multiple carboxylase deficiency, is an autosomal recessive neurocutaneous disorder [7]. The symptoms of biotinidase deficiency can be successfully treated or prevented by administering pharmacological doses of biotin [7], a water-soluble vitamin used widely as a dietary supplement. In children with biotinidase deficiency, doses are considerably higher (5-10 mg per kilogram of body weight per day) [7] than the normal dietary reference intake for children (5–25 μg per kilogram per day) [19]. Biotin has been shown to interfere with many endocrine laboratory assays (including TSH and FT4) [8, 9], which can lead to erroneous or delayed diagnosis of CH. Prior literature has described cases of children receiving an inaccurate diagnosis of hyperthyroidism due to interference with the thyroid function assay from high doses of biotin being given as a therapy for metabolic disease [9, 10]. Our patient with biotinidase deficiency had erroneous thyroid function testing that was suggestive of hyperthyroidism. However, once biotin supplementation was withheld, a true diagnosis of CH was possible.

Thyroid hormones are pivotal for normal physical and neuromotor development during the first years of life. Compliance with L-T4 treatment is one of the main factors that influence the outcome of patients with CH [20]. The therapeutic use of biotin in this infant resulted in false TSH assay measurements so that they appeared in the normal range and delayed the diagnosis of CH. Once the correct diagnosis was made and treatment initiated, the TSH and FT4 levels still remained outside the reference range because of the suboptimal administration of tablet-formulated L-T4, which should have been given in crushed form via a syringe, but instead was being mixed with infant formula. However, changing to L-T4 oral solution improved the ease and consistency of administration and compliance with therapy, and TSH levels subsequently improved.

T21 may cause additional challenges in infants and young children receiving L-T4 treatment due to associated gastrointestinal problems, feeding difficulties, and developmental delays [1]. In addition to the obvious advantage of administering an oral solution instead of a crushed tablet to an infant, L-T4 oral solution has many advantages for this patient population: it has a sweet taste; contains only levothyroxine, glycerol, and water [12]; is free from additional excipients; and does not require a gastric phase of dissolution (before absorption), meaning that it is more readily absorbed than tablets [21]. Compared with the tablet form of LT-4, faster achievement of target TSH values was demonstrated for the oral form and it also allows for easier individualization of the dose [22]. As accurate dosing of L-T4, both at initiation and in the long term, has been recognized as a major challenge in the treatment of CH [22], this case demonstrates the utility of L-T4 oral solution in enabling ease of administration, accurate dosing, and subsequent TSH control in a patient with CH and T21.

In conclusion, this case demonstrates the effectiveness of using L-T4 oral solution to treat a patient with CH and T21.

TABLE 1: Thyroid function tests after diagnosis of biotinidase deficiency.

Weeks of life	Days off biotin	TSH (mIU/mL)		FT4 (ng/dL)	
		Measured	Normal range*	Measured	Normal range*
2	0	3.39	0.71–9.34	5.0	0.7–2.4
3	3	5.1	0.71–9.34	2.4	0.7–2.4
8	4	12.9	0.35–5.5	1.6	0.8–1.9
8.5		Patient started on tablet L-T4 25 μg			
16	3	0.08	0.35–5.5	2.2	0.8–1.9
		Dose of tablet L-T4 reduced to 12.5 μg			
20	3	0.04	0.35–5.5	2.4	0.8–1.9
		Formulation of L-T4 changed to L-T4 oral solution 13 μg daily			
24	4	1.75	0.35–5.5	1.96	0.8–1.9
28	4	3.2	0.35–5.5		0.8–1.9

*Normal ranges shown are those used by the author's institution. FT4, free thyroxine; L-T4, levothyroxine; TSH, thyroid-stimulating hormone.

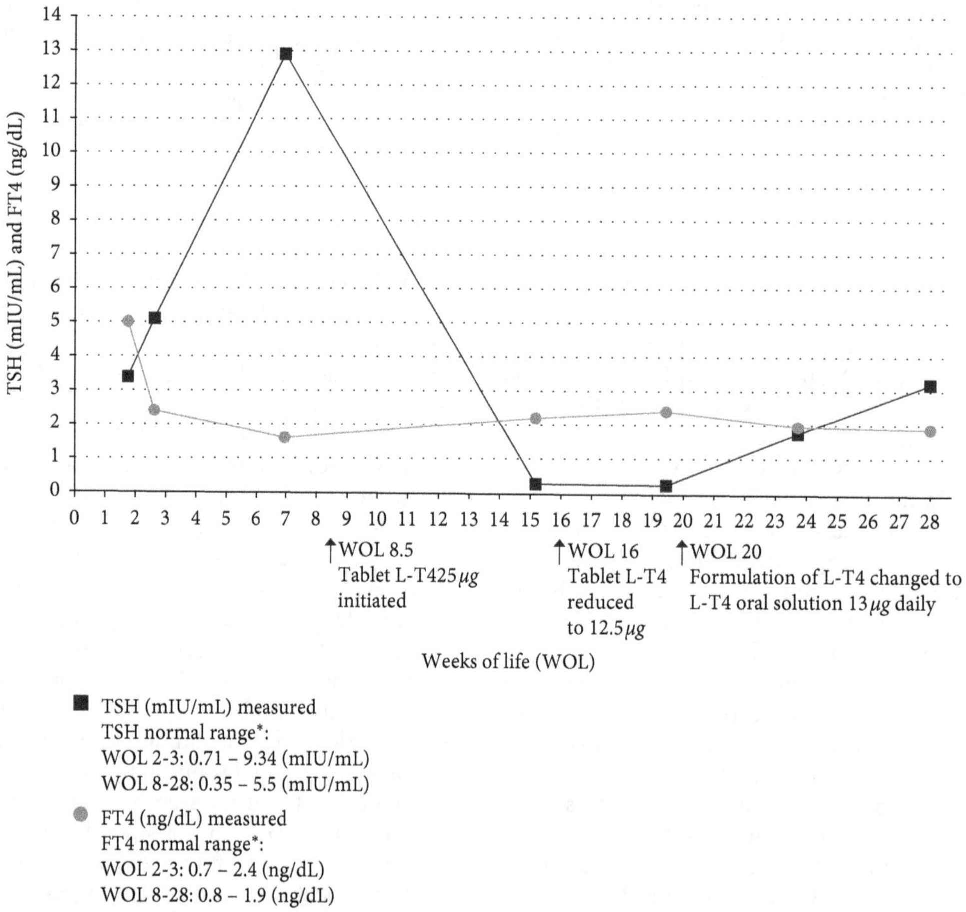

FIGURE 1: Thyroid-stimulating hormone (TSH) and free thyroxine (FT4) timeline. *Normal ranges shown are those used by the author's institution. L-T4, levothyroxine sodium oral solution; WOL, weeks of life.

The use of L-T4 oral solution (Tirosint®-SOL) may improve compliance and consistency of thyroid control in pediatric patients, especially in patients with T21 with/or without CH who have special needs. Also, clinicians should be aware that infants receiving biotin supplementation for biotinidase deficiency will need this therapy to be withheld before screening for CH. Failure to do so can result in erroneous measurement of thyroid levels and delayed diagnosis and treatment of CH.

A limitation of this case report is that we report on a single subject who was followed for a short time. However, this case provides point-of-care evidence that could help to inform practice guidelines and provide practical medical education to other healthcare professionals.

Acknowledgments

The author wishes to acknowledge Diane Kwiatkoski and Karen Wilson Smith of IQVIA for assistance in preparation of this manuscript. Article processing charges and funding for preparation of this manuscript were provided by IBSA Pharma Inc., Parsippany, NJ, USA.

References

[1] G. Holmes, "Gastrointestinal disorders in down syndrome," *Gastroenterology and Hepatology from Bed to Bench*, vol. 7, no. 1, pp. 6–8, 2017.

[2] A. T. Ferreira-Vasques and D. A. Lamônica, "Motor, linguistic, personal and social aspects of children with down syndrome," *Journal of Applied Oral Science*, vol. 23, no. 4, pp. 424–430, 2015.

[3] M. J. Pierce, S. H. LaFranchi, and J. D. Pinter, "Characterization of thyroid abnormalities in a large cohort of children with Down syndrome," *Hormone Research in Paediatrics*, vol. 87, no. 3, pp. 170–178, 2017.

[4] R. Whooten, J. Schmitt, and A. Schwartz, "Endocrine manifestations of Down syndrome," *Current Opinion in Endocrinology, Diabetes and Obesity*, vol. 25, no. 1, pp. 61–66, 2018.

[5] N. H. Amr, "Thyroid disorders in subjects with down syndrome: an update," *Acta Biomedica*, vol. 89, no. 1, pp. 132–139, 2018.

[6] N. Zwaveling-Soonawala, M. E. Witteveen, J. P. Marchal et al., "Early thyroxine treatment in Down syndrome and thyroid function later in life," *European Journal of Endocrinology*, vol. 176, no. 5, pp. 505–513, 2017.

[7] B. Wolf, "Biotinidase deficiency: "if you have to have an inherited metabolic disease, this is the one to have," *Genetics in Medicine*, vol. 14, no. 6, pp. 565–575, 2012.

[8] U.S. Food & Drug Administration, "UPDATE: the FDA warns that biotin may interfere with lab tests: FDA safety communication," 2019, http://www.fda.gov/medical-devices/safety-communications/update-fda-warns-biotin-may-interfere-lab-tests-fda-safety-communication.

[9] S. Charles and M. Blum, "Supplemental biotin and erroneous thyroid diagnoses and management," *Pediatric Dimensions*, vol. 3, no. 1, 2018.

[10] M.-L. Piketty, M. Polak, I. Flechtner, L. Gonzales-Briceño, and J.-C. Souberbielle, "False biochemical diagnosis of hyperthyroidism in streptavidin-biotin-based immunoassays: the problem of biotin intake and related interferences," *Clinical Chemistry and Laboratory Medicine (CCLM)*, vol. 55, no. 6, pp. 780–788, 2017.

[11] J. Jonklaas, A. C. Bianco, A. J. Bauer et al., "Guidelines for the treatment of hypothyroidism: prepared by the American Thyroid Association Task Force on Thyroid Hormone Replacement," *Thyroid*, vol. 24, no. 12, pp. 1670–1751, 2014.

[12] U.S. Food & Drug Administration Website, "Tirosint®-SOL (levothyroxine sodium) oral solution," 2016, https://www.accessdata.fda.gov/drugsatfda_docs/label/2016/206977s000lbl.pdf.

[13] E. Peroni, M. C. Vigone, S. Mora et al., "Congenital hypothyroidism treatment in infants: a comparative study between liquid and tablet formulations of levothyroxine," *Hormone Research in Paediatrics*, vol. 81, no. 1, pp. 50–54, 2014.

[14] A. Cassio, S. Monti, A. Rizzello et al., "Comparison between liquid and tablet formulations of levothyroxine in the initial treatment of congenital hypothyroidism," *The Journal of Pediatrics*, vol. 162, no. 6, pp. 1264–1269, 2013.

[15] J. H. von Heppe, H. Krude, D. L'Allemand, D. Schnabel, and A. Grüters, "The use of L-T4 as liquid solution improves the practicability and individualized dosage in newborns and infants with congenital hypothyroidism," *Journal of Pediatric Endocrinology & Metabolism*, vol. 17, no. 7, pp. 967–974, 2004.

[16] J. Léger, A. Olivieri, M. Donaldson et al., "European Society for Paediatric Endocrinology consensus guidelines on screening, diagnosis, and management of congenital hypothyroidism," *The Journal of Clinical Endocrinology and Metabolism*, vol. 99, no. 2, pp. 363–384, 2014.

[17] A. Grüters, A. Jenner, and H. Krude, "Long-term consequences of congenital hypothyroidism in the era of screening programmes," *Best Practice & Research Clinical Endocrinology & Metabolism*, vol. 16, no. 2, pp. 369–382, 2002.

[18] M. J. Kilberg, I. R. Rasooly, S. H. LaFranchi, A. J. Bauer, and C. P. Hawkes, "Newborn screening in the US may miss mild persistent hypothyroidism," *The Journal of Pediatrics*, vol. 192, pp. 204–208, 2018.

[19] National Institutes of Health Office of Dietary Supplements, Biotin, 2020, https://ods.od.nih.gov/factsheets/Biotin-HealthProfessional/.

[20] V. Eligar, P. Taylor, O. Okosieme, G. Leese, and C. Dayan, "Thyroxine replacement: a clinical endocrinologist's viewpoint," *Annals of Clinical Biochemistry*, vol. 53, no. 4, pp. 421–433, 2016.

[21] C. Yue, C. Scarsi, and M. Ducharme, "Pharmacokinetics and potential advantages of a new oral solution of levothyroxine vs. other available dosage forms," *Arzneimittelforschung*, vol. 62, no. 12, pp. 631–636, 2012.

[22] C. Virili, P. Trimboli, F. Romanelli, and M. Centanni, "Liquid and softgel levothyroxine use in clinical practice: state of the art," *Endocrine*, vol. 54, no. 1, pp. 3–14, 2016.

43

Subacute Thyroiditis Associated with COVID-19

Eugenia Campos-Barrera,[1] Teresa Alvarez-Cisneros,[2] and Mario Davalos-Fuentes[3]

[1]*Hospital Angeles Del Pedregal, Camino de Sta. Teresa 1055-S, Heroes de Padierna, La Magdalena Contreras, Ciudad de Mexico 10700, Mexico*
[2]*Instituto Nacional de Geriatría, Av Contreras 428, San Jeronimo Lidice, Magdalena Contreras, Mexico City 10700, Mexico*
[3]*Instituto Nacional de Rehabilitacion, Arenal de Guadalupe, Tlalpan, Mexico City 14389, Mexico*

Correspondence should be addressed to Eugenia Campos-Barrera; eugecampos81@icloud.com

Academic Editor: Takeshi Usui

Subacute thyroiditis is a self-limiting inflammatory disorder, characterized by neck pain or discomfort, a tender diffuse goiter, and sometimes a transient episode of hyperthyroidism followed by euthyroidism and sometimes hypothyroidism. There is usually a normalization of thyroid function within a few weeks. Subacute thyroiditis has a higher incidence in summer and has been linked to a viral or bacterial upper respiratory postinfection inflammatory response. We hereby describe the case of a previously healthy 37-year-old female presenting with subacute thyroiditis associated with a very mild presentation of COVID-19. As most patients with SARS-Cov-2 are asymptomatic, we suggest to rule out SARS-Cov-2 infection in patients presenting with symptoms suggesting SAT.

1. Case Presentation

On April 10, a previously healthy 37-year-old female experienced odynophagia and anosmia with no other respiratory symptoms. Her laboratory exams confirmed COVID-19 (RT-PCR for SARS-Cov-2) and was prescribed symptomatic treatment for her mild disease improving completely in the following days.

A month after her initial presentation, she presented to the ENT doctor with severe neck pain (8/10) irradiating to the right jaw and ear as well as fatigue. She did not mention any clinical signs of hyperthyroidism (tremor, anxiety, or diaphoresis) but was referred to the endocrinologist with the suspicion of SAT. At this time, her physical exam was significant only for a moderately enlarged tender thyroid gland and neck adenopathies. Her lab test results showed elevated ESR (72 mm/hr) and CRP (66 mg/L), anemia (Hb10.4 g/dL), and normal platelet and leukocyte counts. Her thyroid tests were positive for hyperthyroidism with an undetectable TSH, T4 total 13.5 mcg/dL, T4 free 1.6 ng/dL, and T3 total 211 ng/dL. Anti-Tg and anti-TPO were negative. Thyroid iodine scan showed no radioactive iodine uptake (Figures 1(a) and 1(b)). The diagnosis of subacute thyroiditis (SAT) was confirmed.

2. Outcome and Follow-Up

During her follow-up visit one month after the diagnosis, the patient has remained asymptomatic, but her lab tests are still relevant for anemia, thrombocytopenia, high ESR, and low TSH (0.01 mUI/L).

3. Discussion

The etiology of SAT (subacute granulomatous thyroiditis) is usually viral. The most commonly associated viruses include enterovirus, coxsackievirus, mumps, measles, and adenovirus [1–3]. However, the prevalence of SAT associated with the novel coronavirus seems to be increasing as we are all more aware of its complications [4–7]. The incidence of SAT is 12.1 cases per 100,000/year, and it is more frequent in young women when compared to men (19.1 vs 4.1 per 100,000/year, respectively) [8, 9]. It is characterized by neck pain or discomfort and a tender diffuse goiter associated

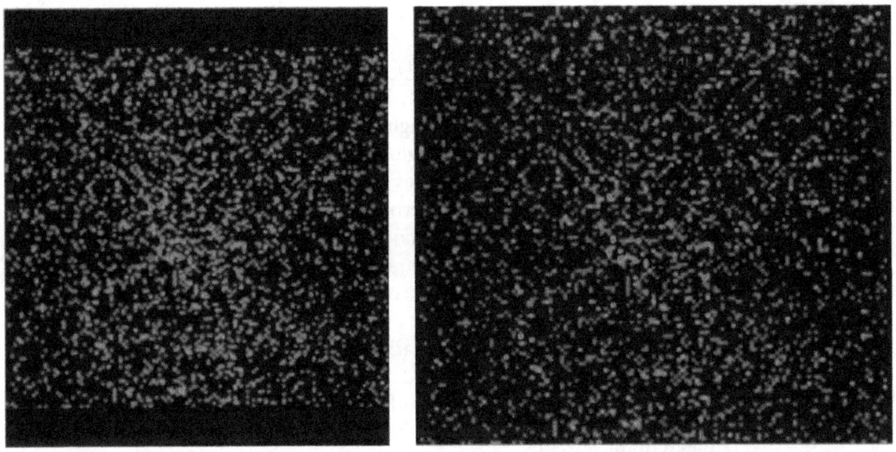

(a) (b)

FIGURE 1: (a, b) The patient's iodine thyroid scan with no uptake by the thyroid gland.

with myalgias, pharyngitis, low-grade fever, and fatigue [1, 10]. Up to 50% experience transient symptoms of thyrotoxicosis followed by euthyroidism, hypothyroidism, and a normalization of thyroid function within 3 months [1]. The incidence is 12.1 cases per 100,000/year with a higher incidence in young females when compared to men (19.1 vs 4.1 per 100,000/year, respectively) [8, 9]. The hallmark laboratory findings of SAT are elevated erythrocyte sedimentation rate (greater than 50 mm/hr) and C-reactive protein (CRP), low TSH concentrations with high free T4 and T3 during the early stages of the illness, and there is also a normal or mildly elevated leukocyte count and mild anemia [1]. Differently from Graves' disease, in SAT, most patients do not experience symptoms of thyroid excess, and T3 is not disproportionally elevated. With regard to antithyroid peroxidase and anti-thyroglobulin antibodies, they are usually undetectable or present at low titers. Imaging studies include a radioiodine or technetium imaging study and a Doppler ultrasound. The radioiodine study will show a low uptake (less than 1–3 percent) or a faint heterogeneous pattern of radionuclide uptake during the hyperthyroid phase. The ultrasound will show a normal or enlarged thyroid but typically, diffusely, or focally hypoechogenic, and the color Doppler sonography will demonstrate low flow.

Accepted treatment for subacute thyroiditis includes anti-inflammatory therapy with nonsteroidal anti-inflammatory drug (NSAID) or prednisone. Patients experiencing bothersome symptoms of hyperthyroidism such as palpitations, anxiety, or tremor benefit from treatment with a beta blocker such as propranolol (40–120 mg). Thionamides should not be used.

SAT is not the only thyroid condition associated with COVID-19, cases of thyroxine thyrotoxicosis have been also described by Muller et al. [6]. All available information on SAT and thyroxine thyrotoxicosis associated with COVID-19 comes from the Italian experience. There are three case reports by Ippolito et al., Brancatella et al., and Ruggeri et al. (see Table 1) and a study focusing on the prevalence of SAT and thyroxine thyrotoxicosis in patients with severe presentation of COVID-19 from an ICU unit by Muller et al. based in Milan (see Table 1) [4–7].

As shown in Table 1, similar to this Mexican case, all individual case reports of SAT associated with SARS-Cov-2 infection have been in women with an age range of 18 to 69. While all Italian cases presented symptoms of thyrotoxicosis, no such findings occurred in the Mexican case. Time between the diagnosis of SARS-Cov-2 and the onset of symptoms ranged from 5 days to one month, and the time between the diagnosis of SAT and recovery ranged from 1 week to 1 month. This differs from the findings of the study by Muller et al. which compared thyroid function tests in patients from the ICU in 2019 (without COVID-19) and patients in the ICU with COVID-19 in 2020 [6]. Findings from this study include that a higher proportion of patients from the ICU presented elevated TSH in 2020, suggesting the presence of SAT associated with SARS-Cov-2. In order to analyze if these findings were consistent with SAT, seven patients with low TSH were followed up for 55 days. While six showed laboratory findings compatible with SAT without ever developing neck pain, imaging studies compatible with SAT were found only in three of the patients. All of these findings suggest that SARS-Cov-2 thyroid infection may occur with or without clinical symptoms.

The pathophysiology of SAT associated with SARS-Cov-2 infection is thought to be similar to the association with other viral conditions, either direct infection or a postviral inflammatory reaction targeting the thyroid of genetically susceptible individuals. Muller et al. suggest that the affinity of SARS-Cov-2 to the thyroid gland is via the ACE2 receptors which are more prevalent in thyroid cells than lung cells. Because of this, clinicians should be aware of the possibility of subacute thyroiditis in patients experiencing SARS-Cov-2 infection. Another consideration is that because of the high prevalence of asymptomatic patients with SARS-Cov-2 infection, patients presenting with SAT should be tested for Sars-Cov-2. On the 21st of May, the Endocrine Society emitted a statement based on the case published by Brancatella et al.

Table 1: Available case reports on SAT associated with COVID-19.

Case	Place	Gender	Age	Presentation	Laboratory findings	Imaging studies	Follow-up
Ippolito et al. [5]	Italy	Female	69	Five days after the diagnosis of COVID-19 pneumonia, she presented with palpitations, insomnia, and agitation. She did not refer neck pain but was under pain killers.	TSH: low; FT4 and FT3: high; anti-thyroglobulin antibodies (TgAb), anti-peroxidase antibodies (TPOAb), and anti-TSH receptor antibodies (TRAb): negative.	Ultrasonography (US): enlarged hypoechoic thyroid with decreased vascularity. No uptake in the thyroid scan using Tc 99-m.	She was given methimazole, but the thyrotoxicosis worsened. She was given steroids, and after 10 days, all laboratory findings and symptoms improved.
Brancatella et al. [4]	Italy	Female	18	Symptoms included fever, neck pain radiated to the jaw, and palpitations 15 days after a SARS-CoV-2-positive oropharyngeal swab.	TSH: undetectable; FT4 and FT3: elevated; TgAb, TPOAb, TRAb, inflammatory markers, and white blood cell count: elevated.	US: bilateral and diffuse hypoechoic areas.	Symptoms improved within 1 week, and thyroid function and labs normalized in 40 days.
Ruggeri et al. [7]	Italy	Female	43	The patient developed neck pain, fatigue, tremors, and palpitation one month after the diagnosis of COVID-19.	TSH: suppressed; FT4 and FT3: elevated; TgAb, TPOAb, and TRAb: undetectable.	US: diffusely enlarged and hypoechogenic thyroid gland. Thyroid scintigraphy with 99mTc-perthecnetate showed markedly reduced uptake.	The patient was treated with oral prednisone, and within 2 weeks, the inflammatory response normalized. Thyroid function tests recovered 4 weeks after steroid treatment.
Campos-Barrera et al.	Mexico	Female	37	Severe neck pain (8/10) irradiating to the right jaw and ear as well as fatigue. She did not mention any clinical signs of hyperthyroidism.	TSH: undetectable; FT4 and FT3: elevated; TgAb, TPOAb, and TRAb: undetectable; elevated ESR and CRP and anemia.	Thyroid iodine scan showed no radioactive iodine uptake.	One month after the diagnosis, the patient remained asymptomatic but her lab tests were still relevant for anemia, thrombocytopenia, high ESR, and low TSH (0.01 mUI/L).

References

[1] E. N. Pearce, A. P. Farwell, and L. E. Braverman, "Thyroiditis," *New England Journal of Medicine*, vol. 348, no. 26, pp. 2646–2655, 2003.

[2] J. H. Lazarus, "Silent thyroiditis and subacute thyroiditis,""Silent thyroiditis and subacute thyroiditis," in *The Thyroid: A Fundamental and Clinical Text*, L. E. Braverman and R. D. Utiger, Eds., p. 577, 7th edition, Lippincott Williams & Wilkins, Philadelphia, PA, USA, 1996.

[3] R. Desailloud and D. Hober, "Viruses and thyroiditis: an update," *Virology Journal*, vol. 6, no. 1, p. 5, 2009.

[4] A. Brancatella, D. Ricci, N. Viola et al., "Subacute thyroiditis after SARS-CoV-2 infection," *The Journal of Clinical Endocrinology and Metabolism*, vol. 105, no. 7, Article ID dgaa276, 2020.

[5] S. Ippolito, F. Dentali, and M. L. Tanda, "SARS-CoV-2: a potential trigger for subacute thyroiditis? Insights from a case report," *Journal of endocrinological investigation*, vol. 43, pp. 1-2, 2020.

[6] I. Muller, D. Cannavaro, and D. Dazzi, "SARS-CoV-2-related atypical thyroiditis," *The Lancet Diabetes & Endocrinology*, vol. 8, no. 9, pp. 739–741, 2020.

[7] R. M. Ruggeri, A. Campennì, M. Siracusa, G. Frazzetto, and D. Gullo, "Subacute thyroiditis in a patient infected with SARS-COV-2: an endocrine complication linked to the COVID-19 pandemic," *Hormones*, 2020.

[8] V. Fatourechi, J. P. Aniszewski, G. Z. E. Fatourechi, E. J. Atkinson, and S. J. Jacobsen, "Clinical features and outcome of subacute thyroiditis in an incidence cohort: olmsted County, Minnesota, study," *The Journal of Clinical Endocrinology & Metabolism*, vol. 88, no. 5, pp. 2100–2105, 2003.

[9] S. H. Golden, K. A. Robinson, I. Saldanha, B. Anton, and P. W. Ladenson, "Prevalence and incidence of endocrine and metabolic disorders in the United States: a comprehensive review," *The Journal of Clinical Endocrinology & Metabolism*, vol. 94, no. 6, pp. 1853–1878, 2009.

[10] E. Nishihara, H. Ohye, N. Amino et al., "Clinical characteristics of 852 patients with subacute thyroiditis before treatment," *Internal Medicine*, vol. 47, no. 8, pp. 725–729, 2008.

Liquid Levothyroxine Formulation Taken during Lunch in Italy: A Case Report and Review of the Literature

Carlo Cappelli, Ilenia Pirola, and Maurizio Castellano

Department of Clinical and Experimental Sciences, SSD Medicina Ad Indirizzo Endocrino-metabolico, University of Brescia, ASST Spedali Civili di Brescia, Brescia 25123, Italy

Correspondence should be addressed to Carlo Cappelli; carlo.cappelli@unibs.it

Academic Editor: Suat Simsek

Levothyroxine (L-T4) is among the most widely prescribed medications in the world, and it is considered by the World Health Organization an essential medicine for basic health care. Replacement therapy has always been considered straightforward although different factors may interfere with intestinal absorption of L-T4, including food, dietary fibre, coffee, drugs, and gastrointestinal diseases. For these reasons, current guidelines recommend that L-T4 should be taken in a fasting state because its absorption is maximised when it is taken on an empty stomach, reflecting the importance of gastric acidity in the absorption process. In addition to sodium L-T4 in tablet form, various formulations (soft-gel capsules and liquid solutions) have become available for clinical use in the last years promising improved absorption. We described a 31-year-old Italian man who took liquid levothyroxine formulation during lunch. He was under replacement therapy with liquid levothyroxine 75 mcg daily for hypothyroidism due to Hashimoto thyroiditis for three years. During confirmation of the L-T4 replacement therapy, the patient stated that he was going to continue to "take liquid levothyroxine during (his) lunch every day." We recommended taking the medication correctly in the morning at least thirty minutes before breakfast and repeating TSH, fT4, and fT3 after three months. The thyroid hormonal profiles taken after 3 and 6 months were comparable to those when the patient was taking the medication during lunch. In conclusion, liquid levothyroxine formulation should be preferred in case of malabsorption or potential malabsorption. Liquid formulation should be preferred due to the possibility of taking it during breakfast, which significantly improves the compliance of patients. Further studies are needed to evaluate the possibility of taking liquid L-T4 during lunch.

1. Introduction

Levothyroxine is among the most widely prescribed medications in the world, and it is considered by the World Health Organization an essential medicine for basic health care [1–3].

The first use of thyroid hormone for the treatment of hypothyroidism was documented in the 1890s, when Bettencourt and Serrano described a patient grafted with an ovine thyroid gland to treat severe hypothyroidism [4]. Synthetic formulations of thyroxine have been available for use since the 1950s although desiccated animal thyroid gland remained the mainstay of therapy until the 1970s [5].

In addition to sodium levothyroxine (L-T4) in tablet form, today various L-T4 formulations (soft-gel capsules and liquid solutions) are being used in most but not all countries for clinical use in the last years [6]. Approximately 60–90% of a tablet L-T4 dose is absorbed within 3 h of ingestion, and the absorption is maximal when it is taken on an empty stomach, reflecting the importance of gastric acidity in the process. Differently, many reports showed that liquid formulations circumvent gastric acidity, improving their absorption even if ingested with breakfast [7–11].

We described a young Italian man who took liquid levothyroxine formulation during lunch.

2. Case Presentation

A 31-year-old male patient was referred to our Department for hypothyroidism on 3 April 2018. His medical history was not significant. He suffered from Hashimoto's thyroiditis and had been under replacement therapy with liquid levothyroxine 75 mcg daily (Tirosint 75 mcg-IBSA®) for three years. Physical examination showed no abnormalities. He exhibited two thyroid hormonal profiles (TSH, fT4, and fT3) taken, respectively, in the previous fifteen days and 6 months by outpatient evaluation (Table 1). The patient underwent thyroid ultrasound that showed an atrophic gland with marked hypoechoic tissue, without nodules (Figure 1). During confirmation of the L-T4 replacement therapy, the patient stated that he was going to continue to "take liquid levothyroxine during (his) lunch every day." The patient said that, only during the first year, he had taken liquid L-T4 at least 30 minutes before breakfast, while in the last two, he had been taking liquid L-T4 with a glass of water during his lunch "for convenience." We recommended taking the medication correctly in the morning at least thirty minutes before breakfast and repeating TSH, fT4, and fT3 after three months. The patient was reassessed on 27 July. He was in good health. The thyroid hormonal profiles are reported in Table 1. No difference in TSH, fT4, and fT3 was observed compared to the values found when the patient took the medication during lunch. New examinations were performed in the same laboratory after 6 months; TSH, fT4, and fT3 were still superimposable with the previous values (Table 1).

3. Discussion

We described for the first time, a patient taking liquid L-T4 during lunch in Italy. There was no change in serum TSH level after changing the timing of L-T4 ingestion to at least 30 minutes before breakfast.

Until ten years ago, the only formulation available was the tablet. Replacement therapy has always been considered straightforward although different factors may interfere with intestinal absorption of L-T4, including food, dietary fibre, coffee, drugs, and gastrointestinal diseases [12]. For these reasons, current guidelines recommend that L-T4 should be taken in a fasting state at least 30 minutes before breakfast or at bedtime (at least three hours after the evening meal) because its absorption is maximised when it is taken on an empty stomach, reflecting the importance of gastric acidity in the absorption process. [13, 14]. Indeed, discordant results on timing of L-T4 administration with respect to main meal are reported [15, 16].

Ten years ago, pharmaceutical companies introduced new levothyroxine formulations (liquid and soft-gel capsules) promising improved absorption. This could be due to the fact that these formulations circumvent the phase of gastric dissolution, which is closely dependent on gastric pH. This is true for liquid formulations because the active ingredient is already dissolved in 85% glycerol and 96% ethanol. Cassio et al. showed that, for the first time in 2013, there is no full bioequivalence between drops and tablets, especially for infants with severe congenital hypothyroidism, suggesting that liquid form could be more effective and/or better absorbed than tablets [17]. The following year, our group observed by chance a series of euthyroid patients who wrongly took liquid L-T4 with coffee at breakfast; after changing the time of intake to 30 min before breakfast, no change in thyroid hormonal profile was observed. This feedback suggested that that liquid T4 can be taken orally at breakfast both with water and with coffee. Taking into account these data, we hypothesized that high temperatures (i.e., coffee temperature) do not alter the molecular properties or stability of L-T4 [10]. This was later clearly demonstrated by Bernareggi and colleagues [18]. Moreover, the TICO study, a double-blind placebo-controlled crossover trial, confirmed that liquid L-T4 can be ingested directly at breakfast, thus potentially improving therapeutic compliance [9], data recently confirmed in more than seven hundred patients [10].

Many other subsequent studies and observations have shown the significant superiority in terms of TSH normalization of the liquid formulation compared to tablets even in different subsets of patients, such as those with or without gastrointestinal malabsorption, submitted to bariatric surgery or taking multiple concomitant drugs [19–24]. Furthermore, the use of liquid L-T4 showed a significantly reduced variability in TSH values, both in young and older people, with a higher number of patients who remained euthyroid during follow-up [25, 26]. This is relevant for at least two reasons: firstly, the simultaneous reduction in risk of developing other disorders mainly associated, but not exclusive, with clinical or subclinical hyperthyroidism, such as atrial fibrillation, osteoporosis, and coronary heart disease [27, 28]; secondly, subjects with stable euthyroidism during replacement L-T4 therapy required fewer blood checks, with a predictable relative reduction in total health care expenditure [29, 30].

Finally, the possibility of taking levothyroxine treatment during breakfast improves quality of life [31] and significantly improves adherence to the treatment [27] as recently reported by two Italian surveys.

Differently from liquid solution, soft-gel capsules contain the drug dissolved in glycerin and enclosed in a gelatinous matrix. This structure should promise protection from variations in gastric pH. In agreement, in vitro research showed that the dissolution profile was more consistent than for tablets in the entire pH range after 60–120 minutes [32]. This has been confirmed in vivo by Fiorni et al., showing a total dissolution time of about 20 minutes [33]. Literature shows that this formulation improves the TSH profile in patients with impaired gastric secretion [34], taking pump inhibitors [35], with central hypothyroidism [36], in post-menopausal woman taking calcium supplements [37] and also a few minutes before breakfast with coffee [38], as compared to tablets. On the contrary, Di Donna et al. demonstrated that there was no difference in L-T4 requirement between soft-gel capsules and tablets in patients without malabsorption although the serum TSH was lower in patients taking soft-gel capsules [39]. To the best of our knowledge only one study, the "TITI" study evaluated whether a soft-gel capsule of L-T4 could also be ingested at breakfast, instead of liquid formulation. The study showed that both the liquid and soft-gel capsule formulations of L-T4 can be taken with breakfast although a significant decrease in fT4 and fT3 was observed 6 months after the switch from liquid to soft-gel capsules [40]. For these

Table 1: Thyroid function tests while taking liquid levothyroxine during lunch and before breakfast at the same daily dose.

	Liquid L-T4 (75 mcg/die) taken during lunch		Liquid L-T4 (75 mcg/die) taken 30 minutes before breakfast	
	6 months before evaluation	15 days before evaluation	After 3 months from evaluation	After 9 months from evaluation
TSH, mIU/L (0.27–4.2)	1.71	1.69	1.80	1.75
fT4, pg/ml (8.0–19.0)	15.7	15.3	15.9	15.6
fT3, pg/ml (2.4–4.7)	3.3	3.1	3.4	3.3

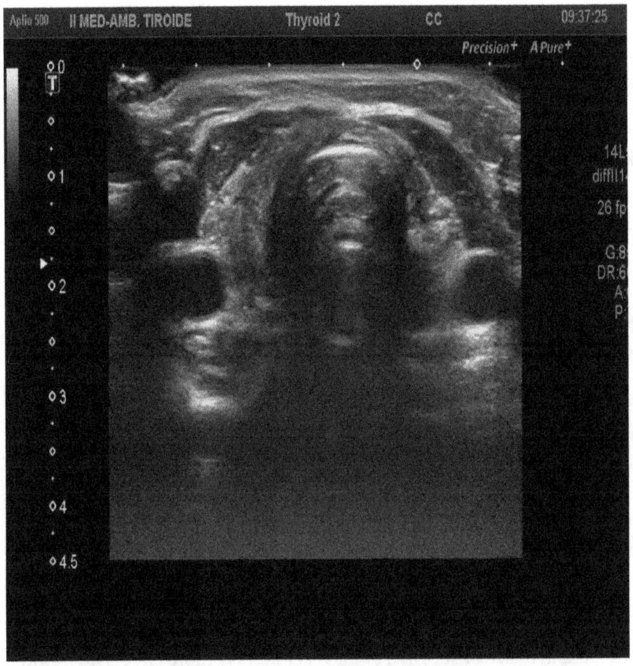

Figure 1: Thyroid ultrasound revealed an atrophic gland without nodules.

reasons, the authors suggested that "liquid L-T4 would be the preferred formulation for patients in whom even small changes in fT4 and fT3 levels are to be avoided." Further studies are needed to clarify this important issue.

4. Conclusion

The new levothyroxine formulation should be preferred in case of malabsorption or potential malabsorption. Liquid formulation should be preferred due to the possibility of taking it during breakfast, which significantly improves the compliance of patients. Further studies are needed to evaluate the possibility of taking liquid L-T4 during lunch.

Acknowledgments

The authors would like to thank the patient for agreeing to participate in this case report and for his contribution to expanding medical knowledge on this topic.

References

[1] F. R. Ernst, P. Barr, R. Elmor et al., "The economic impact of levothyroxine dose adjustments: the CONTROL HE study," *Clinical Drug Investigation*, vol. 37, no. 1, pp. 71–83, 2017.

[2] A. V. Fuentes, M. D. Pineda, and K. C. N. Venkata, "Comprehension of top 200 prescribed drugs in the US as a resource for pharmacy teaching, training and practice," *Pharmacy (Basel)*, vol. 14, no. 6, p. 43, 2018.

[3] World Health Organization, "WHO model list of essential medicines," 2019, http://apps.who.int/iris/bitstream/handle/10665/273826/EML-20-eng.pdf?ua=1.

[4] A.-M. Bettencourt and J.-A. Serrano, *Un Cas De Myxoede`me (Cachexie Pachydermique) Traite´ Par La Greffe Hypodermique Du Corps Thyoı¨de D'un Mouton*, Congres de l'Association Francaise pour l'Avancement des Sciences, Limoges, France, 1890.

[5] B. Bryan, "Levothyroxine: from sheep thyroid injections to synthetic formulations," *The Pharmaceutical Journal*, vol. 291, p. 90, 2013.

[6] B. Biondi and L. Wartofsky, "Treatment with thyroid hormone," *Endocrine Reviews*, vol. 35, no. 3, pp. 433–512, 2014.

[7] P. Trimboli, L. Scappaticcio, A. De Bellis et al., "Different formulations of levothyroxine for treating hypothyroidism: a real-life study," *International Journal of Endocrinology*, vol. 2020, Article ID 4524759, 5 pages, 2020.

[8] M. Castellana, C. Castellana, L. Giovanella, and P. Trimboli, "Prevalence of gastrointestinal disorders having an impact on tablet levothyroxine absorption: should this formulation still be considered as the first-line therapy?" *Endocrine*, vol. 67, no. 2, pp. 281–290, 2020.

[9] C. Cappelli, I. Pirola, L. Daffini et al., "A double-blind placebo-controlled trial of liquid thyroxine ingested at breakfast: results of the TICO study," *Thyroid*, vol. 26, no. 2, pp. 197–202, 2016.

[10] I. Pirola, E. Gandossi, D. Brancato et al., "TSH evaluation in hypothyroid patients assuming liquid levothyroxine at breakfast or 30 min before breakfast," *Journal of Endocrinological Investigation*, vol. 41, no. 11, pp. 1301–1306, 2018.

[11] C. Cappelli, I. Pirola, E. Gandossi, A. Formenti, and M. Castellano, "Oral liquid levothyroxine treatment at breakfast: a mistake?" *European Journal of Endocrinology*, vol. 170, no. 1, pp. 95–99, 2013.

[12] A. M. Formenti, L. Daffini, I. Pirola, E. Gandossi, A. Cristiano, and C. Cappelli, "Liquid levothyroxine and its potential use," *Hormones*, vol. 14, no. 2, pp. 183–189, 2015.

[13] J. Jonklaas, A. C. Bianco, A. J. Bauer et al., "Guidelines for the treatment of hypothyroidism: prepared by the american thyroid association task force on thyroid hormone replacement," *Thyroid*, vol. 24, no. 12, pp. 1670–1751, 2014.

[14] R. Guglielmi, A. Frasoldati, M. Zini et al., "Italian association of clinical endocrinologists statement-replacement therapy

for primary hypothyroidism: a brief guide for clinical practice," *Endocrine Practice*, vol. 22, no. 11, pp. 1319–1326, 2016.

[15] T.-G. Bach-Huynh, B. Nayak, J. Loh, S. Soldin, and J. Jonklaas, "Timing of levothyroxine administration affects serum thyrotropin concentration," *The Journal of Clinical Endocrinology & Metabolism*, vol. 94, no. 10, pp. 3905–3912, 2009.

[16] M. Skelin, T. Lucijanić, A.-M. Liberati-Čizmek et al., "Effect of timing of levothyroxine administration on the treatment of hypothyroidism: a three-period crossover randomized study," *Endocrine*, vol. 62, no. 2, pp. 432–439, 2018.

[17] A. Cassio, S. Monti, A. Rizzello et al., "Comparison between liquid and tablet formulations of levothyroxine in the initial treatment of congenital hypothyroidism," *The Journal of Pediatrics*, vol. 162, no. 6, pp. 1264–1269, 2013.

[18] A. Bernareggi, E. Grata, M. Pinorini, and A. Conti, "Oral liquid formulation of levothyroxine is stable in breakfast beverages and may improve thyroid patient compliance," *Pharmaceutics*, vol. 5, no. 4, pp. 621–633, 2013.

[19] P. Fallahi, S. M. Ferrari, and A. Antonelli, "Oral L-thyroxine liquid versus tablet in patients with hypothyroidism without malabsorption: a prospective study," *Endocrine*, vol. 52, no. 3, pp. 597–601, 2016.

[20] S. Benvenga, F. Di Bari, and R. Vita, "Undertreated hypothyroidism due to calcium or iron supplementation corrected by oral liquid levothyroxine," *Endocrine*, vol. 56, no. 1, pp. 138–145, 2017.

[21] P. Fallahi, S. M. Ferrari, I. Ruffilli, and A. Antonelli, "Reversible normalisation of serum TSH levels in patients with autoimmune atrophic gastritis who received L-T4 in tablet form after switching to an oral liquid formulation: a case series," *BMC Gastroenterology*, vol. 24, no. 16, p. 22, 2016.

[22] P. Fallahi, S. M. Ferrari, S. Camastra et al., "TSH normalization in bariatric surgery patients after the switch from L-thyroxine in tablet to an oral liquid formulation," *Obesity Surgery*, vol. 27, no. 1, pp. 78–82, 2017.

[23] I. Pirola, A. M. Formenti, E. Gandossi et al., "Oral liquid L-thyroxine (L-t4) may be better absorbed compared to L-T4 tablets following bariatric surgery," *Obesity Surgery*, vol. 23, no. 9, pp. 1493–1496, 2013.

[24] R. Vita, F. Di Bari, and S. Benvenga, "Oral liquid levothyroxine solves the problem of tablet levothyroxine malabsorption due to concomitant intake of multiple drugs," *Expert Opinion on Drug Delivery*, vol. 14, no. 4, pp. 467–472, 2017.

[25] R. Negro, R. Valcavi, D. Agrimi, and K. Toulis, "Levothyroxine liquid solution versus tablet for replacement treatment in hypothyroid patients," *Endocrine Practice*, vol. 20, no. 9, pp. 901–906, 2014.

[26] C. Cappelli, I. Pirola, L. Daffini, E. Gandossi, B. Agosti, and M. Castellano, "Thyroid hormonal profile in elderly patients treated with two different levothyroxine formulations: a single institute survey," *European Geriatric Medicine*, vol. 5, no. 6, pp. 382–385, m2014.

[27] B. Biondi, "Natural history, diagnosis and management of subclinical thyroid dysfunction," *Best Practice & Research Clinical Endocrinology & Metabolism*, vol. 26, no. 4, pp. 431–446, 2012.

[28] T. Collet, J. Gussekloo, D. C Bauer et al., "Thyroid studies collaboration, subclinical hyperthyroidism and the risk of coronary heart disease and mortality," *Archives of Internal Medicine*, vol. 172, no. 10, pp. 799–809, 2012.

[29] R. Ferrara, V. Ientile, V. Arcoraci et al., "Treatment pattern and frequency of serum TSH measurement in users of different levothyroxine formulations: a population-based study during the years 2009–2015," *Endocrine*, vol. 58, no. 1, pp. 143–152, 2017.

[30] R. Guglielmi, F. Grimaldi, R. Negro et al., "Shift from levothyroxine tablets to liquid formulation at breakfast improves quality of life of hypothyroid patients," *Endocrine, Metabolic & Immune Disorders - Drug Targets*, vol. 18, no. 3, pp. 235–240, 2018.

[31] C. Cappelli, R. Castello, F. Marini et al., "Adherence to levothyroxine treatment among patients with hypothyroidism: a northeastern Italian survey," *Frontiers in Endocrinology*, vol. 23, no. 9, pp. 699–701, 2018.

[32] D. Pabla, F. Akhlaghi, and H. Zia, "A comparative pH-dissolution profile study of selected commercial levothyroxine products using inductively coupled plasma mass spectrometry," *European Journal of Pharmaceutics and Biopharmaceutics*, vol. 72, no. 1, pp. 105–110, 2009.

[33] G. Fiorini, D. Ribichini, R. Pasquali, and D. Vaira, "In vivo dissolution of levothyroxine soft gel capsules," *Internal and Emergency Medicine*, vol. 11, no. 8, pp. 1151–1152, 2016.

[34] M. G. Santaguida, C. Virili, S. C. D. Duca et al., "Thyroxine softgel capsule in patients with gastric-related T4 malabsorption," *Endocrine*, vol. 49, no. 1, pp. 51–57, 2015.

[35] R. Vita and S. Benvenga, "Tablet levothyroxine (L-T4) malabsorption induced by proton pump inhibitor; a problem that was solved by switching to L-T4 in soft gel capsule," *Endocrine Practice*, vol. 20, no. 3, pp. 38–41, 2014.

[36] S. Benvenga, G. Capodicasa, and S. Perelli, "l-Thyroxine in an oral liquid or softgel formulation ensures more normal serum levels of free T4 in patients with central hypothyroidism," *Frontiers in Endocrinology*, vol. 8, no. 321, pp. 1–6, 2017.

[37] E. Morini, A. Catalano, A. Lasco, N. Morabito, and S. Benvenga, "In thyroxine-replaced hypothyroid postmenopausal women under simultaneous calcium supplementation, switch to oral liquid or softgel capsule L-thyroxine ensures lower serum TSH levels and favorable effects on blood pressure, total cholesterolemia and glycemia," *Endocrine*, vol. 65, no. 3, pp. 569–579, 2019.

[38] R. Vita, G. Saraceno, F. Trimarchi, and S. Benvenga, "A novel formulation of L-thyroxine (L-T4) reduces the problem of L-T4 malabsorption by coffee observed with traditional tablet formulations," *Endocrine*, vol. 43, no. 1, pp. 154–160, 2013.

[39] V. Di Donna, R. M. Paragliola, C. de Waure, G. Papi, A. Pontecorvi, and S. M. Corsello, "Is levothyroxine requirement the same for tablet and soft gel formulations?" *Endocrine*, vol. 59, no. 2, pp. 458–460, 2018.

[40] C. Cappelli, I. Pirola, E. Gandossi et al., "Thyroid hormone profile in patients ingesting soft gel capsule or liquid levothyroxine formulations with breakfast," *International Journal of Endocrinology*, vol. 2016, Article ID 9043450, 5 pages, 2016.

45

Recurrent Thyroid Storm Caused by a Complete Hydatidiform Mole in a Perimenopausal Woman

Anuradha Jayasuriya,[1] **Dimuthu Muthukuda**,[2] **Preethi Dissanayake**,[3] **and Shyama Subasinghe**[3]

[1]*Diabetes and Endocrinology Unit, Colombo South Teaching Hospital, Kalubowila, Colombo, Sri Lanka*
[2]*Diabetes and Endocrinology Unit, Sri Jayewardenepura General Hospital, Nugegoda, Colombo, Sri Lanka*
[3]*Sri Jayewardenepura General Hospital, Nugegoda, Colombo, Sri Lanka*

Correspondence should be addressed to Anuradha Jayasuriya; anuradhajayasuriya@yahoo.com

Academic Editor: Lucy Mastrandrea

Background. Gestational trophoblastic disease (GTD) which includes hydatidiform mole, invasive mole, placental site trophoblastic tumor, and choriocarcinoma is a rare cause of hyperthyroidism due to excess production of placental human chorionic gonadotrophin hormone (hCG) by tumor cells. Molecular mimicry between hCG and thyroid stimulating hormone (TSH) leads to continuous stimulation of TSH receptor by extremely high levels of hCG seen in these tumors. Consequently, biochemical and clinical hyperthyroidism ensues and it is potentially complicated by thyrotoxic crisis which is fatal unless urgent therapeutic steps are undertaken. *Case Description.* We present a 49-year-old perimenopausal woman who presented with recurrent thyroid storm and high output cardiac failure. The initial workup revealed suppressed TSH, high-free thyroxine (FT4), and free triiodothyronine (FT3) levels with increased vascularity of the normal-sized thyroid on ultrasonography. She was managed with parenteral beta blockers, steroids, and high-dose carbimazole. Her lower abdominal tenderness led to further investigations which revealed tremendously elevated beta-hCG and a snow storm appearance on transabdominal ultrasound suggestive of GTD. She underwent curative surgery and was diagnosed with complete hydatidiform mole postoperatively by histology. *Conclusion.* Recurrent thyroid crisis in gestational trophoblastic disease is an exceedingly rare presentation and that is highly fatal. This case highlights the importance of early detection and treatment of the etiology of thyrotoxicosis to eliminate mortality.

1. Introduction

The hormone hCG comprises of an α-subunit and a β-subunit. The former is structurally similar to the α-subunit of luteinizing hormone (LH), follicle-stimulating hormone (FSH), and thyroid-stimulating hormone (TSH) [1]. This similarity in TSH and hCG accounts for the continuous stimulation of TSH receptors in GTD where excessive production of hCG by trophoblastic tumor cells leads to hyperthyroidism.

Epidemiological studies have reported a broad variation in the incidence of GTD including hydatidiform mole (H mole) and choriocarcinoma. Japan and South East Asia have the highest reported incidence of H mole that has been estimated up to be 2 cases in 1000 pregnancies [2].

Molar pregnancy in postmenopausal women is a rare occurrence [3]. To date, there are only a small number of case studies and case series published in the previous literature about the gestational trophoblastic disease and hyperthyroidism [4, 5]. Even rarer are the case reports of thyroid storm and benign trophoblastic disease in perimenopausal women [6]. To our knowledge, our case represents the first description in the world literature of a complete hydatidiform mole (CHM) in a perimenopausal woman presenting with recurrent thyroid storm.

2. Case Report

A 49-year-old mother of 2 children presented with progressively worsening shortness of breath and orthopnea for 3 days. She had been experiencing intermittent fever, anorexia, nausea, and abdominal pain for 1 month, and she had developed sweating, tremors, and palpitations suggestive of hyperthyroidism. Her menstrual history was remarkable for a period of amenorrhoea for 3 months.

On examination, she was dyspneic with bilateral pedal edema. Her blood pressure was 180/110 mmHg, and jugular venous pressure was elevated. There were bibasal crepitations, and abdominal examination revealed a pelvic mass of a 14-week-sized uterus.

Basic investigations including full blood count and renal and liver function tests were normal. Chest X-ray showed diffuse infiltrates with bilateral small pleural effusions. 2D echo findings were compatible with high output cardiac failure. Thyroid functions revealed evidence of thyrotoxicosis with suppressed TSH of 0.009 mIU/mL, elevated free T3 of 10.89 pg/mL, and free T4 of 6.91 ng/dL. There was evidence of hypervascularity in thyroid ultrasonography. She had hyperthermia, atrial fibrillation, severe heart failure, and central nervous system disturbances fulfilling criteria for thyrotoxic crisis [7]. She was urgently commenced on high-dose carbimazole, parenteral beta blockers, and steroids. Because of persistent abdominal pain, ultrasound abdomen was performed which revealed the snow storm appearance that is a unique feature of gestational trophoblastic disease (Figure 1). Her serum beta-hCG level was substantially increased up to 146,092,800 mIU/mL, and contrast CT of abdomen confirmed a uterine mass measuring 12.6 cm × 8.9 cm × 9.0 cm (Figure 2).

Because of extremely high levels of hCG, the working diagnosis was established as choriocarcinoma and, therefore, she was prepared to be sent for chemotherapy at cancer institute of Sri Lanka. While awaiting chemotherapy, she developed the second episode of thyrotoxic crisis. At this point, her beta-hCG titer was 254,532,200 mIU/mL, TSH was0.022 mIU/mL, FT3 was 6.15 pg/mL, and FT4 was 2.89 ng/dL, and she received urgent parenteral furosemide, digoxin, hydrocortisone, and high-dose propylthiouracil.

Preoperative optimization was carried out with antihypertensives (losartan, prazosin, indapamide, and propranolol), antipyretics, and adequate hydration. Cholestyramine and Lugol's iodine were added for further control of her hyperthyroid state. Following stabilization of her thyrotoxic crisis, a transabdominal hysterectomy and bilateral oophorectomy under general anesthesia was performed successfully under intraoperative hydrocortisone and esmolol infusions. Macroscopic appearance of the tumor was compatible with a hydatidiform mole (Figure 3).

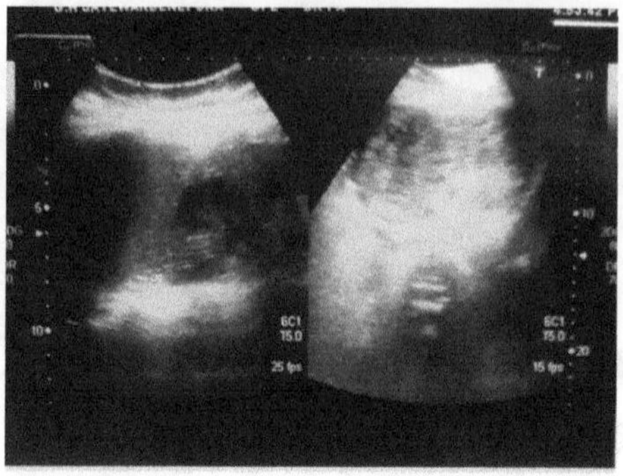

Figure 1: Ultrasound scan of the abdomen showing the typical snow storm appearance of the hydatidiform mole.

The patient was managed by the multidisciplinary team involving the physician, endocrinologist, obstetrician, cardiologist, cardioelectrophysiologist, and anesthesiologist. The tumor was later confirmed by histology as a complete hydatidiform mole without evidence of myometrial invasion.

Following surgery, she became clinically euthyroid and her thyroid functions and hCG level gradually improved over 3 months (Table 1) (Figure 4).

3. Discussion

The usual clinical trial of GTD includes uterine enlargement inconsistent with the period of amenorrhea, hyperemesis gravidarum, and markedly elevated serum hCG level. This patient presented with a period of amenorrhoea, abdominal pain, and irregular vaginal bleeding without vomiting in spite of very high levels of serum beta hCG. Occurrence of symptomatic hyperthyroidism in GTD is not common [7]. On review of the 196 patients with gestational trophoblastic neoplasia treated with chemotherapy in Sheffield since 2005, 14 (7%) had biochemical hyperthyroidism. Of these, only four had evidence of clinical hyperthyroidism [8]. GTD presenting with thyrotoxic crisis in perimenopausal women is extremely rare and restricted to case reports [9]. Although recurrent thyroid storm has been reported in association with thyroid cancer, there were no published literature on GTD presenting with recurrent thyroid crisis [10].

Early recognition of this clinical entity is important due to the complications associated with the hyperthyroid state mostly during surgery. Our patient had hyperthyroidism for 1-month duration, and she developed thyrotoxic crisis complicated with atrial fibrillation and heart failure while awaiting surgery. There has been only few reported cases of atrial fibrillation caused by hyperthyroidism secondary to hydatidiform moles [11]. The use of iodinated substances is a recognized trigger of thyrotoxic crisis (the Jod -Basedow phenomenon) and is reported in association with GTD [12, 13]. Use of iodinated contrast during imaging has possibly contributed to the development of recurrent thyrotoxic crisis in this patient. Because of urgent management with parenteral bata blockers and antithyroid drugs, her perioperative period was uncomplicated. The initial suspicion of choriocarcinoma in this patient can be explained by the fact

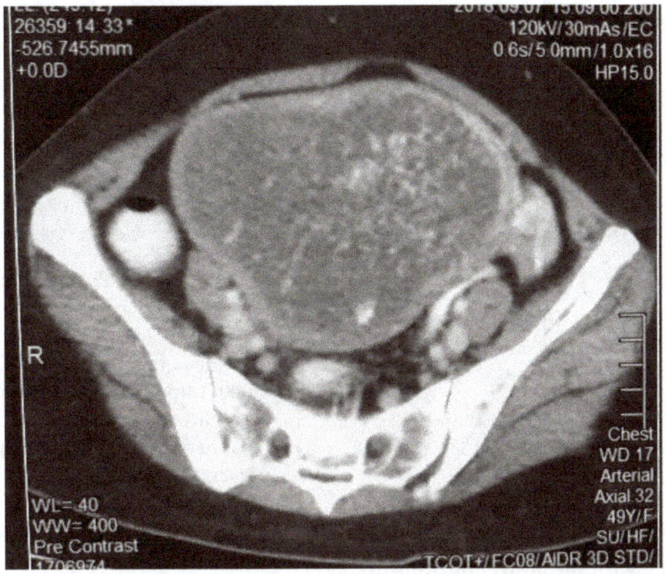

Figure 2: Contrast-enhanced CT appearance of the hydatidiform mole.

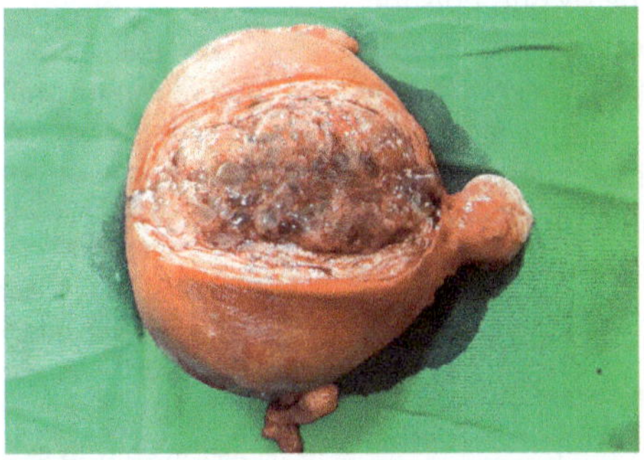

Figure 3: Specimen of the uterus showing the hydatidiform mole along the incision line of myometrium, a large mass of grape-like structures.

Table 1: Evolution of thyroid function.

	Preoperative day		Postoperative day		
	1st episode of thyroid storm	2nd episode of thyroid storm	Day 5	Day 14	Day 60
TSH (mIU/L) (0.27–4.20 mIU/L)	0.009	0.022	0.012	1.38	0.562
Free T4 (ng/dL) (0.93–1.70 ng/dL)	6.91	2.89	1.69	2.64	1.270
Free T3 (pg/mL) (2.3–4.2 pg/mL)	10.89	6.15	1.77	1.17	
FT3/FT4 ratio (10^{-2} pg/ng)	1.576	2.128			

Analytical sensitivity for TSH: 0.008 mIU/mL, FT4: 0.1 ng/dL, and FT3: 0.2 pg/mL. Measured by using a fully automated immunoassay analyzer ADVIA centaur XP.

that extremely high levels of serum hCG correlates better with an underlying choriocarcinoma rather than with an H mole [14].

Serum FT3 to FT4 ratio (FT3/FT4) is a useful tool for the differentiation of the cause of thyrotoxicosis. FT3/FT4 ratio of > 4.4 (10^{-2} pg/ng) strongly supports the diagnosis of Graves' disease, and a lower FT3/FT4 ratio of < 2.73 (10^{-2} pg/ng)) suggests other etiologies for hyperthyroidism [15]. It is a recognized fact that the conversion of T4 to T3 could be impaired in severe thyroid storm [16]. Japanese thyroid association conducted a nationwide survey which revealed that FT3 levels and the FT3/FT4 ratio were

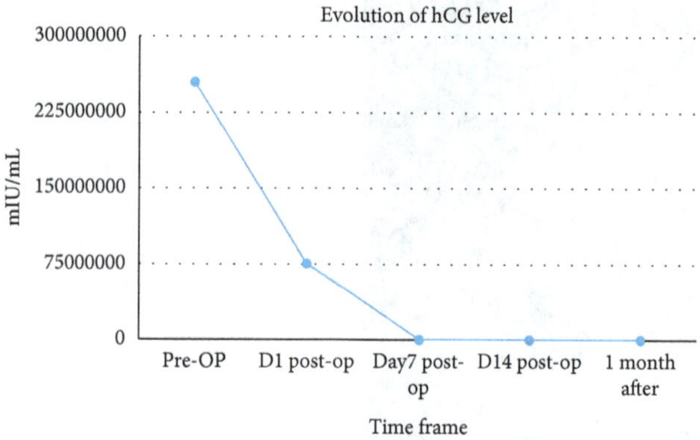

FIGURE 4: Evolution of beta-hCG level over the course of treatment.

inversely proportional to the disease severity in thyroid storm [17]. In both episodes of thyrotoxic crisis, FT3/FT4 < 2.73 (10^{-2} pg/ng) was compatible with the above findings. In the fist episode, higher FT4 and FT3 levels suggest untreated severe hyperthyroidism and FT3/FT4 ratio < 2 (10^{-2}pg/ng) indicate underlying low T3 syndrome associated with euthyroid sick syndrome [18, 19]. During the second episode, comparatively lower FT3 and FT4 concentrations can be caused by antithyroid drug (ATD) therapy. Therefore the difference in the FT3/FT4 ratios at the both episodes of thyroid storm can be explained by multiple factors such as the underlying cause, the precipitant and the severity of thyroid crisis, commencement of ATDs, and non thyroidal illness syndrome.

The definitive management of hydatidiform mole is either surgical evacuation of the molar tissue by hysterectomy or curettage if the patient is willing for further pregnancy. Despite the fact that surgery is curative, it can provoke thyroid crisis which is fatal. Hence perioperative management should be carried out with extreme precautions. There are few reported cases of surgical intervention for trophoblastic disease complicated with thyroid storm [20, 21]. The safety and effectiveness of prophylactic chemotherapy for gestational trophoblastic disease was assessed by several studies, and although prophylactic chemotherapy may reduce the progression of GTD with high malignancy risk, it is not currently recommended because of the adverse effect profile and concerns about drug resistance [22].

This patient underwent hysterectomy and oophorectomy because of the rare possibility of her GTD being malignant. However, it was confirmed by histology to be a benign complete H mole without invasion of surrounding tissues. She was followed up by monitoring of serial hCG levels weekly until negative and then monthly for 6 months.

4. Conclusion

Even though rare, GTD should be considered as an etiology for thyrotoxicosis in women of perimenopausal age. In fact, it is a diagnostic challenge to the clinician, and early recognition and preoperative stabilization with medical management is of paramount importance prior to curative surgery. Complete resection of these tumors leads to dramatic reduction of perioperative morbidity and mortality.

References

[1] L. A. Cole, "Biological functions of hCG and hCG-related molecules," *Reproductive Biology and Endocrinology*, vol. 8, no. 1, p. 102, 2010.

[2] S. Bruce and J. Sorosky, "Gestational trophoblastic disease," 2020, https://www.ncbi.nlm.nih.gov/books/NBK470267.

[3] S. Mehrotra, U. Singh, and S. Chauhan, "Molar pregnancy in postmenopausal women: a rare phenomenon," *BMJ Case Reports*, vol. 2012, 2012.

[4] G. A. Filipescu, O. A. Solomon, N. Clim, A. Milulescu, A. G. Boiangiu, and M. Mitran, "Molar pregnancy and thyroid storm—literature review," *ARS Medica Tomitana*, vol. 23, no. 3, pp. 121–125, 2017.

[5] L. Walkington, J. Webster, B. W. Hancock, J. Everard, and R. E. Coleman, "Hyperthyroidism and human chorionic gonadotrophin production in gestational trophoblastic disease," *British Journal of Cancer*, vol. 104, no. 11, pp. 1665–1669, 2011.

[6] L. Struthmann, M. Günthner-Biller, F. Bergauer, K. Friese, and I. Mylonas, "Complete hydatidiform mole in a perimenopausal woman with a subsequent severe thyriotoxicosis," *Archives of Gynecology and Obstetrics*, vol. 279, no. 3, p. 411, 2009.

[7] H. B. Burch and L. Wartofsky, "Life-threatening thyrotoxicosis: thyroid storm," *Endocrinology and Metabolism Clinics of North America*, vol. 22, no. 2, pp. 263–277, 1993.

[8] H. Düğeroğlu and M. Özgenoğlu, "Thyroid function among women with gestational trophoblastic diseases. A cross-sectional study," *Sao Paulo Medical Journal*, vol. 137, no. 3, pp. 278–283, 2019.

[9] J. D. Kofinas, A. Kruczek, J. Sample, and G. S. Eglinton, "Thyroid storm-induced multi-organ failure in the setting of gestational trophoblastic disease," *The Journal of Emergency Medicine*, vol. 48, no. 1, pp. 35–38, 2015.

[10] H. Raef, T. Dahhan, M. Ahmed, M. Mubarak, T. Rana, and A. Tulba, "Recurrent thyroid storm induced by heretofore unrecognised causes in a patient with thyroid cancer," *BMJ Case Reports*, vol. 2009, 2009.

[11] S. Matsumoto, C. Shingu, S. Hidaka et al., "Anesthetic management of a patient with hyperthyroidism due to hydatidiform mole," *Journal of Anesthesia*, vol. 23, no. 4, pp. 594–596, 2009.

[12] J. B. Stanbury, A. E. Ermans, P. Bourdoux et al., "Iodine-induced hyperthyroidism: occurrence and epidemiology," *Thyroid*, vol. 8, no. 1, pp. 83–100, 1998.

[13] C. E. D. d. Almeida, E. F. Curi, C. R. D. d. Almeida, and D. F. Vieira, "Thyrotoxic crisis associated with gestational trophoblastic disease," *Brazilian Journal of Anesthesiology*, vol. 61, no. 5, pp. 604–609, 2011.

[14] A. Cavaliere, S. Ermito, A. Dinatale, and R. Pedata, "Management of molar pregnancy," *Journal of Prenatal Medicine*, vol. 3, no. 1, pp. 15–17, 2009.

[15] C. Sriphrapradang and A. Bhasipol, "Differentiating Graves' disease from subacute thyroiditis using ratio of serum free triiodothyronine to free thyroxine," *Annals of Medicine and Surgery*, vol. 10, pp. 69–72, 2016.

[16] T. Satoh, O. Isozaki, A. Suzuki et al., "2016 guidelines for the management of thyroid storm from the Japan Thyroid Association and Japan Endocrine Society," *Endocrine Journal*, vol. 63, no. 12, pp. 1025–1064, 2016.

[17] O. Isozaki, T. Satoh, S. Wakino et al., "Treatment and management of thyroid storm: analysis of the nationwide surveys," *Clinical Endocrinology*, vol. 84, no. 6, pp. 912–918, 2016.

[18] R. Nomura, K. Miyai, R. Kuge, T. Okura, M. Goto, and Y. Hasegawa, "Free T3 to free T4 ratio less than 2.0 suggests low T3 syndrome rather than central hypothyroidism from the age of two to eighteen years," *Endocrine Journal*, vol. 64, no. 2, pp. 213–219, 2017.

[19] S. M. Adler and L. Wartofsky, "The nonthyroidal illness syndrome," *Endocrinology and Metabolism Clinics of North America*, vol. 36, no. 3, pp. 657–672, 2007.

[20] E. Erturk, H. Bostan, S. Geze, S. Saracoglu, N. Erciyes, and A. Eroglu, "Total intravenous anesthesia for evacuation of a hydatidiform mole and termination of pregnancy in a patient with thyrotoxicosis," *International Journal of Obstetric Anesthesia*, vol. 16, no. 4, pp. 363–366, 2007.

[21] A. Varela, A. Yuste, R. Villazala, J. Garrido, A. Lorenzo, and E. López, "Spinal anesthesia for emergency abdominal surgery in uncontrolled hyperthyroidism," *Acta Anaesthesiologica Scandinavica*, vol. 49, no. 1, pp. 100–103, 2005.

[22] Q. Wang, J. Fu, L. Hu et al., "Prophylactic chemotherapy for hydatidiform mole to prevent gestational trophoblastic neoplasia," *Cochrane Database of Systematic Reviews*, vol. 9, no. 9, Article ID CD007289, 2017.

HDR Syndrome Accompanying Type 1 Diabetes Mellitus and Hypopituitarism

Mustafa Can, Feridun Karakurt, Muhammed Kocabas, İlker Cordan, Melia Karakose, and Mustafa Kulaksızoglu

Department of Endocrinology and Metabolism, Meram School of Medicine, Necmettin Erbakan University, Konya, Turkey

Correspondence should be addressed to Mustafa Can; can1120can@gmail.com

Academic Editor: Osamu Isozaki

HDR (Hypoparathyroidism, Deafness, and Renal Dysplasia) syndrome is an autosomal dominant disorder characterized by the triad of hypoparathyroidism, sensorineural deafness, and renal disease. Approximately 65% of patients with HDR syndrome have all three of these features, while others have different combinations of these features. We aimed to present a case with primary hypoparathyroidism, hearing loss, and nondiabetic chronic kidney disease and diagnosed as HDR syndrome while being followed up for type 1 diabetes mellitus and hypopituitarism.

1. Introduction

HDR syndrome is an autosomal dominant disorder with a broad clinical spectrum. HDR syndrome is caused by mutations in the GATA3 gene found in the 10p chromosome (10p14) [1–3]. The frequency of the disease is unknown. Patients may present with hypocalcemia, tetany, or convulsion at any age. Other classical features include hearing loss and renal diseases such as nephrotic syndrome, renal dysplasia, hypoplasia or aplasia, pelvicalyceal deformity, vesicoureteral reflux, and chronic renal failure [4–6].

The diagnosis of HDR syndrome is based on clinical findings and can be supported by measurement of parathyroid hormone levels, an audiogram or auditory brainstem response, kidney imaging studies, and kidney biopsy. In addition to classical findings, patients with HDR syndrome may have diseases such as Hirschsprung disease, renal tubular acidosis, autoimmune thyroiditis, and type 1 diabetes mellitus. In this article, we aimed to present a case with primary hypoparathyroidism, hearing loss, and nondiabetic chronic kidney disease and diagnosed as HDR syndrome while being followed up for type 1 diabetes mellitus and hypopituitarism.

2. Case Report

A 28-year-old male patient was admitted to endocrinology outpatient clinic with complaints of impaired balance, hearing loss, and numbness in the hands for a long time. There were type 1 diabetes mellitus, hypopituitarism, and short-term myoclonic jerks after head trauma in his medical history. The drugs he used were insulin aspart, insulin glargine, and carbamazepine. In the family history there was a consanguineous marriage between the parents. His family did not have any history of HDR syndrome. Vital signs upon admission found a blood pressure of 100/70 mmHg, heart rate of 84 beats/min, and body temperature of 36.6°C. He was not mentally retarded. In the neurological examination, the patient was awake, oriented, and cooperative with exam; cranial nerves, motor strength, sensory testing, and proprioception were all intact; only ataxic gait was present. Hair in the face and axillary and inguinal regions was decreased, bilateral testes were small, and gynecomastia was present. All other examinations were normal.

In laboratory examination, the following are found: leukocyte: 8.6 10^3/ml (4-10), hemoglobin: 10.8 gr/dl (12.1-17.2), MCV: 99.7 fL (82.2-99), platelet: 119 10^3/ml (150-400),

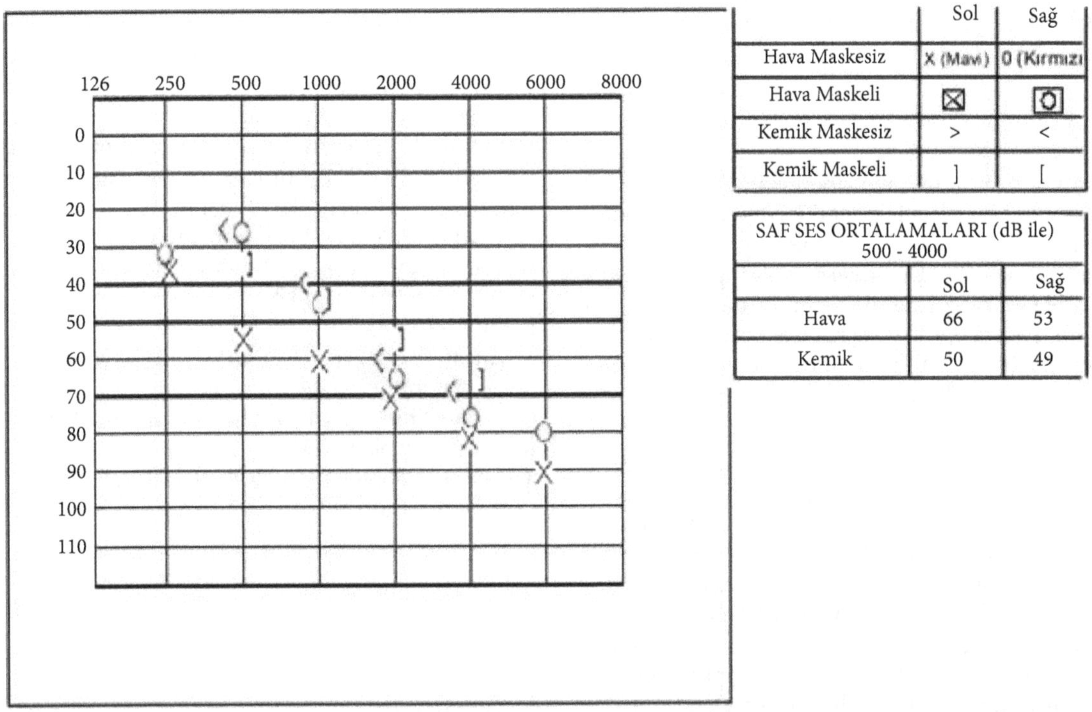

FIGURE 1: Pure tone threshold audiogram shows a moderate mix type in the left ear and sensorineural hearing loss in the right ear at slightly higher frequencies.

glucose: 386 mg/dL (70-100), urea: 80 mg/dL (16.6-48.5), creatinine: 1.9 mg/dL (0.70-1.2), sodium: 161 mmol/L (136-145), potassium: 4.48 mmol/L (3.5-5.1), calcium: 5.68 mg/dL (8.4-10.2), phosphorus: 5.7 mg/dL (2.5-4.5), albumin: 4.02 g/dL (3.5-5.2), HbA1c: 7.6% (4-6), TSH: 1.42 mU/L (0.27-4.2), free T4: 0.546 ng/dL (0.93-1.7), free T3: 1.53 ng/L (2-4.4), iPTH: 19.90 ng/dL (12-88), FSH: 1.3 U/L (1.7 -12), LH: 7.67 IU/L (1.24-8.62), total testosterone: 8.88 ng/dL (249-836), cortisol: 10.15 mcg/dL (6.02-18.4), prolactin: 8.19 mcg/L (4.4- 15.2), B12: 273.2 ng/L (197-771), folic acid: 1.9 mcg/dL (3.89-20), urine analysis Ph: 5.5, density: 1014, microalbumin in spot urine: 0.34 mg/dl (0-2), microprotein in spot urine: 36.3 mg/dl (0-15), creatinine in spot urine: 227.61 (39-259) mg/dl, serum osmolarity: 394 mOsm/KgH2O (285-295), and urine osmolarity: 590 mOsm/KgH2O (50-1200). On abdominal ultrasonography, the size of left kidney was preserved, long axis of right kidney was 8.5 cm, and there was a minimal reduction in cortex thickness and a grade 1 increase in right kidney parenchyma echogenicity. As a result of laboratory and imaging findings, in addition to the diagnosis of type 1 diabetes mellitus and hypopituitarism, chronic kidney disease, primary hypoparathyroidism, and megaloblastic anemia due to folic acid deficiency were detected.

The audiogram showed a moderate mix type sensorineural hearing loss in the left ear and mild sensorineural hearing loss at increased frequencies in the right ear [Figure 1]. There were no pathological findings on eye examination. Bilateral symmetrical calcifications were detected in the basal ganglia, vermis, and cerebellum in brain CT [Figure 2]. There were no pathological findings in the pituitary MRI.

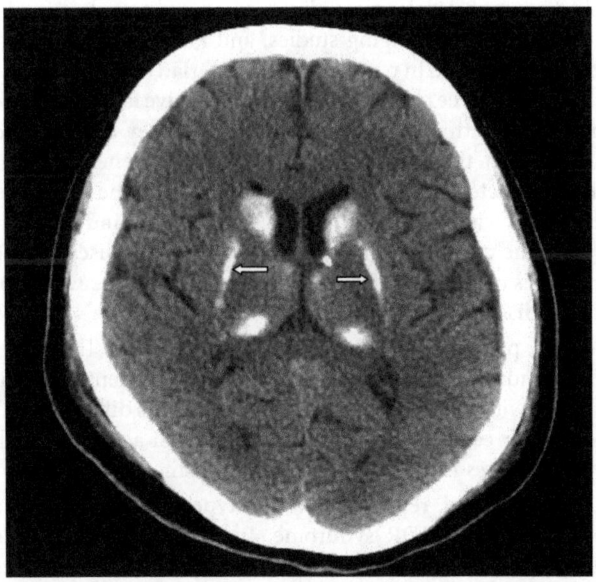

FIGURE 2: Bilateral symmetrical calcifications are seen in the basal ganglia of the brain CT.

HDR syndrome was considered because of the diagnosis of primary hypoparathyroidism, hearing loss, and nondiabetic chronic kidney disease in addition to type 1 diabetes mellitus, hypopituitarism, and epilepsy. The patient's electrolyte and hormone replacement therapies were held. The symptoms and signs improved and the patient was taken to regular follow-up program.

3. Discussion

HDR syndrome is an autosomal dominant disorder. HDR syndrome is caused by mutations in the GATA3 gene found in the 10p chromosome (10p14). The GATA3 gene belongs to the family of double zinc-finger transcription factors involved in the embryonic development of the parathyroid glands, hearing system, kidney, thymus, and central nervous system. The lack of GATA3 mutations and the variability of gene expression lead to phenotypic heterogeneity [1–3].

HDR syndrome can be detected at any age from early childhood to adulthood. The clinical spectrum of HDR syndrome is quite broad and patients may present with clinical findings such as hypocalcemia, tetany, convulsion, hearing loss, nephrotic syndrome, renal dysplasia, hypoplasia or aplasia, vesicoureteral reflux, and chronic renal failure. Ferraris et al. reported that 48 (62.3%) of the 77 patients with HDR syndrome had a complete clinical triad (hypoparathyroidism, sensorineural hearing loss, and kidney disease), 22 (28.6%) had no kidney disease, 2 (2.6%) had no hypoparathyroidism, and 5 (6.5%) had no hearing loss [7].

The diagnosis of HDR syndrome is based on clinical findings and can be supported by measurement of parathyroid hormone levels, an audiogram or auditory brainstem response, kidney imaging studies, and kidney biopsy. Diagnosis is confirmed in patients with HDR triad or patients with two of these three characteristics and a positive family history. In patients with isolated hearing loss or kidney disease who do not meet the above criteria, the GATA3 gene mutation should be detected to confirm the diagnosis [1]. The treatment of patients with HDR syndrome is symptomatic and depends on specific clinical findings and severity of the disease. The prognosis of HDR syndrome is determined by the severity of kidney disease.

Our patient had a complete clinical triad. Therefore, HDR syndrome was diagnosed based on the patient's clinical findings without genetic evaluation. Our case is differentiated from other cases in the literature in terms of accompanying type 1 diabetes mellitus and hypopituitarism.

Muroya et al. reported a case of type 1 diabetes mellitus associated with HDR syndrome. In HDR syndrome, it is thought that GATA 3 haplo insufficiency may cause diabetes mellitus by affecting the function of β cells and/or lymphocytes in patients with predisposition due to the genetic and environmental factors [8]. Pituitary insufficiency may occur due to hereditary and acquired disorders. Clinical signs and symptoms vary according to the lacking hormone, degree of deficiency, and the time of onset. The association of HDR syndrome and hypopituitarism has not been reported previously. This association can be coincidental because hypopituitarism was not detected in patients with GATA 3 mutations before.

A total of 108 cases of HDR syndrome have been reported in the literature; some of them are family reports. A total of 4 cases were reported from our country. In addition to classical findings in patients with HDR syndrome, Hirschsprung disease [9], renal tubular acidosis, autoimmune thyroiditis, hypergonadotropic hypogonadism [10], biliary atresia [11], ichthyosis [12], severe mental retardation [13], congenital choanal atresia [14], psoriasis [15], squamous cell lung carcinoma [16], band keratopathy, pigmentary retinopathy [17], nephrocalcinosis [18], cerebral infarction [19], recurrent cerebral infarction [20], tumoral calcinosis [21], and proliferative glomerulonephritis [22] were reported in previous publications.

In this article, we present the case diagnosed with HDR syndrome while being followed up with type 1 diabetes mellitus and hypopituitarism. Further studies are needed to explain the relationship between GATA3 gene and endocrinopathies such as type 1 diabetes mellitus and hypopituitarism.

References

[1] H. Van Esch, P. Groenen, M. A. Nesbit et al., "GATA3 haplo-insufficiency causes human HDR syndrome," *Nature*, vol. 406, no. 6794, pp. 419–422, 2000.

[2] M.-C. Labastie, M. Catala, J.-M. Gregoire, and B. Peault, "The GATA-3 gene is expressed during human kidney embryogenesis," *Kidney International*, vol. 47, no. 6, pp. 1597–1603, 1995.

[3] T. Hasegawa, Y. Hasegawa, T. Aso et al., "HDR syndrome (hypoparathyroidism, sensorineural deafness, renal dysplasia) associated with del(10)(p13)," *American Journal of Medical Genetics*, vol. 73, no. 4, pp. 416–418, 1997.

[4] A. Y. Barakat, J. B. D'Albora, M. Martin, and P. A. Jose, "Familial nephrosis, nevre deafness, and hypoparathyroidism," *The Journal of Pediatrics*, vol. 91, pp. 61–64, 1977.

[5] R. W. Bilous, G. Murty, D. B. Parkinson et al., "Autosomal dominant familial hypoparathyroidism, sensorineural deafness, and renal dysplasia," *The New England Journal of Medicine*, vol. 327, no. 15, pp. 1069–1074, 1992.

[6] P. Lichtner, R. König, T. Hasegawa, H. Van Esch, T. Meitinger, and S. Schuffenhauer, "An HDR (hypoparathyroidism, deafness, renal dysplasia) syndrome locus maps distal to the DiGeorge syndrome region on 10p13/14," *Journal of Medical Genetics*, vol. 37, no. 1, pp. 33–37, 2000.

[7] S. Ferraris, A. G. Del monaco, E. Garelli et al., "HDR syndrome: a novel 'de novo' mutation in GATA3 gene," *American Journal of Medical Genetics Part A*, vol. 149, no. 4, pp. 770–775, 2009.

[8] K. Muroya, T. Mochizuki, M. Fukami et al., "Diabetes mellitus in a Japanese girl with HDR syndrome and GATA3 mutation," *Endocrine Journal*, vol. 57, no. 2, pp. 171–174, 2010.

[9] M. A. Sepahi, B. Baraty, and F. K. Shooshtary, "HDR syndrome (hypoparathyroidism, sensorineural deafness and renal disease) accompanied by hirschsprung disease," *Iranian Journal of Pediatrics*, vol. 20, no. 1, pp. 123–126, 2010.

[10] A. Taslipinar, L. Kebapcilar, M. Kutlu et al., "HDR syndrome (hypoparathyroidism, sensorineural deafness and renal disease)

accompanied by renal tubular acidosis and endocrine abnormalities," *Internal Medicine*, vol. 47, no. 11, pp. 1003–1007, 2008.

[11] Y. Higuchi, K. Hasegawa, M. Yamashita, Y. Fujii, H. Tanaka, and H. Tsukahara, "HDR syndrome in a Japanese girl with biliary atresia: A case report," *BMC Pediatrics*, vol. 16, no. 1, article 14, 2016.

[12] G. Goodwin, P. P. Hawley, and D. T. Miller, "A case of HDR syndrome and ichthyosis: dual diagnosis by whole-genome sequencing of novel mutations in *GATA3* and *STS* genes," *The Journal of Clinical Endocrinology & Metabolism*, vol. 101, no. 3, pp. 837–840, 2016.

[13] A. Verri, P. Maraschio, K. Devriendt et al., "Chromosome 10p deletion in a patient with hypoparathyroidism, severe mental retardation, autism and basal ganglia calcifications," *Annales de Génétique*, vol. 47, no. 3, pp. 281–287, 2004.

[14] M. Kita, Y. Kuwata, and T. Usui, "Familial congenital choanal atresia with GATA3 associated hypoparathyroidism-deafness-renal dysplasia syndrome unidentified on auditory brainstem response," *Auris Nasus Larynx*, 2018.

[15] S. Aksoylar, Y. Aydinok, E. Serdaroğlu, M. Çoker, F. Özdemir, and F. Özkinay, "HDR (hypoparathyroidism, sensorineural deafness, renal dysplasia) syndrome presenting with hypocalcemia-induced generalized psoriasis," *Journal of Pediatric Endocrinology and Metabolism*, vol. 17, no. 7, pp. 1031–1034, 2004.

[16] M. Kojima, T. Nagano, K. Nakata et al., "Lung squamous cell carcinoma associated with hypoparathyroidism with sensorineural deafness and renal dysplasia syndrome: A case report," *OncoTargets and Therapy*, vol. 11, pp. 1595–1599, 2018.

[17] C. Kim, H. I. L. Cheong, J. H. U. Kim, Y. S. U. Yu, and J. W. O. Kwon, "Presumed atypical HDR syndrome associated with Band Keratopathy and pigmentary retinopathy," *Journal of Pediatric Ophthalmology and Strabismus*, vol. 48, pp. e1–e3, 2011.

[18] O. Bjanid, P. Adamczyk, M. Stojewska et al., "Rare case of nephrocalcinosis in a 14-year-old girl: Answers," *Pediatric Nephrology*, vol. 32, no. 4, pp. 609–613, 2017.

[19] J. D. Mejia, L. Cervantes, H. Puerta, M. Bauer, and A. Diaz, "Neonatal diagnosis of a patient with hypoparathyroidism, sensorineural deafness and renal dysplasia (HDR) syndrome associated with cerebral infarction," *Journal of Pediatric Endocrinology and Metabolism*, vol. 27, no. 9-10, pp. 961–965, 2014.

[20] S. Fujimoto, K. Yokochi, H. Morikawa et al., "Recurrent cerebral infarctions and del(10)(p14p15.1) De novo in HDR (hypoparathyroidism, sensorineural deafness, renal dysplasia) syndrome," *American Journal of Medical Genetics*, vol. 86, no. 5, pp. 427–429, 1999.

[21] R. Hiramatsu, Y. Ubara, T. Tajima et al., "Tumoral calcinosis in a patient with hypoparathyroidism, sensorineural deafness, and renal dysplasia syndrome undergoing hemodialysis," *Clinical Case Reports*, vol. 3, no. 2, pp. 73–75, 2015.

[22] M. Kamezaki, T. Kusaba, T. Adachi et al., "Unusual proliferative glomerulonephritis in a patient diagnosed to have hypoparathyroidism, sensorineural deafness, and renal dysplasia (HDR) syndrome with a novel mutation in the GATA3 gene," *Internal Medicine*, vol. 56, no. 11, pp. 1393–1397, 2017.

Unrecognized Pseudohypoparathyroidism Type 1A as a Cause of Hypocalcemia and Seizures in a 64-Year-Old Woman

Patrizia Del Monte,[1] Carla Micaela Cuttica,[1] Alessandro Marugo,[1] Luca Foppiani,[2] Daniela Audenino,[3] Tomasz Tadeusz Godowicz,[4] Francesca Marta Elli,[5] Giovanna Mantovani,[5] and Emilio Di Maria[6]

[1] *Endocrine Unit, Galliera Hospital, Genoa, Italy*
[2] *Internal Medicine Unit, Galliera Hospital, Genoa, Italy*
[3] *Neurology Unit, Galliera Hospital, Genoa, Italy*
[4] *Neurosurgery Unit, Galliera Hospital, Genoa, Italy*
[5] *Fondazione IRCCS Ca' Granda Ospedale Maggiore Policlinico, Endocrinology and Diabetology Unit, Department of Clinical Sciences and Community Health, University of Milan, Milan, Italy*
[6] *Department of Health Sciences, University of Genoa; Medical Genetics Unit, Galliera Hospital, Genoa, Italy*

Correspondence should be addressed to Patrizia Del Monte; patrizia.del.monte@galliera.it

Academic Editor: Eli Hershkovitz

Pseudohypoparathyroidism type 1A (PHP1A) is usually diagnosed in childhood or early adulthood. We describe the case of a 64-year-old woman admitted to the Neurological Unit for recurrent episodes of loss of consciousness and seizures. Glycemia and ECG were normal, while hypocalcemia was noted. Clinical history revealed carpo-pedal spasm since the age of 30 years, cognitive impairment, hypothyroidism since early adulthood, and menopause at 30 years. She was taking oral calcium and cholecalciferol for chronic hypocalcemia. Physical features suggested Albright's osteodystrophy. Blood calcium was confirmed low, with increased parathyroid hormone, moderate 25OH-vitamin D deficiency, and normal creatinine. Brain CT scan revealed calcifications of the basal ganglia, cortical and subcortical white matter, and cerebellum. Therapy was switched to oral calcitriol, with normalization of calcium levels; levetiracetam was started and no further seizures occurred. The clinical diagnosis of PHP1A was confirmed by molecular analysis, which demonstrated the heterozygous c.568_571del mutation of the *GNAS* gene. Our report illustrates the natural history of a patient with PHP1A, which went undiagnosed until the age of 64 years, with multi-hormonal resistance and clinical sequelae evolving throughout life, and underlines the importance of diagnosing this rare disease, which has a great impact on patients and their family life.

1. Introduction

Pseudohypoparathyroidism (PHP) is a rare congenital disorder, its estimated prevalence being 0.34 - 1.1 in 100.000; it is characterized by impairment of the parathyroid hormone (PTH) signaling pathway, with target organ resistance to the action of PTH [1, 2]. The term PHP comprises several related and highly heterogeneous diseases with genetic/epigenetic causes [3, 4]. PTH exerts its actions by binding to a transmembrane G-protein-coupled receptor, activating cAMP formation. The classical form of PHP, pseudohypoparathyroidism type 1A (PHP1A), which is associated with Albright's hereditary osteodystrophy (AHO), is caused by *de novo* or autosomal dominantly inherited inactivating mutations within the $G_{s\alpha}$-coding *GNAS* gene (20q13.3; OMIM #139320) [5]. The maternal allele is the predominant source of $G_{s\alpha}$-expression in the proximal renal tubule, thyroid, pituitary, and gonads, since paternal $G_{s\alpha}$ expression is silenced in these tissues; in other tissues, however, $G_{s\alpha}$ expression is biallelic. Therefore, an inactivating $G_{s\alpha}$ mutation causes

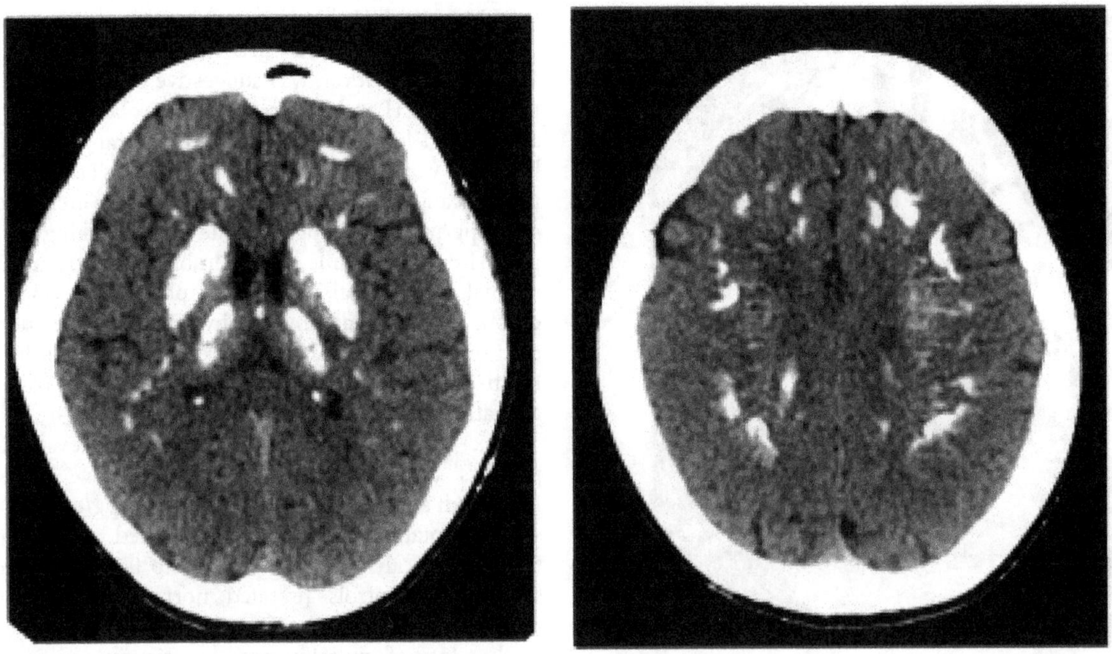

(a) (b)

FIGURE 1: Basal ganglia (a) and subcortical (b) calcifications (CT scan).

PHP1A (AHO clinical features and hormone resistance) in the case of maternal inheritance, while the same mutation on the paternal allele results in AHO clinical features only, a condition known as pseudo-pseudo-hypoparathyroidism (PPHP).

PHP1A patients often develop target-organ resistance to other hormones that act through $G_{s\alpha}$-coupled receptors, particularly TSH; resistance to gonadotrophins and GHRH is also reported.

The disease is usually diagnosed in childhood or early adulthood age, and few studies have addressed its natural history, in which its features evolve during the subject's lifetime. Moreover, to our knowledge, no diagnoses have been made after 60 years of age in patients not studied for known familial disease.

2. Clinical Case

A 64-year-old woman was admitted to the Neurological Unit of our hospital for recent recurrent episodes of loss of consciousness and seizures. Glycemia and ECG were normal, while hypocalcemia was present.

She has a normal brother and both her parents died in old age; her mother had cognitive impairment. Her clinical history evidenced carpo-pedal spasm since the age of 30 years, cognitive impairment, hypothyroidism diagnosed in early adulthood, spontaneous menarche, and oligomenorrhea followed by amenorrhea at the age of 30, which was diagnosed as precocious menopause. She was unmarried and had no pregnancy. She underwent bilateral hip arthroprosthesis at 45 and 50 years of age.

She was taking oral calcium (600 mg daily) and cholecalciferol (400 IU daily) for chronic hypocalcemia, diagnosed about 30 years earlier. She was also on therapy with perindopril for hypertension, atorvastatin for hypercholesterolemia, and L-thyroxine.

Physical examination revealed short stature (145 cm), slight overweight: 52 Kg (BMI: 25 Kg/m^2), round facies, enlarged base of the nose, and brachydactyly. Her blood chemistry evidenced hypocalcemia (7.7 mg/dl, n.v. 8.2-10.2) with increased PTH levels (169 pg/ml, n.v. 15-65 pg/ml, intact PTH immunoassay), moderate 25OH vitamin D deficiency (22 ng/ml; n.v. ≥ 30), normal creatinine (1 mg/dl), and albumin (3.9 g/dl).

Brain computed tomography (CT) revealed calcifications of the basal ganglia, the cortical and subcortical white matter, and the cerebellum (dentate nuclei); subcutaneous pericranial ectopic calcifications were also present (Figures 1, 2, and 3). Hand radiography confirmed shortness of the metacarpal bones and scapho-trapezoidal fusion (not shown). Bone mineral density of the spine and femoral bone was normal. Abdominal ultrasonography did not reveal kidney stones. The clinical picture was suggestive of PHP1A. The patient was therefore promptly switched to 1,25 $(OH)_2$ vitamin D (calcitriol 0.75 mcg daily, in 3 split doses) associated with oral calcium supplementation (1000 mg daily in 2 split doses, after lunch and dinner), with normalization of calcemia (9.2 mg/dl) and a decrease in PTH level (36 pg/ml). Serum phosphate was normal on therapy (4.3 mg/dl), while 24-hour urinary calcium on therapy was above the normal range (321 mg/24 h, n.v. <4 mg/kg/body weight); we do not have a clear explanation for this, since urinary calcium excretion is not normally increased in this condition. However, a

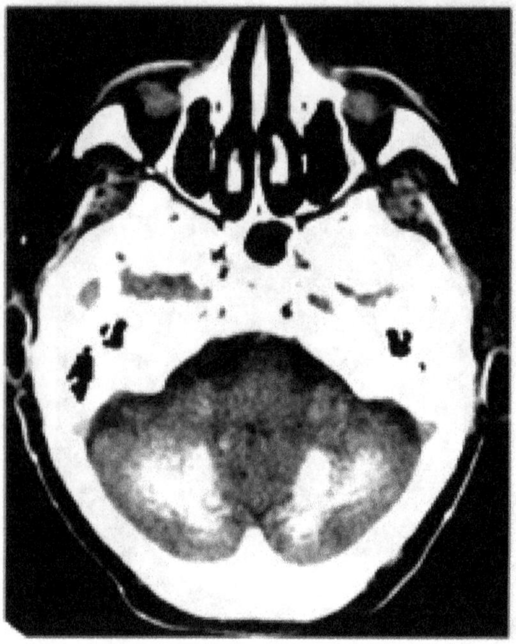

FIGURE 2: Cerebellar calcifications (CT scan).

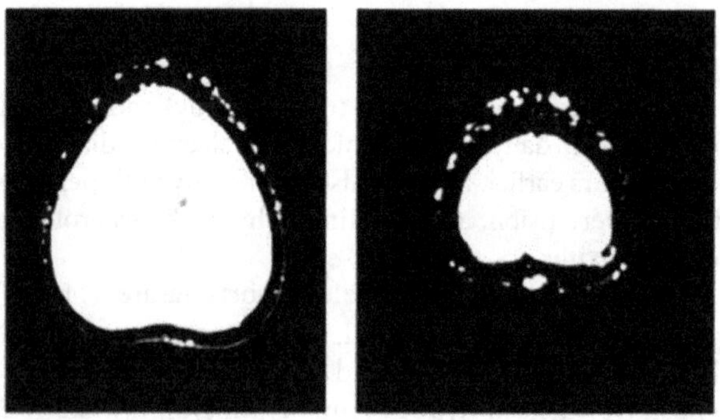

FIGURE 3: Extracranial subcutaneous ectopic calcifications (CT scan).

laboratory assay pitfall or an incorrect urine collection by the patient cannot be ruled out. A further urinary calcium control one month later, however, proved normal (200 mg/24 h). In addition, therapy with levetiracetam (1000 mg daily in 2 split doses) was started, and no further seizures or muscle spasms occurred.

The patient and her family underwent a genetic counseling session and gave informed consent to genetic analysis. Mutation analysis of the *GNAS* gene was performed on DNA extracted from a blood sample by means of Sanger sequencing and MLPA according to standard methods. The analyses revealed a heterozygous c.568_571del (p.Asp190Metfs*13) frameshift mutation. The combination of physical, biochemical, and genetic findings led to the diagnosis of PHP1A.

FT4 and TSH levels were normal during substitutive treatment with L-tiroxine (75 mcg daily). Anti-thyroperoxidase and anti-thyroglobulin antibodies were negative and thyroid ultrasonography was normal, suggesting that TSH resistance was the cause of her hypothyroidism.

LH and FSH levels were in the menopausal range (FSH: 47 mU/ml, LH: 26 mU/ml); the history of premature menopause, however, was suggestive of the development of progressive LH and FSH resistance. Prolactin, basal cortisol, and ACTH levels were in the normal range. Basal growth hormone was 0.63 ng/ml, with IGF-1 levels (129 ng/ml) in the normal range for age. Calcitonin levels were increased (range: 44-92 pg/ml, n.v. <10 pg/ml) (she was not taking any proton-pump inhibitor), while carcinoembryonic antigen (CEA) was normal. Abdominal ultrasonography was normal, as were chest-X-ray and mammography. Our interpretation is that calcitonin resistance was also present, as part of the patient's multi-hormonal resistance due to impairment of the cAMP activation pathway [6, 7].

Six months later, during follow-up evaluation, the patient's calcium level was seen to have increased to 10.6 mg/dl and PTH had decreased to 32 pg/ml; oral calcium supplementation was gradually reduced and then discontinued, and calcitriol was reduced to 0.25 mcg twice daily; subsequent controls revealed normal calcium (10 mg/dl) and slightly increased PTH (72 pg/ml) levels. She had no further loss of consciousness or seizures; on neurological examinations, levetiracetam treatment was confirmed, also on account of the frailty of the patient.

3. Discussion

This is an unusual case of the first diagnosis of PHP type 1 A in a 64-year-old woman, who presented with hypocalcemia and recent recurrent episodes of loss of consciousness and seizures. Combined evaluation of her clinical history, physical features, blood chemistry, and radiological findings suggested this diagnosis. A retrospective interpretation of her history showed how the disease had evolved during the patient's lifetime: in early adulthood, she developed PTH resistance-related hypocalcemia, carpo-pedal spasm, and hypothyroidism due to TSH resistance; around the age of 30 years, she suffered ovarian failure due to FSH and LH resistance; this was followed by bilateral hip disease requiring arthroprosthesis at 45 and 50 years and worsening hypocalcemia, which was unresponsive to cholecalciferol and oral calcium supplementation; finally, recurrent seizures recently ensued. Calcitonin resistance was also present, while IGF-1 was normal. She had no kidney stones; this is in keeping with the observation that urinary calcium levels are not markedly increased in these patients, as the action of PTH is maintained in the distal renal tubule, where GNAS gene expression is biallelic. Switching to calcitriol treatment promptly corrected the woman's hypocalcemia, and she had neither muscle spasms nor seizures on anti-epileptic medication. Both hypocalcemia and the development of multiple cortical and subcortical calcifications could have contributed to the development of seizures.

Based on the patient's clinical characterization, the targeted mutation analysis of the *GNAS* gene identified a known mutation already associated with PHP1A [8], thus allowing the clinical diagnosis to be confirmed. The mutation was presumably inherited from the mother, who was referred to as having cognitive impairment. However, as no sample was available, this hypothesis was not formally confirmed.

In accordance with the recommendations of the recently published first consensus statement on the diagnosis and management of pseudohypoparathyroidism-related disorders [7], the diagnosis should be based on clinical and biochemical characteristics, which will vary according to the age of the patient. The diagnosis of AHO should be based on the presence of major criteria (brachydactyly due to premature fusion of the epiphyses and short stature by adulthood) and additional criteria (stocky build, round facies, and ectopic ossifications). Obesity, dental manifestations, and cognitive impairment are present in a subgroup of patients. In the majority of PHP patients, the main clinical manifestations are symptoms of hypocalcemia due to PTH resistance. In patients with PHP1A, resistance to PTH is usually absent at birth and evolves over time (from the neonatal period to 22 years); the first biochemical abnormalities to appear are increased serum PTH and phosphorous levels, whereas hypocalcemia develops gradually 4-5 years later. Other associated endocrine features that support the diagnosis are as follows: early-onset hypothyroidism due to TSH resistance, which is the most common associated endocrine alteration, being present in nearly 100% of PHP1A patients; hypogonadism (due to FSH and LH resistance); hypercalcitoninemia (due to calcitonin resistance); GH deficiency (due to GHRH resistance).

Owing to the important implications for clinical management, early screening for associated conditions and genetic counselling, the molecular cause of PHP should be promptly identified, in order to confirm the diagnosis and characterize the subtype of the disease. Conversely, no genotype-phenotype correlation can be inferred based on mutation analysis [9]. In a large series, the recurrent c.568_571del mutation detected in our patient was found associated with a wide spectrum of phenotypical features. Namely, PTH levels and serum calcium ranged from 57 to 653 pg/ml (reference range 15-55) and from 1.3 to 2.7 mmol/l (reference range 2.1-2.6), respectively [10].

Few studies have focused on the natural history of this disease and on the outcome of its management. The clinical management of hypocalcemia in PHP patients is based on the administration of the active metabolite of vitamin D calcitriol (1,25$(OH)_2$ vitamin D) as in the case of our patient, who was previously on therapy with cholecalciferol.

Indeed, owing to PTH resistance, 25OH vitamin D cannot be converted by the renal tubule into its biologically active form, 1,25 $(OH)_2$ vitamin D, by PTH-dependent renal 1α-hydroxylase. The goal is to maintain normocalcemia and to keep serum PTH levels in the upper portion of the reference range, thereby avoiding PTH suppression, which can be associated with hypercalciuria and renal calcification. On the other hand, long-term and excessive secondary hyperparathyroidism can result in osteitis fibrosa cystica and dislocation of the femoral capital epiphysis (as may have occurred in our patient, who underwent bilateral hip replacement in adult age). PTH, calcium, and phosphorus should be evaluated every six months during treatment in asymptomatic patients, and more frequently when clinically indicated. Patients and families should be instructed with regard to the symptoms of hypo- and hypercalcemia.

The present case underlines the importance of early diagnosis of pseudohypoparathyroidism, as this is crucial to the appropriate treatment and lifelong management of the disease and its complications, which have a great impact on patients and their families. Appropriate genetic counselling is essential in order to establish effective communication with the family, which in turn allows relevant information to be exchanged and genetic testing to be framed within an integrated clinical path. This is in line with the recent consensus statement [7], which recommends a multidisciplinary approach addressing all aspects of the disease and its potential complications.

Consent

Informed consent was obtained from the patient and her brother.

Acknowledgments

The authors would like to thank Dr. Antonio Castaldi, Neuroradiology Unit, Galliera Hospital, Genoa, Italy, for neuroradiological images.

References

[1] M. Bastepe and H. Jüppner, "Pseudohypoparathyroidism, Albright's hereditary osteodystrophy, and progressive osseous heteroplasia: disorders caused by inactivating GNAS mutations," in *Endocrinology Adult and Pediatric*, L. Jameson and L. De Groot, Eds., pp. 1147–1159, Elsevier, 7th, chapter 66 edition, 2016.

[2] G. Mantovani, "Pseudohypoparathyroidism: Diagnosis and treatment," *The Journal of Clinical Endocrinology & Metabolism*, vol. 96, no. 10, pp. 3020–3030, 2011.

[3] S. Thiele, G. Mantovani, A. Barlier et al., "From pseudohypoparathyroidism to inactivating PTH/PTHrP signalling disorder (iPPSD), a novel classification proposed by the EuroPHP network," *European Journal of Endocrinology*, vol. 175, no. 6, pp. 1–17, 2016.

[4] O. Tafaj and H. Jüppner, "Pseudohypoparathyroidism: one gene, several syndromes," *Journal of Endocrinological Investigation*, vol. 40, no. 4, pp. 347–356, 2017.

[5] G. Mantovani, A. Linglart, I. Garin, C. Silve, F. M. Elli, and G. P. De Nanclares, "Clinical utility gene card for: Pseudohypoparathyroidism," *European Journal of Human Genetics*, vol. 21, no. 6, pp. 698–702, 2013.

[6] V. Vlaeminck-Guillem, M. D'Herbomez, P. Pigny et al., "Pseudohypoparathyroidism Ia and hypercalcitoninemia," *The Journal of Clinical Endocrinology & Metabolism*, vol. 86, no. 7, pp. 3091–3096, 2001.

[7] G. Mantovani, M. Bastepe, D. Monk et al., "Diagnosis and management of pseudohypoparathyroidism and related disorders: first international Consensus Statement," *Nature Reviews Endocrinology*, vol. 14, no. 8, pp. 476–500, 2018.

[8] L. S. Weinstein, P. V. Gejman, P. de Mazancourt, N. American, and A. M. Spiegel, "A heterozygous 4-bp deletion mutation in the Gsα gene (GNAS1) in a patient with albright hereditary osteodystrophy," *Genomics*, vol. 13, no. 4, pp. 1319–1321, 1992.

[9] F. M. Elli, L. deSanctis, B. Ceoloni et al., "Pseudohypoparathyroidism Type Ia and Pseudo-Pseudohypoparathyroidism: The Growing Spectrum of GNAS Inactivating Mutations," *Human Mutation*, vol. 34, no. 3, pp. 411–416, 2013.

[10] S. Thiele, R. Werner, J. Grötzinger et al., "A positive genotype-phenotype correlation in a large cohort of patients with Pseudohypoparathyroidism Type Ia and Pseudo-pseudohypoparathyroidism and 33 newly identified mutations in the GNAS gene," *Molecular Genetics & Genomic Medicine*, vol. 3, no. 2, pp. 111–120, 2015.

48

Desperate Times Call for Desperate Measures: Use of Continuous Subcutaneous 1-34 PTH Infusion for Postsurgical Hypoparathyroidism

Adnan Haider,[1] **Oksana Symczyk**,[1] **Yadel Couso**,[1] **Taylor Cater**,[2] **and Sheree Bryan**[2]

[1]*Department of Endocrinology, West Virginia University, Morgantown, WV, USA*
[2]*Department of Medicine, West Virginia University, Morgantown, WV, USA*

Correspondence should be addressed to Adnan Haider; adnan.haider@hsc.wvu.edu

Academic Editor: Michaï¿½l R. Laurent

Objective. This case highlights use of 1-34 PTH continuous infusion in a patient with postsurgical hypoparathyroidism. *Method.* Clinical presentation and biochemical profile were monitored before and after 1-34 PTH infusion, with notable reduction in pill burden in a patient with postsurgical hypoparathyroidism. *Results.* We present a case of postsurgical hypoparathyroidism following thyroidectomy for Graves disease. The patient was requiring a total of 34 pills daily and, despite medication compliance, her clinical and biochemical control was unsatisfactory. Following initiation of 1-34 PTH in the form of a subcutaneous pump, we were able to stop all calcium supplementation and reduce calcitriol to 0.5 mcg daily. Her current biochemical control as well as quality of life improved significantly on CSPI, calcitriol, and a daily serving of dietary calcium. *Conclusion.* This case highlights the use of 1-34 PTH either as twice-daily dosing or continuous subcutaneous infusion for adult patients with hypoparathyroidism.

1. Introduction

Hypoparathyroidism is a rare endocrine disorder, in contrast to its pathological counterpart primary hyperparathyroidism. In the US and European Union, hypoparathyroidism is classified as an orphan disease. Hypoparathyroidism is the last classical endocrine deficiency for which the missing hormone has become available. Before the use of recombinant PTH in clinical practice, management of hypoparathyroidism was limited to calcium and active vitamin D, often in large doses and with the adverse effect of extraskeletal calcifications. However, without PTH, normal calcium homeostasis, via skeleton, kidney, or central nervous system mechanisms, cannot be restored [1, 2].

It is virtually impossible to manage hypoparathyroidism by providing sufficient calcium via diet alone. Calcium supplements and active vitamin D products are essential. Typically, patients will require 1–2 g of supplemental calcium given in divided doses. Some patients will require higher doses. The FDA approved rhPTH (1-84) for patients with hypoparathyroidism who cannot be controlled on conventional therapy in January 2015, a signal event in the therapeutic history of hypoparathyroidism. 1-84 was especially useful for patients requiring higher doses of oral calcium supplementation (>2.5 g/day or active vitamin D > 1.5 mcg/day). Another indication for 1-84 use is poor control of serum calcium (corrected serum calcium < 7.5 mg/dl or clinical symptomatology of low calcium despite high calcium intake). However, in September 2019, rhPTH (1-84) was recalled due to a potential issue related to particulates originating from the rubber septum of the NATPARA cartridge.

2. Case Presentation

A 34-year-old white female diagnosed with Graves hyperthyroidism was initially treated for about 18 weeks with methimazole without improvement in thyroid levels because of severe endometriosis history, bilateral oophorectomy, and hysterectomy five years before her Graves diagnosis. Her gynecologist did not start hormone replacement therapy on account of her smoking history. Graves orbitopathy and smoking history made RAI ablation contraindicated. She opted for total thyroidectomy to treat her large goiter and associated pressure symptoms. She developed immediate postoperative hypoparathyroidism, presenting with symptomatic hypocalcemia within 24 hours of total thyroidectomy. Pathology reports of the surgical specimen demonstrated diffusely enlarged thyroid along with two parathyroid glands. During hospitalization, she was treated with intravenous calcium gluconate drip and was discharged home on calcium carbonate, vitamin D, and active vitamin D.

Despite her adherence to the discharge regimen, she experienced hypocalcemia symptoms of fatigue and frequent cramping in the hands. She required regular ER visits for symptomatic hypocalcemia. A PICC line was placed due to frequent hospitalizations and the need for calcium monitoring every two weeks. In the six months following her surgery, she required eight ER visits with four overnight stays in the hospital. During hospitalizations, the patient was treated with intravenous calcium gluconate and was discharged on oral calcium and active vitamin D regimen. Postsurgical hypothyroidism remained under reasonable control on a stable levothyroxine dose.

The patient denied the previous history of malabsorption, and celiac disease screening was negative as well. Elevated 24-hour urine calcium before initiation of hydrochlorothiazide was 402 mg/24-hour urine specimen.

The patient's thyroidectomy was performed in August 2019. In September 2019, that 1-84 PTH was recalled and not available for 1-84 PTH naïve patients. At the time of initial consultation in this endocrinology clinic (May 2020), the patient's medications included more than 30 pills daily (Table 1).

The initial plan is summarized in Table 2. Due to the current unavailability of 1-84 PTH (Natpara), it was impossible to start her on Natpara. Because of patient's symptomatic hypocalcemia and frequent hospitalizations despite taking her pills, a decision was made of start 1-34 PTH (Teriparatide) 20 mcg initially as twice-daily subcutaneous injections. Because of the short half-life of 1-34 PTH (Teriparatide) in previous studies, we prescribed twice-daily injections for her.

The patient's calcium dose was reduced by half at the initiation of twice-daily 1-34 dosing, and her calcium levels improved (Figure 1). Her calcium levels improved from 6.4 mg/dl to 7.9 mg/dl on 1-34 PTH, with symptomatic improvement and 50% reduction in pill burden. To further improve her calcium hemostasis, by simulating the physiologic tonic release of PTH, a decision was made to give the teriparatide via a continuous subcutaneous pump. Initially, a dose of 42 mcg/day was infused via an Omnipod pump. At this dose, patient calcium increased from 7.7 mg/dl to 11.2 mg/dl, at which point all calcium supplements and active vitamin D were stopped, and a dose of teriparatide was reduced to 33 mcg/day. Follow-up blood work showed normal calcium and phosphorus levels. With the use of continuous subcutaneous infusion, we observed a 17.5% dose reduction in daily 1-34 PTH and improvement in calcium and phosphorus levels, as shown in Figure 1.

Table 1: List of medications.

List of medications
1. Calcium citrate 500 mg, 2 tablets, four times daily
2. Calcium carbonate 750 mg, 3 tablets, four times daily
3. Calcitriol 0.5 mg, four times daily
4. Calcium acetate 667 mg, 2 tablets. 3 times daily
5. Hydrochlorothiazide 50 mg daily
6. Magnesium citrate 300 mg daily
7. Ergocalciferol 50, 000 IU weekly
8. Levothyroxine 200 mcg daily

Table 2: Plan during initial visit and outcomes.

Plan during initial visit and outcomes
1. Smoking cessation
Stopped smoking 3 weeks after initial consultation
2. Transdermal estradiol patch for postsurgical menopause
Started 2 weeks after smoking cessation
3. I-34 PTH, 20 mcg, twice daily approved by insurance
50% reduction in calcium supplements and active vitamin D
4. Omnipod continuous subcutaneous pump approved
Initial dose: I-34 PTH infusion 42 mcg/24-hour period via Omnipod pump
Dose adjustment: I-34 PTH infusion 33 mcg/24 hour daily plus calcitriol 0.5 mcg daily
All calcium supplements and hydrochlorothiazide were stopped at this time

3. Discussion

Can 1-34 PTH (Teriparatide) provide relief to patients with hypoparathyroidism until 1-84 PTH (NATPARA) is available again?

Will continuous subcutaneous parathyroid infusion of teriparatide provide any advantage in the long run when compared to single daily 1-84 PTH?

A single daily injection of rhPTH improved quality of life, reduced pill burden, and improved calcium levels and hypocalcemia symptomatology in patients with hypoparathyroidism. This agent was especially useful in patients with gastrointestinal dysfunction or following bariatric surgery where unpredictable calcium absorption can make disease management especially challenging. Despite its advantages, rhPTH (1-84) therapy for any length of time can lead to dangerous hypocalcemia once therapy is discontinued: rhPTH (1-84) activates the skeletal system and, as a result, the skeletal bone will continue to accrue calcium, but if treatment is interrupted, hypocalcemia can result [3]. Patients on rhPTH (1-84) are instructed to increase their calcium and active vitamin D to levels that match or surpass the amounts they were taking before starting rhPTH (I-84) therapy.

In the late 1980s, Winer and colleagues demonstrated that 1-34 PTH, an active fragment of PTH, could be used effectively in children and adults with hypoparathyroidism [4]. The short half-life of 1-34 PTH is what makes twice- or

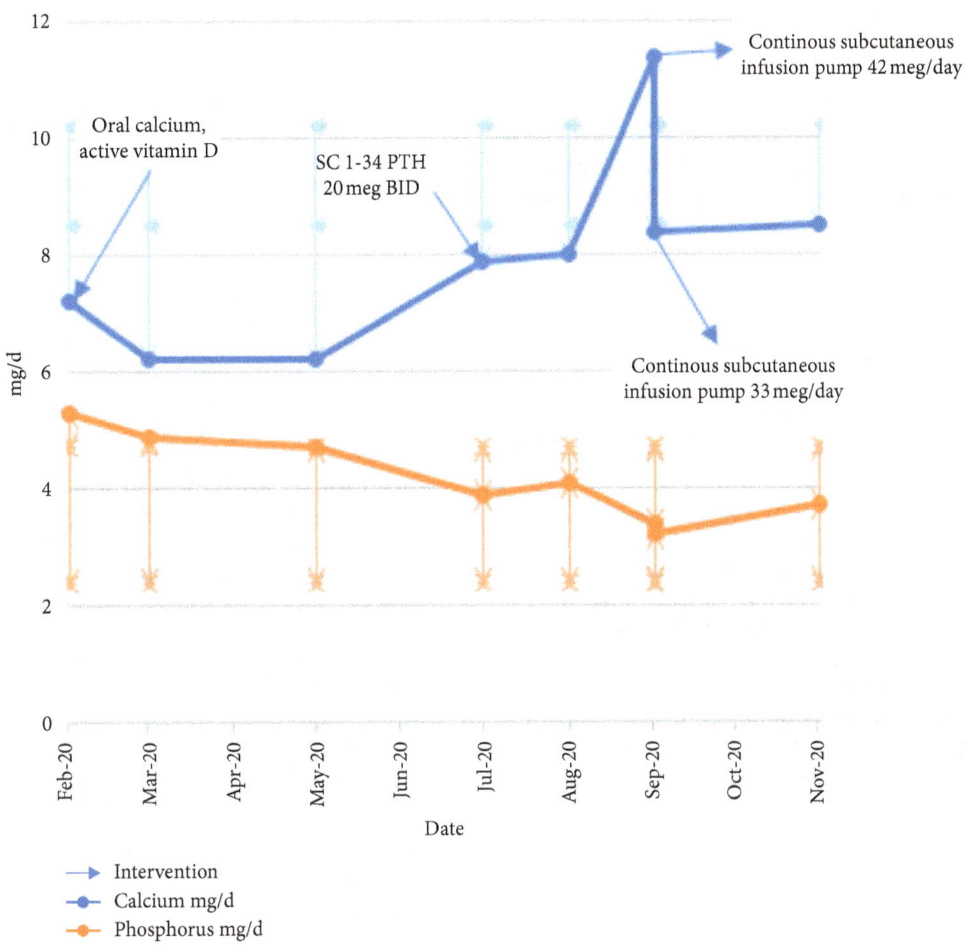

FIGURE 1: Review of her phosphorus and calcium levels prior to oral calcium and vitamin D replacement, to subcutaneous 1-34 PTH therapy, and to CSPI summarized.

thrice-daily dosing more effective in controlling calcium levels. 1-34 PTH improved control of serum calcium and reduced supplementation with calcium and active vitamin D [5, 6].

Andre Palermo studied the effects of 1-34 PTH 20 mcg twice-daily subcutaneous injections in a prospective open-label study. This study showed improvement in calcium levels and reductions in calcium and vitamin D supplementation. No serious adverse events occurred during the study period, no subjects developed nephrolithiasis, and no hypercalcemic events necessitated hospitalization, and over the two years, these patients were using subcutaneous 1-34 PTH injections [6].

Continuous infusion of PTH would mimic the tonic secretory dynamics that represent the majority of secreted PTH under normal circumstances and thus provide advantage over multiple daily injections of 1-34 PTH. Continuous infusion of 1-34 PTH resulted in 65% less rhPTH required to control the serum calcium when compared to a twice-daily injection regimen. Review of the literature indicates that continuous PTH infusion can mimic the tonic release of PTH and can lead to not only better calcium homeostasis but also to reduced total daily dose of 1-34 PTH. Additionally, continuous infusion of 1-34 PTH reduces lower urinary calcium excretion by 50% [7].

Continuous subcutaneous parathyroid infusion (CSPI) allows long-term maintenance of serum and urinary calcium at near-normal values as was demonstrated by Agnes Linglart in three children with hypoparathyroidism [8]. Of significance, CSPI corrected the clinically severe manifestation of hypocalcemia that impeded the children's lives daily.

In rodent studies, all PTH and PTH-related protein molecules, when tested at high doses for prolonged periods, were associated with osteosarcoma [9, 10]. All PTH molecules approved for human use carry with them the black box warning of osteosarcoma. Although the FDA has approved rhPTH (1-84) for long-term use in hypoparathyroidism patients without risk factors for osteosarcoma, restrictions as to the duration of use have not been dictated and so the black box warning persists. Continuous subcutaneous 1-34 PTH for long-term use is valid a concern. However, after non-human primate studies and more than 17 years of human surveillance, no safety signals are evident [11, 12]. Furthermore, osteosarcoma is not a safety signal in human subjects.

Desperate times call for desperate measures. Use of 1-34 PTH, two to three injections daily, or CSPI provides an alternative to 1-84 PTH for patients who are difficult to manage with currently available treatment such as our case patient. Use of CSPI mimics the tonic secretory dynamics that represent the majority of secreted PTH under normal circumstances, a potential advantage in treating hypoparathyroidism.

4. Conclusion

This case highlights the use of 1-34 PTH for postsurgical hypoparathyroidism. Significant biochemical and clinical improvement was achieved. Significant reduction in pill burden was also reduced following initiation on 1-34 PTH injections.

Using CSPI, the total daily dose reduction of 1-34 PTH was observed when compared to twice-daily injections and, at the same time, better biochemical control was noted.

Can 1-34 PTH provide relief to patients with hypoparathyroidism until 1-84 PTH (NATPARA) is available again? The outcome of this case provides hope.

Will CSPI infusion of 1-34 PTH analogue provide any advantage in the long run when compared to single daily 1-84 PTH? A randomized double-blind crossover trial will be the best suited study to answer the two questions and better understand the pathophysiology of hypoparathyroidism.

References

[1] T. B. Usdin, C. Gruber, and T. I. Bonner, "Identification and functional expression of a receptor selectively recognizing parathyroid hormone, the PTH2 receptor," *Journal of Biological Chemistry*, vol. 270, no. 26, pp. 15455–15458, 1995.

[2] A. D. Care and N. H. Bell, "Evidence that parathyroid hormone crosses the blood-brain barrier," in *Calcium Regulation and Bone Metabolism: Basic and Clinical Aspects*, D. V. Conn, R. J. Martin, and J. Meunier, Eds., in *Proceedings of the 9th International Conference on Calcium Regulating Hormones and Bone Metabolism*, p. 540, November, 1986.

[3] M. L. Brandi, J. P. Bilezikian, D. Shoback et al., "Management of hypoparathyroidism: summary statement and guidelines," *The J ournal o f C linical E ndocrinology a nd Metabolism*, vol. 101, no. 6, pp. 2273–2283, 2016.

[4] K. K. Winer, J. A. Yanovski, and G. B. Cutler, "Synthetic human parathyroid hormone 1-34 vs calcitriol and calcium in the treatment of hypoparathyroidism," *JAMA: The Journal of the American Medical Association*, vol. 276, no. 8, pp. 631–636, 1996.

[5] A. Santonati, A. Palermo, E. Maddaloni et al., "Hypoparathyroidism AME Group. PTH (1-34) for surgical hypoparathyroidism: a prospective, open-label investigation of efficacy and quality of life," *The Journal of Clinical Endocrinology & Metabolism*, vol. 100, no. 9, pp. 3590–3597, 2015.

[6] A. Palermo, A. Santonati, G. Tabacco et al., "PTH (1-34) for surgical hypoparathyroidism: a 2-year prospective, open-label investigation of efficacy an d qu ality of li fe," *The Jou rnal of Clinical Endocrinology & Metabolism*, vol. 103, no. 1, pp. 271–280, 2018.

[7] K. K. Winer, B. Zhang, J. A. Shrader et al., "Synthetic human parathyroid hormone 1-34 replacement therapy: a randomized crossover trial comparing pump versus injections in the treatment of chronic hypoparathyroidism," *The Journal of Clinical Endocrinology and Metabolism*, vol. 97, no. 2, pp. 391–399, 2012.

[8] A. Linglart, A. Rothenbuhler, I. Gueorgieva, P. Lucchini, C. Silve, and P. Bougnères, "Long-term results of continuous subcutaneous recombinant PTH (1-34) infusion in children with refractory hypoparathyroidism," *The Journal of Clinical Endocrinology and Metabolism*, vol. 96, no. 11, pp. 3308–3312, 2011.

[9] J. Jolette, C. E. Wilker, S. Y. Smith et al., "Defining a non-carcinogenic dose of recombinant human parathyroid hormone 1-84 in a 2-year study in Fischer 344 rats," *Toxicologic Pathology*, vol. 34, no. 7, pp. 929–940, 2006.

[10] J. L. Vahle, M. Sato, G. G. Long et al., "Skeletal changes in rats given daily subcutaneous injections of recombinant human parathyroid hormone (1-34) for 2 years and relevance to human safety," *Toxicologic Pathology*, vol. 30, no. 3, pp. 312–321, 2002.

[11] C. Cipriani, C. Capriani, D. Irani, and J. P Bilezikian, "Safety of osteoanabolic therapy: a decade of experience," *Journal of Bone and Mineral Research: The Official Journal of the American Society for Bone and Mineral Research*, vol. 27, no. 12, pp. 2419–2428, 2012.

[12] E. B. Andrews, A. W. Gilsenan, K. Midkiff et al., "The US postmarketing surveillance study of adult osteosarcoma and teriparatide: study design and findings from the first 7 years," *Journal of Bone and Mineral Research*, vol. 27, no. 12, pp. 2429–2437, 2012.

A Case of Refractory Hypothyroidism due to Poor Compliance Treated with the Weekly Intravenous and Oral Levothyroxine Administration

Yujiro Nakano,[1] **Koshi Hashimoto**,[2] **Noriaki Ohkiba**,[3] **Hideyuki Okuma**,[1] **Isao Minami**,[1] **Hiromitsu Takahashi**,[4] **Yuji Tanaka**,[5] **Takanobu Yoshimoto**,[1] **and Tetsuya Yamada**[1]

[1]*Department of Molecular Endocrinology and Metabolism, Graduate School of Medical and Dental Science, Tokyo Medical and Dental University, 113-8510, Japan*
[2]*Department of Preemptive and Metabolism, Graduate School of Medical and Dental Science, Tokyo Medical and Dental University, 113-8510, Japan*
[3]*Department of Endocrinology and Metabolism, Kashiwa Municipal Hospital, 277-0825, Japan*
[4]*Department of Pharmacy, Medical Hospital of Tokyo Medical and Dental University, 113-8510, Japan*
[5]*Department of General Medicine, National Defense Medical College Hospital, 359-0042, Japan*

Correspondence should be addressed to Koshi Hashimoto; khashimoto.mem@tmd.ac.jp

Academic Editor: Osamu Isozaki

Refractory hypothyroidism is caused by decreased gut absorption, increased metabolism, and poor compliance. Previous studies suggested that the weekly oral, suppository, or intramuscular administration of levothyroxine (LT4) is an effective treatment for refractory hypothyroidism. However, limited information is currently available on treatment involving the weekly intravenous administration of LT4. We managed a case of refractory hypothyroidism due to poor compliance, for which, by weekly intravenous LT4 administration, LT4 was intravenously administered weekly at a dose of 300 μg without any adverse effects such as acute ischemic heart diseases or liver dysfunction and effectively maintained the euthyroid status for 14 months. The weekly oral administration of LT4 (700 μg) was also safely performed and was as effective as its intravenous administration. We herein present precise clinical course of the present case including pharmacokinetic data during the weekly intravenous and oral administration of LT4 and discuss the safety and efficacy of the treatments.

1. Introduction

Hypothyroidism is one of the most common thyroid disorders, which more frequently affects women, and its incidence increases with age [1]. Its clinical feature ranges from asymptomatic to severe conditions such as myxedema coma [1]. The treatment of hypothyroidism with levothyroxine (LT4) is conventional in clinical practice and average daily doses of 100-200 μg or 1.5-2.2 μg/kg daily are utilized for replacement with TSH normalization or free T4 (FT4) elevation [2]. However, some patients develop refractory hypothyroidism due to malabsorption, pancreatic and liver disorders, drug interactions, polymorphisms in type 2 deiodinase, a high fiber diet, and poor compliance to daily oral LT4 replacement, which is reportedly the most common reason [3]. Although there have been no plausible recommendations for the treatment of refractory hypothyroidism, the weekly oral or intramuscular administration of LT4 may be useful [4, 5].

The intravenous administration of LT4 is commonly used for the medical emergencies such as myxedema coma [6]. However, to date, the safety and efficacy of the weekly intravenous and oral administration of LT4 as alternative ways to treat refractory hypothyroidism remain unknown. We herein precisely present the clinical course of the present case including pharmacokinetic data during the weekly intravenous and oral administration of LT4 and discuss the safety and efficacy of these treatments.

2. Case Presentation

A 41-year-old woman with refractory hypothyroidism was referred to our hospital. She was diagnosed with Graves' disease with thyrotoxicosis at the age of 36 years (thyroid weight: 51.1 g, TSH: <0.001 μU/mL (reference range; 0.4 to 4.0), FT3: 21.85 pg/mL (reference range; 2.36 to 5.00). FT4: 4.00 ng/dL (reference range; 0.88 to 1.67), TSH receptor antibody (TRAb) 22.7 IU/L (reference range; < 2.0)). Neither methimazole, iodine potassium, nor three times of ^{131}I ablation therapy ameliorated thyrotoxicosis. At the age of 39 years, she underwent total thyroidectomy, and oral LT4 replacement was initiated after surgery. Although the dose of LT4 was increased to 650 μg/day (11.8 μg/kg/day), with 150 μg/day of liothyronine (LT3) also being administered, severe hypothyroidism persisted.

She had general fatigue, mild diarrhea, anasarca, hair loss, peripheral coldness, and dry skin. She was hospitalized for further examination to exclude malabsorption.

She was 161.6 cm in height and 55 kg in weight and had a body temperature of 36.3°C. Physical examinations showed a blood pressure of 101/67 mmHg with a heart rate of 56 beats/min, and laboratory findings revealed anemia, mild renal dysfunction, and hypercholesterolemia. Her serum TSH levels were extremely high as 146.8 μIU/mL and FT3 and FT4 levels were undetectable (Table 1). Glucose tolerance (fasting plasma glucose of 71 mg/dL and HbA1c of 5.4%) and adrenal and pituitary hormone levels were within normal ranges. Autoimmune antibodies other than thyroid peroxidase antibody (TPOAb) were all negative (Table 1). Ultrasonic cardiography showed pericardial effusion with normal cardiac output, and electrocardiography revealed a very low voltage and mild bradycardia (data not shown). She was not receiving any concomitant medication that may have interfered with the absorption or metabolism of LT4 [7]. Her serum albumin levels were within normal range, suggesting no evidence of malabsorption (Table 1). Moreover, anemia and hypocalcemia prior to admission to our hospital were successfully treated by the administration of iron and calcium, respectively. *Helicobacter pylori* and other gastrointestinal tract infections were negative. A stool examination was normal. Upper and lower gastrointestinal endoscopies were performed and were also normal. Duodenal biopsy was performed and did not show pathological abnormalities consistent with malabsorptive disorder. After her admission to our hospital, the patient was handed LT4 tablets by nurses every morning; however, her intake was not confirmed.

Since the additional rectal administration of LT4 suppository preparation (100 μg/day) did not ameliorate hypothyroidism, we attempted its intravenous administration to treat refractory hypothyroidism under the permission and approval of the Ethical Committee of Tokyo Medical and Dental University Hospital and written informed consent was obtained from the patient and her father. An intravenous

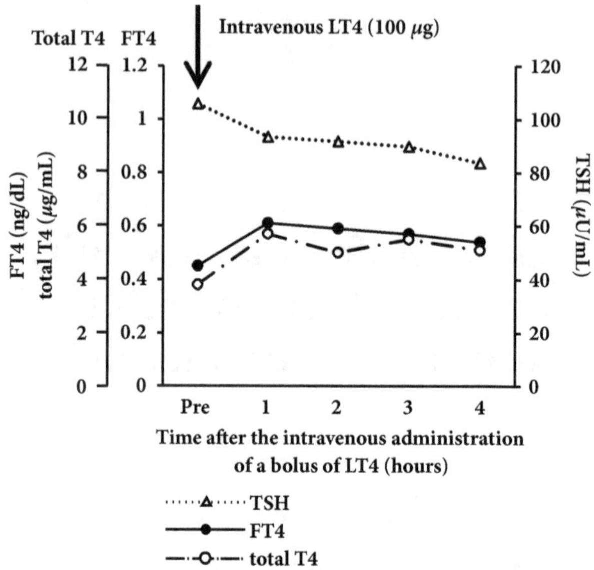

Figure 1: *Serum thyroid hormone and TSH levels after the intravenous administration of a single bolus of LT4 (100 μg).* Serum FT4 and total T4 levels both increased, peaked 1 hour after the administration, and gradually decreased thereafter.

LT4 formula was dispensed in the Department of Pharmacy of the Tokyo Medical and Dental University hospital, following a previously reported prescription [8]. In brief, LT4 sodium salt pentahydrate (Sigma-Aldrich T2501, #6106-07-6) was dissolved by 0.1 N NaOH solution and diluted to a concentration of 200 μg/2 mL by saline. A total of 300 μg of LT4 was then diluted in 50 mL of saline and administered to the patient by intravenous drip infusion in 15 min. Since the patient had suffered from severe hypothyroidism for a long time, we did not really know whether her adrenal function was potentially normal or not. Therefore, prior to the intravenous administration of LT4, we administered 100 mg/day of hydrocortisone (HDC) in an intravenous drip to avoid relative adrenal insufficiency caused by rapid increases in thyroid hormone levels. Six days after the daily intravenous administration HDC, her thyroid hormone levels markedly improved. Therefore, we tapered oral administration of LT4 to 200 μg/day and intravenously a bolus of LT4 was administered (100 μg/day). Following the intravenous administration of a single bolus of LT4 (100 μg/day), her serum FT4 levels were rapidly and markedly increased in 1 hour (Figure 1). At the time of discharge, we decided to administer 200 μg/day of LT4 orally without the intravenous administration. Since we had already administered 100 mg/day of HDC in an intravenous drip for 10 days, we tapered oral administration of HDC to 20 mg/day upon the discharge. However, 7 days after her discharge, her thyroid hormone levels markedly decreased under the prescription. Thus, in the outpatient clinic, we administered 300 μg of LT4 by intravenous bolus injection weekly for several weeks. Then, we examined the time course of serum FT4, FT3 and TSH levels for optimization (Figure 2). Serum FT4 and FT3 levels increased within 3 days of the administration and deceased thereafter

TABLE 1: Changes in parameters following the intravenous (ivLT4) or oral administration of LT4.

Parameter	before ivLT4	after ivLT4	before oral LT4	after oral LT4
Systolic BP (mmHg)	101	142	125	104
Diastolic BP (mmHg)	67	94	78	67
Heart rate (bpm)	56	76	60	83
WBC (/μL)	3400	4600	5000	5300
Hb (g/dL)	8.0	12.6	12.8	11.1
Ht (%)	25.3	37.7	39.4	35.3
PLT (x10000/μL)	12.8	15.1	17.3	18.5
TP (g/dL)	6.6	6.2	7.2	6.9
Alb (g/dL)	3.7	4.3	3.8	3.3
BUN (mg/dL)	25	15	21	18
CRE (mg/dL)	1.29	0.75	1.07	0.97
UA (mg/dL)	5.0	4.3	5.2	4.9
Na (mEq/L)	141	139	141	139
K (mEq/L)	4.2	3.5	3.5	4.2
Cl (mEq/L)	108	106	108	104
Adjusted Ca (mg/dL)	8.3	9.0	8.9	9.1
IP (mg/dL)	4.4	3.9	3.1	3.3
LDH (U/L)	243	167	214	183
AST (U/L)	33	17	23	21
ALT (U/L)	22	13	18	16
γ-GTP (U/L)	28	11	14	12
ALP (U/L)	156	175	188	233
TG (mg/dL)	121	53	73	42
HDL-C (mg/dL)	49	78	109	97
LDL-C (mg/dL)	183	108	219	119
CK (IU/L)	206	55	108	64
CRP (mg/dL)	0.14	0.04	0.02	0.07
TSH (μIU/mL)	146.8	69.22	147.4	34.23
FT3 (pg/mL)	<0.26	1.27	0.26	1.4
FT4 (ng/dL)	<0.02	0.58	0.07	0.68
Total T3 (ng/mL)	<10	42	29	63
Total T4 (μg/mL)	<0.3	3.8	1.9	10.0
Tg (ng/dL)	<0.3	N/A	N/A	N/A
TBG (μg/dL)	33.3	N/A	N/A	N/A
Tg Ab (IU/mL)	11 (ref.<28.0)	N/A	N/A	N/A
TPO Ab (IU/mL)	143 (ref.<16.0)	N/A	N/A	N/A
TR Ab (IU/L)	1.0 (ref.<2.0)	N/A	N/A	N/A
TS Ab (%)	149 (ref.<180)	N/A	N/A	N/A
Fe (μg/dL)	58	65	43	31
UIBC (μg/dL)	263	269	292	377
Ferritin (ng/dL)	38	38	8	7
Folic acid (mg/dL)	3.8	N/A	4.5	4.5
Vit.B12 (mg/dL)	N/A	N/A	1500	1500
GH (ng/mL)	1.53	2.67	N/A	1.68
LH (mIU/mL)	4.0	4.3	N/A	11.6
FSH (mIU/mL)	6.0	5.9	N/A	25.4
PRL (ng/mL)	37.8	8.7	N/A	13.0
ACTH (pg/mL)	25.6	13.2	N/A	17.8
Cortisol (μg/dL)	13.3	10.0	N/A	6.8
IGF-I (ng/mL)	32	72	N/A	68

Parameters were evaluated before and 12 months after weekly intravenous LT4 (300 μg) administration (ivLT4) or before and 6 months after weekly oral LT4 (700 μg) administration (oral LT4). N/A: not applicable. ref: cutoff value or negative. Reference range: TSH; 0.4 to 4.0 μU/mL, FT3; 2.36 to 5.00 pg/mL, FT4; 0.88 to 1.67 ng/dL.

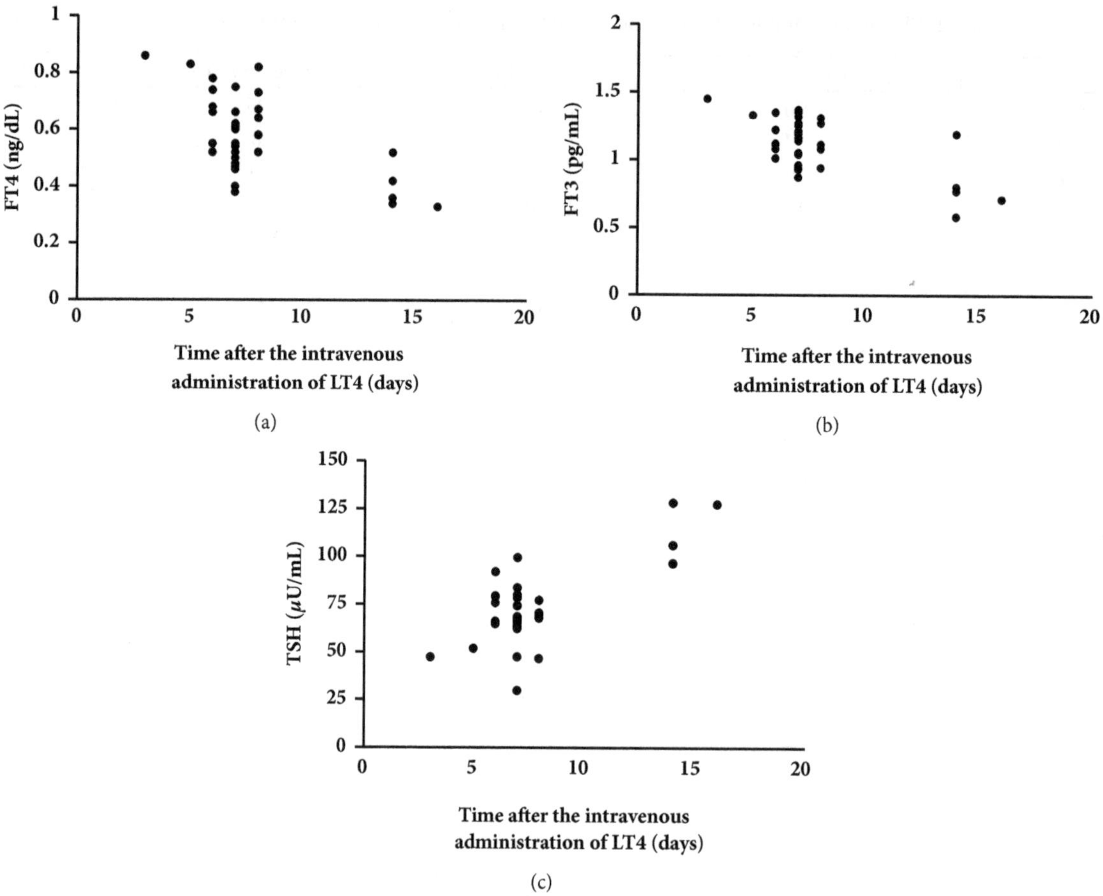

FIGURE 2: *Serum thyroid hormone and TSH levels after the intravenous administration of a single bolus of LT4 (300 μg).* Serum FT4 (a), FT3 (b), and TSH (c) levels were measured several times of the administration.

(Figures 2(a) and 2(b)). Within seven days following the bolus intravenous administration, serum FT4 and FT3 levels remained mostly within normal range. Serum TSH levels increased again 14 days after the intravenous administration of a bolus of LT4 (300 μg) in accordance with the decreases observed in serum FT4 and FT3 levels (Figure 2(c)). Based on these results, we selected the weekly intravenous administration of LT4 (300 μg). Since then, her serum FT4 and FT3 levels had been maintained as low-normal with the weekly intravenous administration of LT4 for 14 months, whereas serum TSH levels had vary (Figure 3). At the time of the intravenous bolus administration of high dose LT4 (300 μg) in the outpatient clinic, since HDC administration was already started, we decided to administer 20 mg/day of PSL orally instead of increasing the dose of HDC to avoid relative adrenal insufficiency. However, no symptom of adrenal insufficiency was found and her plasma ACTH and serum potassium levels decreased, possibly due to the administration of PSL. Therefore, we tapered the dose of PSL to 10 mg/day in a month after the onset of the weekly intravenous administration of LT4 (300 μg). Thereafter, we carefully tapered the daily doses of PSL by 1 mg per month to avoid steroid withdrawal syndrome and subsequently withdrew PSL administration (Figure 3).

Twelve months after weekly intravenous administration of LT4 (300 μg), her hemoglobin levels increased, while serum creatinine, low-dense lipoprotein cholesterol, creatine kinase, and prolactin levels decreased to the normal range. No liver dysfunction or cardiovascular events were detected (Table 1). Under oral administration of 200 μg/day of LT4, we attempted the intravenous administration of LT4 (300 μg) once in two weeks, which resulted in the relapse of severe hypothyroidism, suggesting the pseudomalabsorption of LT4 due to poor compliance (Figure 3). We then attempted the single oral bolus administration (1400 μg) under direct observation instead of the weekly intravenous administration of LT4 [3, 4]. The dose of LT4 selected was 7-fold the usual daily dose, which was 200 μg/day [3, 4]. Following the oral administration of a single bolus of LT4, her serum FT4 levels rapidly elevated within 2 hours (0.52 to 4.56 ng/dL) as shown in Figure 4. Her serum FT4, FT3, and TSH levels were maintained within normal range for 15 days after the single bolus oral administration, and hypothyroidism relapsed thereafter (Figure 4). Based on the results, we employed 700 μg of LT4 for a weekly oral administration protocol, which was 100 μg of LT4 daily, because when we administered 1400 μg of LT4, her FT4 levels after 2 hours were extremely high, which were clearly harmful and had remained elevated for more than one

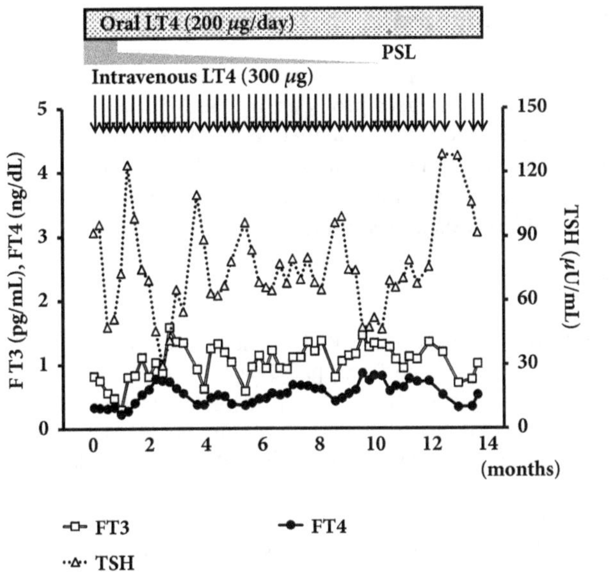

FIGURE 3: *LT4 (300 μg) intravenous administration once in a week and two weeks.* A daily oral LT4 (200 μg/day) replacement was continued. PSL (20 mg/day) was also orally administered at the onset of the weekly intravenous administration of LT4 (300 μg). It was tapered to 10 mg/day in a month after the administration. Thereafter, it was tapered by 1 mg/day per a month and subsequently discontinued 10 months after the intravenous administration of LT4. Twelve months after the intravenous administration of LT4, LT4 was intravenously administered once every two weeks, which resulted in the relapse of severe hypothyroidism with elevated serum TSH levels.

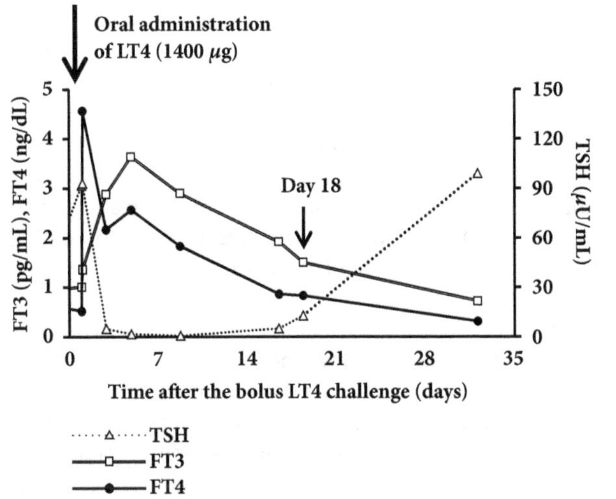

FIGURE 4: *Serum thyroid hormone and TSH levels after the oral administration of a single bolus of LT4 (1400 μg).* Eighteen days after the administration, serum FT4 and FT3 levels were 0.83 ng/dL and 1.5 pg/mL, respectively. Her serum TSH levels were 12.78 μIU/mL.

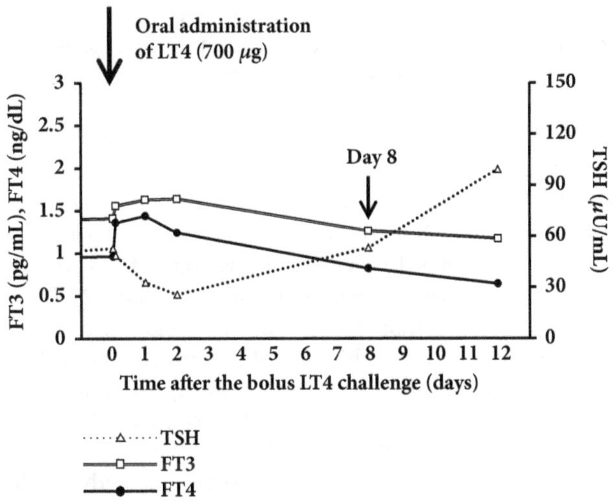

FIGURE 5: *Serum thyroid hormone and TSH levels after the oral administration of a single bolus of LT4 (700 μg).* Eight days after the administration, serum FT4 and FT3 levels were 0.82 ng/dL and 1.26 pg/mL, respectively. Her serum TSH levels were 53.1 μIU/mL.

week. Under the weekly oral administration of 700 μg of LT4, her serum FT4 and FT3 levels were elevated for 2 hours (FT4: 0.96 to 1.36 ng/dL, FT3: 1.41 to 1.56 pg/mL), and TSH levels decreased (52.8 to 48.6 μIU/mL) without liver dysfunction or electrocardiogram abnormalities (Figure 5). Her serum FT4 and FT3 levels were maintained within normal ranges for 8 days after the single bolus oral administration, which demonstrates the relevance of the weekly oral administration of 700 μg of LT4 (Figure 5).

Six months after the weekly oral administration of LT4, her renal and liver dysfunction and lipid profile improved (Table 1). We concluded that she developed severe hypothyroidism due to poor compliance to the daily oral LT4 replacement, even though she denied the poor compliance. Shi is currently being followed up at the psychiatric clinic. To date, her euthyroid status is maintained under the weekly oral administration of LT4 (700 μg) for two years.

3. Discussion

We encountered a severe case of refractory hypothyroidism due to poor compliance to a daily oral LT4 replacement. In the present case, we initially suspected the malabsorption of thyroid hormone. Even though previous doctors gradually increased the dose of LT4, her thyroid hormone levels were not improved and her symptom caused by hypothyroidism was severe. Therefore, presumably followed by the treatment to myxedema coma [9], they decided to coadminister LT4 and LT3. An administration of high dose (150 μg /day) of LT3, which might be potentially dangerous [9, 10], did not increase her free T3 levels (Table 1), suggesting that she was not taking medicine or that LT3 was not absorbed. However, the oral administration of LT4 (1400 μg) under direct observation resulted in increase of serum FT4 levels, which excluded the malabsorption of LT4 and revealed poor compliance to the daily oral LT4 replacement [3].

When HDC was administered prior to the intravenous administration of LT4, her serum FT4 levels markedly increased, possibly because corticosteroid inhibits T4 to T3 conversion. However, the administration of PSL during the weekly intravenous administration of LT4 did not increase her serum FT4 levels.

Due to the relatively long half-life of LT4, the use of a weekly oral LT4 replacement is plausible [11], with previous studies reporting that the weekly oral administration of LT4 is a safe, well-tolerated, and effective therapy for patients with noncompliance [4, 5]. The treatment of hypothyroidism with weekly doses of LT4 has been shown to increase serum FT4 levels within approximately two hours and decrease FT4 levels immediately before the weekly dose [12], which is compatible with our results on the administration of a single bolus of LT4 (1400 μg) (Figure 4). The present results suggest the efficacy, as well as safety of the oral administration of a single bolus of LT4 as a test for possible compliance issues. Our case also showed continuous stable thyroid function with 12.56 μg/kg/week of LT4 being orally administered with no obvious adverse effects, such as liver dysfunction, angina, or thyrotoxicosis. The weekly oral administration of LT4 was previously reported to be safe [3–5, 12]. However, no large-scale clinical trials, particularly those including elderly patients and those with a history of ischemic heart disease, on weekly administration have been performed to date, and, thus, further evidence is required to prove the safety and efficacy of the weekly oral administration of LT4.

On the other hand, there have been no detailed clinical data on the weekly intravenous administration of LT4. Since the intravenous administration of LT4 once in two weeks resulted in severe hypothyroidism in the present case, the pharmacokinetics of LT4 via its intravenous administration may be similar to those via its oral administration [12]. In the present case, we demonstrated that the weekly intravenous administration of LT4 achieves stable normal thyroid hormone levels in the long term (14 months) without severe adverse effects. However, we only reported the results of one case that was treated with the weekly intravenous administration of LT4, which is a limitation. In the present study, we did not perform 24-h electrocardiogram monitoring, ultrasonic cardiography, or bone and muscle parameter measurements, which need to be assessed in future studies. Thus, concrete safety data on the weekly intravenous administration of LT4 were not obtained in the present study.

We treated a case of refractory hypothyroidism due to poor compliance with the weekly administration of LT4 both orally and intravenously, both of which were performed safely and effectively. We provided clinical data to suggest that the weekly intravenous administration of LT4 has potential as an alternative treatment to daily LT4 replacement for cases of refractory hypothyroidism with noncompliance. The oral administration of LT4 to patients on a daily basis represents an ideal treatment. However, the weekly oral or intravenous administration of LT4 may be an alternative for some patients with poor adherence such as the present case.

Acknowledgments

This work was supported in part by the Research Program of Intractable Diseases provided by the Ministry of Health, Labour and Welfare of Japan (Koshi Hashimoto), Grants-in-Aid for Scientific Research (KAKENHI) from the Japan Society for the Promotion of Science (JSPS), and Grant no. JP 26461376 (Koshi Hashimoto).

References

[1] C. G. P. Roberts and P. W. Ladenson, "Hypothyroidism," *The Lancet*, vol. 363, no. 9411, pp. 793–803, 2004.

[2] J. Jonklaas, A. C. Bianco, A. J. Bauer et al., "Guidelines for the treatment of hypothyroidism: prepared by the American thyroid association task force on thyroid hormone replacement," *Thyroid*, vol. 24, no. 12, pp. 1670–1751, 2014.

[3] A. Ramadhan and M. Tamilia, "Treatment-refractory hypothyroidism," *Canadian Medical Association Journal*, vol. 184, no. 2, pp. 205–209, 2012.

[4] S. K. G. Grebe, R. R. Cooke, H. C. Ford et al., "Treatment of hypothyroidism with once weekly thyroxine," *The Journal of Clinical Endocrinology & Metabolism*, vol. 82, no. 3, pp. 870–875, 1997.

[5] J. N. Walker, P. Shillo, V. Ibbotson et al., "A thyroxine absorption test followed by weekly thyroxine administration: A method to assess non-adherence to treatment," *European Journal of Endocrinology*, vol. 168, no. 6, pp. 913–917, 2013.

[6] V. Mathew, R. A. Misgar, S. Ghosh et al., "Myxedema coma: a new look into an old crisis," *Journal of Thyroid Research*, vol. 2011, Article ID 493462, 7 pages, 2011.

[7] M. Skelin, T. Lucijanić, D. Amidžić Klarić et al., "Factors Affecting Gastrointestinal Absorption of Levothyroxine: A Review," *Clinical Therapeutics*, vol. 39, no. 2, pp. 378–403, 2017.

[8] A. Miyauchi, K. Kataoka, Y. Suzuki et al., "Parental replacement of thyroid hormones," *Folia Endocrinologica Japonica (Nihon Naibunpi Gakkai Zasshi)*, vol. 60, no. 1, pp. 23–29, 1984.

[9] Y. Ono, S. Ono, H. Yasunaga, H. Matsui, K. Fushimi, and Y. Tanaka, "Clinical characteristics and outcomes of myxedema coma: Analysis of a national inpatient database in Japan," *Journal of Epidemiology*, vol. 27, no. 3, pp. 117–122, 2017.

[10] T. Yamamoto, J. Fukuyama, and A. Fujiyoshi, "Factors associated with mortality of myxedema coma: report of eight cases and literature survey," *Thyroid*, vol. 9, no. 12, pp. 1167–1174, 1999.

[11] P. Colucci, C. S. Yue, M. Ducharme, and S. Benvenga, "A review of the pharmacokinetics of levothyroxine for the treatment of hypothyroidism," *European Endocrinology*, vol. 9, no. 1, pp. 40–47, 2013.

[12] K. C. Lewandowski, K. Dąbrowska, I. Komorowska-Dudek, and A. Lewiński, "A single bolus of high dose levothyroxine (L-T4) as a test in cases of suspected poor compliance to L-T4 therapy," *Thyroid Research*, vol. 8, no. 1, p. 16, 2015.

50

The Unusual Late-Onset Graves' Disease following Hashimoto's Related Hypothyroidism: A Case Report and Literature Review

Aseel Sukik, Sara Mohamed, Mhd-Baraa Habib, Sundus Sardar, Bashar Tanous, Raad Tahtouh, and Mouhand F. H. Mohamed

Internal Medicine Department, Hamad Medical Corporation, Doha, Qatar

Correspondence should be addressed to Mouhand F. H. Mohamed; dr.m.oraiby@hotmail.com

Academic Editor: Mihail A. Boyanov

Background. The shift of Graves' disease (GD) to Hashimoto's disease- (HD-) related hypothyroidism is well established. However, the opposite is rare. This is likely to the loss of critical thyroid mass available for stimulation by thyroid hormone receptor stimulating antibody, making this shift unusual. Herein, we report a young lady with a late shift from HD into GD and present a scoping literature review. *Case presentation*. We report a twenty-five-year-old lady with a sixteen-year-history of Hashimoto's-related hypothyroidism stable on levothyroxine. While following in the clinic, she started developing thyrotoxic symptoms in the form of anxiety, weight loss, and palpitation. Physical examination was remarkable for mild exophthalmos. The thyroid function test confirmed hyperthyroidism. Levothyroxine-induced hyperthyroidism was initially suspected; however, the symptoms did not improve despite reducing and stopping levothyroxine. Subsequent workup confirmed the diagnosis of GD. *Discussion and Conclusion*. This case highlights a unique association that has significant diagnostic and management implications. This shift should be considered when hyperthyroidism persists despite reducing or stopping levothyroxine. The diagnosis is made utilizing antibody titers and radioiodine update scan. While the management depends on the disease's stage and the treating physician preference, antithyroid agents can be used initially. Following up these patients is essential as the shift can be transient.

1. Introduction

Hashimoto's thyroiditis (HT) and Graves' disease (GD) are autoimmune diseases. They are the leading causes of hypothyroidism and hyperthyroidism, respectively [1, 2]. GD-related hyperthyroidism commonly converts to hypothyroidism following treatment with radioactive iodine treatment or surgery or less commonly shifts to HT-related Hypothyroidism. The latter occurs when the autoimmune response switches from thyroid stimulation to blockade [3].

In contrast, the shift from HT-related hypothyroid state to hyperthyroidism is unusual and has been rarely reported [3]. When a patient on levothyroxine for HT-related Hypothyroidism presents with thyrotoxic symptoms, levothyroxine over-replacement is usually suspected. Nonetheless, the unique possibility of transitioning to GD should be considered. We here describe a case of HT shifting to GD after sixteen years from the initial diagnosis. Additionally, we perform a scoping literature review exploring this unusual entity's mechanism, characteristics, and management.

2. Case presentation

Our patient is a twenty-four-year-old female with a sixteen-year history of HT-related hypothyroidism on oral levothyroxine 100 mcg once daily. She complained of occasional palpitations, nervousness, weight loss, and irregular menses. Thyrotoxicosis was confirmed with a thyroid function test, and levothyroxine dose was reduced. However, the patient continued to exhibit thyrotoxic symptoms even after completely stopping levothyroxine. On examination, the patient was calm but tachycardic and afebrile, and her blood pressure was 116/90 mmHg, weight was 58 kg, and BMI was 21.8. She was noted to have peripheral tremors. Her thyroid exam revealed the presence of diffuse nontender goiter, with

TABLE 1: The patient's laboratory test results.

Test (normal range/unit)	January 2020	November 2019	September 2019	February 2019	November 2017
WBC (4–11 × 10^3/uL)		6.8	7.1	7.4	8.5
RBC (2.8–4.8 × 10^6/uL)		4.8	4.2	4.4	4.3
Hb (12–15 gm/dL)		13.8	12.4	13.1	13.1
Platelets (150–400 × 10^3/uL)		293	325	396	263
Urea (2.7–8 mmol/L)		3.5	3.8	3.4	3.6
Creatinine (44–8 umol/L)		45	48	55	64
Sodium (135–145 mmol/L)		145	143	143	141
Potassium (mmol/L 3.5–5.1)		3.3	3.8	4.7	3.7
Glucose (3.3–5.5 mmol/L)		4.6	5.5	5.8	4.4
ALT (0–33 U/L)		30	34	29	9
AST (0–33 U/L)		26	21	18	14
TSH (0.3–4.2 IU/L)	2.39	<0.01	0.01	<0.01	1.64
Free T3 (3.7–6.4 pmol/L)		7.4	8.3	10.8	
Free T4 (11.6–21.9 pmol/L)	12	23.3	26.4	37.5	19.79

no palpable nodules. Eye examination was only remarkable for mild exophthalmos, and there was no evidence of dermopathy.

Thyroid function revealed depressed TSH <0.01 mIU/L (0.3–4.2) and high T4 26.4 pmol/L (11.6–21.9) (Table 1). Based on the persistence of symptoms despite stopping thyroid hormone supplementations and the presence of ophthalmopathy elements, the rare shift to GD was suspected. Autoimmune workup revealed a strong positive Anti-TSH Receptor (Anti-TSHR) titer, in addition to persistent positivity of previously positive thyroid peroxidase antibody (TPO Ab) and an increasing titer of Antithyroglobulin Ab (Table 2). Thyroid ultrasound revealed slight enlargement of the right lobe and increased vascularity in both lobes. Radioactive iodine uptake scan (RAIU) showed diffuse radiotracer uptake more prominent in the right thyroid lobe (Figure 1). Those findings kept with the shift to GD.

The patient received suppressive therapy with oral carbimazole 20 mg once daily and propranolol. A subsequent follow-up three months later showed normalization of thyroid function and improvement in clinical status.

3. Discussion

GD is the most common cause of hyperthyroidism [1]. It is an autoimmune disorder characterized by the presence of ophthalmopathy, dermopathy, and goiter. TSH receptor antibody is the characteristic for GD with excellent sensitivity and specificity [4]; in some cases, TPO Ab can also be detected. However, TPO Ab is usually the characteristic of HT (>90% of cases) [5]. Both GD and HT share autoimmunity pathogenesis. Although rare, these conditions can coexist [6].

Hypothyroidism follows-up to 20% of GD cases previously treated with antithyroid drugs even after [7, 8] prolonged periods [8]. Thyrotoxic manifestations in the setting of hypothyroidism usually point towards overtreatment that can be managed with modifications in thyroid hormone doses. The shift of HT-related hypothyroidism to GD is a rare entity. This is thought to be due to the critical loss of thyroid mass that can react with TSHR Ab [8]. Although rare, this shift has significant therapeutic implications and, thus, needs timely identification.

We performed a scoping review of the literature to explore this seemingly rare entity's mechanism, frequency, and characteristics. We came across a recent study by Gonzalez-Aguilera et al. [3]. On the retrospective evaluation of 2000 patients attending their clinic, they found 24 (1%) patients transforming from HD to GD. The median duration of the transformation was 18 months, majority cases were females (22/24), only four cases had ophthalmic changes, and all cases were treated initially as medication-induced hyperthyroidism. It was the persistence of symptoms (as in our case) that led to GD's workup and diagnosis. Gonzalez-Aguilera et al. postulated that this shift pathogenesis is either a shift in TSHR Ab from blocking (TSBAb) to stimulating (TSAb) or initially severe thyroid damage causing hypothyroidism that later shifts to hyperthyroidism via stimulating hormones upon thyroid gland recovery. The first explanation is more likely in our case, as she developed GD after sixteen years, which may be a long time for thyroid gland recovery.

Takasu et al. reported the second largest pool of adult patients (8 patients) with extended follow-up [9]. They suggested a classification of this cohort of patients based on the presence of TSAb and the persistence of symptoms to three groups. The first group is transient hyperthyroidism related to GD after hypothyroidism; the second group is persistent GD′-related hyperthyroidism after hypothyroidism. Finally, the third group is persistent hypothyroidism with positive TSAb. In their series, most patients (71%, $n = 5/7$) were transient, not needing specific antithyroid treatment. In two cases, the symptoms persisted, necessitating antithyroid treatment (2/7). One case had positive TSAb, however, without developing hyperthyroidism. Our literature search otherwise revealed additional individual case reports [8, 10–16]. Kamath et al. in 2012 suggested a role for the immunological shift as a possible mechanism, concluding that this theory remains only speculative at this stage [8].

The unilateral GD seen in our patient is relatively rare. It is a condition typical of Graves' symptoms, signs and supporting investigations are present, but radiotracer uptake

Table 2: Autoantibodies' trend during the clinical follow-up.

Antibody	2015	2019
TPO Ab (0–34 IU/ml)	>1000	>600
Antithyroglobulin*	0.93 (<0.6 Units)	585 (0–115 IU/mL)
Anti-TSHR (<1.75 IU/L)	___	12.2

*Different units were used for the antithyroglobulin antibodies test. The first value was indicative of weak positivity; however, the second reading was strongly positive. TPO Ab = thyroid peroxidase antibody, Anti-TSHR = anti-thyroid-stimulating hormone receptor antibody.

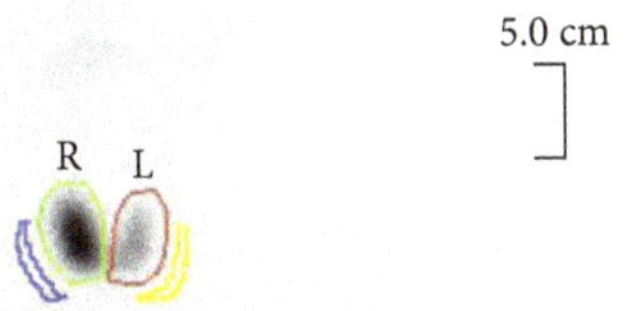

Figure 1: TC-99 THYROID SCINTIGRAPHY demonstrating moderate, asymmetrical enlargement of the thyroid gland, with a larger right lobe. Additionally, the right lobe demonstrates more radiotracer uptake, keeping with unilateral Grave's disease.

is confined more to a single thyroid lobe [16]. Our patient had mild exophthalmos but did not have other typical Grave's orbitopathy features, usually present in almost half of GD patients [17].

Our case report is unique, given that the shift to GD occurred after sixteen years following the initial diagnosis of HD, while in other reported cases, the shift tends to occur earlier in the disease course. This indicates that this shift can occur at any time. TPO Ab remained positive, with the finding of TSHR Ab (TSHR Ab levels were not measured earlier). The patient remained well on follow-up taking antithyroid treatment. Considering the possibility of transient hyperthyroidism state, which is mostly the case in our patient, we will monitor the patient closely for the development of signs or symptoms of hypothyroidism necessitating modifications or cessation of antithyroid treatment.

4. Conclusions

GD should be suspected when HT patients develop thyrotoxic symptoms that do not improve after reducing or stopping levothyroxine. The diagnosis relies upon good history and physical exam followed by supportive antibody titers and radioiodine uptake scan. Our case indicated that HT's shift to GD could be late. This cohort of patients should be followed up closely as the majority may transform back to hypothyroidism.

The patient was started on levothyroxine in October 2019. Abbreviations: WBC = white blood cells, RBC = red blood cells, Hb = hemoglobin, ALT = alanine aminotransferase, AST = aspartate aminotransferase, TSH = thyroid stimulating hormone, *T3* = Triiodothyronine, and *T4* = thyroxine.

Ethical Approval

The hospital's local IRB approved the publication of this case report.

Consent

Consent was obtained from the patient.

Authors' Contributions

The first (AS), second (SM), and the last author (MFHM) contributed equally to the writing and preparation of this article. AS and SM wrote the initial draft and performed the literature review. The draft was reviewed, updated, and supervised by MFHM. AS and MFHM were involved in the patient's care and obtained the written consent. SM constructed the tables. All authors reviewed the initial and final draft critically and approved it for publication.

Acknowledgments

The authors acknowledge the endocrine and medical teams involved in the care of this patient.

References

[1] H. B. Burch and D. S. Cooper, "Management of graves disease a review," *JAMA—Journal of the American Medical Association*, vol. 314, no. 23, pp. 2544–2554, 2015.

[2] D. Dunn and C. Turner, *Hypothyroidism in Women*, pp. 93–98, Elsevier, Amsterdam, Netherlands, 2016.

[3] B. Gonzalez-Aguilera, D. Betea, L. Lutteri et al., "Conversion to graves disease from hashimoto thyroiditis: a study of 24 patients," *Archives of Endocrinology and Metabolism*, vol. 62, no. 6, pp. 609–614, 2018.

[4] G. Barbesino and Y. Tomer, "Clinical utility of TSH receptor antibodies," *Journal of Clinical Endocrinology and Metabolism*, vol. 98, no. 6, pp. 2247–2255, 2013.

[5] P. B. Mehanathan, R. R. Erusan, K. Shantaraman, and S. M. Kannan, "Anti-thyroid peroxidase antibodies in multinodular hashimoto's thyroiditis indicate a variant etiology," *Journal of Thyroid Research*, vol. 2019, Article ID 4892329, 5 pages, 2019.

[6] H. Tamai, Y. Hirota, K. Kasagi et al., "The mechanism of spontaneous hypothyroidism in patients with graves' disease after antithyroid drug treatment," *The Journal of Clinical Endocrinology & Metabolism*, vol. 64, no. 4, pp. 718–722, 1987.

[7] A. Majumder and D. Sanyal, "A case of simultaneous occurrence of Graves' disease and Hashimoto's thyroiditis," *Indian Journal of Endocrinology and Metabolism*, vol. 16, no. Suppl 2, pp. S338–S339, 2012.

[8] C. Kamath, S. Young, K. Kabelis et al., "Thyrotrophin receptor antibody characteristics in a woman with long-standing Hashimoto's who developed Graves' disease and pretibial myxoedema," *Clinical Endocrinology*, vol. 77, no. 3, pp. 465–470, 2012.
[9] N. Takasu, T. Yamada, A. Sato et al., "Graves' disease following hypothyroidism due to hashimoto's disease: studies of eight cases," *Clinical Endocrinology*, vol. 33, no. 6, pp. 687–698, 1990.
[10] A. R. Kafrouni Gerges, S. N. Clark, and H. Shawa, "Hypothyroidism to hyperthyroidism: an immunological pendulum swing from two extreme poles—a case series," *BMJ Case Reports*, vol. 12, no. 4, Article ID e227445, 2019.
[11] R. H. Bishay and R. C. Y. Chen, "Hashimoto's thyroiditis and graves' disease in one patient: the extremes of thyroid dysfunction associated with interferon treatment," *Case Reports in Endocrinology*, vol. 2016, Article ID 6029415, 4 pages, 2016.
[12] E. Ahmad, K. Hafeez, M. F. Arshad, J. Isuga, and A. Vrettos, "Hypothyroidism conversion to hyperthyroidism: it's never too late," *Endocrinology, Diabetes & Metabolism Case Reports*, vol. 2018, no. 1, 2018.
[13] S. Furqan, N. U. Haque, and N. Islam, "Conversion of autoimmune Hypothyroidism to hyperthyroidism," *BMC Research Notes*, vol. 7, no. 1, 2014.
[14] P. M. Bell, D. G. Sinnamon, P. P. A. Smyth et al., "Hyperthyroidism following primary hypothyroidism in association with polyendocrine autoimmunity," *Acta Endocrinologica*, vol. 108, no. 4, pp. 491–497, 1985.
[15] M. T. McDermott, G. S. Kidd, L. E. Dodson, and F. D. Hofeldt, "Case report: hyperthyroidism following hypothyroidism," *The American Journal of the Medical Sciences*, vol. 291, no. 3, pp. 194–198, 1986.
[16] R. Manthri, N. Ajit, S. Vaikakkara, D. Bv, and T. Kalawat, "Unilateral graves' disease: the lesser known," *Indian Journal of Nuclear Medicine*, vol. 34, no. 2, p. 96, 2019.
[17] R. S. Bahn, "Graves' ophthalmopathy [internet]," *New England Journal of Medicine*, vol. 362, 726 pages, 2010.

51

Subacute Thyroiditis Presenting as Idiopathic Intracranial Hypertension

Kanyanatt Boonyatarp,[1] **Kanoksri Samintharapanya**,[2] **Thanawat Vongchaiudomchoke**,[3] **and Nuttaya Wachiraphansakul**[4]

[1]*Department of Internal Medicine, Lampang Hospital, Lampang, Thailand*
[2]*Division of Neurology, Department of Internal Medicine, Lampang Hospital, Lampang, Thailand*
[3]*Division of Nephrology, Department of Internal Medicine, Lampang Hospital, Lampang, Thailand*
[4]*Division of Endocrinology and Metabolism, Department of Internal Medicine, Lampang Hospital, Lampang, Thailand*

Correspondence should be addressed to Nuttaya Wachiraphansakul; iewnuttaya@gmail.com

Academic Editor: Toshihiro Kita

Background. Several case reports have illustrated a rare neurological manifestation, idiopathic intracranial hypertension (IIH), in patients with thyrotoxicosis. However, none were diagnosed with thyroiditis. We report the case of a patient with subacute thyroiditis who presented with severe intractable headache due to IIH. *Case Presentation.* A 36-year-old woman visited Lampang Hospital in February 2021 complaining of neck pain and progressive severe intractable headache. Her vital signs and neurological examination were normal. Thyroid examination revealed a single 1 cm right thyroid nodule. A computed tomography (CT) scan of her brain illustrated diffuse brain edema. However, CT angiography and venography of the brain did not show abnormalities. The opening pressure of the cerebrospinal fluid was elevated (27 cmH_2O). The free triiodothyronine level was 6.19 pg/mL, free thyroxine was 2.32 ng/dL, and thyroid-stimulating hormone was 0.0083 μIU/mL. Anti-Tg was positive at a low titer, but anti-TPO was negative. TRAb was also negative. Methimazole and acetazolamide were prescribed and monitored. The symptoms resolved completely within 2 weeks of onset. Thyroid hormones had returned to normal by 8 weeks. *Conclusion.* This is the first case report of subacute thyroiditis presenting with IIH.

1. Introduction

Thyroiditis is the term used to describe thyroid gland inflammation that arises from any etiology. Therefore, there are variations in the clinical manifestations and course of thyroiditis. Its diagnosis is made by clinical symptoms of thyrotoxicosis with acute destruction of the thyroid gland, which leads to the release of the thyroid hormone into the systemic circulation. Thyroid gland tenderness is commonly found in cases of subacute thyroiditis and infectious thyroiditis but is rarely seen in Hashimoto's thyroiditis. However, no manifestations of idiopathic intracranial hypertension (IIH; also called pseudotumor cerebri) have been reported for the thyrotoxicosis stage. Here, we report the first case of subacute thyroiditis that presents as IIH.

2. Case Presentation

A 36-year-old woman visited Lampang Hospital in February 2021 complaining of a severe progressive intractable headache for 1 week. She also had dull aching shoulder and neck pain on the right side. These symptoms were not relieved with nonsteroidal anti-inflammatory drugs. She had no relevant medical history and was not taking any medications. On physical examination, her body temperature was 36.3°C. No clinical signs of hyperthyroidism were observed. Neurological examination was normal. There was no limitation of extraocular muscle movement, fundoscopic examination did not reveal papilledema, and the visual fields of both eyes were normal. Due to her painful neck, her thyroid function was evaluated on the first day of admission. The

Table 1: Symptoms, laboratory results, and treatment by day of illness, hospital day, and follow-up day.

	Hospital day					Follow-up day			
	1	2	3	4	11	24	38	68	218
Day of illness	D8	D9	D10	D11	D18	D31	D45	D85	D225
Neck pain	■	■	■	■	■				
Headache	■	■	■						
Vomiting	■	■	■						
Body temperature (°C)	36.3	36.7	37.2	36.9	36.9	36.2	37.0	36.5	36.5
Hemoglobin (g/dL)	10.2	9.9	11.3		12.7	12.0	12.9	12.7	
White blood cell count (/cu.mm)	5400	7400	6900		5500	5500	4700	4800	
Neutrophil (%)	76	74	67		61	71	60	55	
Lymphocyte (%)	17	18	22		27	22	32	34	
Platelet count ($\times 10^3$/cu.mm)	287,000	269,000	346,000		399,000	317,000	324,000	273,000	
Free T3 (pg/mL) (1.71–3.71)	6.19				7.07	2.86	2.15	2.07	2.23
Free T4 (ng/dL) (0.70–1.48)	2.32				2.20	1.18	0.66	0.87	0.98
TSH (μIU/mL) (0.350–4.940)	0.0083				0.0040	0.0047	2.18	4.39	3.16
Anti-Tg (IU/mL)	10.13								5.28
Anti-TPO (IU/mL)	<3.00								0.25
TRAb (IU/L)	<0.8								
ESR (mm/hr)		51							6
hs-CRP (mg/L)		41.4							
BUN (mg/dL)	15	15	13		120				
Creatinine (mg/dL)	0.57	0.49	0.70		0.54	0.54			
Sodium (mmol/L)	143	142	138		139	140			
Potassium (mmol/L)	4.1	3.8	3.8		3.8	3.7			
Chloride (mmol/L)	110	111	111		110	107			
Bicarbonate (mmol/L)	28	24	18		16	25			
CSF opening pressure (cmH_2O)	27		18						
Glucose CSF	52								
Protein CSF	23.9								
Color	Colorless								
RBC	No RBC								
Cell count	No cell								
Therapy									
Methimazole	15 mg/day		10 mg/day			5 mg/day			
Acetazolamide	500 mg/day	750 mg/day			500 mg/day × 14 days				

Anti-Tg: antithyroglobulin antibody; anti-TPO: antithyroid peroxidase antibody; BUN: blood urea nitrogen; CSF: cerebrospinal fluid; ESR: erythrocyte sedimentation rate; hs-CRP: high-sensitivity C-reactive protein; T3: triiodothyronine; T4: thyroxine; TRAb: antithyroid receptor antibody.

tests revealed primary hyperthyroidism: a free triiodothyronine level of 6.19 pg/mL (1.71–3.71 pg/mL), a free thyroxine level of 2.32 ng/dL (0.70–1.48 ng/dL), and a thyroid-stimulating hormone level of 0.0083 μIU/mL (0.35–4.94 μIU/mL) (Table 1). The results of a brain computed tomography (CT) scan illustrated a diffuse absence of cortical sulci, which was consistent with diffuse brain edema. Nevertheless, CT angiography and venography of her brain did not demonstrate abnormalities (Figure 1). The opening pressure of the cerebrospinal fluid (CSF) was elevated (27 cmH_2O), and the CSF had normal levels of glucose and protein without cells. The erythrocyte sedimentation rate was high (51 mm/h). A workup was then conducted to determine the cause of thyrotoxicosis. A neck ultrasound showed a single 1 cm right thyroid nodule (Figure 2). However, she did not undergo thyroid scintigraphy due to recent administration of contrast media. While waiting for thyroid antibody results, methimazole (15 mg/day) and acetazolamide (750 mg/day) were prescribed. Potential etiologies of IIH were excluded by blood and CSF analyses (Table 1). Immunological investigation revealed a slightly elevated level of antithyroglobulin antibody (anti-Tg; 10.13 IU/ml). Antithyroid peroxidase antibody (anti-TPO) and antithyroid receptor antibody (TRAb) were both negative. With neck pain accompanied by thyrotoxicosis and a high erythrocyte sedimentation rate, subacute thyroiditis was the most likely diagnosis. Her headache gradually improved without the addition of steroid treatment, and it disappeared after 1 week. Acetazolamide was continued for 2 weeks, and she returned to the euthyroid state. Methimazole was tapered and discontinued after 6 weeks. Six months after the onset of thyrotoxicosis, her thyroid function was still normal, and her thyroid sonographic results did not reveal nodularity. A steady decline in the anti-Tg level was observed over the 6-month period, supporting the diagnosis of subacute thyroiditis (Table 1).

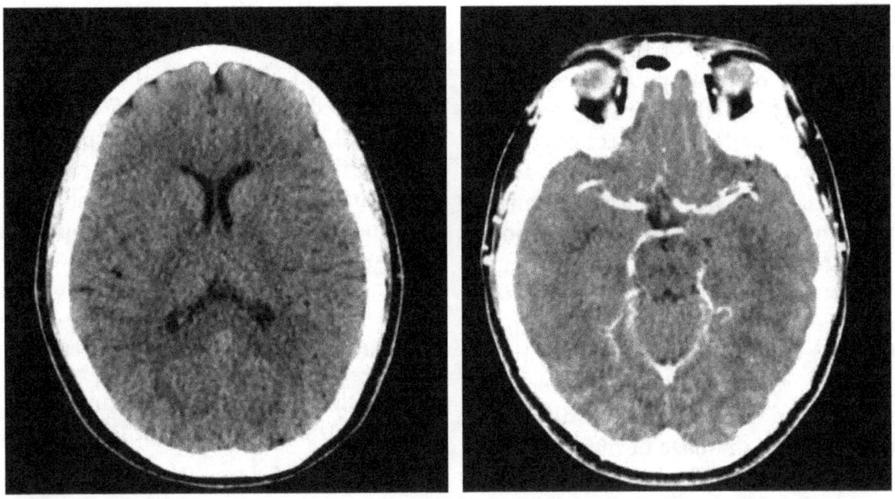

FIGURE 1: Brain computed tomography and venography revealed diffuse absence of cortical sulci without venous obstruction, consistent with diffuse cerebral edema.

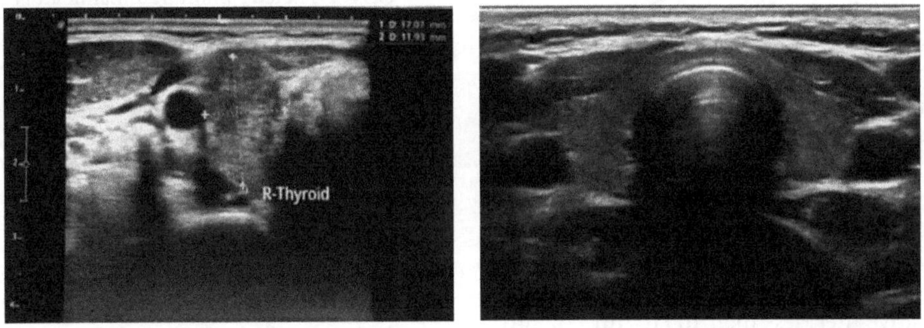

(a) (b)

FIGURE 2: (a) A neck ultrasound showed a solitary 1 cm right thyroid nodule. (b) Follow-up neck ultrasound revealed no nodularity.

3. Discussion and Conclusions

Subacute thyroiditis, also known as de Quervain's thyroiditis, is believed to be caused by postviral inflammation that causes inflammation of the thyroid gland. The clinical course of subacute thyroiditis usually shows 3 consecutive phases that unfold over approximately 6 months. During the first weeks after the onset of symptoms, transient thyrotoxicosis is found as preformed thyroid hormones are released from the damaged gland. Within a few weeks, many patients enter a hypothyroid phase, which is later followed by euthyroid restoration [1]. Tenderness and goiter are common manifestations in most cases [2, 3]. A thyroid antibody workup should be performed to exclude Hashimoto's thyroiditis, which is one of the most common causes of thyroiditis [2]. Differential diagnosis between Graves' disease is also mandatory. In addition, TRAb levels must be measured as treatments for thyroiditis and Graves' disease differ [4].

The presentation in our case involved a painful thyroid enlargement without specific signs of Graves' disease. There was no exposure to contrast media before the first thyroid function workup. The TRAb results were negative. Although a low anti-Tg titer was found, subacute thyroiditis was the most likely diagnosis due to the clinical symptoms and the decrease in the thyroid titer over time.

Aside from tremor and mild agitation, neurological manifestations of thyroiditis are rarely seen. Steroid-responsive encephalopathy, known as Hashimoto encephalopathy, has been reported in individuals with cognitive or neuropsychiatric involvement accompanied by positive anti-TPO [5]. In our case, we demonstrated another neurological manifestation that was found simultaneously with thyroiditis: IIH. This combination of thyroiditis and IIH has not been previously reported.

IIH is not common, with an incidence rate of 0.9 cases per 100,000 population [6]. In nearly 90% of cases, no clearly identifiable etiology could be found. Thus, to make a diagnosis of IIH, other secondary causes of increased intracranial pressure must be investigated and ruled out. Brain magnetic resonance venography should be performed to exclude cerebral venous sinus thrombosis. The most well-known theory of IIH development is venous outflow obstruction or stenosis without thrombosis. Other theories, such as an increased CSF production rate or loss of cerebral autoregulation, have also been proposed [7–9].

There are only a few case reports of thyroid disorders and IIH. Two cases of Graves' disease were reported [10, 11].

Levothyroxine treatment of chronic hypothyroidism in children followed by the development of IIH was also reported [12]. Another 2 cases of levothyroxine treatment accompanied by the occurrence of IIH were reported in 2 patients with thyroid carcinoma after thyroidectomy [13].

Two mechanisms of thyroid hormone action and IIH have been postulated. First, thyroxine replacement might alter CSF flow due to normalization of excess water in body fluid composition, leading to correction of hyponatremia in the chronic hypothyroid state. Normalization of excess fluid in the CSF might alter the dynamics of the CSF and predispose patients to IIH [11]. Second, thyrotoxicosis leads to decreased cerebral vascular resistance, increased cerebral venous blood flow, and elevated venous blood pressure. As a consequence, failure of adequate drainage of the CSF from the subarachnoid space occurs, and IIH develops [11, 14].

In the present case, a postulated second mechanism is that transient overt thyrotoxicosis may have decreased cerebral vascular resistance and increased cerebral venous volume. Genetic susceptibility and structural abnormalities in venous drainage might also have played an important role, but they are still under investigation.

There are limitations to the investigations in this case. First, thyroid scintigraphy and fine-needle aspiration of thyroid tissue were not performed to definitively diagnose subacute thyroiditis. However, the diagnosis of subacute thyroiditis was the most likely cause of thyrotoxicosis in this patient due to the presence of a painful thyroid goiter in the first manifestation. Furthermore, there were no clinical clues of Graves' disease, and the TRAb level was normal. In the literature, a low positive titer (less than 100 IU/mL) of anti-Tg was also reported for subacute thyroiditis [15]. In the future, interval follow-ups of the clinical manifestations and the thyroid antibody levels should be carried out to determine the cause of thyroiditis. Second, to diagnose IIH, brain magnetic resonance venography was not performed in this case to assess cerebral venous drainage as it could detect venous stasis or early venous thrombosis. Brain CT venography was performed instead due to its widespread availability and acceptable sensitivity for detecting venous thrombosis (approximately 90%) [16, 17].

In conclusion, we demonstrated the first case of the thyrotoxicosis phase of thyroiditis with the unusual neurological manifestation of IIH. The mechanism and causal relationship between the 2 conditions are still unclear; however, these might be established by further investigations in the future.

Ethical Approval

This study protocol was reviewed and approved by the Lampang Hospital Ethics Committee (approval no. EC ID 71/64).

Consent

The patient was deidentified and provided written informed consent to publish her case (including publication of images).

Authors' Contributions

KB, TV, and NW designed the study and wrote the manuscript. KB, KS, TV, and NW contributed to data acquisition. KB, KS, and NW interpreted the data. NW was responsible for supervision or mentorship. Each author contributed important intellectual content to the content of this manuscript, and all authors approved the final version of the manuscript.

Acknowledgments

The authors would like to thank Sakda Sathirareuangchai and David Park for English language editing.

References

[1] R. M. Ruggeri, A. Campennì, D. Deandreis et al., "SARS-COV-2-related immune-inflammatory thyroid disorders: facts and perspectives," *Expert Review of Clinical Immunology*, vol. 17, no. 7, pp. 737–759, 2021.

[2] J. Slatosky, B. Shipton, and H. Wahba, "Thyroiditis: differential diagnosis and management," *American Family Physician*, vol. 61, no. 4, pp. 1047–1054, 2000.

[3] G. A. Brent and A. P. Weetman, "Hypothyroidism and thyroiditis," *Williams Textbook of Endocrinology*, Elsevier, Amsterdam, Netherlands, pp. 416–448, 2016.

[4] R. M. Ruggeri, A. Campennì, G. Giuffrida et al., "Endocrine and metabolic adverse effects of immune checkpoint inhibitors: an overview (what endocrinologists should know)," *Journal of Endocrinological Investigation*, vol. 42, no. 7, pp. 745–756, 2019.

[5] R. S. Ransing, K. K. Mishra, and D. Sarkar, "Neuropsychiatric manifestation of Hashimoto's encephalopathy in an adolescent and treatment," *Indian Journal of Psychological Medicine*, vol. 38, no. 4, pp. 357–360, 2016.

[6] A. J. Degnan and L. M. Levy, "Pseudotumor cerebri: brief review of clinical syndrome and imaging findings," *American Journal of Neuroradiology*, vol. 32, no. 11, pp. 1986–1993, 2011.

[7] H. Suzuki, J. Takanashi, K. Kobayashi, K. Nagasawa, K. Tashima, and Y. Kohno, "MR imaging of idiopathic intracranial hypertension," *American Journal of Neuroradiology*, vol. 22, no. 1, pp. 196–199, 2001.

[8] R. I. Farb, I. Vanek, J. N. Scott et al., "Idiopathic intracranial hypertension: the prevalence and morphology of sinovenous stenosis," *Neurology*, vol. 60, no. 9, pp. 1418–1424, 2003.

[9] J. N. P. Higgins, J. H. Gillard, B. K. Owler, K. Harkness, and J. D. Pickard, "MR venography in idiopathic intracranial hypertension: unappreciated and misunderstood," *Journal of Neurology, Neurosurgery & Psychiatry*, vol. 75, no. 4, pp. 621–625, 2004.

[10] E. Coutinho, A. M. Silva, C. Freitas, and E. Santos, "Graves' disease presenting as pseudotumor cerebri: a case report," *Journal of Medical Case Reports*, vol. 5, no. 1, p. 68, 2011.

[11] M. Gutch, A. Bhattacharjee, S. Kumar, and D. Pushkar, "Graves' disease and idiopathic intracranial hypertension," *Medical Journal of Dr. D. Y. Patil University*, vol. 10, no. 3, pp. 290–292, 2017.

[12] C. Van Dop, F. A. Conte, T. K. Koch, S. J. Clark, S. L. Wilson-Davis, and M. M. Grumbach, "Pseudotumor cerebri associ-

ated with initiation of levothyroxine therapy for juvenile hypothyroidism," *New England Journal of Medicine*, vol. 308, no. 18, pp. 1076–1080, 1983.
[13] N. Panza, M. De Rosa, G. Lombardi, and M. Salvatore, "Pseudotumor cerebri and thyroid-replacement therapy in patients affected by differentiated thyroid carcinoma," *Journal of Endocrinological Investigation*, vol. 8, no. 4, pp. 357-358, 1985.
[14] W. Sensenbach, L. Madison, S. Eisenberg, and L. Ochs, "The cerebral circulation and metabolism in hyperthyroidism and myxedema," *Journal of Clinical Investigation*, vol. 33, no. 11, pp. 1434–1440, 1954.
[15] E. Nishihara, N. Amino, T. Kudo et al., "Moderate frequency of anti-thyroglobulin antibodies in the early phase of subacute thyroiditis," *European Thyroid Journal*, vol. 8, no. 5, pp. 268–272, 2019.
[16] P. Chiewvit, S. Piyapittayanan, and N. Poungvarin, "Cerebral venous thrombosis: diagnosis dilemma," *Neurology International*, vol. 3, no. 3, p. e13, 2011.
[17] G. Saposnik, F. Barinagarrementeria, R. D. Brown Jr. et al., "Diagnosis and management of cerebral venous thrombosis: a statement for healthcare professionals from the American Heart Association/American Stroke Association," *Stroke*, vol. 42, no. 4, pp. 1158–1192, 2011.

Permissions

All chapters in this book were first published by Hindawi Publishing Corporation; hereby published with permission under the Creative Commons Attribution License or equivalent. Every chapter published in this book has been scrutinized by our experts. Their significance has been extensively debated. The topics covered herein carry significant findings which will fuel the growth of the discipline. They may even be implemented as practical applications or may be referred to as a beginning point for another development.

The contributors of this book come from diverse backgrounds, making this book a truly international effort. This book will bring forth new frontiers with its revolutionizing research information and detailed analysis of the nascent developments around the world.

We would like to thank all the contributing authors for lending their expertise to make the book truly unique. They have played a crucial role in the development of this book. Without their invaluable contributions this book wouldn't have been possible. They have made vital efforts to compile up to date information on the varied aspects of this subject to make this book a valuable addition to the collection of many professionals and students.

This book was conceptualized with the vision of imparting up-to-date information and advanced data in this field. To ensure the same, a matchless editorial board was set up. Every individual on the board went through rigorous rounds of assessment to prove their worth. After which they invested a large part of their time researching and compiling the most relevant data for our readers.

The editorial board has been involved in producing this book since its inception. They have spent rigorous hours researching and exploring the diverse topics which have resulted in the successful publishing of this book. They have passed on their knowledge of decades through this book. To expedite this challenging task, the publisher supported the team at every step. A small team of assistant editors was also appointed to further simplify the editing procedure and attain best results for the readers.

Apart from the editorial board, the designing team has also invested a significant amount of their time in understanding the subject and creating the most relevant covers. They scrutinized every image to scout for the most suitable representation of the subject and create an appropriate cover for the book.

The publishing team has been an ardent support to the editorial, designing and production team. Their endless efforts to recruit the best for this project, has resulted in the accomplishment of this book. They are a veteran in the field of academics and their pool of knowledge is as vast as their experience in printing. Their expertise and guidance has proved useful at every step. Their uncompromising quality standards have made this book an exceptional effort. Their encouragement from time to time has been an inspiration for everyone.

The publisher and the editorial board hope that this book will prove to be a valuable piece of knowledge for researchers, students, practitioners and scholars across the globe.

List of Contributors

Piyumi Sachindra Alwis Wijewickrama
Endocrinology Unit, National Hospital of Sri Lanka, Colombo 10, 00700, Sri Lanka

Henry N. Rajaratnam
Nawaloka Hospitals PLC, 23, Deshamanya H. K Dharmadasa Mawatha, Colombo 2, 00200, Sri Lanka

Prateek Shukla
Division of Internal Medicine, UConn Health Center, Farmington, CT 06030, USA

Ketan R. Bulsara
University of Connecticut School of Medicine, Farmington, CT 06030, USA
Division of Neurosurgery, UConn Health Center, Farmington, CT 06030, USA

Pooja Luthra
University of Connecticut School of Medicine, Farmington, CT 06030, USA
Division of Endocrinology and Metabolism, UConn Health Center, Farmington, CT 06030, USA

Fadlila Fitriani
Study Program of Specialty, Department of Internal Medicine, Dr. Sardjito General Hospital/ Faculty of Medicine, Public Health and Nursing, Universitas Gadjah Mada, Jl. Kesehatan No. 1 Sekip Sinduadi DIY, Yogyakarta 55284, Indonesia

Vina Yanti Susanti and Mohammad Robikhul Ikhsan
Division of Endocrinology, Department of Internal Medicine, Dr. Sardjito General Hospital/ Faculty of Medicine, Public Health and Nursing, Universitas Gadjah Mada, Jl. Kesehatan No. 1 Sekip Sinduadi DIY, Yogyakarta 55284, Indonesia

Mario S. Campana, Maria Riofrio, Raja S. Jadav and Mattan Rozenek
St. Barnabas Hospital, Department of Internal Medicine, SBH Health System, e Bronx, NY 10457, USA

Pratibha Rana and Patria Alba Aponte
Children's Mercy Hospital, 3101 Broadway Blvd., Kansas City, MO 64111, USA

Ghufran Babar
Department of Pediatric Endocrinology, Children's Mercy Hospital, 3101 Broadway Blvd., Kansas City, MO 64111, USA

Andreas Hillenbrand, Johannes Lemke and Doris Henne-Bruns
Department of General and Visceral Surgery, University Medical Center Ulm, Ulm, Germany

Ambros J. Beer and Vikas Prasad
Department of Nuclear Medicine, University Medical Center Ulm, Ulm, Germany

Sameh Samir Elawady
Faculty of Medicine, Tanta University, Tanta, Egypt

Diwakar Phuyal
Kirtipur Hospital, PHECT Nepal, Kathmandu, Nepal

Rakesh Kumar Shah
Kathmandu Medical College, Kathmandu, Nepal

Lubna Mirza
Norman Endocrinology Associates, Norman, OK, USA

Zeinab Alnahas
Department of Internal Medicine, Cairo University, Cairo 11956, Egypt

Marko Markov and Mohamad H. Horani
Chandler Regional Medical Center, Chandler 85224, Arizona, USA

Rishi Raj, Edilfavia Mae Uy, Matthew Hager and Kamyar Asadipooya
Department of Endocrinology, Diabetes and Metabolism, University of Kentucky, Lexington, KY, USA

Ann Miller and Kristi D. Silver
Division of Endocrinology, Diabetes, and Nutrition, Department of Medicine, University of Maryland School of Medicine, Baltimore, MD, USA

Jan Adelmeyer, Joachim Nils Goebel and Peter Herbert Kann
Philipps-University Marburg, Endocrinology Baldingerstraße, 35043 Marburg, Germany

Alexander Kauka
General Practice Grossseelheim, Grossseelheim 35274, Germany

Ian Jackson, Yazan Addasi, Moeed Ahmed, Bashar Ramadan, Karson Kalian and Jocelyn Taylor
Department of Medicine, Creighton University School of Medicine, Omaha, NE, USA

Noor Addasi
Department of Endocrinology, University of Nebraska Medical Center, Omaha, NE, USA

Ali Nayfeh and Bryan Krajicek
Department of Pulmonary and Critical Care, Creighton University School of Medicine, Omaha, NE, USA

Khalid Bashir
Department of Nephrology, Creighton University School of Medicine, Omaha, NE, USA

Michael Salim
Department of Internal Medicine, Mount Sinai Hospital, Chicago, IL 60608, USA

Mohannad Samy Behairy
Ross University School of Medicine, Bridgetown, Barbados

Elena Barengolts
Department of Medicine, University of Illinois Medical Center and Department of Medicine, Jesse Brown VA Medical Center, Chicago, IL 60612, USA

S. Alrushaid
Kuwait University, Kuwait City, Kuwait

T. Alessa
Division of Endocrinology, Diabetes and Metabolism, Jaber Al-Ahmad Hospital, Kuwait City, Kuwait
Dasman Diabetes Institute, Kuwait City, Kuwait

Ghada Elshimy
Endocrinology, Diabetes and Metabolism Division, Medical College of Georgia, Augusta University, Augusta, GA, USA
Endocrinology Division, University of Arizona College of Medicine, Phoenix, AZ, USA
Endocrinology Division, Phoenix VA Health Care System, Phoenix, AZ, USA

Mahmoud Alsayed
Endocrinology Division, University of Arizona College of Medicine, Phoenix, AZ, USA

Jerome Targovnik
Endocrinology Division, University of Arizona College of Medicine, Phoenix, AZ, USA
Endocrinology Division, Phoenix VA Health Care System, Phoenix, AZ, USA

Gamal Sidarous
Nuclear Medicine Department, University of Arizona College of Medicine, Phoenix, AZ, USA

Kresimira M. Milas
Endocrine Surgery Department, University of Arizona College of Medicine, Phoenix, AZ, USA

Daniele Cappellani, Alessandro Brancatella, Edda Vignali, Domenico Canale, Filomena Cetani and Claudio Marcocci
Department of Clinical and Experimental Medicine, Unit of Endocrinology, University of Pisa, Pisa, Italy

Martin Kaufmann and Glenville Jones
Department of Biomedical and Molecular Sciences, Queen's University, Kingston, ON, Canada

Angelo Minucci and Elisa De Paolis
Fondazione Policlinico Universitario A. Gemelli IRCCS, Roma, Italy

Ettore Capoluongo
Fondazione Policlinico Universitario A. Gemelli IRCCS, Roma, Italy
Universit`a Cattolica del Sacro Cuore, Roma, Italy

Yassine Er-Rahali, Jad Issouani, Colna Antonio Nfad, Souad El Moussaoui and Ahmed Anass Guerboub
Endocrinology Department, Mohammed V Military Academic Hospital, Faculty of Medicine and Pharmacy, Mohammed V-Souissi University, Rabat, Morocco

Mohammed Massine El Hammoumi and El Hassane Kabiri
Thoracic Surgery Department, Mohammed V Military Academic Hospital, Faculty of Medicine and Pharmacy, Mohammed V-Souissi University, Rabat, Morocco

Dhineshreddy Gurala, Kartikeya Rajdev, Roshan Acharya and Saad Habib
Resident, Internal Medicine, Staten Island University Hospital, Northwell Health, Staten Island, NY, USA

Pretty Sara Idiculla
Foreign Medical Graduate, Sree Gokulam Medical College and Research Foundation, Alamthara, India

Michael Krzyzak
Hospitalist, Internal Medicine, Staten Island University Hospital, Northwell Health, Staten Island, NY, USA

Nanik Ram and Saira Furqan
Department of Medicine, Aga Khan University, Stadium Road, Karachi 74800, Pakistan

Sibtain Ahmed
Department of Pathology and Laboratory Medicine, Aga Khan University, Stadium Road, Karachi 74800, Pakistan

B. López-Muñoz and S. Serrano Corredor
Sección de Endocrinología y Nutrición, Hospital General Universitario de Alicante, ISABIAL-FISABIO, Valencia, Spain

L. Greco Bermúdez and M. F. Sánchez de la Fuente
Sección de Anatomía Patológica, Hospital General Universitario de Alicante, ISABIAL-FISABIO, Valencia, Spain

D. Marín-Jiménez
Sección de Anestesiología y Reanimación, Hospital General Universitario de Alicante, Alicante, Spain

A. Franca Capparelli and I. Mascarell Martínez
Sección de Endocrinología y Nutrición, Hospital Vega Baja de Orihuela, Alicante, Spain

Victor Manuel Blanco, Camilo Andrés Páez and Veline Martínez
Internal Medicine Unit, Fundación Valle del Lili, Cra 98 #18-49, Cali 760032, Colombia

Angela María Victoria
Health Sciences Faculty, Universidad Icesi, Fundación Valle del Lili, Cra 98 #18-49, Cali 760032, Colombia

Luis Guillermo Arango and Guillermo Edinson Guzmán
Internal Medicine Unit - Department of Endocrinology, Fundación Valle del Lili, Cra 98 #18-49, Cali 760032, Colombia

Ana María Arrunategui and Juliana Escobar
Pathology Surgery Unit, Fundación Valle del Lili, Cra 98 #18-49, Cali 760032, Colombia

Masaki Matsubara, Tamiko Tamanaha, Hisashi Makino and Kiminori Hosoda
Division of Diabetes and Lipid Metabolism, National Cerebral and Cardiovascular Center, 6-1 Kishibe-Shimmachi, Suita, Osaka 564-8565, Japan

Tomohiro Tanaka, Akinori Wakamiya, Takeshi Aiba and Kengo Kusano
Department of Cardiovascular Medicine, National Cerebral and Cardiovascular Center, 6-1 Kishibe-Shimmachi, Suita, Osaka 564-8565, Japan

Tomonori Tanei
Department of Breast and Endocrine Surgery, Osaka University Graduate School of Medicine, 2-2-E10 Yamadaoka, Suita, Osaka 565-0871, Japan

Farid Gossili and Trine B. Andersen
Department of Nuclear Medicine, Aalborg University Hospital, Aalborg, Denmark

Allan Carlé
Department of Endocrinology, Aalborg University Hospital, Aalborg, Denmark

Helle D Zacho
Department of Nuclear Medicine, Aalborg University Hospital, Aalborg, Denmark
Department of Clinical Medicine, Aalborg University, Aalborg, Denmark

Ayrton Bangolo and Adam Atoot
Department of Internal Medicine, Hackensack Meridian Health Palisades Medical Center, North Bergen, NJ, USA

John Bukasa Kakamba
Endocrine and Metabolic Disorders Department, University Clinics of Kinshasa, Kinshasa, Democratic Republic of the Congo
Department of Endocrinology, University of Liege, Liege, Belgium

Ali Atoot and Syed Sirajuddin
Department of Anesthesia, Hackensack University Medical Center, Hackensack, NJ, USA

Mohammad Jurri and Ashraf Mahmoud
Department of Family Medicine, Hackensack Meridian Health Palisades Medical Center, North Bergen, NJ, USA

Arthur Oliver Lo
University of the East Ramon Magsaysay, Quezon City, Philippines

Kunchang Song
Department of Pathology, Hackensack Meridian Health Palisades Medical Center, North Bergen, NJ, USA

Federico Cappellacci, Fabio Medas, Gian Luigi Canu, Enrico Erdas and Pietro Giorgio Caló
Department of Surgical Sciences, University of Cagliari, "Policlinico Universitario Duilio Casula", 09042 Monserrato, Italy

Maria Letizia Lai
Department of Cytomorphology, University of Cagliari, Cagliari, Italy

Giovanni Conzo
Division of Medical Oncology, Department of Internal and Experimental Medicine "F. Magrassi", School of Medicine, University of Campania "Luigi Vanvitelli", Cagliari, Italy

Iván Emilio de la Cruz Rodríguez, Elsy Sarahí García Montesinos, Guadalupe Vargas Ortega, Lourdes Balcázar Hernández, Victoria Mendoza Zubieta, Victor Hernández Avendaño and Baldomero González Virla
Endocrinology Department. Hospital de Especialidades, Centro M´edico Nacional Siglo XXI, Mexico City 067200, Mexico

María Fernanda Rodríguez-Delgado
Faculty of Medicine, Universidad Nacional Aut´onoma de M´exico, Coordinacion de Servicios a la Comunidad, Programa Comunidad Saludable-Comunidad Solidaria, Mexico City, Mexico

Subash Thapa
Department of Radiology, Nepal Police Hospital, Kathmandu, Nepal

Prakash Khanal
Department of ENT-Head and Neck Surgery, Nepal Police Hospital, Kathmandu, Nepal

Vânia Benido Silva, Maria Teresa Pereira, Sílvia Santos Monteiro and Maria Helena Cardoso
Department of Endocrinology, Centro Hospitalar e Universit´ario do Porto, Porto, Portugal

Carla Leal Moreira
Department of Nephrology, Centro Hospitalar e Universit´ario do Porto, Porto, Portugal

Isabel Inácio
Department of Endocrinology, Centro Hospitalar do Baixo Vouga, Aveiro, Portugal

Maxim Barnett and Asha Rattan
University of Buckingham Medical School, Hunter St, Buckingham MK18 1EG, UK

Farhan Ahmed and Malik Asif Humayun
Milton Keynes University Hospital, Standing Way, Eaglestone, Milton Keynes MK6 5LD, UK

Radu Mihai
Oxford Radcliffe Hospitals NHS Foundation Trust, Old Road, Headington, Oxford OX3 7LH, UK

Young Sil Eom and Pyung Chun Oh
Department of Internal Medicine, Gil Medical Center, Gachon University College of Medicine, Incheon, Republic of Korea

Shraddha Banthia
Department of Endocrinology, Sutherland Hospital, Sydney, NSW, Australia

Malgorzata Monika Brzozowska
Department of Endocrinology, Sutherland Hospital, Sydney, NSW, Australia
The University of New South Wales Sydney, Faculty of Medicine, Sydney, NSW, Australia

Simon Thompson
Department of Chemical Pathology, NSW Health Pathology, Prince of Wales Hospital, Sydney, NSW, Australia

Manisha Narasimhan
Department of Neurology, Sutherland Hospital, Sydney, NSW, Australia
The University of Sydney, Brain and Mind Centre, Sydney, NSW, Australia

James Lee
Department of Neurology, Sutherland Hospital, Sydney, NSW, Australia
Department of Neurology, Royal North Shore Hospital, Sydney, NSW, Australia

Sarah Wing-yiu Poon, Brian Hon-yin Chung, Anita Man-ching Tsang and Grace Wing-kit Poon
Department of Paediatrics and Adolescent Medicine, Queen Mary Hospital, LKS Faculty of Medicine, The University of Hong Kong, Pok Fu Lam, Hong Kong

Narangoda Liyanage Ajantha Shyamali
University of Sri Jayewardenepura, Gangodawila, Nugegoda, Sri Lanka

Chandrike Ponnamperuma
National Hospital of Sri Lanka, Colombo 10, Sri Lanka

Le Yu Khine, Omolola Olajide and Henry Driscoll
Division of Endocrinology, Marshall University, Joan C. Edwards School of Medicine, USA

Dong Won Kim
Division of Internal Medicine, University of Maryland School of Medicine, USA

Chelsey White and Yousef Shweihat
Division of Pulmonary and Critical Care and Sleep Medicine, Marshall University, Joan C. Edwards School of Medicine, USA

Arunava Saha
PGY2 Internal Medicine, Saint Vincent Hospital, Worcester, MA, USA

Sanjita Chittimoju and Nitin Trivedi
Endocrinology and Metabolic Medicine, Saint Vincent Hospital, Worcester, MA, USA

Claire E. Moore
Department of Pediatrics, the Warren Alpert Medical School of Brown, Providence, RI, USA

Sabitha Sasidharan Pillai, Meghan E. Fredette and Monica Serrano-Gonzalez
Department of Pediatrics, the Warren Alpert Medical School of Brown, Providence, RI, USA
Division of Pediatric Endocrinology, Hasbro Children's Hospital, Providence, RI, USA

Juliana Austin
Center for Endocrinology, Diabetes and Metabolism, Children's Hospital Los Angeles, Los Angeles, CA, USA
Department of Pediatrics, Keck School of Medicine, University of Southern California, Los Angeles, CA, USA

Leidy Plaza-Enriquez, P. Khatiwada and A. Sikha
Department of Internal Medicine, Memorial Healthcare System, Hollywood, FL, USA

M. Sanchez-Valenzuela
Internal Medicine Residency, St. Barnabas Hospital, Bronx, NY, USA

Henrik Elenius, Marie Cesa, Corina C. Nava Suarez, Abhishek Nimkar, Prasanta Basak and Nandita Sinha
Montefiore New Rochelle Hospital, 16 Guion Pl, New Rochelle, NY 10801, USA

Zaw Win Htet
Division of Endocrinology, Department of Medicine, National University Hospital, Level 10, NUHS Tower Block, 1E Kent Ridge Road, Singapore

E. Shyong Tai and Samantha Peiling Yang
Division of Endocrinology, Department of Medicine, Yong Loo Lin School of Medicine, National University of Singapore, Level 10, NUHS Tower Block, 1E Kent Ridge Road, Singapore

Abuobeida Ali and Habib Ahmad
Department of Acute Medicine, Pilgrim Hospital, Boston PE21 9QS, UK

Wail Mostafa
Department of Gastroenterology, Pilgrim Hospital, Boston PE21 9QS, UK

Cornelius Fernandez and Nyi Htwe
Department of Endocrinology, Pilgrim Hospital, Boston PE21 9QS, UK

Mojgan Sanjari
Department of Endocrinology, Afzalipour Medical Faculty and Endocrinology and Metabolism Research Center, Institute of Basic and Clinical Physiology Sciences, Kerman University of Medical Sciences, Kerman, Iran

Mohammadreza Shakibi
Rheumatology Department, Afzalipour Medical Faculty and Physiology Research Center, Institute of Neuropharmacology, Kerman University of Medical Sciences, Kerman, Iran

Moeinadin Safavi
Pathology Department, School of Medicine, Kerman University of Medical Sciences, Kerman, Iran
Pathology Department, School of Medicine, Tehran University of Medical Sciences, Tehran, Iran

Matthew M. Feldt
Pediatric Endocrinologist, Children's Mercy Hospital, Kansas City, MO, USA

Eugenia Campos-Barrera
Hospital Angeles Del Pedregal, Camino de Sta. Teresa 1055-S, Heroes de Padierna, La Magdalena Contreras, Ciudad de Mexico 10700, Mexico

Teresa Alvarez-Cisneros
Instituto Nacional de Geriatr´ıa, Av Contreras 428, San Jeronimo Lidice, Magdalena Contreras, Mexico City 10700, Mexico

Mario Davalos-Fuentes
Instituto Nacional de Rehabilitacion, Arenal de Guadalupe, Tlalpan, Mexico City 14389, Mexico

Carlo Cappelli, Ilenia Pirola and Maurizio Castellano
Department of Clinical and Experimental Sciences, SSD Medicina Ad Indirizzo Endocrino-metabolico, University of Brescia, ASST Spedali Civili di Brescia, Brescia 25123, Italy

Anuradha Jayasuriya
Diabetes and Endocrinology Unit, Colombo South Teaching Hospital, Kalubowila, Colombo, Sri Lanka

Dimuthu Muthukuda
Diabetes and Endocrinology Unit, Sri Jayewardenepura General Hospital, Nugegoda, Colombo, Sri Lanka

Preethi Dissanayake and Shyama Subasinghe
Sri Jayewardenepura General Hospital, Nugegoda, Colombo, Sri Lanka

Mustafa Can, Feridun Karakurt, Muhammed Kocabas, Elker Cordan, Melia Karakose and Mustafa KulaksJzoglu
Department of Endocrinology and Metabolism, Meram School of Medicine, Necmettin Erbakan University, Konya, Turkey

Patrizia Del Monte, Carla Micaela Cuttica and Alessandro Marugo
Endocrine Unit, Galliera Hospital, Genoa, Italy

Luca Foppiani
Internal Medicine Unit, Galliera Hospital, Genoa, Italy

Daniela Audenino
Neurology Unit, Galliera Hospital, Genoa, Italy

Tomasz Tadeusz Godowicz
Neurosurgery Unit, Galliera Hospital, Genoa, Italy

Francesca Marta Elli and Giovanna Mantovani
Fondazione IRCCS Ca' Granda Ospedale Maggiore Policlinico, Endocrinology and Diabetology Unit, Department of Clinical Sciences and Community Health, University of Milan, Milan, Italy

Emilio Di Maria
Department of Health Sciences, University of Genoa; Medical Genetics Unit, Galliera Hospital, Genoa, Italy

Adnan Haider, Oksana Symczyk and Yadel Couso
Department of Endocrinology, West Virginia University, Morgantown, WV, USA

Taylor Cater and Sheree Bryan
Department of Medicine, West Virginia University, Morgantown, WV, USA

Yujiro Nakano, Hideyuki Okuma, Isao Minami, Takanobu Yoshimoto and Tetsuya Yamada
Department of Molecular Endocrinology and Metabolism, Graduate School of Medical and Dental Science, Tokyo Medical and Dental University, 113-8510, Japan

Koshi Hashimoto
Department of Preemptive and Metabolism, Graduate School of Medical and Dental Science, Tokyo Medical and Dental University, 113-8510, Japan

Noriaki Ohkiba
Department of Endocrinology and Metabolism, Kashiwa Municipal Hospital, 277-0825, Japan

Hiromitsu Takahashi
Department of Pharmacy, Medical Hospital of Tokyo Medical and Dental University, 113-8510, Japan

Yuji Tanaka
Department of General Medicine, National Defense Medical College Hospital, 359-0042, Japan

Aseel Sukik, Sara Mohamed, Mhd-Baraa Habib, Sundus Sardar, Bashar Tanous, Raad Tahtouh and Mouhand F. H. Mohamed
Internal Medicine Department, Hamad Medical Corporation, Doha, Qatar

Kanyanatt Boonyatarp
Department of Internal Medicine, Lampang Hospital, Lampang, Thailand

Kanoksri Samintharapanya
Division of Neurology, Department of Internal Medicine, Lampang Hospital, Lampang, Thailand

Thanawat Vongchaiudomchoke
Division of Nephrology, Department of Internal Medicine, Lampang Hospital, Lampang, Thailand

Nuttaya Wachiraphansakul
Division of Endocrinology and Metabolism, Department of Internal Medicine, Lampang Hospital, Lampang, Thailand

Index

www.ingramcontent.com/pod-product-compliance
Lightning Source LLC
LaVergne TN
LVHW082126200926
848484LV00008B/2010